ROUTINE BLOOD TESTING

Many laboratory tests include the direction to perform routine blood testing. The protocol for those tests is presented here and is cross-referenced within the many tests requiring them.

Before
- Follow proper patient identification protocols to avoid wrong patient events. Usually name and date of birth are used as two identifiers.
- **PT** Explain the procedure to the patient.
- **PT** Tell the patient if fasting is necessary. (Fasting is most commonly required with glucose and lipid studies.)
- **PT** If fasting is required, instruct the patient not to consume any food or fluids. Only water is permitted. Fasting requirements usually vary from 8 to 12 hours.
- **PT** Instruct the patient to continue taking medications unless told otherwise by the health care provider.

During
- Collect the blood in a properly color-coded test tube (Table A, p. xiii), which indicates the presence or absence of additives. Tube stopper colors may vary with different manufacturers. If uncertain, verify with the laboratory.

After
- Apply pressure or a pressure dressing to the venipuncture site.
- Assess the site for bleeding.

PT = Patient teaching

T0295096

ROUTINE URINE TESTING

Many laboratory tests include the direction to perform routine urine testing. The protocol for those tests is presented here and is cross-referenced within the many tests requiring them.

Before
- Follow proper patient identification protocols to avoid wrong patient events. Usually name and date of birth are used as two identifiers.
- **PT** Explain the procedure to the patient.
- **PT** Inform the patient if food or fluid restrictions are needed.

During
Random, fresh, or spot specimen
PT Instruct the patient to urinate into an appropriate nonsterile container.

24-hour specimen
1. Begin the 24-hour collection by discarding the first specimen.
2. Collect all urine voided during the next 24 hours.
3. Show the patient where to store the urine.
4. Keep the urine on ice or refrigerated during the collection period. Foley bags are kept in a basin of ice. Some collections require a preservative. Check with the laboratory.
5. Post the hours for the urine collection in a prominent place to prevent accidentally discarding a specimen.
6. Instruct the patient to void before defecating so that urine is not contaminated by stool.
7. Remind the patient not to put toilet paper in the urine collection container.
8. Collect the last specimen as close as possible to the end of the 24-hour period. Add this urine to the collection.

After
- Transport the specimen promptly to the laboratory.

PT = Patient teaching

MOSBY'S®
DIAGNOSTIC & LABORATORY TEST REFERENCE

Seventeenth Edition

Kathleen Deska Pagana, PhD, RN
Professor Emeritus
Department of Nursing
Lycoming College
Williamsport, Pennsylvania

Timothy J. Pagana, MD, FACS
Medical Director Emeritus
The Kathryn Candor Lundy Breast Health Center
Susquehanna Health System
Williamsport, Pennsylvania

Theresa Noel Pagana, MD, FAAEM
Emergency Medicine Physician
Greater Philadelphia, Pennsylvania

ELSEVIER

Elsevier
3251 Riverport Lane
St. Louis, Missouri 63043

MOSBY'S® DIAGNOSTIC & LABORATORY
TEST REFERENCE, SEVENTEENTH EDITION   ISBN: 978-0-323-82866-6

Notice

Practitioners and researchers must always rely on their own experience and
knowledge in evaluating and using any information, methods, compounds
or experiments described herein. Because of rapid advances in the medical
sciences, in particular, independent verification of diagnoses and drug
dosages should be made. To the fullest extent of the law, no responsibility
is assumed by Elsevier, authors, editors or contributors for any injury
and/or damage to persons or property as a matter of products liability,
negligence or otherwise, or from any use or operation of any methods,
products, instructions, or ideas contained in the material herein.

Previous editions copyrighted 2023, 2021, 2019, 2017, 2015, 2013, 2011,
2009, 2007, 2005, 2003, 2001, 1999, 1997, 1995, 1992

Senior Content Strategist: Yvonne Alexopoulos
Senior Content Development Manager: Lisa P. Newton
Senior Content Development Specialist: Tina Kaemmerer
Publishing Services Manager: Deepthi Unni
Project Manager: Thoufiq Mohammed
Design Direction: Renee Duenow

Printed in India

Last digit is the print number: 9   8   7   6   5   4   3   2   1

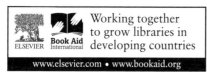

Working together
to grow libraries in
developing countries

ELSEVIER   Book Aid International

www.elsevier.com • www.bookaid.org

It is with admiration and encouragement that we dedicate this book to all those entering health care.

—KDP, TJP, TNP

preface

The 17th edition of *Mosby's® Diagnostic & Laboratory Test Reference* provides the user with an up-to-date, essential reference that allows easy access to clinically relevant laboratory and diagnostic tests. All tests begin on a new page and are listed in alphabetical order by their complete names. The alphabetical format is a strong feature of the book; it allows the user to locate tests quickly without first having to place them in an appropriate category or body system. The User's Guide to Test Preparation and Procedures section outlines the responsibilities of healthcare providers to ensure that the tests are accurately and safely performed. Use of this guide should eliminate the need for test repetition resulting from problems with patient preparation, test procedures, or collection techniques. Information on radiation exposure and risks has been added.

The following information is provided, wherever applicable, for effective diagnostic & laboratory testing:

- **Name of test.** Tests are listed by their complete names. A complete list of abbreviations and alternate test names follows each main entry.
- **Type of test.** This section identifies whether the test is, for example, an x-ray procedure, ultrasound, nuclear scan, blood test, urine test, sputum test, or microscopic examination of tissue.
- **Normal findings.** Where applicable, normal values are listed for the infant, child, adult, and elderly person. Also, where appropriate, values are separated into male and female. It is important to realize that normal ranges of laboratory tests vary from institution to institution. This variability is even more obvious among the various laboratory textbooks. For this reason, we have deliberately chosen not to add a table of normal values as an appendix, and we encourage the user to check the normal values at the institution where the test is performed. This should be relatively easy because laboratory reports include normal values. Results are given in both conventional units and the International System of Units (SI units) where possible.
- **Possible critical values.** These values give an indication of results that are well outside the normal range. These results require healthcare provider notification and usually result in some type of intervention.
- **Test explanation and related physiology.** This section provides a concise yet comprehensive description of each test. It

includes fundamental information about the test itself, specific indications for the test, how the test is performed, what disease or disorder the various results may show, how it will affect the patient or client, and relevant pathophysiology that will enhance understanding of the test.

- **Contraindications.** These data are crucial because they alert healthcare providers to patients to whom the test should not be administered.
- **Potential complications.** This section alerts the user to potential problems that necessitate astute assessments and interventions. For example, if a potential complication is renal failure, the implication may be to hydrate the patient before the test and force fluids after the test.
- **Interfering factors.** This section contains pertinent information, because many factors can invalidate the test or make the test results unreliable.
- **Procedure and patient care.** This section emphasizes the role of nurses and other healthcare providers in diagnostic & laboratory testing by addressing psychosocial and physiologic interventions. Patient teaching priorities are noted with a special icon (**PT**) to highlight information to be communicated to patients. For quick access to essential information, this section is divided into before, during, and after time sequences.
  - ○ **Before.** This section addresses the need to explain the procedure and to allay patient concerns or anxieties. If patient consent is usually required, this is listed as a bulleted item. Other important features include requirements such as fasting, obtaining baseline values, and performing bowel preparations. Radiation risk is addressed with x-rays and nuclear medicine studies.
  - ○ **During.** This section gives specific directions for clinical specimen studies (e.g., urine and blood studies). Diagnostic procedures and their variations are described.
  - ○ **After.** This section includes vital information that the nurse or other healthcare provider should heed or convey after the test. Examples include such factors as maintaining bed rest, encouraging fluid intake, and observing the patient for signs and symptoms of sepsis.
- **Abnormal findings.** As the name implies, this section lists the abnormal findings for each study. Diseases or conditions that may be indicated by increased (▲) or decreased (▼) values are listed where appropriate.

- **Notes.** This blank space at the end of the tests facilitates individualizing the studies according to the institution at which the test is performed. Variations in any area of the test (e.g., patient preparation, test procedure, normal values, postprocedural care) can be noted here.

This logical format emphasizes clinically relevant information. The clarity of this format allows for quick understanding of content essential to both students and healthcare providers. Color has been used to help locate tests and to highlight critical information (e.g., possible critical values). Color is also used in the illustrations to enhance the reader's understanding of many diagnostic procedures (e.g., amniocentesis, bronchoscopy, colposcopy, fetoscopy, transesophageal echocardiography [TEE]).

Standard guidelines for routine blood and urine testing are located on the inside front cover for easy access. A list of abbreviations for test names is included on the book's endpapers.

Appendix A includes a list of studies according to *body system*.

Appendix B provides a list of studies according to *test type*.

Appendix C provides a list of blood tests used for *disease and organ panels*.

Appendix D provides a list of *symbols and units of measurement*.

Finally, a comprehensive index includes the names of all tests, their synonyms and abbreviations, and any other relevant terms found in the tests.

Note the table of *Common Reference Ranges* on the inside front cover. This adds to the user-friendly aspect of this book by quickly identifying common reference ranges. This is a good starting point for students and a quick reference for routine lab values. However, because lab values vary from institution to institution, be sure to use the normal values of the lab performing the test.

We sincerely thank our editors for their enthusiasm and continued support. We are most grateful to the many nurses and other healthcare providers who made the first 16 editions of this book so successful. Thank you so much. This success validated the need for a user-friendly and quick-reference approach to laboratory and diagnostic testing.

We sincerely invite additional comments from current users of this book so that we may continue to provide useful, relevant diagnostic & laboratory test information to users of future editions.

Kathleen D. Pagana
Timothy J. Pagana
Theresa N. Pagana

contents

list of figures

The following guidelines delineate the responsibilities of health-care providers to ensure safety of test procedures and accuracy of test results. Guidelines are described for the following major types of tests: blood, urine, stool, x-ray, nuclear scanning, ultrasound, and endoscopy.

Blood tests

Overview

Blood studies are used to assess a multitude of body processes and disorders. *Appendix C* provides a list of current disease and organ panels.

Guidelines

- Observe universal precautions when collecting a blood specimen.
- Check whether fasting is required. Many studies, such as fasting blood sugar and cholesterol levels, require fasting for a designated period of time. Water is permitted.
- If ordered, withhold medications until the blood is drawn.
- Record the time of day when the blood test is drawn. Some blood test results (e.g., those for cortisol) vary according to a diurnal pattern, and this must be considered when blood levels are interpreted.
- In general, two or three blood tests can be done per tube of blood collected (e.g., two or three chemistry tests from one red-top tube of blood).
- Note the patient's position for certain tests (e.g., renin, because levels are affected by body position).
- Collect the blood in a properly color-coded test tube. Blood collection tubes have color-coded stoppers to indicate the presence or absence of different types of additives (preservatives and anticoagulants). A preservative prevents change in the specimen, and an anticoagulant inhibits clot formation or coagulation. Charts are available from the laboratory indicating the type of tube needed for each particular blood test. A representative chart is shown in Table A.
- Follow the recommended *order of draw* when collecting blood in tubes. Draw specimens into nonadditive (e.g., red-top) tubes before drawing them into tubes with additives. This prevents contamination of the blood specimen with additives that may cause incorrect test results. Fill the tubes in the following order:
  1. Blood culture tubes (to maintain sterility)

2. Nonadditive tubes (e.g., red-top)
3. Coagulation tubes (e.g., blue-top)
4. Heparin tubes (e.g., green-top)
5. Ethylenediaminetetraacetic acid (EDTA) tubes (e.g., lavender-top)
6. Oxalate/fluoride tubes (e.g., gray-top)

- To obtain valid results, do not fasten the tourniquet for longer than 1 minute. Prolonged tourniquet application can cause stasis and hemoconcentration.
- Collect the blood specimen from the arm without an intravenous (IV) device, if possible. IV infusion can influence test results.
- Do not use the arm bearing a dialysis arteriovenous fistula for venipuncture unless the physician specifically authorizes it.
- Because of the risk of cellulitis, do not take specimens from the side on which a mastectomy or axillary lymph node dissection was performed.
- Follow the unit guidelines for drawing blood from an indwelling venous catheter (e.g., a triple-lumen catheter). Guidelines will specify the amount of blood to be drawn from the catheter and discarded before blood is collected for laboratory studies. The guidelines will also indicate the amount and type of solution needed to flush the catheter after drawing the blood to prevent clotting.
- Do not shake the blood specimen. Hemolysis may result from vigorous shaking and can invalidate test results. Use gentle inversions.
- Collect *blood cultures* before the initiation of antibiotic therapy.
- *Skin punctures* can be used for blood tests on capillary blood. Common puncture sites include the fingertips, earlobes, and heel surfaces. Fingertips are often used for small children, and the heel is the most commonly used site for infants.
- After the specimen is drawn, apply pressure or a pressure dressing to the venipuncture site. Assess the site for bleeding.
- If the patient fasted before the blood test, reinstitute the appropriate diet.

Urine tests

Overview

Urine tests are easy to obtain and provide valuable information about many body system functions (e.g., kidney function, glucose metabolism, and various hormone levels). The ability of the

TABLE A   Common blood collection tubes

Top color	Additive	Purpose	Test examples
Red	Clot activator	Allows blood sample to clot Separates the serum for testing	Chemistry Bilirubin Blood urea nitrogen
Red/black	Clot activator and gel for serum separator	Serum separator tube for serum determinatives in chemistry and serology	Chemistry, serology
Royal blue Tan	Heparin/EDTA Heparin/EDTA	Provides low levels of trace elements Contains no lead	Trace metals, toxicology Lead determinatives
Purple or lavender	EDTA	Prevents blood from clotting	Hematology CBC
Gray	Oxalate/fluoride	Prevents glycolysis	Chemistry Glucose
Green	Heparin	Prevents blood from clotting when plasma needs to be tested	Chemistry Ammonia
Blue (light)	Sodium citrate	Prevents blood from clotting when plasma needs to be tested	Prothrombin time Partial thromboplastin time
Black	Sodium citrate	Binds calcium to prevent blood clotting	Westergren ESR
Yellow	Citrate dextrose	Preserves red cells	Blood cultures, blood banking studies

CBC, Complete blood count; *EDTA*, ethylenediaminetetraacetic acid; *ESR*, erythrocyte sedimentation rate.

patient to collect specimens appropriately should be assessed to determine the need for assistance.

Guidelines

- Observe universal precautions in collecting a urine specimen.
- Use the first morning specimen for routine urinalysis because it is more concentrated. To collect a first morning specimen, have the patient void before going to bed and collect the first urine specimen immediately upon rising.
- *Random* urine specimens can be collected at any time. They are usually obtained during daytime hours and without any prior patient preparation.
- If a *culture and sensitivity (C&S)* study is required or if the specimen is likely to be contaminated by vaginal discharge or bleeding, collect a *clean-catch* or *midstream* specimen. This requires meticulous cleansing of the urinary meatus with an antiseptic preparation to reduce contamination of the specimen by external organisms. Then the cleansing agent must be completely removed because it may contaminate the specimen. Obtain the *midstream* collection by doing the following:
  1. Have the patient begin to urinate in a bedpan, urinal, or toilet and then stop urinating. (This washes the urine out of the distal urethra.)
  2. Correctly position a sterile urine container and have the patient void 3 to 4 oz of urine into it.
  3. Cap the container.
  4. Allow the patient to finish voiding.
- One-time *composite* urine specimens are collected over a period that may range anywhere from 2 to 24 hours. To collect a timed specimen, instruct the patient to void and discard the first specimen. This is noted as the *start time* of the test. Instruct the patient to save all subsequent urine in a special container for the designated period. Remind the patient to void before defecating so that urine is not contaminated by feces. Also, instruct the patient not to put toilet paper in the collection container. A preservative is usually used in the collection container. At the end of the specified time period, have the patient void and then add this urine to the specimen container, thus completing the collection process.
- Collection containers for *24-hour urine specimens* should hold 3 to 4 L of urine and have tight-fitting lids. They should be labeled with the patient's name, the starting collection date and time, the ending collection date and time, the name of the test, the preservative, and storage requirements during collection.

- Many urine collections require preservatives to maintain their stability during the collection period. Some specimens are best preserved by being kept on ice or refrigerated.
- *Urinary catheterization* may be needed for patients who are unable to void. This procedure is not preferred because of patient discomfort and the risk of patient infection.
- For patients with an *indwelling urinary catheter*, obtain a specimen by aseptically inserting a needleless syringe into the catheter at a drainage port distal to the sleeve leading to the balloon. Aspirate urine and then place it in a sterile urine container. The urine that accumulates in the plastic reservoir bag should never be used for a urine test.
- Urine specimens from infants and young children are sometimes collected in a disposable pouch called a *U bag*. This bag has an adhesive backing around the opening to attach to the child's perineum. After the bag is in place, check the child every 15 minutes to see if an adequate specimen has been collected.

Stool tests

Overview

The examination of feces provides important information that aids in the differential diagnosis of various gastrointestinal disorders. Fecal studies may also be used for microbiologic studies, chemical determinations, and parasitic examinations.

Guidelines

- Observe universal precautions in collecting a stool specimen.
- Collect stool specimens in a clean container with a fitted lid.
- Do not mix urine and toilet paper with the stool specimen. Both can contaminate the specimen and alter the results.
- Fecal analysis for occult blood, white blood cells, or qualitative fecal fat requires only a small amount of a randomly collected specimen.
- Quantitative tests for daily fecal excretion of a particular substance require a minimum of a 3-day fecal collection. This collection is necessary because the daily excretion of feces does not correlate well with the amount of food ingested by the patient in the same 24-hour period. Refrigerate specimens or keep them on ice during the collection period. Collect stool in a 1-gallon container.
- A small amount of fecal blood that is not visually apparent is termed *occult blood*. Chemical tests using commercially prepared slides are routinely used to detect fecal blood.

Numerous commercial slide tests use guaiac as the indicator. These guaiac tests are routinely done on nursing units and in medical offices.

- Consider various factors (e.g., other diagnostic tests and medications) in planning the stool collection. For example, if the patient is scheduled for x-ray studies with barium sulfate, collect the stool specimen first. Various medications affect the detection of intestinal parasites.
- Some fecal collections require dietary restrictions before the collection.
- Correctly label and deliver stool specimens to the laboratory within 30 minutes after collection. If you are unable to deliver the specimen within 30 minutes, it may be refrigerated for up to 2 hours.

X-ray studies

Overview

Because of the ability of x-rays to penetrate tissues, x-ray studies provide a valuable picture of body structures. X-ray studies can be as simple as a routine chest x-ray image or as complex as dye-enhanced cardiac catheterization. With the concern about radiation exposure, it is important to realize that the patient may question if the proposed benefits outweigh the risks involved.

In CT scanning, computers re-create a three-dimensional, cross-sectional view of body structures after obtaining x-ray information from the entire circumference of the body. The CT scan results from passing x-rays through the body organs at many angles through 360 degrees. The variation in density of each tissue allows for variable penetration of the x-rays. Each degree of density is given a numeric value called a *density coefficient*, which is digitally computed into a shade of gray. The images are recorded digitally.

Radiation dose

There are several units used to quantify amount of radiation absorbed from diagnostic imaging tests. The gray (Gy) is the measure of the amount of energy absorbed per unit mass. Because different organs in the body absorb radiation differently, the sievert (Sv) is often used instead of the gray. The sievert is the biological effect of 1 gray of radiation on human body tissue. The sievert is more helpful in comparing radiation exposure to different parts of the body. Radiation doses in medical imaging are typically measured in millisieverts (mSv) or 1/1000 of a sievert. On average, each person receives about 3 mSv of radiation yearly from natural background radiation.

The roentgen equivalent in man (rem) is an older unit to quantify the amount of radiation absorbed from x-rays. 1 rem is equivalent to 0.01 sievert.

See chart below for average amounts of radiation for adults associated with diagnostic testing.

Risk of radiation

Radiation exposure can cause damage to DNA. The body usually rapidly repairs this damage. Mistakes in DNA repair can lead to chromosomal or gene abnormalities that may be linked to cancer induction. The likelihood of cancer induction secondary to radiation exposure increases as the amount of radiation exposure increases. A person has a 5% increase in developing cancer over his or her lifetime after radiation exposure of 1 Sv or more. There can be a lag of many years between radiation exposure and cancer diagnosis. The average lag time is about 10 years after exposure.

The cumulative radiation dose from diagnostic imaging is very small, and the benefit of proper diagnosis and treatment of disease generally outweighs the risks. However, each patient's current situation and history of radiation must be considered to accurately assess cumulative risks and benefits. Diagnostic procedures with higher radiation doses (e.g., computed tomography [CT] scans) should be clearly justified. Appropriateness Criteria published by the American College of Radiology (acr.org) are helpful in justification of x-ray imaging.

Special consideration should be given to pregnant women and children before ordering x-ray imaging, because the effects of radiation are more profound in fetuses and young children. If a woman is pregnant, the risks versus benefits must be carefully considered. Certain studies with low radiation in which the focus of radiation is not on the fetus are safer. (Lead-containing shields can reduce x-ray exposure to fetuses.) Imaging using higher doses of radiation should be given only if the risk of not making the diagnosis is greater than the radiation risk.

Radiation risks are most significant in early fetal period and are less significant as the pregnancy progresses.

Patients with high body mass indexes should also be given extra consideration before ordering imaging studies. These patients often require greater radiation doses to penetrate body thickness to create acceptable images. Nuclear medicines studies are not affected in the same way. Although the x-ray exposure needed to produce one fluoroscopic image is low, high exposures to patients can occur in lengthy procedures.

Radiation Associated With Diagnostic Testing

Common radiology imaging (XR)	Average adult effective dose[a] (mSv)
Abdomen	0.7
Back (lower)	1.5
Back (upper)	1
Barium enema	8
Bone densitometry (DEXA)	0.001
Cervical spine	0.2
Chest	0.1
Dental	0.005–0.01
Extremity (hands, feet, and so on)	0.001
Fluoroscopy	Per minute
Hip	0.7
Hysterosalpingography	2
Intravenous pyelography (IVP)	3
Mammography	0.4
Neck	0.2
Pelvis	0.6
Skull	0.1
Small bowel follow-through	5
Spine (lumbar)	1.5
Spine (thoracic)	1.0
Upper GI series	6

Common CT imaging	
Abdomen and pelvis	10
Brain (head)	2
Chest	7
Chest (low-dose screening)	2
Coronary angiography	15
CT angiography of the chest	15
Neck	3
Sinuses	0.6
Spine	6
Virtual colonoscopy	10

Nuclear medicine

Bone scan	5
Brain scan	6.9
Cardiac nuclear stress testing	20–40
Gastric emptying scan	0.4
GI bleeding scan	7.8
Liver scan	3.1
Lung scan (ventilation/perfusion)	2
Parathyroid scan	6.7
Renal scan	2.6
Thyroid scan	4.8
Urea breath test	0.003
WBC scan	6.7

Other

Abdominal angiogram	12
Cardiac catheterization (diagnostic)	7
Coronary angiogram (stent)	15
Endoscopic retrograde cholangiopancreatography (ERCP)	4
Fluoroscopic Barium Swallow	1.5
Head and neck angiogram	5
Positron emission tomography (PET)/CT	25
Pulmonary angiography	5

[a]Effective doses are given as an average, and there may be wide variability in dosing depending on particularities of the test in different testing locations.

Guidelines

- Assess the patient for any similar or recent x-ray procedures.
- Evaluate the patient for *allergies to contrast media*. Carefully consider the following points:
  1. Many types of contrast media are used in radiographic studies. The patient should always be assessed for allergies to contrast media before it is administered. Patients at increased risks for allergic reactions include previous intravenous contrast reactions, asthma, multiple true allergies, and those taking beta-blockers. Inform the radiologist if an allergy is suspected. The radiologist may prescribe diphenhydramine and a steroid preparation to be administered before testing.

2. Allergic reactions to contrast media may include flushing, itching, urticaria, bronchospasm, hypotension, and anaphylaxis. In the unusual event of anaphylaxis, the patient is treated with diphenhydramine, steroids, and epinephrine. Oxygen and endotracheal equipment should be on hand for immediate use.

3. After the x-ray procedure, evaluate the patient for a delayed reaction to dye (e.g., dyspnea, rashes, tachycardia, hives). This usually occurs within 2 to 6 hours after the test. Treat with antihistamines or steroids.

- Assess the patient for dehydration or renal disease. Patients with impaired kidney function should be given special consideration before and after receiving iodine-based contrast materials, as renal function may diminish further. Usually BUN and creatinine tests are obtained before administration of contrast media. Hydration may be required before the administration of contrast.

- Assess the patient for diabetes. Patients with diabetes who take metformin are at risk for developing metformin-associated lactic acidosis (MALA). While the incidence of MALA is extremely low, the mortality is 25% to 50%. The American College of Radiology (ACR) recommends that patients taking metformin be classified into one of two categories based on the patient's renal function (as measured by eGFR).

  Category I patients with no evidence of AKI and with eGFR $\geq$30 mL/min/1.73 m^2 have no need to discontinue metformin prior to or following IV iodinated contrast media. Category II patients with acute kidney injury or severe chronic kidney disease (stage IV or stage V; i.e., eGFR<30) should temporarily discontinue metformin for 48 hours following IV iodinated contrast.

- Pregnant women should not have x-ray procedures unless the benefits outweigh the risks.

- Note whether other x-ray studies are being planned; schedule them in the appropriate sequence. For example, x-ray examinations that do not require contrast should precede examinations that do require contrast. X-ray studies with barium should be scheduled after ultrasonography.

- Note the necessary dietary restrictions. Such studies as barium enema and intravenous pyelogram (IVP) are more accurate if the patient is kept NPO (fasting from food and liquids) for several hours before the test.

- Determine whether bowel preparations are necessary. For example, barium enemas and IVPs require bowel-cleansing regimens.

- Determine whether signed consent forms are required. These are necessary for most invasive x-ray procedures.
- Remove metal objects (e.g., necklaces, watches) because they can hinder visualization of the x-ray field.
- Patient aftercare is determined by the type of x-ray procedure. For example, a patient having a simple chest x-ray study will not require postprocedure care. However, invasive x-ray procedures involving contrast dyes (e.g., cardiac catheterization) require extensive nursing measures to detect potential complications.

Nuclear scanning

Overview

With the administration of a radionuclide and subsequent measurement of the radiation of a particular organ, functional abnormalities of various body areas (e.g., brain, heart, lung, bones) can be detected. Because the half-lives of the radioisotopes are short, only minimal radiation exposure occurs.

Guidelines

- Radiopharmaceuticals concentrate in target organs by various mechanisms. For example, some labeled compounds are cleared from the blood and excreted by the kidneys. Some phosphate compounds concentrate in the bone and infarcted tissue. Lung function can be studied by imaging the distribution of inhaled gases or aerosols.
- Note whether the patient has had any recent exposure to radionuclides. The previous study could interfere with the interpretation of the current study.
- Note the patient's age and current weight. This information is used to calculate the dose of radioactive substances.
- Nuclear scans are limited in pregnant women and nursing mothers.
- Many scanning procedures do not require special preparation. However, a few have special requirements. For example, for bone scanning, the patient is encouraged to drink several glasses of water between the time of the injection of the isotope and the actual scanning. For some studies, blocking agents may need to be given to prevent other organs from taking up the isotope.
- For most nuclear scans, a small amount of an organ-specific radionuclide is given orally or injected intravenously. After the radioisotope concentrates in the desired area, the area is scanned. The scanning procedure usually takes place in the nuclear medicine department.

- Instruct the patient to lie still during the scanning.
- Usually encourage the patient to drink extra fluids to enhance excretion of the radionuclide after the test is finished.
- Although the amount of radionuclide excreted in the urine is very low, rubber gloves are sometimes recommended if the urine must be handled. Some hospitals may advise the patient to flush the toilet several times after voiding.

Ultrasound studies

Overview

In diagnostic ultrasonography, high-frequency sound waves are emitted and penetrate the organ being studied. The sound waves bounce back to the sensor and are electronically converted into a picture of the organ. Ultrasonography is used to assess a variety of body areas, including the pelvis, abdomen, breast, heart, and pregnant uterus.

Guidelines

- Many ultrasound procedures require little or no preparation.
- Ultrasound examinations are usually performed in an ultrasound room; however, they can be performed anywhere.
- For ultrasound, a gel lubricant is applied to the skin overlying the desired organ. This is used to enhance sound transmission and reception, because air impedes transmission of sound waves to the body.
- Barium has an adverse effect on the quality of abdominal studies. For this reason, schedule ultrasound of the abdomen before barium studies.
- Large amounts of gas in the bowel obstruct visualization of the bowel. This is because bowel gas is a reflector of sound.

Endoscopy procedures

Overview

With the help of a lighted, flexible instrument, internal structures of many areas of the body (e.g., stomach, colon, joints, bronchi, urinary system, and biliary tree) can be directly viewed. The specific purpose and procedure should be reviewed with the patient.

Guidelines

- Preparation for an endoscopic procedure varies according to the internal structure being examined. For example, examination of the stomach (gastroscopy) will require the passage of an instrument through the esophagus and into the stomach. The patient is kept NPO for 8 to 12 hours before the test to prevent gagging, vomiting, and aspiration. For colonoscopy, an instrument is passed through the rectum and into the colon. Therefore, the bowel must be cleansed and free of fecal material to afford proper visualization. Arthroscopic examination of the knee joint is usually done with the patient under general anesthesia, which necessitates routine preoperative care.

- Schedule endoscopic examinations before barium studies.
- Obtain a signed consent for endoscopic procedures.
- Endoscopic procedures are preferably performed by a physician in a specially equipped endoscopy room or in an operating room. However, some kinds can safely be performed at the bedside.
- Air is instilled into the bowel during colon examinations to maintain patency of the bowel lumen and to afford better visualization. This sometimes causes gas pains.
- In addition to visualization of the desired area, special procedures can be performed. Biopsies can be obtained, and bleeding ulcers can be cauterized. Also, knee surgery can be performed during arthroscopy.
- Specific postprocedure interventions are determined by the type of endoscopic examination performed. All procedures have the potential complication of perforation and bleeding. Most procedures use some type of sedation; safety precautions should be observed until the effects of the sedatives have worn off.
- After colonoscopy and similar studies, the patient may complain of rectal discomfort. A warm tub bath may be soothing.
- Usually keep the patient NPO for 2 hours after endoscopic procedures of the upper gastrointestinal system. Be certain that swallow, gag, and cough reflexes are present before permitting fluids or liquids to be ingested orally.

acetylcholine receptor antibody panel (AChR Ab, Anti–AChR antibody)

Type of test Blood

Normal findings

ACh receptor (muscle) binding antibodies: ≤ 0.02 nmol/L

ACh receptor (muscle) modulating antibodies: 0%-20% (reported as % loss of AChR)

Striational (striated muscle) antibodies: $< 1:60$

Test explanation and related physiology

Myasthenia gravis (MG) is an autoimmune disease caused by antibodies directed toward receptors embedded in the motor endplate of the neuromuscular junction. There are three types of antibodies against muscle AChR that impede neuromuscular transmission by a range of pathogenic mechanisms:

1. *AChR binding antibodies* attach to the AChR and activate the complement system causing destruction of the neuromuscular junction.

2. *AChR modulating antibodies* crosslink receptor subunits and cause the receptors to be degraded in a process known as antigenic modulation. Modulating antibodies are implicated with an increased risk of thymoma.

3. *AChR blocking antibodies* functionally block the binding of acetylcholine to the AChR.

Antibodies to AChR occur in more than 85% of patients with MG. Lower levels are seen in patients with ocular MG only. The presence of these antibodies is virtually diagnostic of MG, but a negative test result does not exclude the disease. The measured titers do not correspond well with the severity of MG. However, antibody levels are particularly useful in monitoring disease and response to therapy. As the patient improves, antibody titers decrease. Patients with MG frequently have thymic abnormalities (thymic hyperplasia or thymoma).

Other non-AChR antibodies can develop in MG. *Lipoprotein receptor-related protein 4 (LRP4)* is another autoantibody that activates muscle-specific tyrosine kinase (MuSK) and AChR clustering and neuromuscular junction formation. *Muscle-specific tyrosine kinase antibody (MuSK-ab)* acts as an antibody against a receptor-associated protein. These antibodies may be positive especially in AChR antibody "negative" patients. *Antistriated muscle antibody* (*striated muscle antibody, IgG*) and *titin antibodies* are directed

TABLE A1 Autoimmune antineural antibodies associated with lung cancer

Antibody	Neurological disease
Acetylcholine receptor ganglionic	Autoimmune autonomic ganglionopathy
Voltage-gated calcium channel P/Q	Lambert-Eaton MG
Voltage-gated calcium channel N	Lambert-Eaton MG
Voltage-gated potassium channel	Limbic encephalitis

against the contractile elements of striated muscle and are found in some adult patients with MG and in most of those with thymoma.

Neoplasms can also be an endogenous source of autoimmune antineural antibodies. See Table A1.

Interfering factors

- False-positive results may occur in patients with amyotrophic lateral sclerosis who have been treated with cobra venom.
- False-positive results may be seen in patients with penicillamine-induced or Lambert-Eaton myasthenic syndrome.
- Patients with autoimmune liver disease may have elevations.

Procedure and patient care

- See inside front cover for Routine Blood Testing.
- Fasting: no
- Blood tube commonly used: red

Abnormal findings

▲ **Increased titer levels**
Myasthenia gravis
Ocular myasthenia gravis
Thymoma

notes

activated clotting time (ACT, Activated coagulation time)

Type of test Blood

Normal findings

70–120 sec

Therapeutic range for anticoagulation: 150–600 sec

(Normal ranges and anticoagulation ranges vary according to type of laboratory procedure and particular therapy.)

Possible critical values

Depend on use for the test and clinical situation

Test explanation and related physiology

The ACT is primarily used to measure the anticoagulant effect of heparin or other direct thrombin inhibitors during cardiac angioplasty, hemodialysis, and cardiopulmonary bypass (CPB) surgery. This test measures the time for whole blood to clot after the addition of particulate activators. It is similar to the *activated partial thromboplastin time* (APTT, p. 557) in that it measures the ability of the *intrinsic* pathway to begin clot formation by activating factor XII (see Figure C3, p. 212). By checking the blood clotting status with ACT, the response to unfractionated heparin therapy can be monitored.

Both the APTT and the ACT can be used to monitor heparin therapy for patients during CPB. However, the ACT has several advantages over the APTT. First, the ACT is more accurate than the APTT when high doses of heparin are used for anticoagulation. This makes it especially useful during clinical situations requiring high-dose heparin, such as during CPB, when high-dose anticoagulation is necessary at levels 10 times those used for venous thrombosis. The APTT is not measurable at these high doses. The accepted goal for the ACT is 400 to 480 seconds during CPB.

Second, the ACT is both less expensive and more easily performed, even at the bedside. This allows for immediate accessibility and decreased turnaround time. The capability to perform the ACT at the point of care makes the ACT particularly useful for patients requiring angioplasty, hemodialysis, and CPB.

A nomogram is often used as a guide to reach the desired level of anticoagulation. This nomogram is used in determining the dose of protamine to neutralize the heparin upon completion of these procedures. The ACT is used in determining when it is safe to remove the vascular access upon completion of these procedures. The benefits of the *modified* ACT test are that it requires a smaller-volume blood specimen; it can be automated; it can use standardized blood/reagent mixing; and it provides faster clotting time results than the conventional ACT. The modified ACT is now used more frequently.

Interfering factors

- The ACT is affected by biologic variables, including hypothermia, hemodilution, and platelet number and function.
- Factors affecting the pharmacokinetics of heparin (e.g., kidney or liver disease) and heparin resistance can affect ACT measurements.
- A clotted specimen can increase ACT measurements.

Procedure and patient care

- See inside front cover for Routine Blood Testing.
- Fasting: no
- Blood tube commonly used: verify with laboratory
- Less than 1 mL of blood is collected and placed in a machine at the bedside. When a clot forms, the ACT value is displayed.
- If the patient is receiving a continuous heparin drip, the blood sample is obtained from the arm without the intravenous catheter.
- The bleeding time will be prolonged because of anticoagulation therapy.
- Assess the patient to detect possible bleeding. Check for blood in the urine and all other excretions, and assess the patient for bruises, petechiae, and low back pain.

Abnormal findings

▲ **Increased levels**
Cirrhosis of the liver
Clotting factor deficiencies
Heparin administration
Lupus inhibitor
Warfarin administration

▼ **Decreased levels**
Thrombosis

notes

adiponectin

Type of test Blood
Normal findings

BMI	Adiponectin (mcg/mL)	
	Male	Female
<25 kg/m²	4–26	5–37
25–30 kg/m²	4–20	5–28
>30 kg/m²	2–20	4–22

Test explanation and related physiology

Adiponectin is an accurate biomarker of the risk for developing metabolic syndrome and type 2 diabetes. Individuals with low adiponectin levels have a three times greater risk for developing metabolic syndrome. Individuals with low levels of adiponectin are up to nine times as likely to develop type 2 diabetes.

Adiponectin is a protein hormone produced and secreted by adipose tissue. Adiponectin is normally found in relatively high concentrations in healthy individuals. Its role in the body is to regulate the metabolism of lipids and glucose, which influences the body's response to insulin and inflammation. Adiponectin levels are inversely correlated with abdominal visceral fat. Visceral fat is associated with insulin resistance, high blood pressure, and high levels of cholesterol, subsequently increasing the risk for metabolic syndrome, diabetes, cardiovascular disease, and benign prostatic hypertrophy. Adiponectin is a biomarker related to type 2 diabetes. If women have lower adiponectin concentration during the first trimester of pregnancy, they are 3.5 times more likely to develop gestational diabetes. Adiponectin levels are an independent predictor of coronary heart disease (CHD) in Caucasian men with no previous history of CHD. Measuring serum concentration of adiponectin is a more reliable indicator of at-risk patients in comparison to conventional methods of determining whether a patient is overweight or obese.

Procedure and patient care

- See inside front cover for Routine Blood Testing.
- Fasting: yes, overnight
- Blood tube commonly used: tiger-top
- After drawing blood, gently invert tube five times immediately.

• Do not shake the specimen because hemolysis will nullify the test results.

Abnormal findings

Benign prostatic hypertrophy
Coronary artery disease
Metabolic syndrome
Obesity
Type 2 diabetes

notes

adrenal steroid precursors (Androstenediones [AD], Dehydroepiandrosterone [DHEA], Dehydroepiandrosterone sulfate [DHEA S], 11-Deoxycortisol, 17-Hydroxyprogesterone, 17-Hydroxypregnenolone, Pregnenolone)

Type of test   Blood

Normal findings

		Male	Female
AD	Tanner stage I	0.04–0.32 ng/mL	0.05–0.51 ng/mL
	Tanner stage II	0.08–0.48 ng/mL	0.15–1.37 ng/mL
	Tanner stage III	0.14–0.87 ng/mL	0.37–2.24 ng/mL
	Tanner stage IV-V	0.27–1.07 ng/mL	0.35–2.05 ng/mL
DHEA	Tanner stage I	0.11–2.37 ng/mL	0.14–2.76 ng/mL
	Tanner stage II	0.37–3.66 ng/mL	0.83–4.87 ng/mL
	Tanner stage III	0.75–5.24 ng/mL	1.08–7.56 ng/mL
	Tanner stage IV-V	1.22–6.73 ng/mL	1.24–7.88 ng/mL
DHEA S	Tanner stage I	7–126 mcg/dL	7–209 mcg/dL
	Tanner stage II	13–241 mcg/dL	28–260 mcg/dL
	Tanner stage III	32–446 mcg/dL	39–390 mcg/dL
	Tanner stage IV-V	65–371 mcg/dL	81–488 mcg/dL

Test explanation and related physiology

Androstenediones (ADs, DHEA, and the sulfuric ester, DHEA S) are precursors of testosterone and estrone and are made in the gonads and the adrenal gland. 11-Deoxycortisol, 17-hydroxyprogesterone, 17-hydroxypregnenolone, and pregnenolone are precursors of cortisol. ACTH stimulates their adrenal secretion. Children with congenital adrenal hyperplasia (CAH) have genetic mutations that cause deficiencies in the enzymes involved in the synthesis of cortisol, testosterone, aldosterone, and estrone. When defects in enzyme synthesis occur along the path of hormone synthesis, the previously listed precursors exist in levels that exceed normal through the increased stimulation of ACTH.

The symptoms of the disorder depend on which steroids are overproduced and which are deficient. As a result, CAH may present with various symptoms, including virilization of the affected female infant, signs of androgen excess in males and females, signs of sex hormone deficiency in males and females, salt-wasting crisis secondary to cortisol and aldosterone deficiency, or hormonal hypertension due to increased mineralocorticoids. A milder, nonclassic form of CAH is characterized by premature puberty, acne, hirsutism, menstrual irregularity, and infertility.

These same precursors can occur in adults due to adrenal or gonadal tumors. Patients with polycystic ovary syndrome (Stein-Leventhal syndrome) have particularly elevated levels of ADs. DHEA S levels are particularly high in patients with adrenal carcinoma.

In patients suspected of CAH, testing for a panel of steroids involved in the cortisol biosynthesis pathway may be performed to establish the specific enzyme deficiency. In most cases, basal concentrations within the normal reference interval rule out CAH. The ratio of the precursor to the final pathway product (with and without ACTH stimulation) may be used to diagnose which enzyme is deficient.

Procedure and patient care

- See inside front cover for Routine Blood Testing.
- Fasting: no
- Blood tube commonly used: serum separator or red
- **PT** Tell the female patient that the specimen should be collected 1 week before or after the menstrual period.
- Indicate the date of the last menstrual period (if applicable) on the laboratory form.

Abnormal findings

▲ **Increased levels**

Adrenal tumor
Congenital adrenal
  hyperplasia
Cushing syndrome
  (some cases)
Ectopic ACTH-producing
  tumors
Ovarian sex cord tumor
Stein-Leventhal
  syndrome

▼ **Decreased levels**

Gonadal failure
Primary or secondary
  adrenal insufficiency

notes

adrenocorticotropic hormone (ACTH, Corticotropin)

Type of test Blood

Normal findings

Adult/elderly:

Male: 19 years and older: 7–69 pg/mL

Female: 19 years and older: 6–58 pg/mL

Children:

Male and female: 10–18 years: 6–55 pg/mL

Male and female: 1 week-9 years: 5–46 pg/mL

Test explanation and related physiology

The ACTH tests the anterior pituitary gland function and provides the greatest insight into the causes of either Cushing syndrome (overproduction of cortisol) or Addison disease (underproduction of cortisol). An elaborate feedback mechanism for cortisol exists to coordinate the function of the hypothalamus, pituitary gland, and adrenal glands. ACTH is an important part of this mechanism. Corticotropin-releasing hormone (CRH) is made in the hypothalamus. This stimulates ACTH production in the anterior pituitary gland. This, in turn, stimulates the adrenal cortex to produce cortisol. The rising levels of cortisol act as negative feedback and curtail further production of CRH and ACTH.

In a patient with Cushing syndrome, an elevated ACTH level can be caused by a pituitary or a nonpituitary (ectopic) ACTH-producing tumor, usually in the lung, pancreas, thymus, or ovary. ACTH levels over 200 pg/mL usually indicate ectopic ACTH production. If the ACTH level is lower than normal in a patient with Cushing syndrome, an adrenal adenoma or carcinoma is probably the cause of the hyperfunction.

In patients with Addison disease, an elevated ACTH level indicates primary adrenal gland failure, as in adrenal gland destruction caused by infarction, hemorrhage, or autoimmunity; surgical removal of the adrenal gland; congenital enzyme deficiency; or adrenal suppression after prolonged ingestion of exogenous steroids. If the ACTH level is lower than normal in a patient with adrenal insufficiency, hypopituitarism is most probably the cause of the hypofunction.

One must be aware that there is a diurnal variation of ACTH levels that corresponds to variation of cortisol levels. Levels in evening (8 PM to 10 PM) samples are usually one-half to two-thirds those of morning (4 AM to 8 AM) specimens. This diurnal variation is lost when disease (especially neoplasm) affects the pituitary or adrenal glands. Likewise, stress can blunt or eliminate this normal diurnal variation.

Interfering factors

- Stress (trauma, pyrogens, or hypoglycemia) and pregnancy can increase levels.
- Recently administered radioisotope scans can affect levels.

Procedure and patient care

- See inside front cover for Routine Blood Testing.
- Fasting: yes
- Blood tube commonly used: green. Verify with lab.
- Evaluate the patient for stress factors.
- Evaluate the patient for sleep pattern abnormalities that can impact the normal diurnal variation.
- Chill the blood tube to prevent enzymatic degradation.
- Place the specimen in ice water and send it to the laboratory immediately. ACTH is very unstable in plasma and should be stored at $-20°$ C to prevent artificially low values.

Abnormal findings

▲ **Increased levels**

Addison disease (primary adrenal insufficiency)

Adrenogenital syndrome (congenital adrenal hyperplasia)

Cushing syndrome (pituitary-dependent adrenal hyperplasia)

Ectopic ACTH syndrome

Stress

▼ **Decreased levels**

Adrenal adenoma or carcinoma

Cushing syndrome

Hypopituitarism

Secondary adrenal insufficiency (pituitary insufficiency)

Steroid administration

notes

adrenocorticotropic hormone stimulation test with cosyntropin (ACTH stimulation test, Cortisol stimulation test)

A

Type of test Blood

Normal findings

Rapid test: cortisol levels increase > 7 mcg/dL higher than baseline
24-hour test: cortisol levels > 40 mcg/dL
3-day test: cortisol levels > 40 mcg/dL

Test explanation and related physiology

This test is performed in patients found to have an adrenal insufficiency. An increase in plasma free or total cortisol levels after the infusion of an ACTH-like drug indicates that the adrenal gland is normal and is capable of functioning if stimulated. In that case, the cause of the adrenal insufficiency would lie within the pituitary gland (hypopituitarism, which is called secondary adrenal insufficiency). If little or no rise in cortisol levels occurs after the administration of the ACTH-like drug, the adrenal gland is the source of the problem and cannot secrete cortisol. This is called primary adrenal insufficiency (Addison disease).

This test can also be used in the evaluation of patients with Cushing syndrome. Patients with Cushing syndrome caused by bilateral adrenal hyperplasia have an exaggerated cortisol elevation in response to the administration of the ACTH-like drug. Those experiencing Cushing syndrome as a result of hyperfunctioning adrenal tumors have little or no increase in cortisol levels over baseline values.

Cosyntropin (Cortrosyn) is a synthetic subunit of ACTH. During this test, cosyntropin is administered to the patient, and the ability of the adrenal gland to respond is measured by plasma cortisol levels.

The *rapid stimulation test* is only a screening test. A normal response excludes adrenal insufficiency. An abnormal response, however, requires a 24-hour to 3-day prolonged ACTH stimulation test to differentiate primary insufficiency from secondary insufficiency. It should be noted that the adrenal gland can also be stimulated by insulin-induced hypoglycemia as a stressing agent. When insulin is the stimulant, cortisol and glucose levels are measured.

Procedure and patient care

- See inside front cover for Routine Blood Testing.
- Fasting: yes
- Blood tube commonly used: red

Rapid test
- Obtain a baseline plasma cortisol level.
- Administer an IV injection of cosyntropin as prescribed.
- Measure plasma cortisol levels 30 and 60 minutes after drug administration.

24-hour test
- Obtain a baseline plasma cortisol level.
- Start an IV infusion of synthetic cosyntropin.
- Administer the solution as prescribed for 24 hours.
- After 24 hours, obtain another plasma cortisol level.

3-day test
- Obtain a baseline plasma cortisol level.
- Administer the prescribed dose of cosyntropin IV over an 8-hour period for 2 to 3 consecutive days.
- Measure plasma cortisol levels at 12, 24, 36, 48, 60, and 72 hours after the start of the test.

Abnormal findings

In adrenal insufficiency

Increase higher than normal response (secondary adrenal insufficiency)
> Hypopituitarism
> Exogenous steroid ingestion
> Endogenous steroid production from a nonendocrine tumor

Normal or lower than normal response (primary adrenal insufficiency)
> Addison disease
> Adrenal infarction/hemorrhage
> Metastatic tumor to the adrenal gland
> Congenital enzyme adrenal insufficiency
> Surgical removal of the adrenal gland

In Cushing syndrome

Increase higher than normal response
> Bilateral adrenal hyperplasia

Normal or lower than normal response
> Adrenal adenoma
> Adrenal carcinoma
> ACTH-producing nonadrenal tumor
> Chronic steroid use

notes

adrenocorticotropic hormone stimulation test with metyrapone (ACTH stimulation test with metyrapone, Metyrapone test)

Type of test   Blood; urine (24-hour)

Normal findings

Blood

11-deoxycortisol increased to > 7 mcg/dL and cortisol < 10 mcg/dL

Urine (24-hour)

Baseline excretion of urinary *17-hydroxycorticosteroid* (17-OCHS) more than doubled

Test explanation and related physiology

Metyrapone is a potent blocker of an enzyme involved in cortisol production. Therefore cortisol production is reduced. When this drug is given, the resulting fall in cortisol production should stimulate pituitary secretion of ACTH by way of a negative feedback mechanism. Cortisol, ACTH, or cortisol precursors (*11-deoxycortisol* and *17-OCHS*) can be detected in the urine or blood. This test is similar to the ACTH stimulation test with *cosyntropin* (p. 11).

In patients with adrenal hyperplasia caused by pituitary overproduction of ACTH, the cortisol precursors are greatly increased, more than expected in normal patients. This is because the normal adrenal–pituitary response mechanism is still intact. No response to metyrapone occurs in patients with Cushing syndrome resulting from adrenal adenoma or carcinoma because the tumors are autonomous and therefore insensitive to changes in ACTH secretion.

This test is also used to evaluate the pituitary reserve capacity to produce ACTH. It can document that adrenal insufficiency exists as a result of pituitary disease (secondary adrenal insufficiency) rather than primary adrenal pathology.

Contraindications

- Patients with possible adrenal insufficiency
- Patients taking glucocorticosteroids

Potential complications

- Addison disease and Addisonian crisis because metyrapone inhibits cortisol production
- Dizziness, sedation, allergic reaction, and bone marrow suppression

Interfering factors
- Recent administration of radioisotopes can affect results.

Procedure and patient care
- Obtain a baseline cortisol level (p. 241) for the blood test.
- See inside front cover for Routine Blood Testing.
- Fasting: no
- Blood tube commonly used: red or green
- See inside front cover for Routine Urine Testing.

During

Blood
- Administer a prescribed dose (based on body weight) of metyrapone at bedtime the night before the blood sample is to be collected. Collect a venous blood sample in a red-top tube in the morning.

Urine
- Obtain a 24-hour urine specimen for the 17-OCHS level as a baseline. Then collect a 24-hour urine specimen for the 17-OCHS level during and again 1 day after the oral administration of a dose of metyrapone, which is given in 5 doses every 4 hours within 24 hours.
- Metyrapone should be administered with a glass of milk to diminish any GI side effects.

After
- Assess the patient for impending signs of Addisonian crisis (muscle weakness, mental and emotional changes, anorexia, nausea, vomiting, hypotension, hyperkalemia, or vascular collapse).
- Note that Addisonian crisis is a medical emergency that must be treated vigorously with replenishing steroids, reversing shock, and restoring circulation.

Abnormal findings
Increased cortisol precursors
Adrenal hyperplasia

No change in cortisol precursors
Adrenal tumor
Ectopic ACTH syndrome
Secondary adrenal insufficiency

notes

age-related macular degeneration risk analysis (ARMD risk analysis, Y402H, and A69S)

Type of test Blood

Normal findings

No mutation noted

Test explanation and related physiology

Age-related macular degeneration (ARMD) is recognized as a leading cause of blindness in the United States. Blurred or distorted vision and difficulty adjusting to dim light are common symptoms. ARMD, both wet and dry types, is considered a multifactorial disorder because it is thought to develop because of an interplay between environmental (smoking) and genetic (gender, ethnicity) risk and protective (antioxidants) factors. At least two genetic variants (Y402H and A69S) have been found to be associated with an increased risk for ARMD. The Y402H and the A69S genetic variants are common polymorphisms in ARMD. An individual with two copies of the Y402H variant in the gene *CFH* and two copies of the A69S variant in the gene *LOC387715* has an approximately 60-fold increased risk for ARMD. This is significant, given how common ARMD is in the general population.

This information can be clinically useful when making medical management decisions (e.g., the use of inflammatory markers) and emphasizing to patients the benefits of smoking cessation and dietary modification. In some cases, genotype information may also assist with clinical diagnosis.

Procedure and patient care

- See inside front cover for Routine Blood Testing.
- Fasting: no
- Blood tube commonly used: lavender or yellow
- PT Tell the patient that results may not be available for a few weeks.

Abnormal findings

Increased risk of ARMD

notes

alanine aminotransferase (ALT, formerly Serum glutamic-pyruvic transaminase [SGPT])

Type of test Blood

Normal findings

Adult/child: 4–42 units/L at 37° C, or 4–36 units/L (SI units)
Elderly: may be slightly higher than adult
Infant: may be twice as high as adult

Test explanation and related physiology

ALT is found predominantly in the liver; lesser quantities are found in the kidneys, heart, and skeletal muscles. Injury or disease affecting the liver parenchyma causes a release of this hepatocellular enzyme into the bloodstream, thus elevating serum ALT levels. Generally, most ALT elevations are caused by liver disease. Therefore this enzyme is not only sensitive but also very specific in indicating hepatocellular disease. In hepatocellular disease other than viral hepatitis, the ALT/AST ratio *(De Ritis ratio)* is less than 1. In viral hepatitis, the ratio is greater than 1. This is helpful in the diagnosis of viral hepatitis.

Interfering factors

- Previous IM injections can cause elevated levels.

Procedure and patient care

- See inside front cover for Routine Blood Testing.
- Fasting: no
- Blood tube commonly used: red
- Patients with liver dysfunction often have prolonged clotting times.

Abnormal findings

▲ **Increased levels**
Cholestasis
Cirrhosis
Hepatic ischemia
Hepatic necrosis
Hepatic tumor
Hepatitis
Hepatotoxic drugs

Infectious mononucleosis
Myocardial infarction
Myositis
Obstructive jaundice
Pancreatitis
Severe burns
Shock
Trauma to striated muscle

notes

aldolase

Type of test   Blood

Normal findings

Adult: 3–8.2 Sibley-Lehninger units/dL or 22–59 mU/L at 37° C (SI units)
Child: approximately two times the adult values
Newborn: approximately four times the adult values

Test explanation and related physiology

Serum aldolase is very similar to the enzymes aspartate aminotransferase AST (SGOT) (p. 105) and CPK (p. 247). Aldolase is an enzyme used in glycolysis (breakdown of glucose). As with AST and creatine phosphokinase, aldolase exists throughout the body in most tissues. This test is most useful for indicating muscular or hepatic cellular injury or disease. The serum aldolase level is very high in patients with muscular dystrophies, dermatomyositis, and polymyositis. Levels also are increased in patients with gangrenous processes, muscular trauma, and muscular infectious diseases (e.g., trichinosis). Elevated levels are also noted in chronic hepatitis, obstructive jaundice, and cirrhosis.

Neurologic diseases causing weakness can be differentiated from muscular causes of weakness with this test. Normal values are seen in patients with such neurologic diseases as poliomyelitis, myasthenia gravis, and multiple sclerosis. Elevated aldolase levels are seen in the primary muscular disorders.

Interfering factors

• Previous IM injections may cause elevated levels.
• Strenuous exercise can cause a transient spike in aldolase.

Procedure and patient care

• See inside front cover for Routine Blood Testing.
• Fasting: verify with laboratory
• Blood tube commonly used: red

Abnormal findings

▲ Increased levels
  Gangrenous processes (e.g., gangrene of the bowel)
  Hepatocellular diseases (e.g., hepatitis)

▼ Decreased levels
  Hereditary fructose intolerance
  Late muscular dystrophy
  Muscle-wasting disease

▲ **Increased levels**

Muscular diseases (e.g., muscular dystrophy, dermatomyositis, and polymyositis)

Muscular infections (e.g., trichinosis)

Muscular trauma (e.g., severe crush injuries)

Myocardial infarction

▼ **Decreased levels**

notes

aldosterone

Type of test Blood; urine (24-hour)

Normal findings

Blood

Supine: 3–10 ng/dL or 0.08–0.3 nmol/L (SI units)

Upright:

    Male: 6–22 ng/dL or 0.17–0.61 nmol/L (SI units)

    Female: 5–30 ng/dL or 0.14–0.8 nmol/L (SI units)

    Results in the elderly many be decreased.

    Child/adolescent:

    Newborn: 5–60 ng/dL

1 week-1 year: 1–160 ng/dL;	5–7 years: 5–50 ng/dL
1–3 years: 5–60 ng/dL;	7–11 years: 5–70 ng/dL
3–5 years: 5–80 ng/dL;	11–15 years: 5–50 ng/dL

Urine (24-hour)

2–26 mcg/24 hr or 6–72 nmol/24 hr (SI units)

Test explanation and related physiology

This test is used to diagnose hyperaldosteronism. Production of aldosterone, a hormone produced by the adrenal cortex, is regulated primarily by the renin-angiotensin system. Secondarily, aldosterone is stimulated by ACTH, low serum sodium levels, and high serum potassium levels. Aldosterone in turn stimulates the renal tubules to absorb sodium (water follows) and to secrete potassium into the urine. In this way, aldosterone regulates serum sodium and potassium levels. Because water follows sodium transport, aldosterone also partially regulates water absorption (and plasma volume).

Increased aldosterone levels are associated with primary aldosteronism, in which a tumor (usually an adenoma) of the adrenal cortex (Conn syndrome) or bilateral adrenal nodular hyperplasia causes increased production of aldosterone. Patients with primary aldosteronism characteristically have hypertension, weakness, polyuria, and hypokalemia.

Increased aldosterone levels also occur with secondary aldosteronism caused by nonadrenal conditions. These include:

- Renal vascular stenosis or occlusion
- Hyponatremia (from diuretic or laxative abuse) or low salt intake
- Hypovolemia
- Pregnancy or use of estrogens
- Malignant hypertension

- Potassium loading
- Edematous states (e.g., congestive heart failure, cirrhosis, nephrotic syndrome)

The aldosterone assay can be done on a 24-hour urine specimen or a plasma blood sample. The advantage of the 24-hour urine sample is that short-term fluctuations are eliminated. Plasma values are more convenient to sample, but they are affected by the short-term fluctuations.

Primary aldosteronism (PA) can be diagnosed by demonstrating very little to no rise in serum renin levels after an *aldosterone stimulation test* (using salt restriction as the stimulant). This is because aldosterone is already maximally secreted by the pathologic adrenal gland. PA can also be diagnosed by the *aldosterone suppression test* which shows failure to suppress aldosterone with saline infusion (1.5–2L of NSS infused between 8PM and 10AM) or with oral salt loading. Aldosterone can also be measured in blood obtained from *adrenal venous sampling.*

In venous adrenal sampling, blood is separately obtained from each adrenal vein. Access to each vein is obtained by *venography.* Measuring aldosterone from each vein will help locate the exact cause of PA. If one adrenal gland has a hyperfunctioning adenoma, aldosterone levels will be elevated only on the affected side. If adrenal hyperplasia is the cause of PA, aldosterone levels will be elevated on both sides.

The *aldosterone-to-renin ratio (ARR)*—that is, the ratio of plasma aldosterone (expressed in ng/dL) to plasma renin activity (PRA, expressed in ng/mL/h)—is the most sensitive means of differentiating primary from secondary causes of hyperaldosteronism. It can be obtained under random conditions of sodium intake. The principle behind this test is that as aldosterone secretion rises, PRA should fall because of sodium retention. Persistent relatively high levels of aldosterone above 30 ng/dL per ng/mL/hour indicate primary aldosteronism. APR is used to screen patients with stage 2 or 3 hypertension, drug-resistant hypertension, or a strong family history of hypertension. One should also be aware that a *Captopril Challenge Test* (p. 643) can also act as a confirmatory test for primary aldosteronism.

Interfering factors

- Strenuous exercise and stress can stimulate adrenocortical secretions and increase aldosterone levels.
- Excessive licorice ingestion can cause decreased levels because it produces an aldosterone-like effect.
- Values are influenced by posture, position, diet, diurnal variation, and pregnancy.

Procedure and patient care

- See inside front cover for Routine Blood Testing.
- Fasting: no
- Blood tube commonly used: serum separator
- **PT** Note that the patient is asked to be in the upright position (at least sitting) for at least 2 hours before the blood is drawn.
- **PT** Explain the procedure for collecting a 24-hour urine sample if urinary aldosterone is ordered. (See inside front cover for Routine Urine Testing.)
- **PT** Give the patient verbal and written instructions regarding dietary restrictions.
- **PT** Have the patient ask the physician whether drugs that alter sodium, potassium, and fluid balance (e.g., diuretics, antihypertensives, steroids, oral contraceptives) should be withheld.

During

- Occasionally, for hospitalized patients, draw the sample with the patient in the supine position *before* he or she rises.
- Obtain the specimen in the morning.
- Note that sometimes a second specimen (upright sample) is collected 4 hours later, after the patient has been up and moving.

After

- Indicate on the laboratory slip if the patient was supine or standing during the venipuncture.
- Handle the blood specimen gently. Rough handling may cause hemolysis and alter the test results.
- Transport the specimen on ice to the laboratory.

Abnormal findings

▲ **Increased levels**

Primary aldosteronism
Adrenal cortical nodular hyperplasia
Aldosterone-producing adrenal adenoma (Conn syndrome)
Bartter syndrome

Secondary aldosteronism
Cushing syndrome
Diuretic ingestion resulting in hypovolemia and hyponatremia

▼ **Decreased levels**

Addison disease
Aldosterone deficiency
Antihypertensive therapy
Hypernatremia
Hypokalemia
Patients on a high sodium diet
Renin deficiency
Steroid therapy
Toxemia of pregnancy

▲ **Increased levels**   ▼ **Decreased levels**

Generalized edema
Hyperkalemia
Hyponatremia
Hypovolemia or
  hemorrhage
Laxative abuse
Malignant hypertension
Oral contraceptives
Pregnancy
Renal arterial stenosis
Stress

notes

alkaline phosphatase (ALP)

Type of test Blood

Normal findings

Adult: 30–120 units/L or 0.5–2 µKat/L
Elderly: slightly higher than adults
Child/adolescent:
    16–21 years: 30–200 units/L
    9–15 years: 60–300 units/L
    2–8 years: 65–210 units/L
    < 2 years: 85–235 units/L

Test explanation and related physiology

Although ALP is found in many tissues, the highest concentrations are found in the liver, biliary tract epithelium, and bone. Detection of this enzyme is important for determining liver and bone disorders. Enzyme levels of ALP are greatly increased in both extrahepatic and intrahepatic obstructive biliary disease and cirrhosis. Reports have indicated that the most sensitive test to indicate metastatic tumor to the liver is ALP.

Bone is the most frequent extrahepatic source of ALP; new bone growth is associated with elevated ALP levels, which explains why ALP levels are high in adolescents. Pathologic new bone growth occurs with osteoblastic metastatic (e.g., breast, prostate) tumors. Paget disease, healing fractures, rheumatoid arthritis, hyperparathyroidism, and normal-growing bones are sources of elevated ALP levels as well.

Isoenzymes of ALP are sometimes used to distinguish between liver and bone diseases. The detection of isoenzymes can help differentiate the source of the pathology associated with the elevated total ALP. ALP_1 is from the liver. ALP_2 is from the bone.

Interfering factors

- Recent ingestion of a meal can increase ALP levels.

Procedure and patient care

- See inside front cover for Routine Blood Testing.
- Fasting: no
- Blood tube commonly used: red
- Note that overnight fasting may be required for isoenzymes.
- Patients with liver dysfunction often have prolonged clotting times.

Abnormal findings

▲ **Increased levels**

Cirrhosis

Healing fracture

Hyperparathyroidism

Intestinal ischemia or infarction

Intrahepatic or extrahepatic biliary obstruction

Metastatic bone tumor

Osteomalacia

Paget disease of bone

Primary or metastatic liver tumor

Rheumatoid arthritis

Rickets

Sarcoidosis

▼ **Decreased levels**

Celiac disease

Excess vitamin B ingestion

Hypophosphatasia

Hypophosphatemia

Hypothyroidism

Malnutrition

Milk-alkali syndrome

Pernicious anemia

Scurvy (vitamin C deficiency)

notes

allergy testing (Allergy blood testing, Allergy skin testing, IgE antibody test, Radioallergosorbent test [RAST])

Type of test: Blood, skin

Blood testing: Total IgE serum

Adult: 0–100 international units/mL

Child:

6–10 years: 0–85 international units/mL

2–5 years: 0–56 international units/mL

0–23 months: 0–13 international units/mL

Skin testing

< 3-mm wheal diameter

< 10-mm flare diameter

Test explanation and related physiology

Measurement of serum IgE is an effective method to diagnose allergy and specifically identify an allergen (the substance to which the person is allergic). Serum IgE levels increase when allergic individuals are exposed to the allergen. Although skin testing can also identify a specific allergen, measurement of serum levels of IgE is helpful when a skin test result is questionable or when the allergen may incite an anaphylactic reaction. IgE is also helpful in cases in which skin testing is difficult (e.g., in patients with dermatographism or widespread dermatitis), and when it is uncomfortable to remove the patient from allergy blocking medications. IgE levels are also used to identify the allergen so that an immunotherapeutic regimen can be developed.

Another type of allergy blood testing is called *Specific IgE blood allergy testing* or *in vitro allergy blood testing.* With this test, the specific allergen can be identified. It is more accurate and safer than skin testing. *IgG antibody allergy blood testing* can also be performed and may provide a more accurate correlation between allergen and allergic symptoms. IgG and IgE antibody testing are often performed in "panels" (e.g., meat or fruit panels). Specific allergen antibody testing should follow a positive panel testing to identify the specific allergen.

Allergy skin testing, in general, is more accurate, simpler to use, and less expensive than blood testing. When properly performed, skin testing is the most convenient and least expensive test for detecting allergic reactions. Skin testing provides useful confirmatory evidence when a diagnosis of allergy is suspected on clinical grounds. In skin testing, a skin wheal (swelling) and redness that follow injection of the specific allergen to which the person is allergic is considered a positive result. This reaction is instigated by IgE and is mediated primarily by histamine. In some patients, a late-phase reaction occurs, which is highlighted by antibody and cellular infiltration into the area.

There are three commonly accepted methods of injecting the allergen into the skin. The first method is called the *prick-puncture test* or *scratch test*. In this method, the allergen is injected into the epidermis. The second method is called the *intradermal test* where the allergen is injected into the dermis (creating a skin wheal). The third method is called the *patch test* where the patient wears a patch containing the allergen for 48 hours to see if there is a delayed allergic reaction. Patients with dermographism can have a false-positive reaction with skin testing. To eliminate these false positives, a "negative control" substance consisting of just the diluent without an allergen is used to compare any reaction. Patients who are immunosuppressed may have a blunted skin reaction even in the face of allergy. To avoid false negatives, a "positive control" substance consisting of a histamine analog is also provided at the time of skin testing. This will cause a wheal and flare response even in the nonallergic patient unless the patient is immunosuppressed.

For inhalant allergens, skin tests are extremely accurate. However, for food allergies, latex allergies, drug sensitivity, and occupational allergies, skin tests are less reliable.

Contraindications
• Patients with a history of prior anaphylaxis

Potential complications
• Anaphylaxis

Interfering factors
• Concurrent diseases associated with elevated IgG levels will cause false-negative results.

Procedure and patient care
Blood
• See inside front cover for Routine Blood Testing.
• Fasting: no
• Blood tube commonly used: serum separator
• Determine whether the patient has recently been treated with allergy blocking medications.

Skin testing
Before
• Evaluate for dermographism by rubbing the skin with a pencil eraser and looking for a wheal at the site of irritation.

- Draw up 0.05 mL of 1:1000 aqueous epinephrine into a syringe in the event of an exaggerated allergic reaction.

During

- The technique varies according to the method chosen for testing.
- In the *Prick-puncture* method, a 25-gauge needle is passed through the allergen-containing droplet and inserted into the epidermal space
- In the *Intradermal method*, the allergen solution is injected into the dermis by creating a skin wheal.
- In the *Patch method*, several patches are applied to the skin.

After

- Evaluate the patient for an allergic response.
- In the event of a systemic reaction from a skin test, a tourniquet should be placed above the testing site, and epinephrine should be administered subcutaneously.
- With a pen, circle the skin testing site and mark the allergen used.
- Observe the patient for 20 to 30 minutes before discharge.

Abnormal findings

Allergic rhinitis
Allergy-related diseases
Angioedema
Asthma
Dermatitis
Drug, food, latex, occupational allergy

notes

alpha$_1$-antitrypsin (A$_1$AT, AAT, Alpha$_1$-antitrypsin phenotyping)

Type of test Blood

Normal findings

85–213 mg/dL or 0.85–2.13 g/L (SI units)

Negative for S or Z phenotype

Test explanation and related physiology

Serum alpha$_1$-antitrypsin (AAT) levels should be obtained when an individual has a family history of early emphysema. AAT mutated genes can be associated with reduced levels of this enzyme. Patients with mutated AAT genes develop severe, disabling lower lung emphysema in the third and fourth decades of life. A similar deficiency is seen in children with cirrhosis and other liver diseases. The severity of these diseases is determined by the ATT phenotype.

Routine serum protein electrophoresis (p. 614) is a good screening test for AAT deficiency because AAT accounts for most of the protein in the alpha$_1$-globulin region. Quantitative serum levels indicate deficiency. If levels are low, ATT phenotyping can be performed. The three major alleles determined by phenotyping are: M (full functioning, normal allele), S (associated with reduced levels of protein), and Z (disease-causing mutation associated with liver disease and premature emphysema). The S and Z alleles account for the majority of the abnormal alleles detected in affected patients.

Inherited AAT deficiency is associated with symptoms earlier in life than acquired AAT deficiency. Inherited AAT is also commonly associated with liver and biliary disease. Individuals of the heterozygous state have diminished or low normal serum levels of AAT. Approximately 5% to 14% of the adult population is in the heterozygous state and is considered to be at increased risk for the development of emphysema. Homozygous individuals have severe pulmonary and liver disease very early in life. AAT phenotyping is particularly helpful when blood AAT levels are suggestive but not definitive.

Deficiencies of AAT can also be acquired. *Acquired* deficiencies of AAT can occur in patients with protein deficiency syndromes (e.g., malnutrition, liver disease, nephrotic syndrome, and neonatal respiratory distress syndrome).

AAT is also an acute-phase reactant that is elevated in the face of inflammation, infection, or malignancy. It is not specific as to the source of the inflammatory process.

Interfering factors
- Levels increase during pregnancy or inflammatory diseases.

Procedure and patient care
- See inside front cover for Routine Blood Testing.
- Fasting: no (verify with laboratory)
- Blood tube commonly used: red

PT If the results show the patient is at risk for developing emphysema, begin patient teaching. Include such factors as avoidance of smoking, infection, and inhaled irritants; proper nutrition; adequate hydration; and education about the disease process of emphysema.

Abnormal findings

▲ **Increased levels**
 Acute inflammatory
  disorders
 Chronic inflammatory
  disorders
 Infection
 Stress
 Thyroid infections

▼ **Decreased levels**
 Cirrhosis (in children)
 Early onset of emphysema
  (in adults)
 Low serum proteins
 (e.g., nephrotic syndrome,
  malnutrition, end-stage
  cancer, protein-losing
  enteropathy)
 Neonatal respiratory
  distress syndrome

notes

alpha defensin test (Synovasure)

Type of test   Fluid analysis

Normal findings

Negative

Test explanation and related physiology

Infections in prosthetic joints can occur any time after the joint replacement surgery. Infection is a common cause of failed arthroplasties. The diagnosis of periprosthetic joint infection (PJI) remains a serious clinical challenge. Treatment may require prolonged use of parenterally administered antibiotics followed by complex surgery. Therefore it is important that diagnosis is accurate and timely. Diagnosis of PJI is often hampered by administration of antibiotics before or during joint fluid sampling (p. 99). These antibiotics can inhibit bacterial growth and cause false-negative results.

PJI is usually considered when joint pain worsens after replacement. Joint fluid analysis is not very reliable because of lack of sensitivity and specificity. Advanced joint fluid stains, serology (IgG, IgM), and molecular testing for bacterial DNA sequencing to identify bacteria or the body's response to bacteria have been developed to aid the diagnosis of PJI. Unfortunately, these tests require significant pretest care of the specimen, are time consuming, and too expensive to apply to the population of those potentially affected by PJI. Other testing, such as C-reactive protein (p. 245) and sed rate (p. 306), are not specific enough. Imaging (i.e., CT scanning), while more reliable has a low specificity.

Alpha defensin is a protein that is produced by WBCs in joint fluid in response to PJI. An immunoassay to identify this biomarker can accurately identify nearly all incidences of PJI. This testing, however, cannot identify the specific infecting agent or its sensitivity to antibiotics. While synchronously occurring inflammatory disease (e.g., rheumatoid arthritis) can confound other testing for PJI, alpha defensin levels are not affected. A positive alpha defensin test result in the presence of a low C-reactive protein may represent a false-positive result and should be questioned.

Interfering factors

- Fresh blood in the synovial fluid can alter test results.

Procedure and patient care

Before

PT Explain the procedure to the patient. Fasting is not required.
• Obtain an informed consent if indicated.

During

• After aseptically cleaning and locally anesthetizing the area, a needle is inserted into the affected joint space to remove fluid.
• A few cubic centimeters of synovial fluid is injected into tubes provided by the central laboratory.
• The specimen is sent to the central laboratory.

After

PT Assess the joint for pain, fever, and swelling. Teach the patient to look for signs of infection at home.
• Apply ice to decrease pain and swelling.

Abnormal findings

PJI

notes

alpha-fetoprotein (AFP, a₁-Fetoprotein)

Type of test Blood

Normal findings

Adult: < 40 ng/mL or < 40 mcg/L (SI units)

Child (< 1 year): < 30 ng/mL

(Ranges are stratified by weeks of gestation and vary according to laboratory.)

Test explanation and related physiology

Alpha-fetoprotein (AFP) is the dominant fetal serum protein in the first trimester of life and diminishes to very low levels by the age of 1 year. It is also normally found in very low levels in the adult.

AFP is an effective screening serum marker for fetal body wall defects. The most notable of these are neural tube defects, which can vary from a small myelomeningocele to anencephaly. If a fetus has an open body wall defect, fetal serum AFP leaks out into the amniotic fluid and is picked up by the maternal serum. AFP from fetal sources can normally be detected in the amniotic fluid or the mother's blood after 10 weeks' gestation. Peak levels occur between 16 and 18 weeks' gestation. Maternal serum reflects the changes in amniotic AFP levels. When elevated maternal serum AFP levels are identified, further evaluation with repeat serum AFP levels, amniotic fluid AFP levels, and ultrasound is warranted.

Elevated serum AFP levels in pregnancy may also indicate multiple pregnancy, fetal distress, fetal congenital abnormalities, or intrauterine death. Low AFP levels after correction for age of gestation, maternal weight, race, and presence of diabetes are found in mothers carrying fetuses with trisomy 21 (Down syndrome). See *maternal screen testing* (p. 501) and *nuchal translucency* (p. 754) for other pregnancy screening tests.

AFP is also used as a tumor marker; see p. 164.

Interfering factors

- Fetal blood contamination, which may occur during amniocentesis, can cause increased AFP levels.

Procedure and patient care

- See inside front cover for Routine Blood Testing.
- Fasting: no
- Blood tube commonly used: red

- If AFP is to be performed on amniotic fluid, follow the procedure and patient care for amniocentesis (p. 39).
- Include the gestational age on the laboratory slip.

Abnormal findings

▲ **Increased maternal AFP levels**

Abdominal wall defects (e.g., gastroschisis or, omphalocele)

Fetal death

Fetal distress or congenital anomalies

Multiple pregnancy

Neural tube defects (e.g., anencephaly, encephalocele, spina bifida, myelomeningocele)

Threatened abortion

▼ **Decreased maternal serum AFP levels**

Fetal wastage

Trisomy 21 (Down syndrome)

▲ **Increased nonmaternal AFP levels**

Embryonal cell or germ cell tumor of the testes

Germ cell or yolk sac cancer of the ovary

Liver cell necrosis (e.g., cirrhosis or, hepatitis)

Other cancers (e.g., stomach, colon, lung, breast, lymphoma)

Primary hepatocellular cancer (hepatoma)

notes

aluminum (Chromium and other Heavy metals)

Type of test Blood

Normal findings

All ages: 0–6 ng/mL
Dialysis patients of all ages: < 60 ng/mL

Test explanation and related physiology

Under normal physiologic conditions, the usual daily dietary intake of aluminum is completely excreted by the kidneys. Patients in renal failure (RF) lose the ability to clear aluminum and are at risk for aluminum toxicity. Aluminum-laden dialysis water and aluminum-based phosphate binder gels designed to decrease phosphate accumulation increase the incidence of aluminum toxicity in RF patients.

Aluminum overload leads to accumulation of aluminum in the brain and bone. Brain deposition has been implicated as a cause of dialysis dementia. In bone, aluminum replaces calcium and disrupts normal osteoid formation.

Serum aluminum concentrations are likely to be increased higher than the reference range in patients with metallic joint prosthesis. *Chromium* and other metals can be detected using similar laboratory techniques.

Interfering factors

• Special evacuated blood collection tubes are required.
• Most of the common evacuated blood collection devices have rubber stoppers that are composed of aluminum silicate.
• Gadolinium- or iodine-containing contrast media that have been administered within 96 hours can alter test results.

Procedure and patient care

• See inside front cover for Routine Blood Testing.
• Fasting: no
• Blood tube commonly used: royal blue or tan
• If the blood sample is sent to a central diagnostic laboratory, results will be available in 7 to 10 days.

Abnormal findings

▲ **Increased levels**
  Aluminum toxicity

notes

amino acid profiles (Amino acid screen)

Type of test Blood; urine

Normal findings

Normal values vary for different amino acids.

Test explanation and related physiology

Amino acids are "building blocks" of proteins, hormones, nucleic acids, and pigments. They can act as neurotransmitters, enzymes, and coenzymes. There are eight essential amino acids that must be provided to the body by the diet. The essential amino acids must be transported across the gut and renal tubular lining cells. The metabolism of the essential amino acids is critical to the production of other amino acids, proteins, carbohydrates, and lipids.

When there is a defect in the metabolism or transport of any one of these amino acids, excesses of their precursors or deficiencies of their "end product" amino acid are evident in the blood and/or urine.

Clinical manifestations of these diseases may be precluded if diagnosis is early and if appropriate dietary replacement of missing amino acids is provided. Usually, urine testing for specific amino acids is used to screen for some of these errors in amino acid metabolism and transport. Blood testing is very accurate. Federal law requires hospitals to test all newborns for inborn errors in metabolism including amino acids. Testing is required for errors in amino acid metabolism such as phenylketonuria (PKU), maple syrup urine disease (MSUD), and homocystinuria (see newborn metabolic screening, p. 523).

A few drops of blood are obtained from the heel of a newborn to fill a few circles on filter paper labeled with names of infant, parent, hospital, and primary physician. The sample is usually obtained on the second or third day of life, after protein-containing feedings (i.e., breast milk or formula) have started.

After a presumptive diagnosis is made, amino acid levels can be detected in blood or amniotic fluid. The genetic defects for many of these diseases are becoming more defined, allowing for even earlier diagnosis to be made in utero.

Interfering factors

- The circadian rhythm affects amino acid levels. Levels are usually lowest in the morning and highest by midday.
- Pregnancy is associated with reduced levels of some amino acids.

Procedure and patient care

- See inside front cover for Routine Blood Testing.
- Fasting: yes
- Blood tube commonly used: red
- A heel stick is done with newborns.
- Obtain a history of the patient's symptoms.
- Obtain a pedigree highlighting family members with amino acid disorders.

During

- Usually a 24-hour random urine specimen is required. See inside front cover for Routine Urine Testing.
- Screening is done on a spot urine using the first voided specimen in the morning.

After

- Generally, genetic counseling is provided before testing and continued after results are obtained.

Abnormal findings

▲ **Increased blood levels**

Specific aminoacidemias
(e.g., glutaric aciduria)
Specific aminoacidopathies
(e.g., PKU, maple syrup disease)

▼ **Decreased blood levels**

Hartnup disease
Nephritis
Nephrotic syndromes

▲ **Increased urine levels**

Specific aminoacidurias
(e.g., cystinuria, homocystinuria)

notes

ammonia level

Type of test Blood

Normal findings

Adult: 10–80 mcg/dL or 6–47 µmol/L (SI units)
Child: 40–80 mcg/dL
Newborn: 90–150 mcg/dL

Test explanation and related physiology

Ammonia is used to support the diagnosis of severe liver diseases (fulminant hepatitis or cirrhosis). There are better tests to determine severe liver disease through algorithms that include testing of gamma-glutamyltransferase activity, total bilirubin, alpha-2-macroglobulin, apolipoprotein A1, haptoglobin, and alanine aminotransferase (ALT) activity in the patient's serum.

Ammonia levels are also used in the diagnosis and follow-up of hepatic encephalopathy. However, in those with cirrhosis, the ammonia level has little, if any, predictive or clinical value in HE for multiple reasons. Ammonia is a byproduct of protein catabolism. Most of the ammonia is made by bacteria acting on proteins present in the gut. By way of the portal vein, ammonia goes to the liver where it is normally converted into urea and then secreted by the kidneys. With severe hepatocellular dysfunction, ammonia cannot be catabolized. Furthermore, when portal blood flow to the liver is altered (e.g., in portal hypertension), ammonia cannot reach the liver to be catabolized. Ammonia levels in the blood rise. Inherited deficiencies of urea cycle enzymes, inherited metabolic disorders of organic acids, and the dibasic amino acids lysine and ornithine are major causes of high ammonia levels in infants and adults. Finally, impaired renal function diminishes excretion of ammonia, and blood levels rise. High levels of ammonia are often associated with encephalopathy and coma.

Interfering factors

- Hemolysis increases ammonia levels because the RBCs contain about three times the ammonia content of plasma.
- Muscular exertion can increase ammonia.
- Cigarette smoking can produce significant increases in levels.
- Ammonia levels may be falsely increased if the tourniquet is too tight for a long period.

Procedure and patient care

- See inside front cover for Routine Blood Testing.
- Fasting: no
- Blood tube commonly used: green
- Note that some institutions require that the specimen be sent to the laboratory in an iced container.
- Avoid hemolysis and send the specimen promptly to the laboratory.
- Patients with liver disease can have prolonged clotting times.

Abnormal findings

▲ **Increased levels**

Asparagine intoxication
Gastrointestinal bleeding with mild liver disease
Gastrointestinal obstruction with mild liver disease
Genetic metabolic disorder of the urea cycle
Hemolytic disease of the newborn (erythroblastosis fetalis)
Hepatic encephalopathy and hepatic coma
Portal hypertension
Primary hepatocellular disease
Reye syndrome
Severe heart failure with congestive hepatomegaly

▼ **Decreased levels**

Essential or malignant hypertension
Hyperornithinemia

notes

amniocentesis (Amniotic fluid analysis)

Type of test Fluid analysis

Normal findings

Weeks' gestation	Amniotic fluid volume (mL)
15	450
25	750
30–35	1500
Full term	> 1500

Amniotic fluid appearance: clear; pale to straw yellow
L/S ratio: ≥ 2:1
Bilirubin: < 0.2 mg/dL
No chromosomal or genetic abnormalities
Phosphatidylglycerol (PG): positive for PG
Lamellar body count: > 30,000
Alpha-fetoprotein: dependent on gestational age and laboratory
    technique
Fetal lung maturity (FLM):
    Mature: < 260 mPOL
    Transitional: 260 to 290 mPOL
    Immature: > 290 mPOL

Test explanation and related physiology

Amniocentesis is performed on pregnant women to gather information about their fetuses. The following can be evaluated by studying the amniotic fluid:

- *Fetal maturity status,* especially pulmonary maturity (when early delivery is preferred). Fetal maturity is determined by analysis of the amniotic fluid in the following manner:
  a. *Lecithin/sphingomyelin (L/S) ratio.* The L/S ratio is a measure of fetal lung maturity. Lecithin is the major constituent of surfactant, an important substance required for alveolar ventilation. If surfactant is insufficient, the alveoli collapse during expiration. This may result in respiratory distress syndrome (RDS). An L/S ratio of 2:1 (3:1 in mothers with diabetes) or greater is a highly reliable indication that the fetal lungs are mature.

    As an alternative to measuring the L/S ratio, the *fetal lung maturity (FLM) test* determines the ratio of surfactant to albumin to evaluate pulmonary maturity.

b. *Phosphatidylglycerol (PG).* Because PG is almost entirely synthesized by mature lung alveolar cells, it is a good indicator of lung maturity.

c. *Lamellar body count.* Lamellar bodies represent the storage form of pulmonary surfactant and are considered a measure of lung maturity. If the count is greater than 30,000, the infant's lungs are mature enough to not experience RDS. If the lamellar body count is less than 10,000, the probability of RDS is high.

d. *Measurement of surfactant activity.* Surfactant activity is a semiquantitative group of tests performed by determining the development and stability of foam when amniotic fluid is shaken in a solution of alcohol. This testing may be called the *tap test,* the *shake test,* or the *foam stability index test.*

e. *Measurement of optical density of amniotic fluid.* A denser fluid (>650 nm) will be associated with greater lung maturity. This testing method is often used as a rapid screening test for fetal lung maturity.

- *Sex of the fetus.* Sons of mothers who are known to be carriers of X-linked recessive traits would have a 50:50 chance of inheritance.
- *Genetic and chromosomal aberrations.* Genetic and chromosomal studies performed on cells aspirated within the amniotic fluid can indicate the existence of many genetic and chromosomal aberrations (e.g., trisomy 21).
- *Fetal status affected by Rh isoimmunization.* Mothers with Rh isoimmunization may have a series of amniocentesis procedures during the second half of pregnancy to assess the level of bilirubin in the amniotic fluid. The quantity of bilirubin is used to assess the severity of hemolysis in Rh-sensitized pregnancy.
- *Hereditary metabolic disorders,* such as cystic fibrosis.
- *Anatomic abnormalities,* such as neural tube closure defects (myelomeningocele, anencephaly, spina bifida). Increased levels of alpha-fetoprotein (AFP) in the amniotic fluid may indicate a neural crest abnormality. Decreased AFP may be associated with increased risk of trisomy 21. See alpha fetoprotein (p. 32).
- *Fetal distress,* detected by meconium staining of the amniotic fluid. There are, however, more accurate and safer methods of determining fetal stress such as the fetal biophysical profile (p. 333).
- *Assessment of amniotic fluid for infection.* Amniocentesis is used to obtain fluid for viral or bacterial culture and sensitivity

when infection is suspected. This is especially helpful if premature membrane rupture is suspected.

- ***Assessment for pre-mature rupture of membranes.*** Through
  amniocentesis, a dye can be injected into the amniotic fluid. If
  this same dye is found in vaginal fluid, rupture of the amniotic
  membrane is documented. This is sometimes referred to as the
  amnio-dye test. There are, however, more practical tests of vaginal fluid to determine membrane rupture. Most commonly,
  the pH of the vaginal fluid is determined using a *Nitrazine
  test* strip. If the test strip turns dark or blue, amniotic fluid is
  present in the vagina, and membrane rupture is documented.
  Also available are immunoassays that use monoclonal antibodies to identify *placental alpha microglobulin-1(PAMG-1).* The
  concentration of PAMG-1 in vaginal fluid is thousands of times
  higher in amniotic fluid than it is in normal vaginal secretions,
  thus allowing differentiation of the two.
- ***Paternity testing.*** DNA from the fetus can be compared to
  DNA from the potential father.

The timing of the amniocentesis varies according to the clinical circumstances.

Chorionic villus sampling (CVS) may be even better than
amniocentesis for karyotyping and genetic analysis. See page 202.

Contraindications

- Patients with abruptio placentae
- Patients with placenta previa
- Patients with a history of premature labor (before 34 weeks of
  gestation unless the patient is receiving antilabor medication)
- Patients with an incompetent cervix or cervical insufficiency
- Patients with anhydramnios

Potential complications

- Abortion
- Abruptio placentae
- Amniotic fluid embolism
- Fetal injury
- Infection (amnionitis)
- Leak of amniotic fluid
- Maternal Rh isoimmunization
- Miscarriage
- Premature labor

Procedure and patient care

Before

PT Explain the procedure to the patient.

- Obtain an informed consent.
- PT Tell the patient that no food or fluid is restricted.
- Record the mother's blood pressure and the fetal heart rate.
- Follow instructions regarding emptying the bladder, which depend on gestational age. Before 20 weeks of gestation, the bladder may be kept full to support the uterus. After 20 weeks, the bladder may be emptied to minimize the chance of puncture.
- Note that the placenta is localized before the study by ultrasound to permit selection of a site that will avoid placental puncture.

During

- Place the patient in the supine position.
- After local anesthetic is provided at the chosen site, access to the amniotic fluid is gained (Figure A1). Five to 10 mL of amniotic fluid is withdrawn and placed in a light-resistant container to prevent breakdown of bilirubin.
- If the amniotic fluid is bloody, the physician must determine whether the blood is maternal or fetal in origin. The *Kleihauer–Betke stain* will stain fetal cells pink.
- Note that this procedure is performed by a physician and takes approximately 20 to 30 minutes.
- Many women are extremely anxious during and after this procedure.

After

- PT Inform the patient that some results may be available in a few days, while others may take a few weeks.
- For women who have Rh-negative blood, administer RhoGAM because of the risk of isoimmunization from the fetal blood.
- Assess the fetal heart rate after the test to detect any ill effects related to the procedure. Compare this value with the preprocedure baseline value.
- Observe the puncture site for bleeding or other drainage.
- PT Instruct the patient to call her physician if she has any amniotic fluid loss, bleeding, temperature elevation, abdominal pain, abdominal cramping, fetal hyperactivity, or unusual fetal lethargy.

Abnormal findings

Abdominal wall closure defects (e.g., gastroschisis, omphalocele)

Genetic or chromosomal aberrations (e.g., sickle cell anemia, thalassemia, trisomy 21 [Down syndrome])

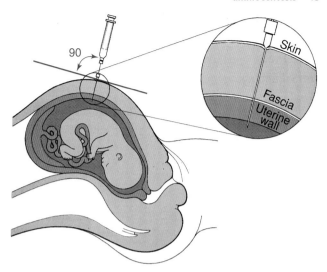

FIG. A1 Amniocentesis. Ultrasound scanning is usually used to determine the placental site and to locate a pocket of amniotic fluid. The needle is then inserted. Three levels of resistance are felt as the needle penetrates the skin, fascia, and uterine wall. When the needle is placed within the uterine cavity, amniotic fluid is withdrawn.

Hemolytic disease of the newborn
Hereditary metabolic disorders (e.g., cystic fibrosis, Tay-Sachs disease, galactosemia)
Immature fetal lungs
Meconium staining
Neural tube closure defects (e.g., myelomeningocele, anencephaly, spina bifida)
Oligohydramnios
Polyhydramnios
Rh isoimmunization
Sex-linked disorders (e.g., hemophilia)

notes

amylase

Type of test Blood; urine

Normal findings

Blood

Adult: 60–120 Somogyi units/dL or 30–220 units/L (SI units)
 Values may be slightly increased during normal pregnancy and in the elderly.
Adolescent: 30–110 units/L
Children: 26–106 units/L
Newborn: 6–65 units/L

Urine (24-hour)

Up to 5000 Somogyi units/24 hr or 6.5–48.1 units/hr (SI units)

Possible critical values

Blood: More than three times the upper limit of normal (depending on the method)

Test explanation and related physiology

Serum amylase is commonly used to diagnose and monitor the treatment of pancreatitis or obstruction of the pancreatic duct flow (as a result of pancreatic carcinoma). Blood vessels draining the free peritoneum and absorbing the lymph pick up the excess amylase. An abnormal rise in the serum level of amylase occurs within 12 hours of the onset of disease. Because amylase is rapidly cleared by the kidneys, serum levels return to normal 48 to 72 hours after the initial insult. Persistent pancreatitis, duct obstruction, or pancreatic duct leak will cause persistent elevated amylase levels.

Although serum amylase is a sensitive test for pancreatic disorders, it is not specific. Other nonpancreatic diseases can cause elevated amylase levels in the serum. For example, in a bowel perforation, intraluminal amylase leaks into the free peritoneum and is picked up by the peritoneal blood vessels. Also, a penetrating peptic ulcer into the pancreas will cause elevated amylase levels. Duodenal obstruction can be associated with less significant elevations in amylase. Because salivary glands contain amylase, elevations can be expected in patients with parotiditis (mumps).

Urine amylase levels rise after the blood levels. Several days after the onset of the disease process, serum amylase levels may be normal, but urine amylase levels are significantly elevated. Urine amylase is particularly useful in detecting pancreatitis late in the disease course.

As with serum amylase, urine amylase is sensitive but not specific for pancreatic disorders. A comparison of the renal clearance ratio of amylase with creatinine provides more specific diagnostic information than either the urine amylase level or the serum amylase level alone. When the *amylase/creatinine clearance* ratio is 5% or more, the diagnosis of pancreatitis can be made with certainty.

Interfering factors
- Serum lipemia may falsely decrease amylase levels.
- IV dextrose solutions can cause a false-negative result.

Procedure and patient care
- See inside front cover for Routine Blood Testing.
- Fasting: no
- Blood tube commonly used: red
- See inside front cover for Routine Urine Testing.

Abnormal findings
▲ **Increased levels**
Acute cholecystitis
Acute or chronic relapsing pancreatitis
Cryoglobulinemia
Diabetic ketoacidosis
Duodenal obstruction
Ectopic pregnancy
Necrotic or perforated bowel
Osteogenic sarcoma
Parotiditis (mumps)
Penetrating or perforated peptic ulcer
Pulmonary infarction
Rheumatoid diseases

notes

amyloid beta protein precursor, soluble (sBPP, APP, and Tau protein, AB42/AB40 ratio)

Type of test Cerebrospinal fluid (CSF) analysis

Normal findings

> 450 units/L

Test explanation and related physiology

This test is performed on patients who become increasingly demented and confused. It is a test used to help diagnose Alzheimer disease (AD) and other neurodegenerative diseases. Amyloid protein is an amino-acid peptide that is broken off a larger amyloid precursor protein (beta APP). These beta amyloid proteins, AB42, AB40, and their ratio (AB42/AB40), have been shown to be neurotrophic and neuroprotective. Beta amyloid is deposited on the brain in the form of plaques in patients with AD. It has been discovered that these plaques contain damaged nerve cells in a compacted core of beta amyloid protein. As a result of this deposition, levels of beta amyloid are decreased in the cerebrospinal fluid or blood of patients with AD and other forms of dementia. Research has demonstrated the diagnostic potential of this biochemical marker for AD.

Tau protein is another biochemical marker for AD. There is a general consensus that CSF levels of tau are significantly increased in patients with AD as well as Pick disease, corticobasal degeneration, supranuclear palsy, multisystem atrophy, and a recently recognized category of disorders known as tauopathies. These tests are performed on CSF or blood.

At this time, there is little or no consensus on the use of screening tests for diagnosing early AD. However, plasma biomarker combinations such as *AT(N) Biomarkers* where A (amyloid), T (tau), and N (neurodegeneration biomarker) are considered strong *biomarkers of Alzheimer disease*. Other panels include apolipoprotein E (p. 464). PET scanning with amyloid and or Tau imaging (p. 590) has shown promise for the diagnosis of AD. Pittsburgh Agent B (PIB) appears to reliably detect brain amyloid due to the accumulation of AB42 within plaques which may help discern AD from other dementia disorders.

Procedure and patient care

Before

PT Explain the procedure to the patient.

• Refer to the instructions for a lumbar puncture and CSF examination (p. 474).

During
- Collect a CSF specimen as per the lumbar puncture discussion.

After
- Follow the postprocedure guidelines after a lumbar puncture.

Abnormal findings
▼ **Decreased levels**
   Alzheimer disease

notes

angiotensin

Type of test Blood

Normal findings

Angiotensin I: ≤ 25 pg/mL
Angiotensin II: 10–60 pg/mL

Test explanation and related physiology

Renin is an enzyme that is released by the juxtaglomerular apparatus of the kidneys. Its release is stimulated by hypokalemia, hyponatremia, decreased renal blood perfusion, or hypovolemia. Renin stimulates the release of angiotensinogen. Angiotensin-converting enzyme (ACE) metabolizes angiotensinogen to angiotensin I and subsequently to angiotensin II and III. Angiotensin then stimulates the release of catecholamines, antidiuretic hormone, ACTH, oxytocin, and aldosterone. Angiotensin is also a vasoconstrictor. Angiotensin is used to identify renovascular sources of hypertension.

Interfering factors

See renin, p. 642

Procedure and patient care

- See inside front cover for Routine Blood Testing.
- Fasting: no
- Blood tube commonly used: lavender
- PT Instruct the patient to maintain a normal diet with a restricted amount of sodium (~ 3 g/day) for 3 days before the test.
- PT Instruct the patient to check with a healthcare provider about discontinuing any medications that may interrupt renin activity.
- Record the patient's position, dietary status, and time of day.
- Place the tube of blood on ice and immediately send it to the laboratory.

Abnormal findings

▲ **Increased levels**
Essential hypertension
Malignant hypertension
Renovascular
  hypertension

▼ **Decreased levels**
Congenital adrenal
  hyperplasia
Primary hyperaldosteronism
Steroid therapy

notes

angiotensin-converting enzyme (ACE, Serum angiotensin-converting enzyme [SACE])

A

Type of test Blood

Normal findings

8–53 U/L

Test explanation and related physiology

ACE is used to detect and monitor the clinical course of sarcoidosis. It is also used to differentiate sarcoidosis from other granulomatous diseases and to differentiate between active and dormant sarcoid disease.

Elevated ACE levels are found in a high percentage of patients with sarcoidosis. This test is used primarily in patients with sarcoidosis to evaluate the severity of disease and the response to therapy. Levels are especially high with active pulmonary sarcoidosis and can be normal with inactive (dormant) sarcoidosis. Elevated ACE levels also occur in conditions other than sarcoidosis, including Gaucher disease (a rare familial lysosomal disorder of fat metabolism), leprosy, alcoholic cirrhosis, active histoplasmosis, tuberculosis, Hodgkin disease, myeloma, scleroderma, pulmonary embolism, and idiopathic pulmonary fibrosis. ACE is elevated in the CSF of patients with neurosarcoidosis.

Interfering factors

- Patients younger than 20 normally have very high levels.
- Hemolysis or hyperlipidemia may falsely decrease ACE levels.

Procedure and patient care

- See inside front cover for Routine Blood Testing.
- Fasting: no
- Blood tube commonly used: red

Abnormal findings

▲ Increased levels

Active histoplasmosis	Leprosy
Alcoholic cirrhosis	Myeloma
Amyloidosis	Primary biliary cirrhosis
Diabetes mellitus	Pulmonary embolism
Gaucher disease	Sarcoidosis
Hodgkin disease	Scleroderma
Hyperthyroidism	Tuberculosis
Idiopathic pulmonary fibrosis	

notes

anion gap (AG, R factor)

Type of test Blood

Normal findings

16 ± 4 mEq/L (if potassium is used in the calculation)

12 ± 4 mEq/L (if potassium is not used in the calculation)

Test explanation and related physiology

The anion gap (AG) is the difference between the cations and the anions in the extracellular space that is routinely calculated in the laboratory (i.e., AG = [sodium + potassium] − [chloride + bicarbonate]). In some laboratories, the potassium is not measured because the level of potassium in acid-base abnormalities varies. The normal value of the AG is adjusted downward if potassium is eliminated from the equation. The AG, although not real physiologically, is created by the small amounts of anions in the blood (e.g., lactate, phosphates, sulfates, organic anions, and proteins) that are not measured.

This calculation is most often helpful in identifying the cause of metabolic acidosis. As such acids as lactic acid or ketoacids accumulate in the bloodstream, bicarbonate neutralizes them to maintain a normal pH within the blood. Mathematically, when bicarbonate decreases, the AG increases. In general, most metabolic acidotic states are associated with an increased AG. The higher the gap is above normal, the more likely that the metabolic acidotic state is associated with the AG. Proteins can have a significant effect on AG. As albumin (usually negatively charged) increases, AG will increase.

A decreased AG is very rare but can occur when there is an increase in unmeasured (calcium or magnesium) cations. A reduction in anionic proteins (nephrotic syndrome) will also decrease AG. Except for hypoproteinemia, conditions that cause a reduced or negative AG are relatively rare compared with those associated with an elevated AG.

Interfering factors

- Hyperlipidemia may cause undermeasurement of sodium and falsely decrease AG.
- Normal values of AG vary according to different normal values for electrolytes, depending on laboratory methods.

Procedure and patient care

- See inside front cover for Routine Blood Testing.

- Fasting: no
- Blood tube commonly used: red or green
- If the patient is receiving an IV infusion, obtain the blood from the opposite arm.
- The sodium, potassium, chloride, and bicarbonate levels are determined by an automated multichannel analyzer.

Abnormal findings

▲ **Increased levels**

Alcoholic ketoacidosis
Diabetic ketoacidosis
Hypoaldosteronism
Increased gastrointestinal
  losses of bicarbonate
  (e.g., diarrhea or fistulae)
Lactic acidosis
Renal failure
Renal tubular acidosis
Starvation

▼ **Decreased levels**

Bromide (cough syrup)
  toxicity
Chronic vomiting or
  gastric suction
Excess alkali ingestion
Hyperaldosteronism
Hypoproteinemia
Lithium toxicity
Multiple myeloma

notes

anticentromere antibody test (Centromere antibody)

Type of test Blood

Normal findings

Negative (if positive, serum will be titrated)

Weak positive: positive at the screening titer (1:40 for human epithelial type 2 cells [HEp-2 cells]) (1:20 for kidney cells)

Moderately positive: one dilution higher than screening titer

Strong positive: two dilutions higher than screening titer

Test explanation and related physiology

A centromere is the region of the chromosome referred to as the *primary constriction* that divides the chromosome into *arms*. During cell division, the centromere exists in the *pole* of the mitotic spindle.

Anticentromere antibodies are a form of *antinuclear antibodies*. They are found in a very high percentage of patients with CREST syndrome, a variant of scleroderma. CREST syndrome is characterized by calcinosis, Raynaud's phenomenon, esophageal dysfunction, sclerodactyly, and telangiectasia. Anticentromere antibodies, on the contrary, are present in only a small minority of patients with scleroderma, a disease that is difficult to differentiate from CREST syndrome. No correlation exists between antibody titer and severity of CREST syndrome.

Procedure and patient care

- See inside front cover for Routine Blood Testing.
- Fasting: no
- Blood tube commonly used: red

Abnormal findings

Positive results

CREST syndrome

notes

A

antichromatin antibody test (Antinucleosome antibody [anti-NCS], Antihistone antibody test [anti-HST, AHA])

Type of test Blood

Normal findings

Antinucleosome antibodies

No antibodies present in < 1:20 dilution

Antihistone antibody

None detected: < 1.0 units
Inconclusive: 1.0–1.5 units
Positive: 1.6–2.5 units
Strong positive: > 2.5 units

Test explanation and related physiology

There are several chromatin antinuclear antibodies associated with autoimmune diseases. Nucleosome (NCS) represents the main autoantigen-immunogen in systemic lupus erythematosus (SLE), and these specific antibodies are an important marker of the disease activity. *Antinucleosome (anti-NCS; antichromatin)* antibodies play a key role in the pathogenesis of SLE. Nearly all patients with SLE have anti-NCS antibodies. Anti-NCS antibodies show the highest correlation with disease activity. Anti-NCS antibodies also show strong association with renal damage associated with SLE. Anti-NCS autoantibodies are more prevalent than anti-DNA in SLE patients.

Histone antibodies are present in about 20% to 55% of idiopathic SLE and 80% to 95% of drug-induced lupus erythematosus. There are several subtypes of *antihistone antibodies (AHAs)*. In drug-induced lupus erythematosus, a specific AHA (anti-[(H2A-H2B)-DNA] IgG) is produced, whereas in most of the other associated diseases the AHAs are of other varying specificities.

Procedure and patient care

- See inside front cover for Routine Blood Testing.
- Fasting: no
- Blood tube commonly used: red or gold

Abnormal findings

▲ **Increased levels**

Drug-induced lupus erythematosus
Other autoimmune diseases
Systemic lupus erythematosus

> **anticyclic citrullinated peptide antibody** (Cyclic citrullinated peptide antibody, CCP IgG anti-CCP) and anti-mutated citrullinated vimentin (anti-MCV)

Type of test Blood

Normal findings

< 20 units/mL

Test explanation and related physiology

Anti-CCP is known more formally as *anticyclic citrullinated peptide antibody*. The citrullinated peptide antigen is formed by the intermediary conversion of the amino acid ornithine to arginine. Anti-CCP appears early in the course of rheumatoid arthritis (RA). When the citrulline antibody is detected in a patient's blood, there is a high likelihood that the patient has RA. Anti-CCP is therefore useful in the diagnosis of patients with unexplained joint inflammation, especially when the traditional blood test, rheumatoid factor (RF; p. 648), is negative or lower than 50 units/mL.

Many patients with early RA may not have elevation of RF, making the diagnosis difficult in the initial stage. The diagnosis of RA can be made, even if RF is negative, if the anti-CCP is elevated. This is particularly important because aggressive treatment in the early stages of RA prevents progression of joint damage. Anti-CCP may occur years before any clinical onset of arthritis or significant elevation of anti-CCP. At a cutoff of 5 units/mL, the sensitivity and specificity of anti-CCP for RA are 67.5% and 99.3%, respectively. RF has a sensitivity of 66.3% and a lower specificity (82.1%) than anti-CCP. When the two antibodies are used together, the specificity for diagnosing RA is 99.1%.

The presence of anti-CCP in RA indicates a more aggressive and destructive form of the disease. It is also a marker for disease progression.

Procedure and patient care

• See inside front cover for Routine Blood Testing.
• Fasting: no
• Blood tube commonly used: red

Abnormal findings

▲ **Increased levels**

Rheumatoid arthritis

antidiuretic hormone (ADH, Vasopressin)

Type of test Blood

Normal findings

ADH: 1–5 pg/mL or 1–5 ng/L (SI units)

ADH suppression test (water load test):

    65% of water load excreted in 4 hours

    80% of water load excreted in 5 hours

    Urine osmolality (in second hour) ≤ 100 mmol/kg

    Urine to serum (U/S) osmolality ratio > 100

    Urine specific gravity < 1.003

Test explanation and related physiology

ADH, also known as *vasopressin*, is formed by the hypothalamus and is stored in the posterior pituitary gland. It controls the amount of water resorbed by the kidneys. ADH release is stimulated by an increase in serum osmolality or a decrease in intravascular blood volume. Physical stress, surgery, and even high levels of anxiety may also stimulate ADH release. With a release of ADH, more water is resorbed from the kidneys. This increases the amount of free water in the bloodstream and causes a very concentrated urine. With low ADH levels, water is allowed to be excreted, thereby producing hemoconcentration and a more dilute urine.

Diabetes insipidus (DI) results when ADH secretion is inadequate or when the kidney is unresponsive to ADH stimulation. Inadequate ADH secretion is usually associated with central neurologic abnormalities (neurogenic DI), such as trauma, tumor, inflammation of the brain (hypothalamus), or surgical ablation of the pituitary gland. Patients with DI excrete large volumes of free water within a dilute urine. Their blood is hemoconcentrated, causing them to have a strong thirst.

Primary renal diseases may make the renal collecting system less sensitive to ADH stimulation (nephrogenic DI). Again, in this instance, a dilute urine created by excretion of high volumes of free water may occur. To differentiate neurogenic DI from nephrogenic DI or from primary polydipsia, a *water deprivation test (ADH stimulation test)* is performed. During this test, water intake is restricted, and urine osmolality is measured before and after vasopressin is administered. In neurogenic DI, there is no rise in urine osmolality with water restriction, but there is a rise after vasopressin administration. In nephrogenic DI, there is no rise in urine osmolality after water deprivation or vasopressin administration. The diagnosis indicated by this test can be corroborated by a serum ADH level. In neurogenic DI and primary polydipsia, ADH levels are low. In nephrogenic DI, ADH levels are high.

High serum ADH levels are also associated with the syndrome of inappropriate antidiuretic hormone (SIADH) secretion. In response to the inappropriately high level of ADH secretion, water is resorbed by the kidneys greatly in excess of normal amounts. Thus the patient becomes very hemodiluted and the urine concentrated. Blood levels of important serum ions diminish, causing severe neurologic, cardiac, and metabolic alterations. SIADH can be associated with pulmonary diseases (e.g., tuberculosis, bacterial pneumonia), severe stress (e.g., surgery, trauma), CNS tumor, or infection. Ectopic secretion of ADH from neoplasm (paraneoplastic syndrome) can cause SIADH. The most common tumors associated with SIADH include carcinomas of the lung and thymus, lymphomas, leukemia, and carcinomas of the pancreas, urologic tract, and intestine. Patients with myxedema or Addison disease also can experience SIADH.

The *water load test (ADH suppression test)* is used to differentiate SIADH from other causes of hyponatremia or edematous states. Usually this test is done concomitant with measurements of urine and serum osmolality. Patients with SIADH will excrete none or very little of the water load. Furthermore, their urine osmolality will never be less than 100, and the urine/serum ratio is greater than 100. Patients with other hyponatremia, edematous states, or chronic renal diseases will excrete up to 80% of the water load and will develop midrange osmolality results.

Interfering factors

- Patients with dehydration, hypovolemia, and stress may have increased ADH levels.
- Patients with overhydration, decreased serum osmolality, and hypervolemia may have decreased ADH levels.
- A glass syringe or collection tube causes degradation of ADH.

Procedure and patient care

- See inside front cover for Routine Blood Testing.
- Fasting: yes
- Blood tube commonly used: red
- Evaluate the patient for physical or emotional stress.
- Collect a venous blood sample in a *plastic* red-top tube with the patient in the sitting or recumbent position.

- The *water load* test necessitates a baseline serum sodium before water administration. Urine is later collected for specific gravity and osmolality. Blood is collected for osmolality.

Abnormal findings

▲ **Increased levels**

Acute porphyria

Dehydration

Hypovolemia

Nephrogenic diabetes insipidus caused by primary renal diseases

Postoperative days 1–3

Severe physical stress (e.g., trauma, pain, prolonged mechanical ventilation)

Syndrome of inappropriate antidiuretic hormone (SIADH)

▼ **Decreased levels**

Decreased serum osmolality

Hypervolemia

Neurogenic (or central) diabetes insipidus

Primary polydipsia

Surgical ablation of the pituitary gland

notes

anti-DNA antibody test (Anti–deoxyribonucleic acid antibodies, Antibody to double-stranded DNA, Anti–double-stranded DNA, Anti–ds-DNA, DNA antibody, Native double-stranded DNA)

Type of test Blood
Normal findings
Negative: < 5 international units/mL
Intermediate: 5–9 international units/mL
Positive: ≥ 10 international units/mL

Test explanation and related physiology
The anti-DNA test is useful for the diagnosis and follow-up of systemic lupus erythematosus (SLE). This antibody is found in approximately 65% to 80% of patients with active SLE and rarely in other diseases. The anti-DNA titer decreases with successful therapy and increases with an exacerbation of SLE, especially with the onset of lupus glomerulonephritis.

The anti-DNA IgG antibody is a subtype of the *antinuclear antibodies (ANAs)* (p. 71). If the ANAs are negative, there is no reason to test for anti-DNA antibodies. There are two types of anti-DNA antibodies. The first and most popular is the antibody against double-stranded DNA (anti–ds-DNA). The second type is the antibody against single-stranded DNA (anti–ss-DNA), which is less sensitive and specific for SLE but is positive in other autoimmune diseases.

Interfering factors
• A radioactive scan performed within 1 week before the test may alter the test results.

Procedure and patient care
• See inside front cover for Routine Blood Testing.
• Fasting: no
• Blood tube commonly used: red

Abnormal findings
▲ Increased levels
  Biliary cirrhosis
  Chronic hepatitis
  Collagen vascular disease (e.g., systemic lupus erythematosus)
  Infectious mononucleosis

notes

antiextractable nuclear antigens (Anti-ENAs, Antibodies to extractable nuclear antigens, Antihistidyl transfer synthase [anti–Jo-1], Antiribonucleoprotein [anti-RNP], Anti-Smith [anti-SM])

Type of test   Blood

Normal findings

Negative

Test explanation and related physiology

The anti-ENAs are used to assist in the diagnosis of systemic lupus erythematosus (SLE) and mixed connective tissue disease (MCTD) and to eliminate other rheumatoid diseases.

Anti-ENAs are a type of *antinuclear antibody* to certain nuclear antigens that consist of RNA and protein. The ENA antigen is sometimes referred to as *saline-extracted antigen*. The most common ENAs are *Smith (SM)* and *ribonucleoprotein (RNP)*.

The *antinuclear Smith (anti-SM)* antibody is present in about 30% of patients with SLE and in about 8% of patients with MCTD. However, it is not present in patients with most other rheumatoid-collagen diseases.

The *antinuclear ribonucleoprotein (anti-RNP)* antibody is reported in nearly 100% of patients with MCTD and in about 25% of patients with SLE, discoid lupus, and progressive systemic sclerosis (scleroderma). In high titer, anti-RNP is suggestive of MCTD.

The *antihistidyl transfer synthase (anti–Jo-1)* antibodies occur in patients with autoimmune interstitial pulmonary fibrosis and in a minority of patients with aggressive autoimmune myositis.

There are two other antibodies to ENAs. Anti–SS-A and anti–SS-B are described on p. 81 and are used mainly in the diagnostic evaluation of Sjögren syndrome.

Procedure and patient care

- See inside front cover for Routine Blood Testing.
- Fasting: no
- Blood tube commonly used: red

Abnormal findings

▲ Increased anti-SM antibodies

  Systemic lupus erythematosus

▲ **Increased anti-RNP antibodies**
  Discoid lupus scleroderma
  Mixed connective tissue disease
  Systemic lupus erythematosus

▲ **Increased anti–Jo-1 antibodies**
  Autoimmune myositis
  Pulmonary fibrosis

notes

antifactor Xa (Anti-Xa)

Type of test Blood

Normal findings

Adults and children > 8 weeks

Therapeutic ranges of heparin:
  LMWH: 0.5–1.2 IU/mL
  UFH: 0.3–0.7 IU/mL
Prophylactic ranges of heparin:
  LMWH: 0.2–0.5 IU/mL
  UFH: 0.1–0.4 IU/mL

Children <8 weeks

Therapeutic ranges:
  Standard heparin (UFH): 0.3 to 0.7 IU/mL
  LMWH: 0.5 to 1 IU/mL (specimen drawn 4–6 hours after subcutaneous injection)
Prophylactic range:
  LMWH: 0.1 to 0.3 IU/mL

Test explanation and related physiology

Through its action on the protein antithrombin, heparin interferes with the clotting process by accelerating the inhibition of coagulation factors Xa and IIa. The plasma Anti-Xa assay (see secondary hemostasis, Figure C3, p. 212) is used to monitor patients on low molecular weight heparins (LMWHs) (e.g., enoxaparin or rivaroxaban) or unfractionated standard heparin (UFH). Although UFH is commonly monitored by means of the APTT (p. 557), the APTT can underestimate the degree of heparin anticoagulation in patients with a high factor VIII level or suspected heparin resistance (also evaluated by APC; p. 325). In these situations, the measurement of a plasma anti-Xa level may provide a more accurate assessment of anticoagulation. Reference ranges for anti-Xa levels vary depending on the laboratory performing the test. When a person is not taking heparin, anti-Xa concentrations should be zero or undetectable.

When used to monitor LMWHs, anti-Xa levels are usually ordered as a "peak" test. They are collected 3 to 4 hours after a LMWH dose is given when the blood level is expected to be the highest. Random and "trough" anti-Xa tests may also be ordered when there are concerns that a LMWH may be accumulating in patients with renal failure.

As with all heparins, protamine sulfate can inhibit the drug action. The following formula is useful for calculating the dose of protamine sulfate required to neutralize UFH based upon the anti-Xa level:

Anti Xa (IU/mL) X Plasma volume (mL/kg) = dose of Protamine
Sulfate (mg)

Interfering factors
• Accurate testing requires indication of which LMWH is being administered.

Procedure and patient care
• See inside front cover for Routine Blood Testing.
• Fasting: no
• Blood tube commonly used: blue
• If the patient is receiving heparin by intermittent injection, plan to draw the blood specimen 30 minutes to 1 hour before the next dose of heparin.
• If the patient is receiving continuous heparin, draw the blood at any time.
• When it is used to monitor LMWHs, the specimen is collected 3 to 4 hours after a LMWH dose is administered.
• Apply pressure to the venipuncture site. Remember, if the patient is receiving anticoagulants or has coagulopathies, the bleeding time will be increased.
• Assess the patient to detect possible bleeding. Check for blood in the urine and all other excretions and assess the patient for bruises, petechiae, and low back pain.
• If severe bleeding occurs, note that the anticoagulant effect of heparin can be reversed by parenteral administration of protamine sulfate.

Abnormal findings
▲ **Increased levels**
  Hemophilia
  Heparin administration
  Heparin resistance
  Lupus anticoagulant
  Renal failure

notes

antiglomerular basement membrane antibodies
(Anti-GBM antibody, AGBM, Glomerular basement antibody, Goodpasture antibody)

A

Type of test   Blood; microscopic examination of tissue

Normal findings

Tissue

Negative: no immunofluorescence noted on the renal or lung tissue basement membrane

Blood: EIA (enzyme immunoassay)

Negative: < 20 units
Borderline: 20 to 100 units
Positive: > 100 units

Test explanation and related physiology

This test is used to detect the presence of circulating glomerular basement membrane (GBM) antibodies commonly present in autoimmune-induced nephritis (Goodpasture syndrome).

Goodpasture syndrome is an autoimmune disease characterized by the presence of antibodies circulating against antigens in the basement membrane of the renal glomerular and the pulmonary alveoli. These immune complexes activate the complement system and thereby cause tissue injury. Patients with this problem usually display a triad of glomerulonephritis (hematuria), pulmonary hemorrhage (hemoptysis), and antibodies to basement membrane antigens.

Lung or renal biopsies are required to obtain tissue. Serum assays are faster and more reliable methods for diagnosing Goodpasture syndrome.

Procedure and patient care

- See inside front cover for Routine Blood Testing.
- Fasting: yes
- Blood tube commonly used: red
- **PT** If a lung biopsy (p. 480) or renal biopsy (p. 636) will be used to collect the specimen, explain these procedures.

Abnormal findings

Positive

Autoimmune glomerulonephritis
Goodpasture syndrome
Lupus nephritis

notes

antiglycan antibodies (Crohn's disease prognostic panel, Multiple sclerosis antibody panel)

Type of test Blood

Normal findings

Negative

Test explanation and related physiology

Antiglycan antibodies are immunologically directed to sugar-containing components on the surface of cells (particularly erythrocytes). Antibodies to glycans can be instigated by bacterial, fungal, and parasite infections. The use of glycan arrays for systematic screening of patients with multiple sclerosis (MS) and inflammatory bowel disease (particularly Crohn's disease) has been helpful in differentiating these diseases. Furthermore, these antibodies are used to determine treatment and prognosis.

Anti-Saccharomyces cerevisiae antibody (ASCA), antilaminaribioside carbohydrate antibody (ALCA), antimannobioside carbohydrate antibody (AMCA), and antichitobioside carbohydrate antibody (ACCA) are used to evaluate Crohn's disease and to differentiate Crohn's colitis from ulcerative colitis. When all are positive, Crohn's disease is much more likely than ulcerative colitis.

Other antiglycan antibodies are specific for MS patients.

Procedure and patient care

- See inside front cover for Routine Blood Testing.
- Fasting: no
- Blood tube commonly used: lavender, pink, or green

Abnormal findings

▲ **Increased levels**

Crohn's disease

Multiple sclerosis

notes

antiliver/kidney microsomal type 1 antibodies
(Anti-LKM-1 antibodies)

Type of test Blood

Normal findings

≤ 20 units (negative)
20.1–24.9 units (equivocal)
≥ 25 units (positive)

Test explanation and related physiology

Autoimmune liver disease (e.g., autoimmune hepatitis and primary biliary cirrhosis) is characterized by the presence of autoantibodies, including smooth muscle antibodies (SMA) (p. 78), antimitochondrial antibodies (AMA) (p. 66), and antiliver/kidney microsomal antibodies type 1 (anti–LKM-1). Subtypes of autoimmune hepatitis (AIH) are based on autoantibody reactivity patterns.

Anti–LKM-1 antibodies serve as a serologic marker for AIH type 2 and typically occur in the absence of SMAs and antinuclear antibodies. Patients with AIH type 2 more often tend to be young and female and have a severe form of disease that responds well to immunosuppressive therapy.

Patients with chronic hepatitis resulting from hepatitis C can also have elevated anti–LKM-1 antibodies. The diagnosis of autoimmune liver disease cannot be made on antibody testing alone. In many instances, autoimmune liver disease panel testing is performed.

Procedure and patient care

- See inside front cover for Routine Blood Testing.
- Fasting: no
- Blood tube commonly used: serum separator
- **PT** Explain the value of performing the test in the morning.
- Blood may be sent to a reference laboratory. Results are available in about 1 week.

Abnormal findings

▲ **Increased levels**
  Autoimmune hepatitis

notes

antimitochondrial antibody (AMA)

Type of test Blood

Normal findings

No antimitochondrial antibodies (AMAs) at titers > 1:5 or < 0.1 units

Test explanation and related physiology

The AMA is used primarily to aid in the diagnosis of primary biliary cirrhosis. AMA is an anticytoplasmic antibody directed against a lipoprotein in the mitochondrial membrane. Normally the serum does not contain AMA at a titer greater than a ratio of 1 to 5. AMA appears in most patients with primary biliary cirrhosis. This disease occurs predominantly in young and middle-aged women. It has a slow, progressive course marked by elevated liver enzymes, especially alkaline phosphatase and gamma-glutamyl transpeptidase (pp. 23 and 361) and positive AMA. Liver biopsy (p. 468) is usually required to confirm the diagnosis. There are subgroups of AMA. The M-2 subgroup is very specific for primary biliary cirrhosis.

Procedure and patient care

- See inside front cover for Routine Blood Testing.
- Fasting: no
- Blood tube commonly used: red

Abnormal findings

▲ Increased levels

Acute infectious hepatitis

Autoimmune hepatitis (e.g., scleroderma, systemic lupus erythematosus)

Chronic active hepatitis

Drug-induced cholestasis

Extrahepatic obstruction

Primary biliary cirrhosis

Syphilis

Systemic lupus erythematosus

notes

antimyocardial antibody

Type of test Blood

Normal findings

Negative (if positive, serum will be titrated)

Test explanation and related physiology

This test is used to detect an autoimmune source of myocardial injury and disease. Antimyocardial antibodies (AMAs) may be detected in rheumatic heart disease, cardiomyopathy, postthoracotomy syndrome, and postmyocardial infarction syndromes. This test is used both in the detection of an autoimmune cause for these conditions and for monitoring their response to treatment. Antibodies against heart muscle are found in about 20% to 40% of postcardiac surgery patients and in a smaller number of postmyocardial infarction patients. These antibodies are usually associated with a pericarditis that follows the myocardial injury associated with cardiac surgery or myocardial infarction (Dressler syndrome). AMA has also been detected with cardiomyopathy.

Procedure and patient care

- See inside front cover for Routine Blood Testing.
- Fasting: no
- Blood tube commonly used: red

Abnormal findings

▲ **Increased levels**

Cardiomyopathy
Postmyocardial infarction
Postthoracotomy syndrome
Rheumatic fever
Rheumatic heart disease
Streptococcal infection

notes

antineutrophil cytoplasmic antibody (ANCA)

Type of test   Blood

Normal findings

Components	Reference interval
Antineutrophil cytoplasmic antibody, IgG	<1:20: Not significant
Myeloperoxidase antibody	Negative: ≤ 19 AU/mL Equivocal: 20–25 AU/mL Positive: ≥ 26 AU/mL
Serine protease 3 antibody	Negative: ≤ 19 AU/mL Equivocal: 20–25 AU/mL Positive: ≥ 26 AU/mL

Test explanation and related physiology

ANCAs are directed against cytoplasmic components of neutrophils. This test is used to assist in the diagnosis of granulomatous vascular diseases, such as Wegener granulomatosis (WG). It also is useful in tracking the course of the disease, monitoring the response to therapy, and providing early detection of relapse. WG is a regional systemic vasculitis in which the small arteries of the kidneys, lungs, and upper respiratory tract (nasopharynx) are damaged by a granulomatous inflammation.

When ANCAs are detected with indirect immunofluorescence microscopy, two major patterns of staining are present: cytoplasmic ANCA (c-ANCA) and perinuclear ANCA (p-ANCA). Specific immunochemical assays demonstrate that c-ANCA consists mainly of antibodies to proteinase 3 (PR3), and p-ANCA consists of antibodies to myeloperoxidase (MPO). Using the antigen-specific immunochemical assay to characterize ANCA (rather than the pattern of immunofluorescence microscopy) is more specific and more clinically relevant; therefore the terms *proteinase 3-ANCA (PR3-ANCA)* and *myeloperoxidase-ANCA (MPO-ANCA)* are used.

The PR3 autoantigen is highly specific (95%–99%) for WG. When the disease is limited to the respiratory tract, the PR3 is positive in about 65% of patients. Nearly all patients with WG limited to the kidney do not have positive PR3. When WG is inactive, the percentage of positive PR3 drops to about 30%.

The MPO autoantigen is found in 50% of patients with WG centered in the kidney. It also occurs in patients with non-WG glomerulonephritis, such as microscopic polyangiitis (MPA).

P-ANCA antibodies can also differentiate various forms of inflammatory bowel disease. (See also antiglycan antibodies, p. 64). P-ANCA antibodies are found in 50% to 70% of patients with ulcerative colitis (UC) but in only 20% of patients with Crohn's disease (CD).

Procedure and patient care

- See inside front cover for Routine Blood Testing.
- Fasting: no
- Blood tube commonly used: verify with laboratory

Abnormal findings

▲ **Increased levels**

Active viral hepatitis
Autoimmune hepatitis
Churg-Strauss vasculitis
Crohn's disease
Idiopathic crescentic glomerulonephritis
Microscopic polyarteritis
Primary sclerosing cholangitis
Ulcerative colitis
Wegener granulomatosis

notes

antinuclear antibody (ANA)

Type of test   Blood

Normal findings

Negative at 1:40 dilution

Test explanation and related physiology

ANA is a group of antinuclear antibodies used to diagnose systemic lupus erythematosus (SLE) and other autoimmune (rheumatic) diseases (Box A1). Some of the antibodies in this group are specific for SLE, and others are specific for other autoimmune diseases. ANA can be tested as a specific antibody or as a group with nonspecific antigens (Box A2). The former is more specific, but testing ANA with less specific antigens may be an excellent preliminary test for those suspected of having autoimmune diseases.

Because almost all patients with SLE develop autoantibodies, a negative ANA test result nearly excludes the diagnosis. Positive results occur in most patients with this disease; however, many other rheumatic diseases (see Box A1 and Table A2) are also associated with ANA.

ANA shows up on indirect immunofluorescence as fluorescent patterns in cells that are fixed to a slide and are evaluated under a UV microscope. Different patterns are associated with a variety of autoimmune disorders. When combined with a more specific subtype of ANA (see Table A3), the pattern can increase specificity of the ANA subtypes for the various autoimmune

---

BOX A1   Diseases associated with antinuclear antibodies
Autoimmune hepatitis Autoimmune thyroiditis Dermatomyositis Juvenile rheumatoid arthritis Mixed connective tissue disease Polymyositis Primary biliary cirrhosis Raynaud's disease Rheumatoid arthritis Scleroderma Sjögren syndrome Systemic lupus erythematosus

A

BOX A2 Antinuclear antibodies

Antichromatin antibodies
  Anti-DNA antibodies
    Anti–ds-DNA antibodies
    Anti–ss-DNA antibodies
  Antihistone antibodies
  Antinucleosome antibodies
Anti-ENA antibodies
  Antihistidyl antibodies
  Antinuclear RNP antibodies
  Antinuclear Smith (SM) antibodies
Anti-RNA antibodies
Anti–SS-A (Ro)
Anti–SS-B (La)

TABLE A2 Autoimmune disease and positive ANAs

Autoimmune disease	Positive antibodies
Chronic active hepatitis	ASMA
Drug-induced SLE	ANA
Mixed connective tissue disease	ANA, RNP, RF, ss-DNA
Primary biliary cirrhosis	AMA
Raynaud's disease	ACA, Scl-70
Rheumatoid arthritis	RF, ANA, RANA, RAP
Scleroderma	ANA, Scl-70, RNA, ds-DNA, ARA, ATA
Sjögren syndrome	RF, ANA, SS-A, SS-B
SLE	ANA, SLE prep, ds-DNA, ss-DNA, anti-DNP, SS-A
Thyroiditis	Antimicrosomal, antithyroglobulin

diseases. An example of a positive result might be: "Positive at 1:320 dilution with a homogeneous pattern."

As the disease becomes less active because of therapy, the ANA titers can be expected to fall. In this text, the more commonly used ANA subtypes are separately discussed. Most SLE patients have a positive ANA test result. If a patient also has symptoms of SLE (e.g., arthritis, rash, autoimmune thrombocytopenia), then he or she probably has SLE.

TABLE A3   Immunofluorescent patterns

Characteristics	Diseases
Homogeneous (Entire nucleus is stained)	Mixed connective tissue disease SLE
Speckled (Small fluorescent dots)	Mixed connective tissue disease Polymyositis Rheumatoid arthritis Scleroderma Sjögren syndrome SLE
Centromere (30–60 dots throughout the nucleus in resting)	Limited SLE
Nucleolar (Fluorescent large dots localized to chromosomes)	Polymyositis Scleroderma

Procedure and patient care

- See inside front cover for Routine Blood Testing.
- Fasting: no
- Blood tube commonly used: red

Abnormal findings

▲ **Increased levels**

Chronic hepatitis
Cirrhosis
Dermatomyositis
Infectious mononucleosis
Leukemia
Myasthenia gravis
Other immune diseases
Periarteritis (polyarteritis) nodosa
Raynaud's disease
Rheumatoid arthritis
Scleroderma
Sjögren syndrome
Systemic lupus erythematosus

notes

antiparietal cell antibody (APCA)

Type of test Blood

Normal findings

Negative

Test explanation and related physiology

Parietal cells exist in the proximal stomach and produce hydrochloric acid and intrinsic factor. Intrinsic factor is necessary for the absorption of vitamin B_{12} (p. 805). Antiparietal cell antibodies (APCAs) are found in most patients with pernicious anemia. Nearly 60% of these patients also have antiintrinsic factor antibodies. It is thought that these antibodies contribute to the destruction of the gastric mucosa. APCA is also found in patients with atrophic gastritis, gastric ulcers, and gastric cancer.

APCA is present in other autoimmune-mediated diseases such as thyroiditis, myxedema, juvenile diabetes, Addison disease, and iron-deficiency anemia. Nearly 10% to 15% of the normal population has APCA. As one ages, the incidence of having APCA increases (especially with relatives having pernicious anemia).

APCA can crossreact with other antibodies, especially anticellular and antithyroid antibodies. Titer levels greater than 1:240 are considered positive.

Procedure and patient care

- See inside front cover for Routine Blood Testing.
- Fasting: no
- Blood tube commonly used: red

Abnormal findings

▲ **Increased levels**

Addison disease

Atrophic gastritis

Hashimoto thyroiditis

Insulin-dependent diabetes mellitus

Myxedema

Pernicious anemia

notes

anti-PM/Scl-75 and anti-PM/Scl-100 antibodies
(PM/Scl-75 and PM/Scl-100 antibodies)

Type of test Blood

Normal findings

Negative

Test explanation and related physiology

Anti-PM/Scl antibodies are present in patients with an overlap syndrome of polymyositis (PM) and scleroderma (systemic sclerosis [SSc]). Only 2.5% of SSc patients exhibit anti-PM/Scl antibodies, but these antibodies are a part of commonly performed panels designed to detect and classify autoimmune diseases.

Anti-PM/Scl antibodies are a heterogeneous group of autoantibodies directed at several proteins of the nucleolar PM/Scl macromolecular complex. The two main autoantigenic protein components were identified and termed *PM/Scl-75* and *PM/Scl-100* based on their apparent molecular weights. Anti-PM/Scl-100 may be positive in autoimmune interstitial lung disease (or pulmonary fibrosis associated with SSc). Anti-PM/Scl-100 is often associated with Raynaud's phenomenon and arthritis in these patients. Anti-PM/Scl-75 may be a bit more common in SSc than anti-PM/Scl-100. Also it is more often associated with patients who have gastrointestinal effects of scleroderma.

Procedure and patient care

- See inside front cover for Routine Blood Testing.
- Fasting: No
- Blood tube commonly used: Gold

Abnormal findings

Limited scleroderma (CREST)
Polymyositis
Sclerodermatomyositis (overlap syndrome)
Systemic scleroderma

notes

A

anti-RNA polymerase antibody (anti-RNA polymerase I, II, III, RNAP, ARA)

Type of test Blood

Normal findings

≤19 units	Negative
20–39 units	Weak positive
40–80 units	Moderate positive
≥81 units	Strong positive

Test explanation and related physiology

Anti-RNA polymerase antibodies (ARAs) are an aid to the diagnosis of systemic sclerosis (SSc). They are a marker of very rapid onset of disease and skin thickening progression in SSc.

There are three classes of RNA polymerase antibodies (RNAPs I, II, and III). Anti-RNA polymerase III antibodies are a specific marker for SSc associated with severe disease characterized by major organ and cutaneous involvement. A rapid onset of SSc (within 6 months from Raynaud's phenomenon onset) is found in patients with ARA. The clinical specificity for SSc is excellent. Clinical features associated with ARA include diffuse cutaneous scleroderma, a high total skin score, and a trend toward high prevalence of renal crisis. A negative ARA result does not rule out the possibility of SSc. *Anti-topoisomerase 1 (ATA)* is another autoantibody associated with the presence of pulmonary fibrosis in patients with SSc.

Procedure and patient care

* See inside front cover for Routine Blood Testing.
* Fasting: no
* Blood tube commonly used: gold

Abnormal findings

Scleroderma

notes

antiscleroderma antibody (Scl-70 antibody, Anti-topoisomerase I, Scleroderma antibody, RNA polymerase III antibody)

Type of test Blood

Normal findings

Scl-70 antibody
> <1 U (negative)
> ≥1 U (positive)

RNA polymerase III antibody
> <20 U (negative)
> 20–39.9 U (weak positive)
> 40–80 U (moderate positive)
> >80 U (strong positive)

Test explanation and related physiology

This antibody is diagnostic for systemic scleroderma (SSc) and is present in 45% of patients with that disease. *Scl-70* antibody (also called Anti-topoisomerase I) is an *antinuclear antibody* (p. 70). PSS is a multisystem disorder characterized by inflammation with subsequent fibrosis of the small blood vessels in skin and visceral organs, including the heart, lungs, kidneys, and gastrointestinal tract. A collagen-like substance is also deposited into the tissue of these organs.

The absence of this antibody does not exclude the diagnosis of SSc. The antibody is rather specific for SSc but is occasionally seen in other autoimmune diseases.

RNA polymerase III antibodies are found in 11% to 23% of patients with SSc. SSc patients who are positive for *RNA polymerase III* antibodies form a distinct serologic subgroup and usually may not have any of the other antibodies typically found in SSc patients, such as anticentromere (p. 52) or anti-Scl70.

Anti-RNA polymerase III antibodies (ARA) are a specific marker for SSc, associated with severe disease characterized by major organ and diffuse cutaneous involvement. Patients with isolated ARA have a more rapid disease onset. A positive result supports a possible diagnosis of systemic sclerosis. This autoantibody is also strongly associated with an increased risk of acute renal crisis. Because less than 30% of the SSc patients have ARA, a negative result does not rule out the possibility of systemic sclerosis. However, the overall mortality is no worse when the disease is associated with positivity of this autoantibody.

See other SSc antibodies (**Anti-PM/Scl-75 and anti-PM/Scl-100 antibodies**) and **anticentromere antibodies**.

Procedure and patient care
- See inside front cover for Routine Blood Testing.
- Fasting: no
- Blood tube commonly used: red

Abnormal findings
Positive results
CREST syndrome
Scleroderma

notes

antismooth muscle antibody (ASMA)

Type of test Blood

Normal findings

No antismooth muscle antibodies (ASMAs) at titers > 1:20

Test explanation and related physiology

The ASMA is used primarily to aid in the diagnosis of auto-immune chronic active hepatitis (CAH), which has also been referred to as *lupoid* CAH. ASMA is an *anticytoplasmic antibody* directed against actin, a cytoskeletal protein. Normally the serum does not contain ASMA at a titer greater than 1:20. ASMA is the most commonly recognized autoantibody in the setting of CAH. It appears in 70% to 80% of patients with CAH. Some types of CAH do not have positive ASMA antibodies.

ASMA is not specific for CAH and can be positive in patients with viral infections, malignancy, multiple sclerosis, primary biliary cirrhosis, and *Mycoplasma* infections. Usually the titer of ASMA is low in these diseases. With CAH, the titer is usually higher than 1 to 160. The titers are not helpful in prognosis nor do they indicate disease response to therapy.

Procedure and patient care

- See inside front cover for Routine Blood Testing.
- Fasting: no
- Blood tube commonly used: red

Abnormal findings

▲ **Increased levels**

Chronic active hepatitis
Intrinsic asthma
Malignancy
Mononucleosis hepatitis
Multiple sclerosis
Primary biliary cirrhosis
Viral hepatitis

notes

antispermatozoal antibody (Sperm agglutination and inhibition, Sperm antibodies, Antisperm antibodies, Infertility screen)

Type of test   Fluid analysis; blood

Normal findings

< 50% binding

Test explanation and related physiology

The antispermatozoal antibody test is an infertility test used to detect the presence of sperm antibodies. Antibodies directed toward sperm antigens can result in diminished fertility. This test is used in the evaluation of an infertile couple usually after a postcoital test result is positive. For fertilization to occur, the sperm head must first attach to the *zona pellucida* of the egg. Sperm antibodies interfere with this binding. IgA antisperm antibodies attached to the sperm tail are associated with poor motility and poor penetration of cervical mucus. IgG antisperm antibodies are associated with blockage of sperm-ovum fusion. Semen and serum may contain sperm antibodies. Semen is the preferred specimen type for men. Serum is the preferred specimen type in females.

Positives are reported as percentage of sperm with positive bindings, the class of antibody involved (IgG, IgA, and IgM), and the site of binding (head, midpiece, tail, and/or tail tip). Greater than 50% binding is usually required to significantly lower a patient's fertility.

Not only is this test indicated for male infertility studies, but it is also used as a follow-up test when sperm agglutination is noted in the ejaculate. It is also used in men with a history of testicular trauma, biopsy, vasectomy reversal, genital tract infection, or obstructive lesions of the male ductal system. Antisperm antibodies may be found in the blood of men with blocked efferent ducts of the testes and in 30% to 70% of men who have had a vasectomy. Resorption of sperm from the blocked ducts results in the formation of autoantibodies to sperm as a result of sperm antigens interacting with the immune system. High titers of IgG autoantibodies are often associated with postvasectomy degeneration of the testes, which explains why 50% of males remain infertile after successful repair of a previous vasectomy.

Procedure and patient care

- See inside front cover for Routine Blood Testing.
- Fasting: no
- Blood tube commonly used: red

Sperm specimen

PT Inform the man that a semen specimen should be collected after avoiding ejaculation for at least 3 days.

• Give the patient the proper container for the collection.

PT If the specimen is to be collected at home, be certain the patient is told that it must be taken to the laboratory for testing within 2 hours after collection.

• Collect venous blood samples from both the male and the female patient.

• For a vaginal mucus specimen, collect 1 mL of cervical mucus and place it in a plastic vial.

PT Instruct the couple on how to obtain the test results.

Abnormal findings

Blocked efferent ducts in the testes
Infertility
Testicular trauma
Vasectomy

notes

anti–SS-A (RO), anti–SS-B (LA), and anti–SS-C antibodies (Anti-Ro, Anti-La, Sjögren antibodies)

Type of test Blood

Normal findings

SS-A (Ro) antibodies, IgG
    < 1 U (negative)
    ≥ 1 U (positive)
SS-B (La) antibodies, IgG
    < 1 U (negative)
    ≥ 1 U (positive)

Test explanation and related physiology

These three antinuclear antibodies are considered *antiextractable nuclear antigens* (p. 59) and are used to diagnose Sjögren syndrome. Ro, La, and SS-C antibodies are subtypes of *antinuclear antibodies (ANAs);* they react to nuclear antigens extracted from human B lymphocytes. Sjögren syndrome is an immunogenic disease characterized by progressive destruction of the lacrimal and salivary exocrine glands, leading to mucosal and conjunctival dryness. This disease can occur by itself (primary) or in association with other autoimmune diseases such as systemic lupus erythematosus (SLE), rheumatoid arthritis (RA), and scleroderma. In the latter case, it is referred to as secondary Sjögren syndrome.

Anti–SS-A antibodies may be found in approximately 60% to 70% of patients with primary Sjögren syndrome. Anti–SS-B antibodies may be found in approximately half of patients with primary Sjögren syndrome. When anti–SS-A and anti–SS-B antibodies are both positive, Sjögren syndrome can be diagnosed. These antibodies are only occasionally found when secondary Sjögren syndrome is associated with RA. In fact, anti–SS-B is found only in primary Sjögren syndrome. However, anti–SS-C is positive in about 75% of patients with RA or patients with RA and secondary Sjögren syndrome. Therefore these antibodies are also useful in differentiating primary from secondary Sjögren syndrome.

Anti–SS-A can also be found in 25% of patients with SLE. This is particularly useful in ANA-negative cases of SLE because these antibodies are present in the majority of such patients. Anti–SS-B is rarely found in SLE, however. In general, the higher the titer of anti-SS antibodies, the more likely that Sjögren syndrome exists and the more active the disease is. As Sjögren syndrome becomes less active with therapy, the anti-SS antibody titers can be expected to fall.

Procedure and patient care

- See inside front cover for Routine Blood Testing.
- Fasting: no
- Blood tube commonly used: red

Abnormal findings

Positive

ANA-negative systemic lupus erythematosus
Neonatal lupus
Rheumatoid arthritis
Sjögren syndrome

notes

antithrombin activity and antigen assay (Antithrombin III [AT-III] activity/assay, Functional antithrombin III assay, Heparin cofactor, Immunologic antithrombin III, Serine protease inhibitor)

Type of test Blood

Normal findings

Antithrombin activity:

    Older than 6 months to adult: 80%-130%

    Newborn: 35%-40%

Antithrombin antigen assay:

    Plasma: > 50% of control value

    Serum: 15%-34% lower than plasma value

    Immunologic: 17–30 mg/dL

    Functional: 80%-120%

Values vary according to laboratory methods.

Test explanation and related physiology

AT-III inhibits the serine proteases involved in coagulation (II, X, IX, XI, XII). In normal homeostasis, coagulation results from a balance between AT-III and thrombin. A deficiency of AT-III increases coagulation or the tendency toward thrombosis. A hereditary deficiency of AT-III is characterized by a predisposition toward thrombus formation. This is passed on as an autosomal dominant abnormality. Individuals with hereditary AT-III deficiency typically develop thromboembolic events in their early twenties. These thrombotic events are usually venous.

Acquired AT-III deficiency may be seen in patients with cirrhosis, liver failure, advanced carcinoma, nephrotic syndrome, disseminated intravascular coagulation (DIC), protein-losing enteropathies, and acute thrombosis. AT-III is also decreased as much as 30% in pregnant women and women who take estrogens. Antithrombin activity testing is ordered, along with other tests for hypercoagulable disorders (e.g., protein C and protein S, and lupus anticoagulant), when a patient has been experiencing recurrent venous thrombosis.

AT-III provides most of the anticoagulant effect of heparin. Heparin increases antithrombin activity by a thousandfold. Patients who are deficient in AT-III may be heparin resistant and require unusually high doses for an anticoagulation effect. In general, patients respond to heparin if more than 60% of normal AT-III levels exist.

There are two tests for AT-III. The first is a *functional* assay and measures AT-III activity. The second *quantifies* the AT-III antigen. The antithrombin activity test is performed before the antigen test to evaluate whether the total amount of functional antithrombin activity is normal. Antithrombin activity is the primary (screening) antithrombin assay. If antithrombin activity is normal, AT-III is not the cause of the hypercoagulable state. If antithrombin activity is abnormal, antithrombin antigen should be quantified.

Procedure and patient care

- See inside front cover for Routine Blood Testing.
- Fasting: no
- Blood tube commonly used: light blue or red
- Patients receiving heparin therapy may develop a hematoma at the venipuncture site.

Test results and clinical significance

▲ **Increased levels**
Acute hepatitis
Kidney transplant
Obstructive jaundice
Vitamin K deficiency

▼ **Decreased levels**
Disseminated intravascular coagulation (DIC)
Hepatic disorders (especially cirrhosis)
Hereditary familial deficiency of AT-III
Hypercoagulation states (e.g., deep vein thrombosis)
Nephrotic syndrome
Protein-wasting diseases (malignancy)

notes

antithyroglobulin antibody (Thyroid autoantibody, Thyroid antithyroglobulin antibody, Thyroglobulin antibody, Thyroid antigen thyroglobulin)

Type of test   Blood

Normal findings
< 116 IU/mL

Test explanation and related physiology

This test is used as a marker for autoimmune thyroiditis and related diseases. Thyroglobulin autoantibodies bind thyroglobulin (Tg), which is a major thyroid-specific protein that plays a crucial role in thyroid hormone synthesis, storage, and release. Tg remains in the thyroid follicles until hormone production is required. Tg is not secreted into the systemic circulation under normal circumstances. However, follicular destruction through inflammation (Hashimoto thyroiditis or chronic lymphocytic thyroiditis and autoimmune hypothyroidism), hemorrhage (nodular goiter), or rapid disordered growth of thyroid tissue (as may be observed in Graves disease or follicular cell-derived thyroid neoplasms) can result in leakage of Tg into the bloodstream. This results in the formation of autoantibodies to Tg in some individuals.

The anti-Tg test is usually performed in conjunction with the antithyroid peroxidase antibody test (p. 87) and is an important companion test for thyroglobulin.

Interfering factors
- Normal individuals, especially elderly women, may have anti-Tg antibodies.

Procedure and patient care
- See inside front cover for Routine Blood Testing.
- Fasting: no
- Blood tube commonly used: red

Abnormal findings
▲ **Increased levels**
   Autoimmune hemolytic anemia
   Hashimoto thyroiditis
   Hypothyroidism

▲ **Increased levels (continued)**

Myxedema
Pernicious anemia
Rheumatoid arthritis
Rheumatoid-collagen disease
Thyroid carcinoma
Thyrotoxicosis

notes

antithyroid peroxidase antibody (Anti-TPO, TPO-Ab, Antithyroid microsomal antibody, Thyroid autoantibody)

Type of test Blood

Normal findings

Titer < 9 IU/mL

Test explanation and related physiology

This test is primarily used in the differential diagnosis of thyroid diseases. Thyroid microsomal antibodies are commonly found in patients with various thyroid diseases. They are present in most patients with Hashimoto thyroiditis. Microsomal antibodies are produced in response to microsomes escaping from the thyroid epithelial cells surrounding the thyroid follicle. These escaped microsomes then act as antigens and stimulate the production of antibodies. These immune complexes initiate inflammatory and cytotoxic effects on the thyroid follicle.

Although many different thyroid diseases are associated with elevated antimicrosomal antibody levels, the most frequent is chronic thyroiditis (Hashimoto thyroiditis in adults and lymphocytic thyroiditis in children and young adults).

Procedure and patient care

- See inside front cover for Routine Blood Testing.
- Fasting: no
- Blood tube commonly used: red

Abnormal findings

▲ **Increased levels**

Hashimoto thyroiditis

Hypothyroidism

Myxedema

Pernicious anemia

Rheumatoid arthritis

Rheumatoid-collagen disease

Thyroid carcinoma

Thyrotoxicosis

notes

apt test (Downey test, Qualitative fetal hemoglobin stool test, Stool for swallowed blood)

Type of test Stool

Normal findings

No fetal blood present.
Maternal blood may be present.

Test explanation and related physiology

Blood in the stool of a newborn must be rapidly evaluated. Furthermore, some serious diseases present as rectal bleeding in newborns. Much more commonly, however, newborns may simply be defecating maternal blood that was swallowed during birth or breastfeeding.

The Apt test is performed on the stool specimen to differentiate maternal from fetal blood in the stool. Fetal hemoglobin is resistant to denaturation; adult hemoglobin (hemoglobin A) is not. This test can be performed on stool, a stool-stained diaper, amniotic fluid, or vomitus.

Procedure and patient care

Before

PT Explain the procedure to the newborn's parents.
- Assess the vital signs of the newborn with possible intestinal bleeding.

During
- Obtain an adequate stool or vomitus specimen.
- In the laboratory, 1% NaOH is added to the specimen. Maternal blood turns brown; newborn blood stays red or pink.

After
- If maternal blood is present, examine the mother for nipple erosion or cracking.
- If newborn blood is present, begin close observation and support during further diagnostic procedures.

Abnormal findings

Active gastrointestinal bleeding
Necrotizing enterocolitis

notes

arterial blood gases (ABGs, blood gases)

Type of test Blood

Normal findings

pH
Adult/child: 7.35–7.45
Newborn: 7.32–7.49
2 months-2 years: 7.34–7.46
pH (venous): 7.31–7.41

P_{CO_2}
Adult/child: 35–45 mm Hg
Child < 2 years: 26–41 mm Hg
P_{CO_2} (venous): 40–50 mm Hg

HCO_3
Adult/child: 21–28 mEq/L
Newborn/infant: 16–24 mEq/L

P_{O_2}
Adult/child: 80–100 mm Hg
Newborn: 60–70 mm Hg
P_{O_2} (venous): 40–50 mm Hg

O_2 saturation
Adult/child: 95%-100%
Elderly: 95%
Newborn: 40%-90%

O_2 content
Arterial: 15–22 vol %
Venous: 11–16 vol %

Base excess
0 ± 2 mEq/L

Alveolar to arterial O_2 difference
< 10 mm Hg

Possible critical values

pH: <7.25, >7.55
PCO_2: < 20, > 60
HCO_3: < 15, > 40
PO_2: < 40
O_2 saturation: 75% or lower
Base excess: ± 3 mEq/L

Test explanation and related physiology

Measurement of ABGs provides valuable information in assessing and managing a patient's respiratory (ventilation) and metabolic (renal) acid-base and electrolyte homeostasis. It is also used to assess adequacy of oxygenation. ABGs are used to monitor patients on ventilators, to monitor critically ill nonventilator patients, to establish preoperative baseline parameters, and to enlighten electrolyte therapy.

pH

The pH is inversely proportional to the actual hydrogen ion concentration. Therefore as the hydrogen ion concentration decreases, the pH increases and vice versa. (Table A4).

P_{CO_2}

The P_{CO_2} is a measure of the partial pressure of CO_2 in the blood. P_{CO_2} is a measurement of ventilation capability. The faster and more deeply one breathes, the more CO_2 is blown off and P_{CO_2} levels drop. Therefore P_{CO_2} is referred to as the *respiratory* component in acid-base determination. See Table A5.

Bicarbonate (HCO_3)

Most of the CO_2 content in the blood is HCO_3. The bicarbonate ion is a measure of the *metabolic (renal/kidney)* component of the acid-base equilibrium. It is regulated by the kidneys. This ion can be measured directly by the bicarbonate value or indirectly by the CO_2 content (p. 167). HCO_3 is elevated in metabolic alkalosis and decreased in metabolic acidosis (see Table A5). The kidneys also are used to compensate for primary respiratory acid-base derangements. (see Table A5.)

P_{O_2}

This is an indirect measure of the oxygen content of arterial blood. The P_{O_2} level is decreased in patients who:

- Are unable to oxygenate the arterial blood because of O_2 diffusion difficulties (e.g., pneumonia)
- Have premature mixing of venous blood with arterial blood (e.g., in congenital heart disease)
- Have underventilated and overperfused pulmonary alveoli (Pickwickian syndrome or patients with significant atelectasis)

O_2 saturation

Oxygen saturation is an indication of the percentage of hemoglobin saturated with O_2. When 92% to 100% of the hemoglobin carries O_2, the tissues are adequately provided with O_2 in most circumstances. At O_2 saturation levels of 70% or

TABLE A4 Normal values for arterial blood gases and abnormal values in uncompensated acid-base disturbances

Acid-base disturbances	pH	Pco$_2$ (mm Hg)	HCO$_3$ (mEq/L)	Common causes
None (normal values)	7.35–7.45	35–45	22–26	
Respiratory acidosis	↓	↑	Normal	Respiratory depression (drugs, central nervous system trauma) Pulmonary disease (pneumonia, chronic obstructive pulmonary disease, respiratory underventilation)
Respiratory alkalosis	↑	↓	Normal	Hyperventilation (emotions, pain, respirator overventilation)
Metabolic acidosis	↓	Normal	↓	Diabetes, shock, renal failure, intestinal fistula
Metabolic alkalosis	↑	Normal	↑	Sodium bicarbonate overdose, prolonged vomiting, nasogastric drainage

TABLE A5   **Acid-base disturbances and compensatory mechanisms**

Acid-base disturbance	Mode of compensation
Respiratory acidosis	Kidneys will retain increased amounts of HCO_3 to increase pH.
Respiratory alkalosis	Kidneys will excrete increased amounts of HCO_3 to lower pH.
Metabolic acidosis	Lungs blow off CO_2 to raise pH.
Metabolic alkalosis	Lungs retain CO_2 to lower pH.

lower, the tissues are unable to extract enough O_2 to carry out their vital functions.

Pulse oximetry is a noninvasive method of determining O_2 saturation (p. 539).

O_2 content

This is a calculated number that represents the amount of O_2 in the blood. Nearly all O_2 in the blood is bound to hemoglobin. O_2 content decreases with the same diseases that diminish Po_2.

Base excess or deficit

This number is calculated using the pH, Pco_2, and hematocrit. It represents the amount of buffering anions in the blood. HCO_3 is the largest of these. Others include hemoglobin, proteins, and phosphates. Base excess is a way to take all these anions into account when determining acid-base treatment based on the *metabolic* component. Negative base excess (deficit) indicates a metabolic acidosis (e.g., lactic acidosis). A positive base excess indicates metabolic alkalosis or compensation to prolonged respiratory acidosis.

Alveolar (A) to arterial (a) O_2 difference (A-a gradient)

This is a calculated number that indicates the difference between alveolar (A) O_2 and arterial (a) O_2. The normal value is less than 10 mm Hg (torr). If the A-a gradient is abnormally high, there is either a problem in diffusing O_2 across the alveolar membrane (thickened edematous alveoli) or unoxygenated blood is mixing with the oxygenated blood.

Contraindications

- Patients with a negative Allen test result
- Patients with arteriovenous fistula proximal to the access site
- Patients with severe coagulopathy

Interfering factors

- O$_2$ saturation can be falsely increased with the inhalation of carbon monoxide.

Procedure and patient care

Before

PT Explain the procedure to the patient.

PT Tell the patient that an arterial puncture is associated with more discomfort than a venous puncture.

- Notify the laboratory before drawing ABGs so that the equipment can be calibrated before the blood sample arrives.
- Perform the *Allen test* to assess collateral circulation.
- To perform the Allen test, make the patient's hand blanch by obliterating both the radial and the ulnar pulses, and then release the pressure over the ulnar artery only. If flow through the ulnar artery is good, flushing will be seen immediately. The Allen test is then positive, and the radial artery can be used for puncture.
- If the Allen test is negative (no flushing), repeat it on the other arm.
- If both arms give a negative result, choose another artery for puncture.

During

- Note that arterial blood can be obtained from any area of the body in which strong pulses are palpable, usually from the radial, brachial, or femoral artery.
- Cleanse the arterial site.
- Use a small gauge needle to collect the arterial blood in an air-free heparinized syringe.
- Expel any air bubbles in the syringe.
- Note that an arterial puncture is performed by laboratory technicians, respiratory-inhalation therapists, nurses, or physicians in approximately 10 minutes.

After

- Place the arterial blood on ice and immediately take it to the chemistry laboratory for analysis.
- Apply pressure or a pressure dressing to the arterial puncture site for 3 to 5 minutes to avoid hematoma formation.
- Assess the puncture site for bleeding. Remember that an artery rather than a vein has been stuck.

Abnormal findings

▲ **Increased pH (alkalosis)**
Metabolic alkalosis
Aldosteronism
Chronic and high-volume
   gastric suction
Chronic vomiting
Hypochloremia
Hypokalemia
Mercurial diuretics

Respiratory alkalosis
Acute and severe
   pulmonary diseases
Anxiety neuroses
Carbon monoxide
   poisoning
Chronic heart failure
Cystic fibrosis
Pain
Pregnancy
Pulmonary emboli
Shock

▼ **Decreased pH (acidosis)**
Metabolic acidosis
Ketoacidosis
Lactic acidosis
Renal failure
Severe diarrhea

Respiratory acidosis
Respiratory failure

▲ **Increased P_{CO_2}**
Chronic obstructive
   pulmonary disease
   (COPD)
Head trauma
Overoxygenation in a
   patient with COPD
Oversedation
Pickwickian syndrome

▼ **Decreased P_{CO_2}**
Anxiety
Hypoxemia
Pain
Pregnancy
Pulmonary emboli

▲ **Increased HCO_3**
Aldosteronism
Chronic and high-volume
   gastric suction
Chronic vomiting
COPD
Use of mercurial diuretics

▼ **Decreased HCO_3**
Acute renal failure
Chronic and severe
   diarrhea
Chronic use of loop
   diuretics
Diabetic ketoacidosis
Starvation

▲ **Increased Po$_2$,
increased O$_2$ content**
Hyperventilation
Increased inspired O$_2$
Polycythemia

▼ **Decreased Po$_2$,
decreased O$_2$ content**
Anemias
Adult respiratory distress
   syndrome
Atelectasis
Atrial or ventricular cardiac
   septal defects
Bronchospasm
Emboli
Inadequate O$_2$ in inspired
   air (suffocation)
Mucus plug
Pneumothorax
Pulmonary edema
Restrictive lung disease
Severe hypoventilation (e.g.,
   oversedation, neurologic
   somnolence)

notes

arteriography (Angiography)

Type of test X-ray with contrast

Normal findings

Normal arterial vasculature

Test explanation and related physiology

With the injection of radiopaque contrast material, arteries can be visualized to determine arterial anatomy and to detect vascular disease. Blood flow dynamics, arterial occlusive disease, or vascular anomalies are easily seen. With the use of *digital subtraction angiography* (DSA), bony structures can be obliterated from the picture, thereby improving the image of the artery.

- Renal angiography permits evaluation of renal artery blood flow dynamics. Arteriosclerotic narrowing (stenosis) of the renal artery is well demonstrated with this study. The angiographic location of the stenotic area is helpful if considering surgery.
- Lower extremity arteriography allows for accurate identification and location of aneurysms or occlusions within the abdominal aorta and lower extremity arteries. Embolic occlusion can also be detected here. Likewise, arterial traumas, such as lacerations or intimal tears (laceration of the inner arterial lining), appear as total or near-total obstruction of the flow of dye. Arterial vascular balloon dilation and stenting can be performed.
- Cerebral, pulmonary, and coronary arteriography are separately discussed in this book.

Contraindications

- Patients with allergy to intravenous contrast
- Patients who are pregnant, unless the benefits outweigh the risks
- Patients with renal dysfunction. See page 231.
- Patients with a bleeding propensity

Potential complications

- Hemorrhage from the arterial puncture site
- Arterial embolism from dislodgment of an arteriosclerotic plaque
- Soft tissue infection around the puncture site
- Dissection of the intimal lining of the artery causing complete or partial arterial occlusion
- Pseudoaneurysm development as a result of failure of the puncture site to seal

Procedure and patient care

Before

PT Explain the procedure to the patient. See p. xviii for radiation exposure and risks.

- Obtain written and informed consent for this procedure.

PT Inform the patient that a warm flush may be felt when the contrast is injected. This lasts only a few seconds.

- Assess the possibility of allergies to iodinated contrast media.
- Determine whether the patient has been taking anticoagulants.
- Keep the patient NPO for 2 to 8 hours before testing.
- Mark the site of the patient's distal peripheral pulses with a pen before arterial catheterization.
- If the patient does not have peripheral pulses before arteriography, document that fact so that arterial occlusion will not be suspected on the postangiogram assessment.
- If the patient has diminished renal function, consider IV hydration to minimize further renal damage.

PT Instruct the patient to void before the study because the contrast can act as an osmotic diuretic.

During

- After appropriate shave/prep and local anesthesia, a catheter is threaded under fluoroscopic visualization through an access artery into the desired position.
- Through the catheter, iodinated contrast material is injected and images are obtained.
- Note that this procedure is usually performed by an angiographer (radiologist) in approximately 1 hour.

PT Tell the patient that the most significant discomfort is the puncture necessary for arterial access.

PT Remind the patient of the discomfort of lying on a hard x-ray table for a long period.

After

- A pressure dressing is applied to the puncture site.
- Assess the distal arterial pulse in the extremity used for vascular access and compare it with the preprocedure baseline.
- Observe the arterial puncture site frequently for bleeding.
- Keep the patient on bed rest for up to 8 hours after the procedure to allow for complete sealing of the arterial puncture site. If a vascular closure product is used, the patient may ambulate within 2 hours.
- Note and compare the color and temperature of the extremity with that of the uninvolved extremity.

PT Instruct the patient to drink fluids to prevent dehydration caused by the diuretic action of the contrast.
• Evaluate the patient for delayed allergic reaction.
PT Instruct the patient to report any signs of numbness, tingling, pain, or loss of function in the involved extremity.

Abnormal findings
Arteriography of the peripheral vascular system
Aneurysm
Arteriosclerotic occlusion
Embolus occlusion
Primary arterial diseases (e.g., fibromuscular dysplasia, Buerger disease)

Kidney arteriography
Atherosclerotic narrowing of the renal artery
Fibrodysplasia of the renal artery
Renal vascular causes of hypertension

notes

arthrocentesis with synovial fluid analysis

Type of test Fluid analysis

Normal findings

Appearance	Clear, straw colored, no blood
RBC	None
WBC	$0-150/mm^3$
WBC differential	
Neutrophils	7%
Lymphocytes	24%
Monocytes	48%
Macrophages	10%
Glucose	Equal to fasting blood glucose
Protein	1–3 dL
LDH	< 25 mg/dL
Uric acid	6–8 mg/dL
Gram stain	Negative

Test explanation and related physiology

Arthrocentesis is performed to establish the diagnosis of joint infection, arthritis, crystal-induced arthritis (gout and pseudogout), synovitis, or neoplasms involving the joint. This procedure is also used to identify the cause of joint inflammation or effusion and to inject antiinflammatory medications (usually corticosteroids) into a joint space.

Arthrocentesis is performed by inserting a sterile needle into the joint space of the involved joint to obtain synovial fluid for analysis. Aspiration may be performed on any major joint such as the knee, shoulder, hip, elbow, wrist, or ankle.

The fluid sample is examined. Normal joint fluid is clear, straw colored, and quite viscous. Viscosity is reduced in patients with inflammatory arthritis. Viscosity can be roughly estimated by forcing some synovial fluid from a syringe. Fluid of normal viscosity forms a "string" more than 5 cm long (*string sign*); fluid of low viscosity as seen in inflammation drips in a manner similar to water. A Gram stain and culture of the fluid is usually performed.

The *mucin clot test* correlates with the viscosity and is an estimation of hyaluronic acid–protein complex integrity. This test is performed by adding acetic acid to joint fluid. The formation of a tight, ropy clot indicates qualitatively good mucin and the presence of adequate molecules of intact hyaluronic acid. The mucin clot is poor in quality and quantity in the presence of an inflammatory joint disease such as rheumatoid arthritis (RA). By itself, synovial fluid should not spontaneously form a fibrin clot (clot without the addition of acetic acid) because normal joint fluid does not contain fibrinogen. If, however, bleeding into the joint (from trauma or injury) has occurred, the synovial fluid will clot.

The synovial fluid glucose value is usually within 10 mL/dL of the fasting serum glucose value. For proper interpretation, the synovial fluid glucose and serum glucose samples should be drawn simultaneously after the patient has fasted for 6 hours. The synovial fluid glucose level falls with increasing severity of inflammation. Although lowest in septic arthritis, a low synovial glucose level also may be seen in patients with rheumatoid arthritis. The synovial fluid is also tested for protein, uric acid, and lactate levels. Increased uric acid levels indicate gout. Increased protein and lactate levels indicate bacterial infection or inflammation.

Cell counts are also performed on the synovial fluid. An increased WBC count with a high percentage of neutrophils supports the diagnosis of acute bacterial infectious arthritis. Leukocytes can also occur in other conditions such as acute gouty arthritis and rheumatoid arthritis.

Bacterial and fungal cultures are usually requested and performed when infection is suspected. The administration of antibiotics before arthrocentesis may diminish growth of bacteria from synovial fluid cultures and confound results. Smears for acid-fast stains for tubercle bacilli are also performed on the synovial fluid. Synovial fluid is also examined under polarized light for the presence of crystals, which permits differential diagnosis between gout and pseudogout.

The synovial fluid is also analyzed for complement levels (p. 226). Complement levels are decreased in patients with systemic lupus erythematosus, rheumatoid arthritis, or other immunologic arthritis. These decreased joint complement levels are caused by consumption of the complement induced by the antigen-antibody immune complexes within the joint cavity.

One of the most important tests routinely performed on synovial fluid is the microscopic examination for crystals. For example, urate crystals indicate gouty arthritis. Calcium pyrophosphate crystals are found in pseudogout. Cholesterol crystals occur in rheumatoid arthritis.

Contraindications

- Patients with skin or wound infections near the needle puncture because of the risk of sepsis

Potential complications

- Joint infection
- Hemorrhage in the joint area

Procedure and patient care

Before

PT Explain the procedure to the patient.
- Obtain an informed consent if indicated.
- The physician may request that the patient be kept NPO after midnight on the day of the test.

During

- Have the patient lie on his or her back with the joint fully extended.
    1. The site chosen for aspiration is cleaned and anesthetized.
    2. A needle is inserted into the joint space and fluid is aspirated for analysis. Corticosteroid or other medications can be injected.
    3. Sometimes a peripheral venous blood sample is taken to compare chemical tests on the blood with chemical studies on the synovial fluid.
- Note that a physician performs this procedure in an office or at the patient's bedside in approximately 20 minutes.
PT Tell the patient that the only discomfort associated with this test is the injection of the local anesthetic.
- Be aware that joint-space pain may worsen after fluid aspiration, especially in patients with acute arthritis.

After

PT Assess the joint for any pain, fever, or swelling. Teach the patient to look for signs of infection at home.
PT Apply ice to decrease pain and swelling and instruct the patient to continue this at home.
PT Tell the patient to avoid strenuous use of the joint for the next several days.
PT Teach the patient to walk on crutches if indicated.
PT Instruct the patient to look for signs of bleeding into the joint (significant swelling, increasing pain, or joint weakness).
PT Inform the patient when driving is permitted.

Abnormal findings

Gout
Infection
Joint effusion
Neoplasm

Osteoarthritis
Pseudogout
Rheumatoid arthritis
Septic arthritis
Synovitis
Systemic lupus erythematosus

notes

arthroscopy

Type of test Endoscopy

Normal findings

Normal ligaments, menisci, and articular surfaces of the joint

Test explanation and related physiology

Arthroscopy is an endoscopic procedure that allows direct visual examination of a joint space with a specially designed endoscope. Although this technique can visualize many joints of the body, it is most often used to evaluate the knee for meniscus cartilage or ligament injury. It is also used in the differential diagnosis of acute and chronic disorders of the knee (e.g., arthritic inflammation vs. injury). The shoulder is commonly visualized for injury to the rotator cuff.

Physicians can perform corrective surgery through the endoscope. Diagnostic arthroscopy is performed less often because of the availability and accuracy of MRI of the joints (p. 490). Other joints that can be evaluated by the arthroscope include the tarsal, ankle, knee, hip, carpal, wrist, and temporomandibular joints.

Contraindications

- Patients with ankylosis
- Patients with local skin infections near the joint
- Patients who have recently had an arthrogram

Potential complications

- Infection
- Hemarthrosis
- Swelling
- Thrombophlebitis
- Joint injury
- Synovial rupture

Procedure and patient care

Before

PT Explain the procedure to the patient.
- Ensure that the physician has obtained written consent for this procedure.
- Follow the routine preoperative procedure of the institution.
- Keep the patient NPO after midnight on the day of the test.
PT Instruct the patient who will use crutches after the procedure regarding the appropriate crutch gait.

- Shave the hair in the area 6 inches above and below the joint before the test (if ordered).

During

- After general or nerve block anesthesia, a tourniquet is placed on the patient's leg.
- The arthroscope (a lighted instrument) is inserted into the joint space through a small incision to visualize the inside of the knee joint. Although the entire joint can be viewed from one puncture site, additional punctures may be required for any reparative work.
- Note that this procedure is performed in the operating room by an orthopedic surgeon in approximately 60 minutes.

After

PT Instruct the patient to elevate the knee when sitting and to avoid overbending the knee, so that swelling is minimized.

PT Inform the patient that he or she can usually walk with the assistance of crutches; however, this depends on the extent of the procedure and the physician's protocol.

PT Tell the patient to minimize use of the joint for several days.

- Apply ice to reduce pain and swelling and instruct the patient to continue this at home.

Abnormal findings

Chondromalacia
Cyst (e.g., Baker)
Degenerative arthritis
Meniscal disease
Osteochondritis dissecans
Osteochondromatosis
Patellar disease/fracture
Rheumatoid arthritis
Synovitis
Torn cartilage/ligament

notes

aspartate aminotransferase (AST; Formerly called serum glutamic-oxaloacetic transaminase [SGOT])

Type of test Blood

Normal findings

Adult: 0–35 units/L or 0–0.58 µKat/L (SI units); females tend to have slightly lower values than males

Elderly: values slightly higher than adult values

Children:

12–18 years: 10–40 units/L

6–12 years: 10–50 units/L

3–6 years: 15–50 units/L

< 3 years: 15–60 units/L

0–5 days: 35–140 units/L

Test explanation and related physiology

Because AST exists within the liver cells, diseases that affect the hepatocytes cause elevated levels of this enzyme. This test is used in the evaluation of suspected hepatocellular diseases. The amount of elevation depends on the time after the injury that the blood is drawn. AST is cleared from the blood in a few days. Serum AST levels become elevated 8 hours after cell injury, peak at 24 to 36 hours, and return to normal in 3 to 7 days. If the cellular injury is chronic, levels will be persistently elevated.

In acute hepatitis, AST levels can rise to 20 times the normal value. In acute extrahepatic obstruction (e.g., gallstones), AST levels quickly rise to 10 times the normal value and fall swiftly. In cirrhotic patients, the level of AST depends on the amount of active inflammation.

Serum AST levels are often compared with alanine aminotransferase (ALT, p. 16) levels. The AST-to-ALT ratio is usually greater than 1.0 in patients with alcoholic cirrhosis, liver congestion, or metastatic tumor of the liver. Ratios less than 1.0 may be seen in patients with acute hepatitis, viral hepatitis, or infectious mononucleosis.

Interfering factors

- Exercise may cause increased levels.
- Pyridoxine deficiency (beriberi or pregnancy), severe long-standing liver disease, uremia, or diabetic ketoacidosis may cause decreased levels.

Procedure and patient care

- See inside front cover for Routine Blood Testing.
- Fasting: no
- Blood tube commonly used: red
- If possible, avoid giving the patient any IM injection because increased enzyme levels may result.
- Record the exact time and date when the blood test is performed. This aids in the interpretation of the temporal pattern of enzyme elevations.

Abnormal findings

▲ **Increased levels**

Liver diseases
Drug-induced liver injury
Hepatic cirrhosis
Hepatic infiltrative process
 (e.g., tumor)
Hepatic metastasis
Hepatic necrosis (initial stages
 only)
Hepatic surgery
Hepatitis
Infectious mononucleosis with
 hepatitis

Skeletal muscle disveases
Heat stroke
Multiple traumas
Primary muscle diseases (e.g.,
 myopathy, myositis)
Progressive muscular dystrophy
Recent convulsions
Recent noncardiac surgery
Severe, deep burns
Skeletal muscle trauma

Other diseases
Acute hemolytic anemia
Acute pancreatitis
Acute renal disease

▼ **Decreased levels**
Acute renal disease
Beriberi
Chronic renal dialysis
Diabetic ketoacidosis
Pregnancy

notes

barium enema (BE, Lower GI series)

B

Type of test X-ray with contrast

Normal findings

Normal filling, contour, patency, and positioning of barium in the colon

Test explanation and related physiology

The BE study consists of a series of x-rays with contrast to visualize the colon. It is used to demonstrate the presence and location of polyps, tumors, and diverticula. Anatomic abnormalities (e.g., malrotation) also can be detected. Therapeutically, the BE may be used to reduce nonstrangulated ileocolic intussusception in children.

In many instances, air is insufflated into the colon after the instillation of barium. With air contrast, the colonic mucosa can be much more accurately visualized. This is called an *air-contrast BE* and is more accurate than single contrast barium enema. With the use of colonoscopy and CT Scans (p. 231), BE is rarely performed.

Contraindications

- Patients suspected of a perforation of the colon
  In these patients, diatrizoate (Gastrografin), a water-soluble contrast medium, is used.
- Patients with megacolon because barium can worsen this condition

Potential complications

- Colonic perforation, especially when the colon is weakened by inflammation, tumor, or infection
- Barium fecal impaction

Interfering factors

- Barium within the abdomen from previous barium tests
- Significant residual stool within the colon may be confused with polyps.

Procedure and patient care

Before

- **PT** Explain the procedure to the patient. See p. xviii for radiation exposure and risks.
- Assist the patient with the bowel preparation, which varies among institutions.

- Because this procedure is rarely performed, we encourage the reader to follow the local healthcare instructions.

During

- Note the following procedural steps:
  1. The test begins with placement of a rectal balloon catheter.
  2. The balloon on the catheter is inflated tightly against the anal sphincter to hold the barium within the colon.
  3. The patient is asked to roll into multiple positions.
  4. The barium is dripped into the rectum by gravity.
  5. The barium flow is monitored fluoroscopically.
  6. The colon is examined as the barium flow progresses through the large colon and into the terminal ileum.

After

- Ensure that the patient defecates as much barium as possible.
- **PT** Inform the patient that bowel movements will be white. When all the barium has been expelled, the stool will return to a normal color.

Abnormal findings

Colonic fistula
Colonic stenosis
Colon volvulus
Diverticula
Extrinsic compression of the colon from an abscess/tumor
Hernia
Inflammatory bowel diseases (e.g., ulcerative colitis, Crohn disease)
Intussusception
Malignant tumor
Malrotation of the gut
Perforated colon
Polyps

notes

barium swallow

Type of test X-ray with contrast

Normal findings

Normal size, contour, filling, patency, and positioning of the esophagus

Test explanation and related physiology

The barium swallow provides a more thorough examination of the esophagus than most upper GI series (p. 765). Defects in normal filling and narrowing of the barium column indicate tumor, strictures, or extrinsic compression from extraesophageal tumors or an abnormally enlarged heart and great vessels. Varices, hiatal hernia, Schatzki rings, and diverticula (Zenker or epiphrenic) can be seen as well.

In patients with esophageal reflux, the radiologist may identify reflux of the barium from the stomach back into the esophagus. Muscular abnormalities (e.g., achalasia, diffuse esophageal spasm) can be detected by a barium swallow.

Contraindications

- Patients with evidence of bowel obstruction
- Patients with a perforated viscus or ruptured esophagus
- Patients who are unable to cooperate for the test

Potential complications

- Barium-induced fecal impaction

Interfering factors

- Food within the esophagus prevents adequate visualization.

Procedure and patient care

Before

PT Explain the procedure to the patient. See p. xviii for radiation exposure and risks.

PT Instruct the patient not to take anything by mouth for at least 8 hours before testing. Usually the patient is kept NPO after midnight on the day of the test.

- Assess the patient's ability to swallow. If the patient tends to aspirate, inform the radiologist.

During

- Note the following procedural steps:

1. The fasting patient is asked to swallow the contrast medium. If an esophageal leak is suspected, a water soluble contrast (diatrizoate) is used.
2. As the patient drinks the contrast through a straw, the x-ray table is tilted to the near-erect position.
3. The patient is asked to roll into various positions so that the entire esophagus can be adequately visualized.
4. With digital fluoroscopy, the radiologist follows the barium column through the entire esophagus.

PT Tell the patient that no discomfort is associated with this test.

After

PT Inform the patient of the need to evacuate all the barium. Cathartics are recommended. Initially stools are white but should return to a normal color with complete evacuation.

Abnormal findings

Achalasia
Cancer
Chalasia
Diverticula
Esophageal motility disorders (e.g., presbyesophagus, diffuse esophageal spasm)
Extrinsic compression from extraesophageal tumors, cardiomegaly, or aortic aneurysm
Lower esophageal rings
Peptic esophageal ulcers
Peptic or corrosive esophagitis
Scarred strictures
Total or partial esophageal obstruction
Varices

notes

basic metabolic profile (BMP, Chemistry panel, Chem 7, Sequential multiple analysis [SMA] 7, SMAC 7, Chemistry Screen)

The BMP is a frequently ordered panel of eight tests that provides information about the patient's metabolism, kidney function, blood glucose level, electrolytes, and acid-base balance. Depending on the reason for the test, blood may be drawn after fasting or on a random basis. Abnormal results can indicate the need for further testing. The tests are listed below and discussed separately:

Electrolytes
- Potassium (p. 595)
- Chloride (p. 196)
- Calcium (p. 159)
- CO_2 (carbon dioxide, bicarbonate [HCO_3], p. 167)

Kidney tests
- BUN (p. 134)
- Creatinine, serum (p. 249)

Glucose (p. 386)

Test results can be displayed as shown in Figure B1. For accuracy, check the normal ranges at the institution or lab where the test was performed.

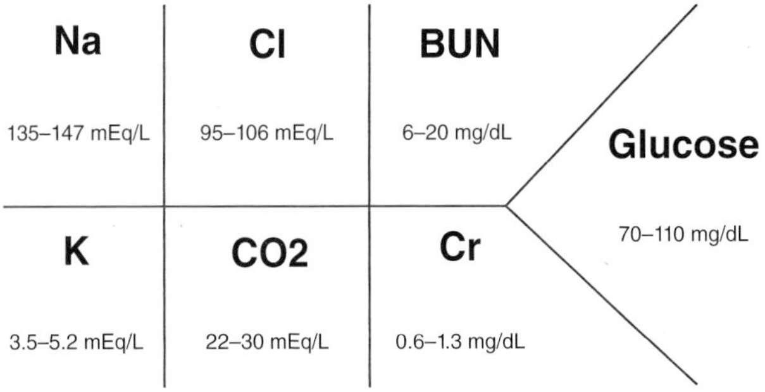

Na	Cl	BUN	
135–147 mEq/L	95–106 mEq/L	6–20 mg/dL	**Glucose**
K	**CO2**	**Cr**	70–110 mg/dL
3.5–5.2 mEq/L	22–30 mEq/L	0.6–1.3 mg/dL	

FIG. B1 Basic metabolic profile.

Bence Jones protein (Free kappa and lambda light chains)

Type of test Urine

Normal findings

Kappa total light chain: < 0.68 mg/dL
Lambda total light chain: < 0.4 mg/dL
Kappa/lambda ratio: 0.7–6.2

Test explanation and related physiology

The detection of Bence Jones protein in the urine most commonly indicates multiple myeloma (especially when the urine levels are high). The test is used to detect and monitor the treatment and clinical course of multiple myeloma and other similar globulin diseases.

Bence Jones proteins are monoclonal light-chain portions of immunoglobulins found in most patients with multiple myeloma. They also may be associated with tumor metastases to the bone, chronic lymphocytic leukemias, lymphoma, macroglobulinemia, and amyloidosis.

Immunoglobulin light chains are usually cleared from the blood through the renal glomeruli and are reabsorbed in the proximal tubules; thus urine light-chain concentrations are normally very low or undetectable. The production of large amounts of monoclonal light chains, however, can overwhelm this reabsorption mechanism. Because the Bence Jones protein is rapidly cleared from the blood by the kidneys, it may be very difficult to detect in the blood; therefore urine is used for this study. Normally urine should contain no Bence Jones proteins. Proteins in the urine are best identified by *protein electrophoresis* of the urine and then are identified and quantified *(immunofixation)*.

Interfering factors

• Dilute urine may yield a false-negative result.

Procedure and patient care

• See inside front cover for Routine Urine Testing.

PT Instruct the patient to collect an early morning specimen of at least 50 mL of uncontaminated urine in a container. It may be helpful to know the amount of these proteins excreted over 24 hours. If so, a 24-hour collection is ordered.

- Immediately transport the specimen to the laboratory. If it cannot be taken to the laboratory immediately, refrigerate it. Heat-coagulable proteins can decompose, causing a false-positive test.

Abnormal findings

▲ **Increased levels**

Amyloidosis

Chronic lymphocytic leukemia

Cryoglobulinemia

Lymphoma

Multiple myeloma (plasmacytoma)

Osteogenic sarcoma

Rheumatoid diseases

Various metastatic tumors

Waldenström macroglobulinemia

notes

beta-hydroxybutyrate (Beta-hydroxybutyric acid)

Type of test   Blood

Normal findings

< 0.4–0.5 mmol/L

Possible critical values

> 3 mmol/L

Test explanation and related physiology

Beta-hydroxybutyrate is the main metabolic product in ketoacidosis. The most clinically relevant application of serum β-hydroxybutyrate determination involves the diagnosis, management, and monitoring of diabetic ketoacidosis (DKA).

β-hydroxybutyrate is the most abundant ketone body produced during DKA. During states of insulin deficiency, lipolysis of the adipose tissue provides a huge fatty acid load to the liver. Fatty acids are initially metabolized to acetyl-coenzyme A, which cannot enter the citric acid cycle in the mitochondria of the cell due to oxaloacetate deficiency. Thus acetyl-coenzyme A is diverted to ketones through the activity of several enzymes, producing acetoacetate. Acetoacetate is then reduced to 3-β-hydroxybutyrate by 3-β-hydroxybutyrate dehydrogenase.

Elevated levels are diagnostic of DKA, but in the absence of concomitant hyperglycemia, alcoholic ketoacidosis is suspected.

Procedure and patient care

- See inside front cover for Routine Blood Testing.
- Fasting: No
- Blood tube commonly used: Red
- Point-of-care devices can measure levels in a single drop of capillary blood within 30 seconds.

Abnormal findings

Elevated Levels

Alcoholic ketoacidosis

Diabetic ketoacidosis

Fasting, starvation, ketogenic diets

Growth hormone deficiency

High-fat diet

Lactation

Salicylate poisoning

notes

11 beta-prostaglandin F(2) alpha

Type of test Urine

Normal findings

> 1000 ng/24 hours

Test explanation and related physiology

Measurement of 11 beta-prostaglandin F(2) alpha in urine is useful in the evaluation of patients suspected of having systemic mastocytosis (systemic mast cell disease [SMCD]). SMCD is characterized by mast cell infiltration of extracutaneous organs (usually the bone marrow). Focal mast cell lesions in the bone marrow are found in approximately 90% of adult patients with SMCD.

Prostaglandin D(2) (PGD[2]) is generated by human mast cells, activated alveolar macrophages, and platelets. Although the most definitive test for SMCD is bone marrow biopsy (p. 139), measurement of mast cell mediators such as beta prostaglandin in urine is advised for the initial evaluation of suspected cases. Elevated levels of 11 beta-prostaglandin F(2) alpha in urine are not specific for SMCD and may be found in patients with angioedema, diffuse urticaria, or myeloproliferative diseases in the absence of diffuse mast cell proliferation.

Procedure and patient care

- See inside front cover for Routine Urine Testing.

Abnormal findings

▲ **Increased levels**

Systemic mast cell disease (SMCD)

notes

bile acids (Cholic acid, Chenodeoxycholic acid, Deoxycholic acid, Ursodeoxycholic acid)

Type of test Blood

Normal findings

Cholic acid (CA): 0–1.9 µmol/L
Chenodeoxycholic acid (CDC): 0–3.4 µmol/L
Deoxycholic acid (DCA): 0–2.5 µmol/L
Ursodeoxycholic acid (UDC): 0–1 µmol/L
Total: 0–10 µmol/L

Test explanation and related physiology

Primary bile acids are formed in the liver from cholesterol, conjugated primarily to glycine and taurine, stored and concentrated in the gallbladder, and secreted into the intestine after the ingestion of a meal. In the intestine, the bile acids emulsify ingested fats and promote fatty digestion. During absorption of fat, nearly all of the bile acids are reabsorbed. The bile acids are then carried through the portal system to the liver. The hepatic clearance of bile acids from portal blood maintains serum concentrations at low levels in normal people.

Elevated fasting serum levels are due to impaired hepatic clearance and are a sensitive indicator of liver diseases, including cirrhosis, hepatitis, cholestasis, portal vein thrombosis, Budd–Chiari syndrome, cholangitis, Wilson disease, intrahepatic cholestasis of pregnancy and hemochromatosis. This test is also helpful in monitoring patients receiving bile acid therapy, such as cholic acid, deoxycholic acid, or ursodeoxycholic acid.

Interfering factors

• Meals: Gallbladder contraction will result in an extra load of bile acids being excreted into the intestine and reabsorbed. Thus higher concentrations are expected.

Procedure and patient care

• See inside front cover for Routine Blood Testing.
• Fasting: Yes
• Blood tube commonly used: Red

Abnormal findings

▲ **Increased bile acids**
Cholestasis
Cirrhosis
Metabolic diseases of
  conjugated bile acids
Portal vein obstruction
Primary hepatocellular
  diseases

▼ **Decreased Bile Acids**
Malabsorption
Metabolic abnormalities in
  bile acid synthesis

B

notes

bilirubin

Type of test Blood

Normal findings

Adult/elderly/child:

Total bilirubin: 0.3–1 mg/dL or 5.1–17 µmol/L (SI units)

Indirect bilirubin: 0.2–0.8 mg/dL or 3.4–12 µmol/L (SI units)

Direct bilirubin: 0.1–0.3 mg/dL or 1.7–5.1 µmol/L (SI units)

Newborn:

Total bilirubin: 1–12 mg/dL or 17.1–205 µmol/L (SI units)

Possible critical values

Total bilirubin

Adult: > 12 mg/dL

Newborn: > 15 mg/dL

Test explanation and related physiology

Bilirubin metabolism begins with the breakdown of red blood cells (RBCs) in the reticuloendothelial system (Figure B2). Hemoglobin is released from RBCs and broken down to heme and globin molecules. Heme is then catabolized to form biliverdin, which is transformed into bilirubin. This form of bilirubin is called *unconjugated (indirect) bilirubin*. In the liver, indirect bilirubin is conjugated with a glucuronide, resulting in *conjugated (direct) bilirubin*. The conjugated bilirubin is then excreted from the liver cells and into the bile ducts and then into the bowel.

Jaundice is the discoloration of body tissues caused by abnormally high blood levels of bilirubin. This yellow discoloration is recognized when the total serum bilirubin exceeds 2.5 mg/dL.

Physiologic jaundice of the newborn occurs if the newborn's liver is immature and does not have enough conjugating enzymes.

When the jaundice is recognized either clinically or chemically, it is important (for therapy) to differentiate whether it is predominantly caused by unconjugated or conjugated bilirubin. This in turn will help differentiate the etiology of the defect. In general, jaundice caused by hepatocellular dysfunction (e.g., hepatitis) results in elevated levels of unconjugated bilirubin. Jaundice resulting from extrahepatic obstruction of the bile

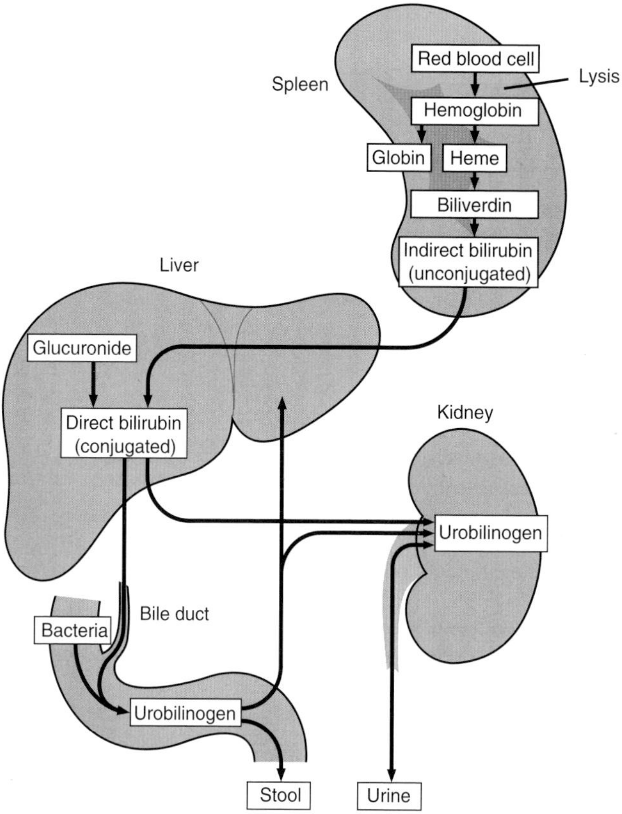

FIG. B2 Bilirubin metabolism and excretion. The spleen, liver, kidneys, and gastrointestinal tract contribute to this process.

ducts (e.g., gallstones or tumor blocking the bile ducts) results in elevated conjugated bilirubin levels; this type of jaundice usually can be resolved surgically or endoscopically.

The total serum bilirubin level is the sum of the conjugated (direct) and unconjugated (indirect) bilirubin. Normally the unconjugated bilirubin makes up 70% to 85% of the total bilirubin. In patients with jaundice, when more than 50% of the bilirubin is conjugated, it is considered a conjugated hyperbilirubinemia from gallstones, tumors, inflammation, scarring, or obstruction of the extrahepatic ducts. Unconjugated hyperbilirubinemia exists when less than 15% to 20% of the total bilirubin is conjugated. Diseases that typically cause this form of jaundice include accelerated erythrocyte (RBC) hemolysis or hepatitis.

Interfering factors

- Blood hemolysis and lipemia can produce erroneous results.

Procedure and patient care

- See inside front cover for Routine Blood Testing.
- Fasting: verify with laboratory
- Blood tube commonly used: red
- Use a heel puncture for blood collection in infants.
- Do *not* shake the tube; inaccurate test results may occur.
- Protect the blood sample from bright light.

Abnormal findings

▲ **Increased levels of conjugated (direct) bilirubin**
Cholestasis from drugs
Dubin–Johnson syndrome
Extensive liver metastasis
Extrahepatic duct obstruction
Gallstones
Rotor syndrome

▲ **Increased levels of unconjugated (indirect) bilirubin**
Cirrhosis
Crigler–Najjar syndrome
Gilbert syndrome
Hemolytic anemia/jaundice
Hemolytic jaundice
Hepatitis
Large-volume blood transfusion
Neonatal hyperbilirubinemia
Pernicious anemia
Resolution of a large hematoma
Sepsis
Sickle cell anemia
Transfusion reaction

notes

biomarkers for acute kidney injury

Type of test Blood

Normal findings

No rise in biomarkers from baseline.

Test explanation and related physiology

There are several biomarkers that can predict acute kidney injury (AKI) and chronic kidney disease (CKD). These are particularly important in patients who have serious nonrenal disease (e.g., heart surgery, renal transplant, sepsis). They can also predict drug-induced AKI with a lead-time of 2–3 days allowing for therapeutic interventions.

Neutrophil gelatinase-associated lipocalin (NGAL, Lipocalin-2), tissue inhibitor of metalloproteinase-2 (TIMP2) and insulin-like growth factor binding protein-7 (IGFBP7) are some of the markers being used to predict AKI. Other markers of AKI include *Cystatin C (p. 250), Kidney injury molecule-1, microalbumin (p. 511), macroglobulin (p. 513), and N-acetyl-β-glucosaminidase*. These biomarkers can be detected in both urine and blood within 2 hours of a renal insult. They can be measured in the urine or blood and are inversely related to GFR.

Procedure and patient care

- See inside front cover for Routine Blood Testing.
- Fasting: no
- Blood tube commonly used: red
- Collect urine specimens at the same time each day for consecutive days.
- Results are compared with previous day's testing.

Abnormal findings

▲ **Increased levels**

Primary or secondary renal disease

notes

bladder cancer indicators (Bladder tumor antigen [BTA], Nuclear matrix protein 22 [NMP22])

Type of test Urine

Normal findings

BTA: < 14 units/mL
NMP22: < 10 units/mL
FISH: No chromosomal amplification or deletions noted

Test explanation and related physiology

The use of bladder tumor indicators may provide a more accurate non-invasive method of diagnosing recurrent bladder cancer.

Bladder tumor antigen (BTA) and *nuclear matrix protein 22 (NMP22)* are proteins produced by bladder tumor cells and deposited into the urine. Normally none or very low levels of these proteins are found in the urine. When levels of bladder cancer tumor markers are normal, cystoscopy rarely yields positive results. When these markers are elevated, bladder tumor recurrence is strongly suspected and cystoscopy is indicated to confirm bladder cancer recurrence.

NMP22 may also be a good screening test for patients at increased risk for developing bladder cancer. However, these markers can be elevated in other circumstances (i.e., recent urologic surgery, urinary tract infection, calculi). Cancers involving the ureters and renal pelvis may also be associated with increased BTA and NMP22.

A bladder cytology test is available that can be used in the early detection of bladder cancer recurrence. Cytology becomes more sensitive when an immunocytofluorescence technique is added based on monoclonal antibodies to two antigens: a *mucin glycoprotein* and a *carcinoembryonic antigen (CEA)*. These antigens are expressed by tumor cells found in patients with bladder cancer and are exfoliated in the urine.

Interfering factors

- These proteins are very unstable. If the urine is not immediately stabilized, false negatives may occur.
- Active infection (including sexually transmitted diseases) of the lower urologic tract and urinary tract infections can cause false elevations.
- BPH and Kidney or bladder calculi can cause false elevations.

Procedure and patient care

- See inside front cover for Routine Urine Testing.
- **PT** Tell the patient that no fasting is required.
- A urine specimen should be collected, preferably from the first void of the day.
- The specimen should be transported to the laboratory immediately to avoid deterioration of the cells.
- If a time delay is required, the specimen should be refrigerated.

Abnormal findings

Bladder cancer
Nonbladder urologic cancer (e.g., ureters, renal pelvis)

notes

bleeding scan (Gastrointestinal bleeding scan, Abdominal scintigraphy, GI scintigraphy)

Type of test Nuclear scan

Normal findings

No collection of radionuclide in GI tract

Test explanation and related physiology

The GI bleeding scan is a test used to localize the site of bleeding in patients who are having active GI hemorrhage. The scan also can be used in patients who have suspected intraabdominal hemorrhage from an unknown source.

Arteriography has limitations in its evaluation of GI bleeding. Arteriography can determine the site of bleeding only if the rate of bleeding exceeds 0.5 mL/min for detection. The GI bleeding scan has several advantages over arteriography. It can detect bleeding if the rate is greater than 0.05 mL/min. Also, with the use of ^{99m}Tc-labeled red blood cells (RBCs), delayed images (as long as 24 hours) can be obtained, indicating the site of an intermittent or extremely slow intestinal bleed.

A GI scintigram is sensitive in locating the area of GI bleeding; however, it is not very specific in pinpointing the exact site or cause of bleeding. It is important to realize that this test can take 1 to 4 hours to obtain useful information. An unstable patient may need to go to surgery in minutes.

Contraindications

- Patients who are pregnant or lactating, unless the benefits outweigh the risks
- Medically unstable patients

Interfering factors

- Barium in the GI tract may mask a small source of bleeding.

Procedure and patient care

Before

PT Explain the procedure to the patient. See p. xviii for radiation exposure and risks.

PT Inform the patient that no pretest preparation is required.

PT Assure the patient that only a small amount of nuclear material will be administered.

PT Instruct the patient to notify the nuclear medicine technologist if he or she has a bowel movement during the test. Blood in the GI tract can act as a cathartic.

During
- Note the following procedural steps:
  1. ^{99m}Tc-labeled sulfur colloid is administered intravenously to the patient. If ^{99m}Tc-labeled RBCs are to be used, 3 to 5 mL of the patient's own blood is combined with the ^{99m}Tc and reinjected into the patient.
  2. Immediately after administration of the radionuclide, the patient is placed under a scintillation camera.
  3. Multiple images of the abdomen are obtained at short intervals (5–15 minutes).
  4. Detection of radionuclide in the abdomen indicates the site of bleeding. If no bleeding sites are noted in the first hour, the scan may be repeated at hourly intervals for as long as 24 hours.
- Note that areas of the bowel hidden by the liver or spleen may not be adequately evaluated by this procedure. Also, the rectum cannot be easily evaluated because other pelvic structures (e.g., the bladder) obstruct the view.
- Note that this test is usually performed in approximately 60 minutes by a technologist in nuclear medicine.

PT Tell the patient that the only discomfort associated with this study is the injection of the radioisotope.

After

PT Assure the patient that only tracer doses of radioisotopes have been used and that radiation precautions are not necessary.

Abnormal findings

Angiodysplasia
Aortoduodenal fistula
Diverticulosis
Inflammatory bowel disease
Polyps
Tumor
Ulcer

notes

blood culture and sensitivity

Type of test Blood

Normal findings

Negative

Test explanation and related physiology

Blood cultures are obtained to detect the presence of bacteria in the blood (bacteremia). An episode of bacteremia is usually accompanied by chills and fever; thus the blood culture should be drawn when the patient manifests these signs to increase the chances of growing bacteria on the cultures. It is important that at least two culture specimens be obtained from two different sites. If one produces bacteria and the other does not, the bacteria in the first culture may be a contaminant and not the infecting agent. When both cultures grow the infecting agent, bacteremia exists and is caused by the organism that is growing in the culture.

If the patient is receiving antibiotics during the time that the cultures are drawn, the laboratory should be notified. Resin may be added to the culture medium to negate the antibiotic effect in inhibiting growth of the offending bacteria in the culture. If cultures are to be performed while the patient is on antibiotics, the blood culture specimen should be taken shortly before the next dose of the antibiotic is administered. All cultures preferably should be performed before antibiotic therapy is initiated.

Culture specimens drawn through an IV catheter are frequently contaminated, and tests using them should not be performed unless catheter sepsis is suspected. Most organisms require approximately 24 hours to grow in the laboratory, and a preliminary report can be given at that time. Often, 48 to 72 hours is required for growth and identification of the organism. Anaerobic organisms may take longer to grow.

Interfering factors

• Contamination of the blood specimen, especially by skin bacteria, may occur.

Procedure and patient care

Before

PT Explain the procedure to the patient.

PT Tell the patient that no fasting is required.

During

- Carefully prepare the venipuncture site with povidone-iodine (Betadine). Allow the skin to dry.
- Clean the tops of the Vacutainer tubes or culture bottles with povidone-iodine and allow them to dry. Some laboratories suggest cleaning with 70% alcohol after cleaning with povidone-iodine and air drying.
- Collect approximately 10 to 15 mL of venous blood by venipuncture from each site in a 20-mL syringe.
- Discard the needle on the syringe and replace it with a second sterile needle before injecting the blood sample into the culture bottle.
- Inoculate the anaerobic bottle first if both anaerobic and aerobic cultures are needed.
- Mix gently after inoculation.
- Label the specimen with the patient's name, date, and time.
- Record the collection site and any medications that may affect test results.

After

- Transport the culture bottles immediately to the laboratory (or at least within 30 minutes).
- Notify the physician of any positive results so that appropriate antibiotic therapy can be initiated.

Abnormal findings

Bacteremia

notes

blood smear (Peripheral blood smear, Red blood cell [RBC] morphology, RBC smear)

Type of test Blood

Normal findings

Normal quantity of red and white blood cells (RBCs, WBCs) and platelets

Normal size, shape, and color of RBCs

Normal WBC differential count

Normal size and granulation of platelets

Test explanation and related physiology

Examination of the peripheral blood smear can provide a significant amount of information concerning drugs and diseases that affect erythrocytes (RBCs), leukocytes (WBCs), or platelets. Furthermore, other congenital and acquired diseases can be diagnosed. When special stains are applied to the blood smear, leukemia, infection, infestation, and other diseases can be identified.

All three hematologic cell lines—RBCs, platelets, and WBCs—can be examined. In the peripheral blood, five different types of WBCs can routinely be identified: neutrophils, eosinophils, basophils, lymphocytes, and monocytes. The first three are also referred to as *granulocytes*. Please see the discussion in bone marrow biopsy (p. 139) for more information concerning the various elements of blood.

Microscopic examination of the RBCs can reveal variations in RBC size (anisocytosis), shape (poikilocytosis), color, or intracellular content (Box B1). Classification of RBCs according to these variables is most helpful in identifying the causes of anemia and the presence of other diseases.

Microscopic examination of thick (screening) and thin (diagnostic) blood smears is helpful in the diagnosis of *Malaria*, a mosquito-borne disease caused by *Plasmodium* species.

The WBCs are examined for total quantity, differential count, and degree of maturity. An increased number of immature WBCs may indicate leukemia or infection. A decreased WBC count indicates a failure of marrow to produce WBCs (because of drugs, chronic disease, neoplasia, or fibrosis), peripheral destruction, or sequestration.

Platelet examination

A laboratory technologist can estimate platelet number. Platelets are small cell fragments that do not contain a nucleus.

BOX B1 Microscopic examination of red blood cells

RBC size abnormalities
Microcytes (small RBCs)
• Iron deficiency
• Thalassemia
• Hemoglobinopathies
Macrocytes (larger size)
• Vitamin B_{12} or folic acid deficiency
• Reticulocytosis secondary to increased erythropoiesis (RBC production)
• Occasional liver disorder

RBC shape abnormalities
Spherocytes (small and round)
• Hereditary spherocytosis
• Acquired immunohemolytic anemia
Elliptocytes (crescent)
• Iron deficiency
• Hereditary elliptocytosis
Codocytes or target cells (thin cells with less hemoglobin)
• Hemoglobinopathies
• Thalassemia
Echinocytes (Burr cells)
• Uremia
• Liver disease

RBC color abnormalities
Hypochromic (pale)
• Iron deficiency
• Thalassemia
Hyperchromasia (more colored)
• Concentrated hemoglobin, usually caused by dehydration

RBC intracellular structure
Nucleated (normoblasts). (Mature RBCs are round with a small central
pallor without any intracellular structures. They do not have a nucleus.
Immature RBCs [reticulocytes] do contain intracellular RNA. Immature
nucleated cells are not normally found in the peripheral blood and
indicate increased RBC synthesis.)
• Anemia
• Chronic hypoxemia
• Normal for an infant
• Marrow-occupying neoplasm or fibrotic tissue
Basophilic stippling (refers to bodies enclosed or included in the
cytoplasm of the RBCs)
• Lead poisoning
• Reticulocytosis
Howell–Jolly bodies (small, round remnants of nuclear material remaining
within the RBC)
• After a surgical splenectomy
• Hemolytic anemia
• Megaloblastic anemia
• Functional asplenia (after splenic infarction)

The contents of the granules in a platelet are released to promote clotting.

Procedure and patient care

Before

PT Explain the procedure to the patient.

PT Tell the patient that no fasting is required.

During

- Collect a drop of blood from a finger stick or heel stick and place it on a slide.
- If necessary, perform a venipuncture and collect the blood in a lavender-top tube.
- Note that a blood smear is first studied with an automated cytometer programmed to recognize abnormal blood cell shapes and other variations. An evaluation smear is performed by a technologist. Low counts may be hand counted to ensure accuracy. The most accurate smear requires review by a pathologist.

After

- Apply pressure to the venipuncture site.

Abnormal findings

See Box B1 in the Test explanation and related physiology section.

notes

blood typing (Blood group microarray testing)

Type of test Blood

Normal findings

Compatibility

Test explanation and related physiology

With blood typing, ABO and Rh antigens can be detected in the blood of prospective blood donors and potential blood recipients. This test is also used to determine the blood type of expectant mothers and newborns. A description of the ABO system, Rh factors, and blood crossmatching is reviewed here.

ABO system

Human blood is grouped according to the presence or absence of A or B antigens. The surface membranes of group A red blood cells (RBCs) contain A antigens; group B RBCs contain B antigens; group AB RBCs have both A and B antigens; and group O RBCs have neither A nor B antigens. In general, a person's serum does not contain antibodies to match the surface antigen on their RBCs. That is, persons with group A antigens (type A blood) will not have anti-A antibodies; however, they will have anti-B antibodies. The converse is true for persons with group B antigens. Group O blood will have both anti-A and anti-B antibodies (Table B1). These antibodies against A and B blood group antigens are formed in the first 3 months of life after exposure to similar antigens on the surface of naturally occurring bacteria in the intestine.

TABLE B1   Blood typing

Blood type (ABO, Rh)	Antigens present	Antibodies possibly present	Percent of general population
O, +	Rh	A, B	35
O, −[a]	None	A, B, Rh	7
A, +	A, Rh	B	35
A, −	A	B, Rh	7
B, +	B, Rh	A	8
B, −	B	A, Rh	2
AB, +[b]	A, B, Rh	None	4
AB, −	A, B	Rh	2

[a]Universal donor.
[b]Universal recipient.

Blood transfusions are actually transplantations of tissue (blood) from one person to another. It is important that the recipient not have antibodies to the donor's RBCs. If this were to occur, there could be a hypersensitivity reaction, which can vary from mild fever to anaphylaxis with severe intravascular hemolysis.

Persons with group O blood are considered *universal donors* because they do not have antigens on their RBCs. People with group AB blood are considered *universal recipients* because they have no antibodies to react to the transfused blood.

Rh factor

The presence or absence of Rh antigens on the RBC's surface determines the classification of Rh positive or Rh negative. After ABO compatibility, Rh factor is the next most important antigen affecting the success of a blood transfusion. The major Rh factor is $Rh_o(D)$. There are several minor Rh factors. If $Rh_o(D)$ is absent, the minor Rh antigens are tested. If negative, the patient is considered *Rh negative (Rh−)*.

Rh− persons may develop antibodies to Rh antigens if exposed to Rh-positive (Rh+) blood by transfusions or fetal–maternal blood mixing. All women who are pregnant should have a blood typing and Rh factor determination. If the mother's blood is Rh−, the father's blood should also be typed. If his blood is Rh+, the woman's blood should be examined for the presence of Rh antibodies (by the indirect Coombs test; p. 237). Hemolytic disease of the newborn can be prevented by Rh typing during pregnancy. If the mother is Rh−, she should be advised that she is a candidate for RhoGAM (Rh immunoglobulin that "neutralizes" the Rh antigen) after the birth. RhoGAM can reduce the chance of fetal hemolytic problems during subsequent pregnancies.

Other blood typing systems

There are nine different gene codes for blood groups assayed. Most are minor and not clinically significant. However, in certain clinical circumstances, these minor blood group antigens and acquired antigens can become significant. This may occur with frequent blood transfusions or in patients with leukemia or lymphoma.

Blood crossmatching

Although typing for the major ABO and Rh antigens is no guarantee that a reaction will not occur, it does greatly reduce the possibility of such a reaction. Many potential minor antigens are not routinely detected during blood typing. If allowed to go unrecognized, these minor antigens also can initiate a blood transfusion reaction. Therefore blood is not only typed but also crossmatched to identify a mismatch of blood caused by minor antigens. Crossmatching includes an indirect Coombs test. Only blood products containing RBCs need to be crossmatched. Plasma products do not need to be crossmatched but should be ABO compatible because other cells (WBCs and platelets) have ABO antigens.

Finally, one must be aware of graft-versus-host disease (GVHD) in which donor lymphocytes included in the blood transfusion may engraft and multiply in the recipient.

Procedure and patient care
- See inside front cover for Routine Blood Testing.
- Fasting: no
- Blood tube commonly used: red. Verify with laboratory.

Abnormal findings
See Test explanation and related physiology section.

notes

blood urea nitrogen (BUN, urea nitrogen)

Type of test Blood

Normal findings

Adult: 10–20 mg/dL or 3.6–7.1 mmol/L (SI units)
Elderly: may be slightly higher than those of adult
Child: 5–18 mg/dL
Infant: 5–18 mg/dL
Newborn: 3–12 mg/dL
Cord: 21–40 mg/dL

Possible critical values

> 100 mg/dL (indicates serious impairment of renal function)

Test explanation and related physiology

The BUN measures the amount of urea nitrogen in the blood. Urea is formed in the liver as the end product of protein metabolism. BUN is directly related to the metabolic function of the liver and the excretory function of the kidney. It serves as an index of the function of these organs. Patients who have elevated BUN levels are said to have azotemia.

Nearly all renal diseases cause inadequate excretion of urea, which causes the blood concentration to rise above normal. BUN also increases in conditions other than primary renal disease. For example, when excess amounts of protein are available for hepatic catabolism (from gastrointestinal [GI] bleeding), large quantities of urea are made. BUN may be affected by hydration status.

BUN is interpreted in conjunction with the creatinine test (p. 249). These tests are referred to as *renal function studies*.

The BUN/creatinine ratio is a good measurement of kidney and liver function. The normal adult range is 6 to 25, with 15.5 being the optimal adult value for this ratio.

Interfering factors

• Changes in protein intake may affect BUN levels.
• Advanced pregnancy may cause increased BUN levels.
• Overhydration and underhydration will affect BUN levels.
• GI bleeding can cause increased BUN levels.

Procedure and patient care

• See inside front cover for Routine Blood Testing.
• Fasting: no

- Blood tube commonly used: red

Abnormal findings

▲ **Increased levels**

Prerenal causes
Alimentary tube feeding
Burns
Congestive heart failure
Dehydration
Excessive protein catabolism
Excessive protein ingestion
GI bleeding
Hypovolemia
Myocardial infarction
Sepsis
Shock
Starvation

Renal causes
Nephrotoxic drugs
Renal disease (e.g.,
   glomerulonephritis,
   pyelonephritis, acute tubular
   necrosis)
Renal failure

Postrenal azotemia
Bladder outlet obstruction
Ureteral obstruction

▼ **Decreased levels**

Liver failure
Negative nitrogen
   balance (e.g.,
   malnutrition or
   malabsorption)
Nephrotic syndrome
Overhydration caused
   by fluid overload
   or syndrome of
   inappropriate
   antidiuretic hormone
   (SIADH)
Pregnancy

notes

bone densitometry (Bone mineral content [BMC], Bone mineral density [BMD], DEXA scan)

Type of test X-ray

Normal findings

Normal: < 1 standard deviation below normal (> –1)
Osteopenia: 1 to 2.5 standard deviations below normal (–1 to –2.5)
Osteoporosis: > 2.5 standard deviations below normal (< –2.5)

Test explanation and related physiology

Bone densitometry is used to determine bone mineral content (BMC) and density (BMD) to diagnose osteoporosis as early as possible. It is also used to monitor patients who are undergoing treatment for osteoporosis. *Osteoporosis* and *low bone mass* are terms used for bones that become weakened and fracture easily. Bone densitometry can provide early and accurate measurements of bone strength based on BMD.

Several groups of bones are routinely evaluated. The lumbar spine is one of the best representatives of cancellous bone. The radius is the most frequently studied cortical bone. The proximal hip (neck of the femur) is the best representative of mixed (cancellous and cortical) bone. However, specific bone sites can be evaluated if they are particularly symptomatic.

Dual-energy x-ray absorptiometry (DEXA) is the method most commonly used. Because DEXA uses two photons, more energy is produced so that bones (spine and hip [femoral neck]) surrounded by a lot of soft tissue can be more easily penetrated.

Several other methods are available to measure BMD. *Quantitative computed tomography (QCT)* uses CT technology to measure central bones, especially the spine. *Ultrasound absorption (quantitative ultrasound)* can be used to measure peripheral bones (heel [calcaneus], patella, or midtibia).

BMD is usually reported in terms of standard deviation (SD) from mean values. T scores compare the patient's results to a group of young healthy adults. Z scores compare the patient's results to a group of age-matched controls. The World Health Organization has defined *low bone mass* as a BMD value greater than 1 SD below peak bone mass levels in young women and *osteoporosis* as a value greater than 2.5 SD below that same measurement scale. Positive T scores indicate a normal BMD. Negative T scores indicate reduced BMD. *Vertebral fracture assessment (VFA)* can be performed utilizing the images generated by the DEXA scan.

BMD testing is an important part of routine screening testing for postmenopausal women. In general, BMD is recommended every 2 years to screen for osteoporosis. Women and men with known osteoporotic fractures, hyperparathyroidism, or administration of long-term steroid therapy may benefit from annual BMD testing.

Interfering factors

- Barium may falsely increase the density of the lumbar spine. BMD measurements should not be performed for about 10 days after barium studies.
- Calcified abdominal aortic aneurysm may falsely increase BMD of the spine.
- Internal fixation devices of the hip or radius will falsely increase BMD of those bones.
- Metal jewelry or other objects may falsely increase BMD.
- Previous fractures or severe arthritis changes of the bone can falsely increase BMD.
- Metallic clips placed in the vertebrae of patients who have had previous abdominal surgery can falsely increase BMD.
- Prior bone scans, MRI, or CT scans can falsely decrease BMD because the photons generated from the bone (as a result of the previously administered bone scan radionuclide) will be detected by the scintillator detector.

Procedure and patient care

Before

- **PT** Explain the procedure to the patient. See p. xviii for radiation exposure and risks.
- **PT** Tell the patient that no fasting or sedation is required.
- **PT** Instruct the patient to remove all metallic objects (e.g., belt buckles, zippers, coins, keys) that might be in the scanning path.

During

- Note the following procedural steps:
  1. The patient lies supine on an imaging table, with his or her legs supported and placed on a padded box to flatten the pelvis and lumbar spine.
  2. Under the table, a photon generator is slowly and successively passed under the lumbar spine.
  3. A scintillator (gamma or x-ray) detector/camera is passed over the patient in a manner parallel to that of the generator. An image of the lumbar spine and hip bone is obtained by the scintillator camera and projected onto a computer monitor.

4. Next, the appropriate foot is applied to a brace that internally rotates the nondominant hip, and the procedure is repeated over the hip. A similar procedure is performed for radius evaluation.
5. When the radius is examined, the nondominant arm is preferred unless there is a history of fracture to that bone.

- Note that the data are interpreted and reported by a radiologist or a physician trained in nuclear medicine.
- Note that BMD studies take about 30 minutes to perform and are free of any discomfort. Only minimal radiation is used for this procedure.
- Note that there are numerous types of bone densitometry machines. Peripheral units that quickly scan the finger, heel, or forearm are often used to identify patients at risk for osteoporosis. Abnormal results are followed up with the more comprehensive table procedure previously described.

After

- No special care is required.

Abnormal findings

Low bone mass
Osteoporosis

notes

B

bone marrow biopsy (Bone marrow examination, Bone marrow aspiration)

Type of test Microscopic examination of tissue

Normal findings

Active erythroid cell line, myeloid and lymphoid cell lines, and megakaryocyte (platelet) production. See range of cell types below.

Cell type	Range (%)
Neutrophilic series	49.2–65
Myeloblasts	0.2–1.5
Promyelocytes	2.1–4.1
Myelocytes	8.2–15.7
Eosinophilic series	1.2–5.3
Myelocytes	0.2–1.3
Metamyelocytes	0.4–2.2
Bands	0.2–2.4
Segmented	0.0–1.3
Basophilic and mast cells	0.0–0.2
Erythrocyte series	18.4–33.8
Pronormoblasts	0.2–1.3
Basophilic	0.5–2.4
Polychromatophilic	17.9–29.2
Orthochromatic	0.4–4.6
Monocytes	0.0–0.8
Lymphocytes	11.1–23.2
Plasma cells	0.4–3.9
Megakaryocytes	0.0–0.4
Reticulum cells	0.0–0.9
Myeloid to erythrocyte (M/E) ratio	2:1–4:1

Normal iron content is demonstrated by staining with Prussian blue.

Test explanation and related physiology

Bone marrow examination is an important part of the evaluation of patients with hematologic diseases. Indications for bone marrow examination include the following:

- To evaluate anemias, leukopenia, or thrombocytopenia
- To diagnose leukemia, myelodysplastic syndromes, myeloproliferative neoplasms, and plasma cell dyscrasia

- To document abnormal iron stores
- To document bone marrow infiltrative diseases (e.g., neoplasm, infection, or fibrosis)
- To stage lymphomas or other cancers

The bone marrow is located in the central fatty core of cancellous bone (particularly sternum, rib, and pelvis). There, the blood-forming cells produce blood cells and release them into the circulation.

Examination of bone marrow reveals the number, size, and shape of the RBCs, WBCs, and megakaryocytes (platelet precursors) as these cells evolve through their various stages of development in the bone marrow. Samples of bone marrow can be obtained by aspiration, bone marrow biopsy, or surgical removal. Microscopic examination of the marrow biopsy includes determination of the presence of infiltrative diseases (fibrosis or neoplasms, both primary and metastatic). Estimation of iron storage is performed.

For the estimation of cellularity, the specimen is examined and the relative quantity of each cell type is determined. Leukemias or leukemoid drug reactions are suspected when increased numbers of leukocyte precursors are present. Physiologic marrow leukemoid compensation is also seen with infection. Decreased numbers of marrow leukocyte precursors occur in patients with myelofibrosis, metastatic neoplasia, or agranulocytosis/aplastic anemia; in elderly patients; and after radiation therapy or chemotherapy. Some drugs or infections can diminish leukocyte production.

Increased numbers of marrow RBC precursors occur with polycythemia vera or as physiologic compensation to blood loss (hemorrhage or hemolysis). Decreased numbers of marrow RBC precursors occur with erythroid hypoplasia after chemotherapy, infection (parvovirus), aplastic anemia, radiation therapy, administration of other toxic drugs, iron administration, or marrow replacement by fibrotic tissue or neoplasms.

Increased numbers of platelet precursors (megakaryocytes) can be the result of compensation to platelet loss from a recent hemorrhage. They are also seen in some forms of acute and chronic myeloid leukemias. This increase also may be compensatory in patients with platelet sequestration (secondary hypersplenism associated with portal hypertension) or platelet destruction (idiopathic thrombocytopenic purpura). Platelet counts decrease, and the marrow compensates by increasing production. Decreased numbers of megakaryocytes occur in patients who have had radiation therapy, chemotherapy, or other drug therapy and in patients with neoplastic or fibrotic marrow infiltrative diseases. Patients with aplastic anemia also have decreased numbers of megakaryocytes.

B

Increased numbers of lymphocyte precursors occur in chronic, viral, or mycoplasmal infections (e.g., mononucleosis), lymphocytic leukemia, and lymphoma. Plasma cells and lymphocytes are increased in patients with plasma cell dyscrasia, lymphomas, hypersensitivity states, autoimmune disease, chronic infections, and other chronic inflammatory diseases.

Estimation of cellularity also can be expressed as a ratio of myeloid precursors to erythroid precursors (M/E ratio). The normal M/E ratio is approximately 3:1.

Contraindications

- Patients with acute coagulation disorders, because of the risk of excessive bleeding
- Patients who cannot remain still during the procedure

Potential complications

- Hemorrhage, especially if the patient has a coagulopathy
- Infection, especially if the patient is leukopenic

Procedure and patient care

Before

PT Explain the procedure to the patient.
- Obtain a written informed consent for this procedure.
- Encourage the patient to verbalize fears because many patients are anxious concerning this study. Conscious sedation may be required.
- Assess the results of the coagulation studies. Report any evidence of coagulopathy to the physician. Platelets should be greater than 20,000, and international normalized ratio (INR) should be less than 1.5.

PT Instruct the patient to remain very still throughout the procedure.

During

PT Inform the patient that during bone marrow aspiration, most patients feel pain or a burning sensation during lidocaine infiltration and pressure when the syringe plunger is withdrawn for aspiration.
- Note the following procedural steps for *bone marrow aspiration:*
  1. The skin prepping is usually begun as described in step 1 below for bone marrow biopsy.

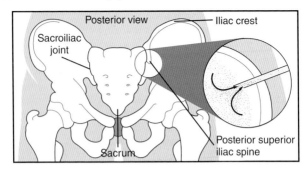

FIG. B3 Bone marrow aspiration. Samples of the bone marrow are taken from along the posterior superior iliac spine.

2. For aspiration, an Illinois- or Jamshidi-type large-bore needle is used.
3. When inside the marrow, a syringe is used to aspirate marrow contents (Figure B3).
4. Several small-volume (0.5–2 mL) samples of bone marrow are aspirated.
5. The aspirate is placed in an appropriate blood specimen collecting test tube depending on the test requested.

• Note the following procedural steps for *bone marrow biopsy:*
1. The skin and soft tissues overlying the posterior superior spine of the iliac bone are prepped and draped. A small skin incision is made in that area after local anesthesia is provided.
2. A Jamshidi needle (or other specialized needle) is positioned into the bone.
3. The aspiration specimen is obtained first. With repositioning of the needle (to avoid aspiration artifact), the biopsy specimen is obtained and placed in a formalin fixative. It is then sent to the pathology laboratory for analysis.
4. Bilateral bone marrow biopsies may be performed for staging of lymphoma or other neoplasms.

After
• Apply pressure to the puncture site to arrest any bleeding.
• Apply an adhesive bandage.
• Observe the puncture site for bleeding. Ice packs may be used to minimize bleeding.
• Assess for tenderness and erythema, which may indicate infection. Report this to the physician.

- Normally, place the patient in the supine position at bed rest for 30 to 60 minutes after the test. This provides pressure on the biopsy site.
- Note that some patients complain of tenderness at the puncture site for several days after this study. Mild analgesics may be ordered.

Abnormal findings

Acquired immunodeficiency syndrome (AIDS)
Agranulocytosis
Anemia
Bone marrow aplasia
Chronic inflammatory disease
Hodgkin lymphoma
Infection (e.g., viral, bacterial, fungal)
Lymphoblastic leukemia
Metastatic neoplasm
Myelodysplastic syndromes
Myeloid leukemia
Myeloproliferative neoplasms
Non-Hodgkin lymphoma
Plasma cell dyscrasia
Red cell aplasia

notes

bone scan

Type of test   Nuclear scan

Normal findings

No evidence of abnormality

Test explanation and related physiology

The bone scan permits examination of the skeleton after IV injection of a radionuclide material. The major reason a bone scan is performed is to detect metastatic cancer to the bone. Bone scans are also useful in staging primary bone tumors. Bone scans may be serially repeated to monitor tumor response to antineoplastic therapy.

Bone scans also provide valuable information in the evaluation of patients with trauma or unexplained pain. Bone scanning is more sensitive than routine x-ray images in detecting small and difficult-to-find fractures.

Although the bone scan is extremely sensitive, unfortunately it is not very specific. Fractures, infections, tumors, and arthritic changes all appear similar in this scan.

Contraindications

- Patients who are pregnant, unless the benefits outweigh the risk of fetal damage
- Patients who are lactating

Interfering factors

- Recent x-rays using barium can interfere with test results.

Procedure and patient care

Before

PT   Explain the procedure to the patient. See p. xviii for discussion of radiation exposure and risks.

PT   Tell the patient that no fasting or sedation is required.

PT   Inform the patient that the injection of the radionuclide may cause slight discomfort, nausea, or vomiting.

During

- The patient receives an IV injection of radionuclide and images of the bones are obtained.
- The patient may be repositioned in the prone and lateral positions during the test.

- Note that this scan is performed by a nuclear medicine technician in 30 to 60 minutes. It is interpreted by a physician trained in nuclear medicine imaging.

PT Inform patients that lying on the hard scanning table can be uncomfortable.

After

- Because only tracer doses of radionuclide are used, no radiation precautions need to be taken.
PT Assure the patient that the radioactive substance is usually excreted from the body within 6 to 24 hours.
PT Encourage the patient to drink fluids to aid in the excretion of the radioactive substance.

Abnormal findings

Arthritis
Bone necrosis
Fracture
Osteomyelitis
Paget disease of bone
Primary or metastatic tumor of the bone
Renal osteodystrophy

notes

bone turnover markers (BTMs, N-telopeptide [NTx], N-terminal propeptide of type 1 collagen [P1NP], Bone collagen equivalents [BCEs], Osteocalcin [bone G1 a protein, BGP, osteocalc], Pyridinium [PYD] crosslinks, Bone-specific alkaline phosphatase [BSAP], C-telopeptide [CTx])

Type of test Blood; urine

Normal findings

Results vary greatly with age.

N-telopeptide

Urine (nm BCE*/mm creatinine)
   Male: 21–83
   Female, premenopausal: 17–94
   Female, postmenopausal: 26–124
Serum (nm BCE*)
   Male: 5.4–24.2
   Female: 6.2–19
(*BCE = bone collagen equivalents)

C-telopeptide

Urine (ng/mL)
   Adults: 1.03 ± 0.41
   Children: 8 ± 3.37
Serum (pg/mL)
   Male: 60–700
   Female, premenopausal: 40–465
   Female, postmenopausal: 104–1008

N-terminal propeptide of type I procollagen, serum (mcg/L)
   Male: 22–87
   Female, premenopausal: 19–83
   Female, postmenopausal: 16–96

Osteocalcin, serum (ng/mL)
Adult (> 22 years)
   Male: 5.8–14
   Female: 3.1–14.4

Pyridium, urine (nm/mm)
   Male: 10.3–33.6
   Female: 15.3–33.6

Bone-specific alkaline phosphatase, serum (mcg/L)
    Male: 6.5–20.1
    Female, premenopausal: 4.5–16.9
    Female, postmenopausal: 7–22.4

Test explanation and related physiology

While bone mineral density scan is the most effective method to screen women to determine bone fracture risk, improved results associated with treatments for osteoporosis are slow to identify with scans.   Bone turnover markers (BTMs), on the other hand, provide more rapid measurements of improved bone density and, therefore, are used to monitor the effectiveness and compliance of treatment. BTMs may be helpful in secondary diseases such as hyperparathyroidism, hyperthyroidism, vitamin D deficiency, and certain blood cancers.

Most BTMs display marked diurnal variation, peaking between midnight and 8 am and reaching a trough in the early afternoon. Specimens for BTMs should be obtained in the morning. BTMs are generally high in growing children, reflecting active skeletal growth and modeling. BTMs are not recommended for fracture risk assessment.

N- and C-telopeptides (NTx and CTx) are good indicators of bone resorption.

N-terminal propeptide of type 1 collagen (P1NP), like NTx, is directly proportional to the amount of new bone formation by increased osteoblastic activity.

Osteocalcin, or *bone G1a protein (BGP),* enters the circulation during bone resorption and bone formation; it is a good indicator of bone metabolism. Increased levels are associated with bone mineral density loss.

Pyridinium (PYD) is a urinary test indicating bone resorption.

Bone-specific alkaline phosphatase (BSAP) is an isoenzyme of alkaline phosphatase (p. 23) and is an indicator of the metabolic status of osteoblasts and bone formation.

Interfering factors

- Because most BTMs are excreted by the kidneys, renal disease may be associated with high levels and not an indication of bone metabolism.
- Bodybuilding treatments, such as testosterone, can cause reduced levels of NTx.

Procedure and patient care

Blood

- See inside front cover for Routine Blood Testing.
- Fasting: yes
- Blood tube commonly used: verify with laboratory
- Collect a venous blood sample in a red-top tube for NTx and/or a lavender- or green-top tube for osteocalcin. Check with the laboratory for guidelines with other markers.
- It is important to obtain baseline levels before instituting therapy.

Urine

- See inside front cover for Routine Urine Testing.
- Preferably, obtain a double-voided specimen.
- Collect the first urine specimen 30 to 40 minutes before the time the specimen is needed.
- Discard this first specimen.
- Give the patient a glass of water to drink.
- At the requested time, obtain a second specimen.

Abnormal findings

▲ **Increased levels**
Acromegaly
Advanced bone tumors
   (primary or metastatic)
Hyperparathyroidism
Hyperthyroidism
Osteoporosis
Paget disease of bone

▼ **Decreased levels**
Cortisol therapy
Effective antiresorptive
   therapy
Hypoparathyroidism
Hypothyroidism

notes

bone x-ray

Type of test X-ray

Normal findings

No evidence of fracture, tumor, infection, or congenital abnormalities

Test explanation and related physiology

Radiographic images of the long bones are usually taken when the patient has complaints about a particular body area. Fractures or tumors are readily detectable by x-ray studies. In patients who have a severe or chronic infection overlying a bone (osteomyelitis), an x-ray may detect the infection involving that bone. X-ray studies of the long bones also can detect joint destruction and bone spurring as a result of persistent arthritis. Growth patterns can be followed by serial x-rays of a long bone, usually the wrists and hands. Healing of a fracture can be documented and followed. X-rays of the joints reveal the presence of joint effusions and soft tissue swelling as well. Calcifications in the soft tissue indicate chronic inflammatory changes of the nearby bursa or tendons. Soft tissue swelling also can be seen on these bone x-rays. Because the cartilage and tendons are not directly visualized, cartilage fractures, sprains, or ligamentous injuries cannot be seen.

At least two x-rays at 90-degree angles are required so that the bone region being studied can be visualized from two different angles (usually anterior to posterior and lateral). Some bone studies (e.g., skull, spine, hip) require oblique views to visualize all the parts that need to be seen.

Interfering factors

- Jewelry or clothing can obstruct radiographic visualization of part of the bone to be evaluated.
- Prior barium studies can diminish the full radiographic visualization of some of the bones surrounding the abdomen (e.g., spine and pelvis).

Procedure and patient care

Before

PT Explain the procedure to the patient. See p. xviii for radiation exposure and risks.
- Handle carefully any injured parts of the patient's body.

PT Instruct the patient that he or she will need to keep the extremity still while the x-ray image is being taken. This can sometimes be difficult, especially when the patient has severe pain associated with a recent injury.

PT Tell the patient that no fasting or sedation is required.

During

- Note that, in the x-ray department, the patient is asked to place the involved extremity in several positions. An x-ray image is taken of each position.
- Note that this test is routinely performed by a radiologic technologist within several minutes.

PT Tell the patient that no discomfort is associated with this test, except possibly from moving an injured extremity.

After

- Administer an analgesic for relief of pain if indicated.

Abnormal findings

Abnormal growth pattern

Bone spurring

Congenital bone disorders (e.g., achondroplasia, dysplasia, dysostosis)

Foreign bodies

Fractures

Infection or osteomyelitis

Joint destruction (arthritis)

Joint effusion

Osteoporosis or osteopenia

Tumors (osteogenic sarcoma, Paget disease, myeloma, or metastatic)

notes

B

brain scan (Cisternogram, Cerebral blood flow)

Type of test Nuclear scan

Normal findings

No areas of altered radionuclide uptake within the brain

Test explanation and related physiology

The usefulness of a nuclear brain scan is narrow compared with computed tomography (CT), magnetic resonance imaging (MRI), and positron emission tomography (PET) scans of the brain. Primarily, a nuclear brain scan is used to indicate complete and irreversible cessation of brain function (brain death).

Procedure and patient care

Before

PT Explain the procedure to the patient. See p. xviii for radiation exposure and risks.

During

- Note the following procedural steps:
    1. After administration of the radioisotope, the patient is placed in the supine position for planar and single-photon emission computed tomography (SPECT) images.
    2. When cerebral flow studies are performed, the counter is immediately placed over the head.
    3. The counts are recorded in timed sequence to follow the isotope during its first flow through the brain.
- Note that this study is performed by a technologist in nuclear medicine in approximately 45 minutes.

After

PT Inform the patient that no precautions are needed to prevent radioactive exposure to others.

Abnormal findings

Cerebral death

Cerebral neoplasm

Cerebral vascular stenosis/occlusion

CSF leakage

Hydrocephalus

notes

brain trauma indicator (BTI, Concussion biomarkers, Ubiquitin carboxy-terminal hydrolase L1 [UCH-L1], Glial fibrillary acidic protein [GFAP])

Type of test   Blood

Normal findings

UCH-L1 $\leq$ 327 pg/mL
GFAP $\leq$ 22 pg/mL

Test explanation and related physiology

Traumatic brain injury (TBI) caused by external physical force disrupts normal brain function and can result in temporary or permanent coma. When TBI is suspected, a neurological assessment using the 15-point Glasgow Coma Scale, a thorough neurological examination, and commonly a computed tomography (CT) scan of the head are done. Because 90% of patients with mild TBI have a negative CT scan, use of a blood test for determining the possibility of serious TBI is helpful.

BTIs are a measurement of serum levels of ubiquitin C-terminal hydrolase-L1 (UCH-L1) and glial fibrillary acidic protein (GFAP). These proteins are released from the brain into the bloodstream and can be measured within 12 hours of TBI.

Concussion biomarkers generally have excellent diagnostic sensitivity but poor specificity compared to CT, the accepted gold standard reference test. Nearly all patients with TBI noted on CT scan of the head will have an elevated level of either protein. Less than 1% of patients with normal levels of both proteins will have a positive CT scan of the head.

Interfering factors

- Levels of proteins vary with age. The test is considered accurate only for individuals who are over 18 years of age.

Procedure and patient care

- See inside front cover for Routine Blood Testing.
- Fasting: No
- Blood tube commonly used: Gold

Abnormal findings

Brain trauma injury

notes

bronchoscopy

Type of test   Endoscopy

Normal findings

Normal larynx, trachea, bronchi, and alveoli

Test explanation and related physiology

Bronchoscopy permits endoscopic visualization of the larynx, trachea, and bronchi by either a flexible fiberoptic bronchoscope or a rigid bronchoscope. There are many diagnostic and therapeutic uses for bronchoscopy.

Diagnostic uses of bronchoscopy include:

- Direct visualization of the tracheobronchial tree for abnormalities (e.g., tumors, inflammation, strictures)
- Biopsy of tissue from observed lesions
- Aspiration of deep sputum for culture, sensitivity, and cytology determinations
- Direct visualization of the larynx for identification of vocal cord paralysis if present

Therapeutic uses of bronchoscopy (Interventional bronchoscopy) include:

- Aspiration of retained secretions
- Control of bleeding within the bronchus
- Removal of foreign bodies that have been aspirated
- Brachytherapy, which is endobronchial radiation therapy using an iridium wire placed via the bronchoscope
- Palliative laser obliteration of bronchial neoplastic obstruction
- Access for ultrasound
- Placement of stents to open the airway

Transbronchial needle aspiration can be directed by the use of *endobronchial ultrasound*. This technique is particularly helpful in staging lung cancers and identifying sarcoidosis, lymphomas, and infections.

Laryngoscopy is often performed through a short bronchoscope to allow inspection of the larynx and paralaryngeal structures. Cancers, polyps, inflammation, and infections of these structures can be identified. The vocal cord motion can be evaluated also. Anesthesiologists use laryngoscopy to visualize the vocal cord structures on patients who are difficult to intubate for general anesthesia.

Contraindications

- Patients with hypercapnia and severe shortness of breath who cannot tolerate interruption of high-flow oxygen
- Tracheal stenosis may make it difficult to pass the scope.

Potential complications

- Aspiration
- Bronchospasm
- Fever
- Hemorrhage (after biopsy)
- Hypoxemia
- Laryngospasm
- Pneumothorax

Procedure and patient care

Before

PT Explain the procedure to the patient. Allay any fears and allow the patient to verbalize any concerns.
- Obtain informed consent for this procedure.
- Keep the patient NPO for 4 to 8 hours before the test to reduce the risk of aspiration.
PT Instruct the patient to perform good mouth care to minimize the risk of introducing bacteria into the lungs.
- Remove and safely store the patient's dentures, glasses, or contacts before administering the preprocedure medications.
- Administer the preprocedure medications as ordered.
PT Reassure the patient that he or she will be able to breathe during this procedure.
PT Instruct the patient not to swallow the local anesthetic sprayed into the throat. Provide a basin for expectoration.

During

- Note the following procedural steps for *fiberoptic bronchoscopy:*
  1. This test is performed by a pulmonary specialist or a surgeon at the bedside or in an appropriately equipped room.
  2. The patient's nasopharynx and oropharynx are anesthetized topically with lidocaine spray before insertion of the bronchoscope.
  3. The patient is placed in a sitting or supine position, and the tube is inserted through the nose or mouth and into the pharynx (Figure B4).
  4. After the tube is passed into the larynx and through the glottis, more lidocaine is sprayed into the trachea to prevent the cough reflex.

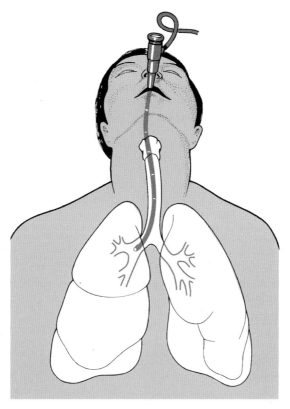

FIG. B4 Bronchoscopy. A bronchoscope is inserted through the trachea and into the bronchus.

    5. The tube is passed farther, well into the trachea, bronchi, and first- and second-generation bronchioles, for systematic examination of the bronchial tree.
    6. Biopsy specimens and washings are taken if pathology is suspected.
- Note that this procedure is performed by a physician in approximately 30 to 45 minutes.
- PT Tell the patient that because of sedation, no discomfort is usually felt.

After

PT   Instruct the patient not to eat or drink anything until the tracheobronchial anesthesia has worn off and the gag reflex has returned, usually in approximately 2 hours.

- Observe the patient's sputum for hemorrhage if biopsy specimens were removed. A small amount of blood streaking may be expected and is normal for several hours after the procedure. Large amounts of bleeding can cause a chemical pneumonitis.

- Observe the patient closely for evidence of impaired respiration or laryngospasm. The vocal cords may go into spasms after intubation.

PT   Inform the patient that postbronchoscopy fever often develops within the first 24 hours. High, persistent fever should be reported immediately.

- If a tumor is suspected, collect a postbronchoscopy sputum sample for a cytology determination.

PT   Inform the patient that warm saline gargles and lozenges may be helpful if a sore throat develops.

PT   Inform the patient that biopsy or culture reports will be available in 2 to 7 days.

Abnormal findings

Abscess
Cancer
Foreign body
Hemorrhage
Infection
Inflammation
Strictures
Tuberculosis

notes

calcitonin (Human calcitonin [HCT], Thyrocalcitonin)

Type of test Blood

Normal findings

Basal (plasma)

Males: ≤ 19 pg/mL or ≤ 19 ng/L (SI units)

Females: ≤ 14 pg/mL or ≤ 14 ng/L (SI units)

Calcium infusion (2.4 mg/kg)

Males: ≤ 190 pg/mL or ≤ 190 ng/L

Females: ≤ 130 pg/mL or ≤ 130 ng/L

Pentagastrin injection (0.5 mcg/kg)

Males: ≤ 110 pg/mL or ≤ 110 ng/L

Females: ≤ 30 pg/mL or ≤ 30 ng/L

Procalcitonin < 2 ng/mL

Test explanation and related physiology

Calcitonin is a hormone secreted by the parafollicular or C-cells of the thyroid gland. Its secretion is stimulated by elevated serum calcium levels. The purpose of calcitonin is to contribute to calcium homeostasis.

This test is usually used in the evaluation of patients with or suspected medullary carcinoma of the thyroid (p. 165). C-cell hyperplasia, a benign calcitonin-producing disease, is also associated with elevated calcitonin levels.

Equivocal elevations in calcitonin levels should be followed with further provocative testing using pentagastrin or calcium to stimulate calcitonin secretion. *Pentagastrin stimulation* involves an intravenous (IV) infusion with blood samples drawn before the injection and at 90 seconds, 2 minutes, and 5 minutes after the infusion. The *calcium infusion test* can be performed in a variety of ways but is most commonly administered with baseline and 5- and 10-minute postinfusion blood levels.

Elevated levels of calcitonin also may be seen in people with cancer of the lung, breast, or pancreas. This is probably a form of paraneoplastic syndrome in which there is an ectopic production of calcitonin by the nonthyroid cancer cells.

Interfering factors

- Levels are often elevated in pregnancy and in newborns.

Procedure and patient care

- See inside front cover for Routine Blood Testing.
- Fasting: yes

- Blood tube commonly used: green or red
- Collect a venous sample of blood in a heparinized green-top tube or a chilled red-top tube according to the laboratory's protocol.
- The specimen should be placed on ice immediately. The blood may be frozen and sent to a reference laboratory.

PT Tell the patient that results may not be available for several days.

Abnormal findings

▲ **Increased levels**

Alcoholic cirrhosis
Breast carcinoma
C-cell hyperplasia
Medullary carcinoma of the thyroid
Oat cell carcinoma of the lung
Pancreatic cancer
Pernicious anemia
Primary hyperparathyroidism
Secondary hyperparathyroidism because of chronic renal failure
Thyroiditis
Zollinger–Ellison syndrome

notes

calcium (Total/ionized calcium, Ca, Serum calcium)

Type of test Blood; urine

Normal findings

Age	mg/dL	mmol/L
Total calcium		
Adult*	9–10.5	2.25–2.62
Child	8.8–10.8	2.2–2.7
10 days-2 years	9–10.6	2.3–2.65
Umbilical	9–11.5	2.25–2.88
< 10 days	7.6–10.4	1.9–2.6
Ionized calcium		
Adult	4.5–5.6	1.05–1.3
2 months-18 years	4.8–5.52	1.2–1.38
Newborn	4.2–5.58	1.05–1.37

* In elderly individuals, values tend to decrease.

Possible critical values

Total calcium: < 6 or > 13 mg/dL
Ionized calcium: < 2.2 or > 7 mg/dL

Test explanation and related physiology

The serum calcium test is used to evaluate parathyroid function and calcium metabolism by directly measuring the total amount of calcium in the blood. Determination of serum calcium is used to monitor patients with renal failure, renal transplantation, hyperparathyroidism, and various malignancies. It is also used to monitor calcium levels during and after large-volume blood transfusions.

About half the total calcium in the blood exists in its free (ionized) form, and about half exists in its protein-bound form (mostly with albumin). The serum calcium level is a measure of both. As a result, when the serum albumin level is low (as in malnourished patients), the serum calcium level will also be low. As a rule of thumb, the total serum calcium level decreases by approximately 0.8 mg for every 1-g decrease in the serum albumin level. Serum albumin should be measured with serum calcium.

When the serum calcium level is elevated on at least three separate determinations, the patient is said to have *hypercalcemia*.

The most common cause of hypercalcemia is hyperparathyroidism. Malignancy, the second most common cause of hypercalcemia, can cause elevated calcium levels in two main ways. First, tumor metastasis (myeloma, lung, breast, renal cell) to the bone can destroy the bone, causing resorption and pushing calcium into the blood. Second, the cancer (lung, breast, renal cell) can produce a PTH-like substance that drives the serum calcium up (ectopic PTH). Excess vitamin D ingestion can increase serum calcium by increasing renal and GI absorption. Granulomatous infections, such as sarcoidosis and tuberculosis, are associated with hypercalcemia.

Hypocalcemia occurs in patients with hypoalbuminemia. Large blood transfusions are associated with low serum calcium levels because the citrate additives used in banked blood for anticoagulation bind the free calcium in the recipient's bloodstream. Intestinal malabsorption, renal failure, rhabdomyolysis, alkalosis, and acute pancreatitis (caused by saponification of fat) are also known to be associated with low serum calcium levels.

Urinary calcium can also be measured. Excretion of calcium in the urine is increased in all patients with hypercalcemia. Urinary calcium levels are decreased in patients with hypocalcemia. The test is helpful in determining the cause of recurrent nephrolithiasis.

Interfering factors

- Vitamin D intoxication may cause increased calcium levels.
- Excessive ingestion of milk may cause increased levels.
- Serum pH can affect calcium values. A decrease in pH causes increased calcium levels.
- Prolonged tourniquet time will lower pH and falsely increase calcium levels.
- There is normally a small diurnal variation in calcium, with peak levels occurring around 9 PM.
- Hypoalbuminemia is artifactually associated with decreased levels of total calcium.

Procedure and patient care

- See inside front cover for Routine Blood Testing.
- Fasting: verify with laboratory
- Blood tube commonly used: red

Abnormal findings

▲ **Increased levels
(hypercalcemia)**

Acromegaly
Addison disease
Granulomatous infections
   (e.g., sarcoidosis and
   tuberculosis)
Hyperparathyroidism
Hyperthyroidism
Lymphoma
Metastatic bone tumor
Milk-alkali syndrome
Nonparathyroid PTH-
   producing tumor (e.g.,
   lung or renal carcinoma)
Paget disease of bone
Prolonged immobilization
Vitamin D intoxication

▼ **Decreased levels
(hypocalcemia)**

Alkalosis
Fat embolism
Hypoalbuminemia
Hyperphosphatemia
   secondary to renal failure
Hypoparathyroidism
Malabsorption
Osteomalacia
Pancreatitis
Renal failure
Rickets
Vitamin D deficiency

notes

caloric study (Oculovestibular reflex study, Caloric stimulation)

Type of test Electrodiagnostic

Normal findings

Nystagmus with irrigation

Test explanation and related physiology

Caloric studies are used to evaluate the vestibular portion of the eighth cranial nerve (acoustic nerve) by irrigating the external auditory canal with hot or cold water. This is considered a part of a complete neurologic examination. Normally stimulation with cold water causes rotary nystagmus (involuntary rapid eye movement) away from the ear being irrigated; hot water induces nystagmus toward the side of the ear being irrigated. If the labyrinth is diseased or CN VIII is not functioning (e.g., from tumor compression), no nystagmus is induced. This study aids in the differential diagnosis of abnormalities that may occur in the vestibular system, brainstem, or cerebellum.

Contraindications

- Patients with a perforated eardrum
- Cold air may be substituted for the fluid, although this method is much less reliable.
- Patients with an acute disease of the labyrinth (e.g., Ménière syndrome)

Procedure and patient care

Before

PT Explain the procedure to the patient.

PT Instruct the patient to avoid solid foods before the test to reduce the incidence of vomiting.

During

- Although the exact procedures for caloric studies vary, note the following steps in a typical test:
    1. Before the test, the patient is examined for the presence of nystagmus, postural deviation (Romberg sign), and past-pointing. This examination provides the baseline values for comparison during the test.
    2. The ear canal should be examined and cleaned before testing to ensure that the water will freely flow to the middle ear area.

3. If using electro-oculography (EOG) or video-oculography (VOG), electrodes or goggles are placed around the eyes to measure eye movement during the test.

4. The ear on the suspected side is irrigated first because the patient's response may be minimal.

5. After an emesis basin is placed under the ear, the irrigation solution is directed into the external auditory canal until the patient complains of nausea and dizziness or nystagmus is seen. Usually this occurs in 20 to 30 seconds.

6. If after 3 minutes no symptoms occur, the irrigation is stopped.

7. The patient is tested again for nystagmus, past-pointing, and Romberg sign.

8. After approximately 5 minutes, the procedure is repeated on the other side.

• Note that this procedure is usually performed by a physician or technician in approximately 15 minutes.

PT Tell the patient that he or she will probably experience nausea and dizziness during the test.

After

• Usually place the patient on bed rest for approximately 30 to 60 minutes until nausea or vomiting subsides.

• Ensure patient safety related to dizziness.

Abnormal findings

Acoustic neuroma
Brainstem inflammation, infarction, or tumor
Cerebellar inflammation, infarction, or tumor
CN VIII neuritis or neuropathy
Vestibular or cochlear inflammation or tumor

notes

cancer tumor markers (Tumor markers [TMs], Tumor-associated markers)

Type of test Blood

Normal findings

Normal values vary per laboratory

Test explanation and related physiology

Tumor markers are produced by cancer cells or by other cells of the body in response to cancer. Most TMs are made by normal cells as well as by cancer cells; however, they are overproduced by cancers. These substances can be found in the blood, urine, stool, tumor tissue, or other tissues or bodily fluids. Most TMs are proteins. However, changes in tumor cell RNA and DNA are also used as TMs. Many different TMs have been characterized. Some are associated with only one type of cancer, but others are associated with two or more cancer types.

Tumor markers are generally not used for cancer screening because they are not sensitive or specific enough. Neither are they used to diagnose cancers. Prostate-specific antigen(PSA), CA-125, and a few other TMs are being used very carefully in screening, but, alone, the cost-effectiveness is questionable.

Tumor marker levels may be measured before treatment to help doctors plan the appropriate therapy. In some types of cancer, the level of a tumor marker reflects the stage of the disease and/or the patient's prognosis. Pretreatment TM scan be used to establish a baseline level against which posttreatment TMs can be compared in order to determine the effectiveness of therapy. A decrease in the level of a TM or a return to the TM's normal level may indicate that the cancer is responding to treatment, but no change or an increase may indicate no response.

Tumor markers may also be measured during cancer follow-up evaluations to check for recurrent disease. Table C1 lists the most commonly used markers.

Procedure and patient care

- See inside front cover for Routine Blood Testing.
- Fasting: no
- Blood tube commonly used: varies by test and laboratory
- Test results may not be available for 7 to 10 days.

TABLE C1 Tumor markers and their associated cancers

Tumor marker	Associated cancer
Anaplastic lymphoma kinase (ALK gene)	Non–small cell lung cancer Lymphoma
Alpha-fetoprotein (AFP)	Liver Germ cell tumors
BCR-ABL fusion gene (Philadelphia chromosome)	Chronic myeloid leukemia Acute lymphoblastic leukemia Acute myelogenous leukemia
Beta 2 microglobulin	Liver Germ cell tumors
BRAF V600 mutations	Cutaneous melanoma Colorectal
C-kit/CD117	Gastrointestinal stromal tumor Melanoma
CA15-3/CA27.29	Breast
CA19-9	Pancreas Biliary Stomach
CA-125	Ovary
Calcitonin	Medullary thyroid carcinoma
Carcinoembryonic antigen (CEA)	Colon Other gastrointestinal tumors Breast
CD20	Non-Hodgkin lymphoma
Chromogranin A	Neuroendocrine
Chromosomes 3, 17, and 9p21	Bladder
Cyclin D1 (CD1)	HPV associated tumors
Cytokeratin fragment 21-1	Lung
Des-gamma-carboxy prothrombin	Liver
Fibrin/fibrinogen	Bladder
Human epididymis protein 4 (HE4)	Ovary, testicle, uterus, liver
Human chorionic gonadotropin (HCG)	Choriocarcinoma, Uterine cancer Germ cell tumors
Immunoglobulins	Multiple myeloma Waldenström macroglobulinemia

Continued

TABLE C1 Tumor markers and their associated cancers—cont'd

Tumor marker	Associated cancer
Inhibin A	Germ cell tumors of ovary
Ki-67	Most epithelial cancers and lymphomas
KRAS	Colorectal
	Non-small cell lung cancer
Lactate dehydrogenase (LDH)	Germ cell tumors
	Leukemia
	Melanoma
	Brain
Minichromosome maintenance protein (MCM2)	HPV associated tumors
Neuron-specific enolase (NSE)	Small cell lung cancer
	Neuroblastoma
Nuclear matrix protein 22	Bladder
Plasminogen activator inhibitor (PAI-1)	Breast
Programmed death ligand 1 (PD-L1)	Non-small cell lung cancer
Prostate-specific antigen (PSA)	Prostate
Retinoblastoma protein (pRb)	HPV associated tumors
Squamous cell carcinoma (SCC) antigen	Squamous cell carcinoma of the cervix, oral cavity, esophagus, lung, anal canal, and skin
Thyroglobulin	Thyroid
Urokinase plasminogen activator (uPA)	Breast

Abnormal findings

▲ **Increased levels**
 Benign disease
 Cancer (primary and metastatic)

notes

carbon dioxide content (CO₂ content, CO₂ combining power)

C

Type of test   Blood

Normal findings

Adult/elderly: 23–30 mEq/L or 23–30 mmol/L (SI units)
Child: 20–28 mEq/L
Infant: 20–28 mEq/L
Newborn: 13–22 mEq/L

Possible critical values

< 6 mEq/L

Test explanation and related physiology

The CO_2 content is a measure of CO_2 in the blood. In the peripheral venous blood, this assists in evaluation of the pH status of the patient and in evaluation of electrolytes. The serum CO_2 test is usually included with other assessments of electrolytes. It is usually done with a multiphasic testing machine that also measures sodium, potassium, chloride, blood urea nitrogen (BUN), and creatinine.

It is important not to get this test confused with P_{CO_2}. This CO_2 content measures the H_2CO_3, the dissolved CO_2, and the bicarbonate ion (HCO_3) that exists in the serum. Because the amounts of H_2CO_3 and dissolved CO_2 in the blood are so small, CO_2 content is an indirect measure of the HCO_3 anion. The HCO_3 anion is second in importance to the chloride ion in electrical neutrality (negative charge) of extracellular and intracellular fluid; its major role is in acid–base balance.

Levels of HCO_3 are regulated by the kidneys. Increases cause alkalosis, and decreases cause acidosis. See further discussion of this test as it is performed on arterial blood (p. 89). When CO_2 content is measured in the laboratory with other serum electrolytes, air affects the specimen, and the CO_2 partial pressure can be altered. Therefore venous blood specimens are not very accurate for true CO_2 content or HCO_3 determination. This test is used mostly as a rough guide to the patient's acid–base balance.

Interfering factors

- Underfilling the tube with blood allows CO_2 to escape from the serum specimen and may significantly decrease HCO_3 values.

Procedure and patient care

- See inside front cover for Routine Blood Testing.
- Fasting: no
- Blood tube commonly used: red or green

Abnormal findings

▲ **Increased levels**

Aldosteronism
Emphysema
Gastric suction
Metabolic alkalosis
Severe diarrhea
Severe vomiting
Starvation

▼ **Decreased levels**

Diabetic ketoacidosis
Metabolic acidosis
Renal failure
Salicylate toxicity
Shock
Starvation

notes

carboxyhemoglobin (COHb, Carbon monoxide)

Type of test Blood

Normal findings

Saturation of hemoglobin
  Nonsmoker: < 3%
  Smoker: ≤ 12%
  Newborn: ≥ 12%

Possible critical values

> 20%

Test explanation and related physiology

This test is used to detect carbon monoxide poisoning. It measures the amount of serum COHb, which is formed by the combination of carbon monoxide (CO) and hemoglobin (Hb). CO combines with Hb 200 times more readily than oxygen (O_2) can combine with Hb; thus fewer Hb bonds are available to combine with O_2. Furthermore, when CO occupies the O_2 binding sites, Hb is changed to bind the remaining O_2 more tightly. This greater affinity of CO for Hb and this change in O_2 binding strength do not allow O_2 to pass readily from RBCs to tissue. Less O_2 is therefore available for tissue cell respiration. This results in hypoxemia.

This test can also be used to evaluate patients with complaints of headache, irritability, nausea, vomiting, and vertigo, who unknowingly may have been exposed to CO. Its greatest use, however, is in patients exposed to smoke inhalation, exhaust fumes, and fires.

Procedure and patient care

- See inside front cover for Routine Blood Testing.
- Fasting: no
- Blood tube commonly used: lavender or green
- Obtain the patient's history for possible sources of CO.
- Assess the patient for signs and symptoms of mild CO toxicity (e.g., headache, weakness, dizziness, malaise, dyspnea) and moderate to severe CO toxicity (e.g., severe headache, bright red mucous membranes, cherry-red blood).
- Usually the patient receives high concentrations of O_2 to displace the COHb.
- **PT** Encourage respirations to clear CO.

Abnormal findings

Carbon monoxide poisoning

notes

cardiac catheterization (Coronary angiography, Ventriculography)

Type of test X-ray with contrast

Normal findings

Normal heart-muscle motion, normal coronary arteries, normal great vessels, and normal intracardiac pressures and volumes

Test explanation and related physiology

Cardiac catheterization is used to visualize the heart chambers, arteries, and great vessels. It is used most often to evaluate patients with chest pain. Patients with positive stress test results are also studied to locate the region of coronary occlusion. This test is also used to determine the effects of valvular heart disease. Right heart catheterization is performed to calculate cardiac output and to measure right heart pressures. Right heart catheterization is also used to identify pulmonary emboli.

Cardiac output and other measures of cardiac functions can be determined. Cardiac catheterization is indicated for the following reasons:

- To identify, locate, and quantitate the severity of atherosclerotic, occlusive coronary artery disease
- To evaluate the severity of acquired and congenital cardiac valvular or septal defects
- To detect congenital cardiac abnormalities, such as transposition of great vessels and patent ductus arteriosus
- To evaluate the success of surgery or balloon angioplasty
- To evaluate cardiac muscle function
- To identify and quantify ventricular aneurysms
- To detect disease of the great vessels, such as atherosclerotic occlusion or aneurysms within the aortic arch
- To evaluate and treat patients with acute myocardial infarction
- To insert a catheter to monitor right-sided heart pressures, such as pulmonary artery pressure and pulmonary wedge pressure (See Table C2.)
- To perform dilation of stenotic coronary arteries (angioplasty), place coronary artery stents, or perform laser atherectomy

In right-sided heart catheterization, usually the jugular, subclavian, brachial, or femoral vein is used for vascular access. In left-sided heart catheterization, usually the right femoral artery is cannulated; alternatively, however, the radial or brachial artery may be chosen (Figure C1). As the catheter is

TABLE C2 Pressures and volumes used in cardiac monitoring

Pressures/volumes	Description	Normal values
Pressures		
Routine blood pressure	Routine brachial artery pressure	90–140/60–90 mm Hg
Systolic left ventricular pressure	Peak pressure in the left ventricle during systole	90–140 mm Hg
End-diastolic left ventricular pressure	Pressure in the left ventricle at the end of diastole	4–12 mm Hg
Central venous pressure	Pressure in the superior vena cava	2–14 cm H_2O
Pulmonary wedge pressure	Pressure in the pulmonary venules, an indirect measurement of left atrial pressure and left ventricular end-diastolic pressure	Left atrial: 6–15 mm Hg
Pulmonary artery pressure	Pressure in the pulmonary artery	15–28/5–16 mm Hg
Aortic artery pressure	Same as routine blood pressure	
Volumes		
End-diastolic volume (EDV)	Amount of blood present in the left ventricle at the end of diastole	50–90 mL/m²
End-systolic volume (ESV)	Amount of blood present in the left ventricle at the end of systole	25 mL/m²
Stroke volume (SV)	Amount of blood ejected from the heart in one contraction (SV = EDV − ESV)	45 ± 12 mL/m²
Ejection fraction (EF)	Proportion (fraction) of EDV ejected from the left ventricle during systole (EF = SV/EDV)	0.67 ± 0.07

Continued

TABLE C2   Pressures and volumes used in cardiac monitoring—cont'd

Pressures/volumes	Description	Normal values
Volumes		
Cardiac output (CO)	Amount of blood ejected by the heart in 1 minute	3–6 L/min
Cardiac index (CI)	Amount of blood ejected by the heart in 1 minute per square meter of body surface area (CI = CO/body surface area)	2.8–4.2 L/min/m² for a patient with 1.5 m² of body surface area

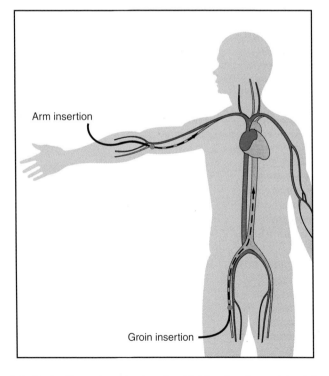

FIG. C1 Cardiac catheterization. Brachial (arm) or femoral (groin) arterial insertion for cardiac catheterization.

placed into the great vessels of the heart chamber, pressures are monitored and recorded. Blood samples for analysis of O_2 content are also obtained. After pressures are obtained, angiographic visualization of the heart chambers, valves, and coronary arteries is achieved with the injection of radiographic contrast.

A significant portion of patients with signs and symptoms of myocardial ischemia have no obstructive coronary artery disease (CAD). Some of these patients may have endothelial or microvascular dysfunction, with associated adverse cardiovascular outcomes. By evaluating epicardial and microvascular function, *functional coronary angiography (FCA)* can establish diagnosis in these patients. With the administration of intracoronary acetylcholine or intravenous adenosine, multiple measurements of coronary flow reserve (CFR) and hyperemic microvascular resistance (HMR) are obtained.

Percutaneous transluminal coronary angioplasty and *intracoronary stents* are therapeutic procedures that can be performed during cardiac catheterization in some medical facilities.

Likewise, *atherectomy* of coronary arterial plaques can be performed to more permanently open some of the hard, atheromatous plaques.

Contraindications

There are no absolute contraindications for cardiac catheterization. Some relative contraindications include:
- Allergy to contrast media
- Acute renal failure
- Acute stroke
- Severe uncontrolled hypertension
- Uncompensated congestive heart failure
- Severe coagulopathy
- Cardiac arrhythmias

Potential complications
- Cardiac arrhythmias (dysrhythmias)
- Perforation of the heart myocardium
- Catheter-induced embolic stroke or myocardial infarction
- Complications associated with the catheter insertion site
- Infection at the catheter insertion site
- Pneumothorax after subclavian vein catheterization
- Lactic acidosis in patients who are taking metformin and receiving contrast. Metformin should be held the day of the test to prevent this complication.

Procedure and patient care

Before

PT Explain the procedure to the patient. See p. xviii for radiation exposure and risks.

• Obtain written permission from the fully informed patient.

PT Allay the patient's fears and anxieties regarding this test.

PT Instruct the patient to abstain from oral intake for at least 4 to 8 hours before the test.

• Prepare the catheter insertion site as per protocol.

• Mark the patient's peripheral pulses with a pen before catheterization. This will facilitate postcatheterization assessment.

• Provide appropriate precatheterization sedation as ordered.

PT Instruct the patient to void before the procedure.

• Remove all valuables and dental prostheses.

• Obtain IV access.

During

• Take the patient to the cardiac catheterization laboratory.

• Note the following procedural steps:
  1. The chosen catheter insertion site is prepared and draped in a sterile manner.
  2. The desired vessel is punctured, and the angiographic catheter is threaded through the sheath over a guidewire.
  3. When the catheter is in the desired location, the appropriate cardiac pressures and volumes are measured.
  4. Cardiac ventriculography is performed with controlled injection of contrast.
  5. Each coronary artery is catheterized. Cardiac angiography is then carried out with a controlled injection of contrast.
  6. During the injection, x-ray images are obtained.
  7. The patient's vital signs must be monitored constantly.
  8. After obtaining all the required information, the catheter is removed, and a vascular closure device may be placed.
  9. A chemical vascular closure device designed to seal the arterial puncture is often placed.

• Note that this test is usually performed by a cardiologist in approximately 1 hour.

PT Tell the patient that during the injection, he or she may experience a severe hot flush. This is uncomfortable but lasts only 10 to 15 seconds.

• Note that some patients have a tendency to cough as the catheter is placed into the pulmonary artery.

After

- Monitor the patient's vital signs to check for bleeding.
- Apply pressure to the site of vascular access.
- Keep the patient on bed rest for 4 to 8 hours to allow for complete sealing of the arterial puncture.
- Keep the affected extremity extended and immobilized with sandbags to decrease bleeding.
- Assess the puncture site for signs of bleeding, hematoma, or absence of pulse.
- Compare the patient's pulses with preprocedure baseline values.
- PT Encourage the patient to drink fluids to maintain adequate hydration. Dehydration may be caused by the diuretic action of the dye. Monitor urinary output.
- PT Instruct the patient to report any signs of numbness, tingling, pain, or loss of function in the involved extremity.

Abnormal findings

Acquired or congenital septal defects and valvular abnormalities

Anatomic variation of the cardiac chambers and great vessels

Anomalies in pulmonary venous return

Aortic root arteriosclerotic or aneurysmal disease

Cardiomyopathy

Coronary artery occlusive disease, aneurysm, fistula

Intracardiac tumor

Pulmonary emboli and hypertension

Ventricular aneurysm, mural thrombi

notes

> **cardiac nuclear scan** (Myocardial perfusion scan, Myocardial perfusion imaging, Myocardial scan, Cardiac scan, Heart scan, Thallium scan, MUGA scan, Isonitrile scan, Sestamibi cardiac scan, Cardiac flow studies, and Nuclear stress test)

Type of test Nuclear scan

Normal findings

Heterogeneous uptake of radionuclide throughout the myocardium of the left ventricle

Left ventricular end-diastolic volume ≤ 70 mL

Left ventricular end-systolic volume ≤ 25 mL

Left ventricular ejection fraction $> 50\%$

Right ventricular ejection fraction $> 40\%$

Normal cardiac wall motion

No muscle wall thickening

Test explanation and related physiology

A cardiac perfusion scan measures the coronary blood flow at rest and during exercise. It is often used to evaluate the cause of chest pain. It may be done after a coronary ischemic event to evaluate coronary patency or heart muscle function.

In this test, a radionuclide is injected intravenously into the patient. Myocardial perfusion images are then obtained while the patient is lying down under a single-photon emission computed tomography (SPECT) camera that generates a picture of the radioactivity coming from the heart. This scan can be performed at rest or with exercise such as treadmill or bicycling *(myocardial nuclear stress testing)*. Medications may be administered that duplicate the effect of exercise stress testing. Vasodilators (dipyridamole, adenosine, and regadenoson) or chronotropic agents (dobutamine) are commonly used.

The uptake of these agents is proportional to the myocardial coronary flow. At rest, a coronary stenosis must exceed 90% of the normal diameter before blood flow is impaired enough to see it on the perfusion scan. With exercise stress testing, however, stenosis of 50% becomes obvious. Myocardial perfusion scans can be synchronized by gating the images with the cardiac cycle and thereby allowing the visualization and evaluation of cardiac muscle function. Prior muscle injury is demonstrated by reduced muscle wall motion. Most times, nuclear myocardial scans include both perfusion and gated wall motion images.

Cardiac nuclear imaging when gated to the cardiac cycle *(multigated acquisition scan [MUGA], gated blood pool scan)* can provide an accurate measure of ventricular function through the calculation of the *ventricular ejection fraction*. In this scan, the patient's red blood cells (RBCs) are tagged with technetium. Ventricular volumes can be calculated and used to accurately calculate the amount of blood that is ejected from the ventricle with each contraction (ejection fraction). Patients with cardiomyopathies (ischemic, infiltrative, inflammatory), cardiac transplant, or drug-induced cardiac muscle toxicity (from doxorubicin or Herceptin) require frequent evaluation of ventricular ejection fraction.

Contraindications

- Patients who are uncooperative or medically unstable
- Patients with severe cardiac arrhythmia
- Patients who are pregnant (unless the benefits outweigh the risks) because of the risk of fetal exposure to radionuclides.

Interfering factors

- Myocardial trauma
- Cardiac flow studies can be altered by excessive alterations in chest pressure (as exists with excessive crying in children).
- Recent nuclear scans (e.g., thyroid or bone scan)

Procedure and patient care

Before

PT Explain the procedure to the patient. See p. xviii for radiation exposure and risks.

PT Instruct the patient that a short fasting period may be required, especially when using sestamibi or tetrofosmin.

PT Tell the patient that the only discomfort is the venipuncture required for injection of the radioisotope.

- Be sure that all jewelry is removed from the chest wall.
- Obtain a consent form if stress testing is to be performed.

During

- Take the patient to the nuclear medicine department. Depending on the type of nuclear myocardial scan, each scanning protocol is different.
- Note the following general procedural steps:
  1. One or more IV injections of radionuclide are given.
  2. Electrocardiographic (ECG) leads may be applied.
  3. Depending on the radionuclide used, scanning is performed 15 minutes to 4 hours later.
  4. The SPECT camera is placed at the level of the precordium.
  5. If a single gamma camera is used, the patient is placed in a supine position and then may be repositioned to the

lateral position or in the right and left oblique positions. In some departments, the detector can be rotated around the patient, who remains in the supine position.

6. The gamma ray scanner records the image of the heart, and an image is immediately developed.

7. For an exercise stress test, additional radionuclide is injected during exercise when the patient reaches a maximum heart rate. The patient then lies on a table, and scanning is done. A repeat scan may be done 3 to 4 hours later.

• Note that myocardial scans are usually performed in less than 30 minutes by a nuclear medicine technician.

• If nuclear cardiac stress testing is performed, follow the routine protocol described on p. 179.

After

PT Inform the patient that because only tracer doses of radioisotopes are used, no precautions need to be taken against radioactive exposure to personnel or family.

PT Instruct the patient to drink fluids to aid in the excretion of the radioactive substance.

• Apply pressure or a pressure dressing to the venipuncture site.

• Assess the venipuncture site for bleeding.

• If stress testing was performed, evaluate the patient's vital signs at frequent intervals (as indicated).

• Remove any applied ECG leads.

Abnormal findings

Coronary artery occlusive disease

Decreased cardiac output

Decreased myocardial function associated with ischemia, myocarditis, cardiomyopathy, or congestive heart failure

notes

cardiac stress testing (Exercise stress testing; Nuclear stress testing; Echo stress testing)

C

Type of test   Electrodiagnostic; nuclear

Normal findings

Patient able to obtain and maintain maximal heart rate of 85% for predicted age and gender with no cardiac symptoms or ECG change. No cardiac muscle wall dysfunction present.

Test explanation and related physiology

Stress testing is used in the following situations:

- To evaluate chest pain in a patient suspected of having coronary disease
- To determine the limits of safe exercise during a cardiac rehabilitation program or to assist patients with cardiac disease in maintaining good physical fitness
- To detect labile or exercise-related hypertension
- To detect intermittent claudication in patients with suspected vascular occlusive disease in the extremities
- To evaluate the effectiveness of treatment in patients who take antianginal or antiarrhythmic medications
- To evaluate the effectiveness of cardiac intervention (e.g., bypass grafting or angioplasty)

Stress testing is a noninvasive study that provides information about the patient's cardiac function. In stress testing, the heart is stressed in some way and then evaluated during the stress. Changes indicating ischemia suggest coronary occlusive disease. By far the most commonly used method is *exercise stress testing*. *Chemical stress testing* methods are becoming more commonly used because of their safety and increased accuracy. A third method, less commonly used, is *pacer stress testing*.

During *exercise stress testing*, the ECG, heart rate, and blood pressure are monitored while the patient engages in some type of physical activity (stress). The treadmill test is the most frequently used because it is the most easily standardized and reproducible.

The usual goal of exercise stress testing is to increase the heart rate to just below maximal levels or to the *target heart rate*. Usually this target heart rate is 80% to 90% of the maximal heart rate. The test is usually discontinued if the patient reaches that target heart rate or develops any symptoms or ECG changes. The maximal heart rate is determined by a chart that takes into account the patient's age and gender. (Target rate is about 220 minus the patient's age.) Patients taking calcium channel blockers and sympathetic blockers have a lower-than-expected maximal heart rate.

Exercise stress testing is based on the principle that occluded arteries will be unable to meet the heart's increased demand for blood during the testing. This may become obvious with symptoms (e.g., chest pain, fatigue, dyspnea, tachycardia, cardiac arrhythmias [dysrhythmias], fall in blood pressure) or ECG changes (e.g., ST-segment variance > 1 mm, increasing premature ventricular contractions, or other rhythm disturbances).

When exercise testing is not advisable or the patient is unable to exercise at a level adequate to stress the heart (e.g., patients with an orthopedic, arthritic, neurologic, vascular, or pulmonary limitation), *chemical stress testing* is recommended. Although chemical stress testing is less physiologic than exercise testing, it is safer and more controllable. *Dipyridamole* is a coronary vasodilator. If one coronary artery is significantly occluded, the coronary blood flow is diverted to the opened vessels. *Adenosine* works similarly to dipyridamole. *Dobutamine* is another chemical that can stress the heart. Dobutamine stimulates the heart muscle function. The normal heart muscle increases (augments) its contractility (wall motion). Ischemic muscle has no augmentation. In fact, in time the ischemic area becomes hypokinetic. Infarcted tissue is akinetic. In chemical stress testing, the stressed heart is evaluated by nuclear scanning or echocardiography.

Pacing is another method of stress testing. In patients with permanent pacemakers, the rate of capture can be increased to a rate that would be considered a cardiac stress. The heart is then evaluated electrodiagnostically or with nuclear scanning or echocardiography.

Contraindications
- Patients with unstable angina
- Patients with severe aortic valvular heart disease
- Patients who have recently had a myocardial infarction
- Patients with severe congestive heart failure
- Patients with severe left main coronary artery disease

Potential complications
- Fatal cardiac arrhythmias
- Severe angina
- Myocardial infarction
- Fainting

Interfering factors
- Heavy meals before testing can divert blood to the GI tract.
- Nicotine from smoking can cause coronary artery spasm.

- Caffeine blocks the effect of dipyridamole.
- Medical problems, such as left ventricular hypertrophy, hypertension, valvular heart disease, left bundle-branch block, severe anemia, hypoxemia, and chronic pulmonary disease, can affect results.

Procedure and patient care

Before

PT Explain the procedure to the patient.

PT Instruct the patient to abstain from eating, drinking, and smoking for 4 hours before testing.

PT Obtain informed consent.

PT Instruct the patient to bring comfortable clothing and athletic shoes for exercise. Slippers are not acceptable.

PT Inform the patient if any medications should be discontinued for a time period before testing. If patients use an inhaler, instruct them to bring it with them and tell the staff.

- Obtain a pretest ECG.
- Apply and secure appropriate ECG electrodes.

During

- Note that a physician usually is present during stress testing.
- After the patient begins to exercise, adjust the treadmill machine settings to apply increasing levels of stress.

PT Encourage patients to verbalize any symptoms.

- Note that during the test the ECG tracing and vital signs are monitored continuously.
- Terminate the test if the patient complains of chest pain, exhaustion, dyspnea, fatigue, or dizziness.
- Note that testing usually takes approximately 45 minutes.

After

- Place the patient in the supine position to rest after the test.
- Monitor the ECG tracing and record vital signs at poststress intervals until recordings and values return to pretest levels.
- Remove electrodes and paste.

PT Tell the patient when the test results will be available.

Abnormal findings

Arrhythmias
Coronary artery occlusive disease
Exercise-related hypertension or hypotension
Intermittent claudication

notes

carotid artery duplex scanning (Carotid ultrasound)

Type of test Ultrasound

Normal findings

Carotid artery free of antatomic abnormalities, plaques and stenosis

Test explanation and related physiology

This Doppler ultrasound test is performed to identify occlusive disease in the carotid artery or its branches. It is mostly performed on patients with neurologic symptoms to assess for risks for stroke. It is also used to evaluate carotid bruits and to assess patients before coronary artery bypass surgery.

Carotid duplex scanning is a noninvasive ultrasound test used to detect occlusive disease of the carotid artery. It is called "duplex" because it combines B-mode ultrasound imaging and Doppler ultrasound. The degree of occlusion is measured in percentage of the entire lumen that is occluded. Focal increases in blood flow velocity indicate high-grade carotid stenosis. The peak systolic velocity is the most frequently used measurement to gauge the severity of the stenosis. Most patients who are considered for surgical treatment have 70% or greater stenosis.

Carotid duplex ultrasound is less precise in determining stenoses of less than 50% compared with stenoses of higher degrees. Imaging may be limited by patient body habitus. Transcranial Doppler can be used in conjunction with carotid duplex to improve its accuracy and help identify significant carotid disease by evaluating more proximal anatomy. It examines the major intracerebral arteries through the orbit and at the base of the brain.

Procedure and patient care

Before

PT Explain the procedure to the patient.

PT Tell the patient that no special preparation is required.

PT Assure the patient that the test is painless.

During

- Place the patient in the supine position with the head supported to prevent lateral motion.
- Note the following procedural steps:
  1. A water-soluble gel is used to couple the sound from the transducer to the skin surface.
  2. Images of the carotid artery and pulse waveform are obtained.

- Note that this test is performed by an ultrasound technologist in the ultrasound or radiology department in approximately 15 to 30 minutes.

After

- Remove the water-soluble gel from the patient.

C

Abnormal findings

Carotid artery aneurysm
Carotid artery occlusive disease

notes

cell-free maternal DNA testing (Prenatal cell-free DNA screening, Noninvasive prenatal testing [NIPT], cell-free DNA in maternal blood, cf DNA screening)

Type of test Blood

Normal findings

Low risk of chromosomal abnormality

Test explanation and related physiology

Trisomy 21 (Down syndrome), trisomy 18 (Edwards syndrome), and trisomy 13 (Patau syndrome) are the three most common chromosomal abnormalities affecting live births. Although 1 in 450 live births has one of these aneuploidy abnormalities, trisomy 21 is the most common. Abnormal findings on pelvic ultrasonography of the fetus, including fetal nuchal translucency or thickness (p. 754) along with biochemical markers (e.g., hCG, p. 425; PAAP-A, p. 600), can identify pregnancies at high risk for these chromosomal defects. The definitive diagnosis requires chorionic villus sampling (CVS; p. 202) and amniocentesis (p. 39), which are invasive and increase the risk for miscarriage.

Cell-free (cf) DNA from the placental fetal cells circulates in maternal blood. This DNA can be extracted and, through advanced laboratory techniques of targeting genomic sequencing, allows 99% of the cases of trisomy to be detected. False-positive rates instigating unnecessary invasive testing are less than 1%. This testing can be performed as early as 10 weeks of gestation but is typically done between 10 and 22 weeks. Because of newer laboratory techniques of multiplexing, results can be available in about 1 week.

In 2012, the American College of Obstetricians and Gynecologists (ACOG) and the Society for Maternal-Fetal Medicine (SMFM) issued a joint committee opinion that supported noninvasive prenatal testing that uses cell-free fetal DNA for women at increased risk for having a baby with a chromosomal abnormality (Box C1).

Testing of high-risk pregnant women may be done in several ways:

- cf DNA test in the first trimester with ultrasonography
- cf DNA test in the second trimester without ultrasonography
- A combination of both

> **BOX C1   Women at high risk for having children with chromosomal abnormalities**
>
> - Maternal age 35 years or older at delivery
> - Fetal ultrasonographic findings indicating an increased risk for trisomy
> - History of pregnancy with trisomy
> - Positive maternal screen result
> - Other translocation abnormalities with increased risk of trisomy

Procedure and patient care

- See inside front cover for Routine Blood Testing.
- Fasting: no
- Blood tube commonly used: red
- PT Encourage all women undergoing cf DNA to have genetic counseling.
- PT Results should be reviewed with the patient, and the risks, benefits, and alternatives to further testing should be explained.

Abnormal findings

Duchenne muscular dystrophy
Hemophilia
Trisomy 13 (Patau syndrome)
Trisomy 18 (Edwards syndrome)
Trisomy 21 (Down syndrome)

notes

cell surface immunophenotyping (Flow cytometry cell surface immunophenotyping, Lymphocyte immunophenotyping, AIDS T-lymphocyte cell markers, CD4 marker, CD4/CD8 ratio, CD4 percentage)

Type of test Blood

Normal findings

Cells	Percent	No. of cells/μL
T-cells	60–95	800–2500
T-helper (CD4) cells	60–75	600–1500
CD8 T-cells	25–30	300–1000
B-cells	4–25	100–450
Natural killer cells	4–30	75–500

CD4/CD8 ratio: > 1

Test explanation and related physiology

This test is used to detect the progressive depletion of CD4 T-lymphocytes, which is associated with an increased likelihood of clinical complications from acquired immunodeficiency syndrome (AIDS). It is also used to confirm the diagnosis of acute myelocytic leukemia (AML) and to differentiate AML from acute lymphocytic leukemia (ALL).

CD4 (T-helper cells) and CD8 (T-suppressor cells) are examples of T-lymphocytes. T-lymphocytes, and especially CD4 counts, when combined with HIV viral load testing (p. 417) are, used to determine the time to initiate antiviral therapy. Successful antiviral therapy is associated with an increase in CD4 counts. Worsening of disease or unsuccessful therapy is associated with decreasing T-lymphocyte counts.

There are three related measurements of CD4 T-lymphocytes. The first measurement is the *total CD4 count*. This is measured in whole blood and is the product of the white blood cell (WBC) count, the lymphocyte differential count, and the percentage of lymphocytes that are CD4 T-cells. The second measurement, the *CD4 percentage*, is a more accurate prognostic marker. The third prognostic marker, which is also more reliable than the total CD4 count, is the *CD4-to-CD8 ratio*.

Of the three T-cell measurements, the total CD4 count is the most variable. With the CD4 percentage and the CD4-to-CD8 ratio, very little diurnal variation and laboratory error exist. The Multicenter AIDS Cohort Study suggests that the latter two measurements are more accurate than the total CD4 count. However, because the total CD4 count was originally thought to be the best marker, this test was used in many of the studies that now form the basis for practice recommendations.

CD4 measurement is a prognostic marker that can indicate whether a patient infected with HIV is at risk for developing opportunistic infections. The measurement of CD4 levels is used to decide whether to initiate *Pneumocystis jirovecii* pneumonia prophylaxis and antiviral therapy and for determining the prognosis of patients with HIV.

Both immunodeficiency and the dosage of immunosuppressive medications used after organ transplant are also monitored with the use of this cell surface immunophenotyping. Lymphomas and other lymphoproliferative diseases are now classified and treated according to the predominant lymphocyte type identified.

Interfering factors
- Diurnal variation occurs.
- A recent viral illness can decrease total T-lymphocyte counts.
- Nicotine and very strenuous exercise have been shown to decrease lymphocyte counts.

Procedure and patient care
- See inside front cover for Routine Blood Testing.
- Fasting: no
- Blood tube commonly used: green or purple
- Never recap needles.
- Keep the specimen at room temperature. Do not refrigerate.
- The specimen must be evaluated within 24 hours.
- PT Instruct the patient to observe the venipuncture site for infection.
- PT Encourage the patient to discuss his or her concerns regarding the prognostic information obtained by these results.
- Do not give test results over the phone.

Abnormal findings

▲ **Increased counts**
Leukemias
Lymphoma

▼ **Decreased counts**
Immunodeficiency diseases
Organ transplant patients

notes

ceruloplasmin (Cp)

Type of test Blood

Normal findings

Adults: 23–50 mg/dL or 230–500 mg/L (SI units)
Neonates: 2–13 mg/dL or 20–130 mg/L (SI units)

Test explanation and related physiology

The primary use of Cp is in the diagnosis of preclinical states of Wilson disease. Cp is an alpha$_2$-globulin that binds copper for transport within the bloodstream after it is absorbed from the gastrointestinal (GI) tract. Cp levels are decreased in most instances of Wilson disease, which is an inherited disorder. Patients who are homozygous for this disease make very little Cp. This results in high levels of unbound copper which is toxic to tissues. The copper is deposited in the eye, brain, liver, and kidney. Wilson disease is fatal unless early treatment is instituted. If this disease is identified before significant copper deposits affect major organs, the ravages of the disease can be avoided. Young adults with hepatitis, cirrhosis, or recurrent neuromuscular incoordination (signs compatible with Wilson disease) should also have this test.

Cp is also an acute-phase reactant protein that becomes elevated during stress, infection, and pregnancy. However, it rises more slowly than other acute-phase reactants, such as C-reactive protein and erythrocyte sedimentation rate.

Interfering factors

- Values are increased during pregnancy.

Procedure and patient care

- See inside front cover for Routine Blood Testing.
- Fasting: no
- Blood tube commonly used: red

Abnormal findings

▲ **Increased levels**

Acute inflammatory reaction
Biliary cirrhosis
Cancer
Copper intoxication
Pregnancy
Thyrotoxicosis

▼ **Decreased levels**

Kwashiorkor
Menkes (kinky-hair) syndrome
Nephrotic syndrome
Normal infants (6 months)
Sprue
Starvation
Wilson disease

notes

cervical biopsy (LEEP procedure, Cone biopsy)

Type of test   Microscopic examination

Normal findings

Normal squamous cells

Possible critical values

Cancer cells

Test explanation and related physiology

When a Pap smear reveals an *epithelial cell abnormality* or when a pelvic examination reveals a possible abnormality in the cervix, a biopsy of that structure is performed. There are several different methods of biopsy, all of which obtain an increasing amount of tissue. Cervical biopsy procedures include the following:

A *simple cervical biopsy*, sometimes called a *punch biopsy*, removes a small piece of tissue from the surface of the cervix. This is often performed during colposcopy (p. 223).

An *endocervical biopsy (endocervical curettage)* removes tissue from high in the cervical canal by scraping with a sharp instrument.

Loop electrosurgical excision procedure (LEEP) uses a thin, low-voltage electrified wire loop to cut out abnormal tissue on the cervix and high in the endocervical canal (sometimes called a *large loop excision of the transformation zone [LLETZ]*).

A *cone biopsy (conization)* is a more extensive form of a cervical biopsy. It is called a cone biopsy because a cone-shaped wedge of tissue is removed from the cervix. Both normal and abnormal cervical tissues are removed. This can be performed by LEEP, surgical knife (scalpel), or carbon dioxide laser.

Contraindications

- Patients with active menstrual bleeding
- Patients who are pregnant

Potential complications

- After the surgery, a small number of women may have significant bleeding that requires vaginal packing or a blood transfusion.

Procedure and patient care

Before

PT Explain the procedure to the patient.
- Obtain informed consent if required by the institution.

During
- Note the following procedural steps:
  1. The patient is placed in the lithotomy position, and a vaginal speculum is used to expose the vagina and cervix.
  2. The cervix is cleansed with a 3% acetic acid solution or antiseptic to remove excess mucus and cellular debris and to accentuate the difference between normal and abnormal epithelial tissues.
  3. Medication is injected to numb the cervix *(cervical block)*.
  4. With the instrument chosen by the doctor, a punch biopsy, endocervical biopsy, LEEP, or cone biopsy is performed.
- Note that the physician performs the procedure in approximately 30 minutes.
- Whereas cone biopsy is done in the operating room, the other procedures can be performed in the doctor's office.

After
- PT Inform the patient that it is normal to experience some vaginal bleeding/discharge.
- PT Tell the patient to avoid sexual intercourse for 3 to 4 weeks.
- PT Inform the patient not to douche for 3 to 4 weeks.
- PT Tell the patient how to obtain the test results.

Abnormal findings

Cervical carcinoma *in situ*
Cervical intraepithelial neoplasia
Chronic cervical infection
Endocervical adenocarcinoma
Invasive cervical carcinoma

notes

chest x-ray (CXR)

Type of test X-ray

Normal findings

Normal lungs and surrounding structures

Test explanation and related physiology

The CXR is important in a complete evaluation of the pulmonary and cardiac systems. Much information can be provided by this radiographic study. One can identify or follow:

- Tumors of the lung (primary and metastatic), heart (myxoma), chest wall (soft tissue sarcomas), and bony thorax (osteogenic sarcoma)
- Inflammation of the lung (pneumonia), pleura (pleuritis), and pericardium (pericarditis)
- Fluid accumulation in the pleura (pleural effusion), pericardium (pericardial effusion), and lung (pulmonary edema)
- Air accumulation in the lung (chronic obstructive pulmonary disease) and pleura (pneumothorax)
- Fractures of the bones of the thorax or vertebrae
- Diaphragmatic hernia
- Heart size, which may vary depending on cardiac function
- Calcification, which may indicate large-vessel deterioration or old lung granulomas
- Location of centrally placed IV access devices

Most CXRs are taken with the patient standing. The sitting or supine position also can be used, but images taken with the patient in the supine position will not demonstrate fluid levels. A *posteroanterior (PA)* view, with the x-rays passing through the back of the body (posterior) to the front of the body (anterior), is taken first. Then a *lateral* view, with the x-rays passing through the patient's side, is taken.

Oblique views may be taken with the patient turned at different angles as the x-rays pass through the body. *Lordotic* views provide visualization of the apices (rounded upper portions) of the lungs and are usually for detection of tuberculosis. *Decubitus* images are taken with the patient in the recumbent lateral position to localize fluid, which becomes dependent within the pleural space (pleural effusion).

Chest x-ray studies are best performed in the radiology department. Studies using a portable x-ray machine may be done at the bedside and are often performed on critically ill patients who cannot leave the nursing unit.

Contraindications

- Patients who are pregnant unless the benefits outweigh the risks

Interfering factors

- Conditions (e.g., severe pain) that prevent the patient from taking and holding a deep breath
- Scarring from previous lung surgery, which makes interpretation difficult
- Obesity, which requires more x-rays to penetrate the body to provide a quality image

Procedure and patient care

Before

PT Explain the procedure to the patient. See p. xviii for radiation exposure and risks.

PT Tell the patient that no fasting is required.

PT Instruct the patient to remove clothing to the waist and to put on an x-ray gown.

PT Inform the patient to remove all metal objects (e.g., necklaces, pins) so that they do not block visualization of part of the chest.

PT Tell the patient that he or she will be asked to take a deep breath and hold it while the images are taken.

During

PT After the patient is correctly positioned, tell him or her to take a deep breath and hold it until the images are taken.

- Note that x-ray images are taken by a radiologic technologist in several minutes.

PT Inform the patient that no discomfort is associated with chest radiography.

After

- Note that no special care is required after the procedure.

Abnormal findings

Lung
Atelectasis
Chronic obstructive
   pulmonary
   disease
Congenital lung diseases
   (hypoplasia)
Foreign bodies (chest,
   bronchus,
   or esophagus)
Lung abscess
Lung tumor (primary or
   metastatic)
Pleural effusion
Pleuritis
Pneumonia
Pneumothorax
Pulmonary edema
Tuberculosis

Heart
Cardiac enlargement
Pericardial effusion
Pericarditis

notes

Chest wall
Fracture (ribs or thoracic
   spine)
Metastatic tumor to the bony
thorax
Osteogenic sarcoma
Soft tissue sarcoma
Thoracic spine scoliosis

Diaphragm
Diaphragmatic or
   hiatal hernia

Mediastinum
Aortic calcinosis
Dilated aorta
Enlarged lymph nodes
Lymphoma
Substernal thyroid
Thymoma
Widened mediastinum

C

Chlamydia

Type of test   Blood; microscopic examination

Normal findings

Negative culture
Antibodies:
  Chlamydophila pneumoniae
    IgG: < 1:64
    IgM: < 1:10
  Chlamydophila psittaci
    IgG: < 1:64
    IgM: < 1:10
  Chlamydia trachomatis
    IgG: < 1:64
    IgM: < 1:10
Nucleic acid detection: negative

Test explanation and related physiology

There are many *Chlamydia* species that cause various diseases within the human body. *Chlamydophila psittaci* causes respiratory tract infections, headache, altered mentation, and hepatosplenomegaly. It occurs as a result of close contact with infected birds. *Chlamydophila pneumoniae,* another species, causes pneumonia. *Chlamydophila trachomatis* infection is probably the most frequently occurring sexually transmitted disease in developed countries. Infections of the genitalia, pelvic inflammatory disease, urethritis, cervicitis, salpingitis, and endometritis are most common. *C. trachomatis* may also infect the conjunctiva, pharynx, urethra, and rectum and cause lymphogranuloma venereum. The second serotype of *C. trachomatis* causes the eye disease *trachoma,* which is the most common form of preventable blindness. A third serotype produces genital and urethral infections different from lymphogranuloma. Most women colonized with *Chlamydia* are asymptomatic.

Tests are performed on swabs from the conjunctiva, nasopharynx, urethra, urine, rectum, vagina, or cervix.

Interfering factors

- Women presently having routine menses
- Patients undergoing antibiotic therapy

Procedure and patient care

Before

PT Explain the procedure to the patient.

During

- For *Chlamydia* antibody testing, collect venous blood in a red-top tube. Acute and convalescent serum should be drawn 2 to 3 weeks apart.
- Sputum cultures (p. 682) are used to check for *C. psittaci* respiratory infections.
- A conjunctival smear is obtained by swabbing the eye lesion with a cotton-tipped applicator or scraping with a sterile ophthalmic spatula and smearing on a clean glass slide.
- Note the following procedural steps for *cervical culture:*
  1. The patient should refrain from douching and bathing in a tub before the cervical culture is performed.
  2. The patient is placed in the lithotomy position.
  3. A nonlubricated vaginal speculum is inserted to expose the cervix.
  4. Excess mucus is removed using a cleaning swab.
  5. A second sterile, cotton-tipped swab is inserted into the endocervical canal and moved from side to side for 30 seconds to obtain the culture.
  6. The swab is then placed into an appropriate transport tube.
- Note the following procedural steps for *urethral culture:*
  1. The urethral specimen should be obtained from the man before voiding within the previous hour.
  2. A culture is taken by inserting a thin sterile swab with rotating movement about 3 to 4 cm into the urethra.
- Note the following procedural steps for a *urine specimen:*
  1. The patient should not have urinated for at least 1 hour before specimen collection.
  2. The patient should collect the first portion (first part of stream) of a random voided urine into a sterile, plastic, preservative-free container.
  3. Transfer 2 mL of urine into the urine specimen collection tube using the disposable pipette provided.
- Note that these tests are performed by a physician, nurse, or other health-care provider in several minutes.

PT Tell the patient these procedures cause minimal discomfort.

After

- Treat patients who have positive smears with antibiotics.

PT Tell affected patients to have their sexual partners examined.

Abnormal findings

Chlamydia infection

notes

chloride, blood (CL)

Type of test Blood

Normal findings

Adult/elderly: 98–106 mEq/L or 98–106 mmol/L (SI units)
Child: 90–110 mEq/L
Newborn: 96–106 mEq/L
Premature infant: 95–110 mEq/L

Possible critical values

< 80 or > 115 mEq/L

Test explanation and related physiology

This test is performed as a part of multiphasic testing in what is usually called electrolytes, Astra-7, chemprofile, metabolic panel, kidney profile, comprehensive profile, SMA 12, or SMA 6. By itself, not much information is obtained. However, with interpretation of the other electrolytes, chloride can give an indication of acid–base balance and hydrational status.

Hypochloremia and hyperchloremia rarely occur alone and are usually part of parallel shifts in sodium or bicarbonate levels. Signs and symptoms of hypochloremia include hyperexcitability of the nervous system and muscles, shallow breathing, hypotension, and tetany. Signs and symptoms of hyperchloremia include lethargy, weakness, and deep breathing.

Interfering factors

- Excessive infusions of saline can result in increased chloride levels.

Procedure and patient care

- See inside front cover for Routine Blood Testing.
- Fasting: no
- Blood tube commonly used: red or green

Abnormal findings

▲ **Increased levels (hyperchloremia)**

Anemia
Cushing syndrome
Dehydration
Eclampsia
Excessive infusion of normal saline
Hyperparathyroidism
Hyperventilation
Kidney dysfunction
Metabolic acidosis
Multiple myeloma
Renal tubular acidosis
Respiratory alkalosis

▼ **Decreased levels (hypochloremia)**

Addison disease
Aldosteronism
Burns
Chronic gastric suction
Chronic respiratory acidosis
Congestive heart failure
Diuretic therapy
Hypokalemia
Metabolic alkalosis
Overhydration
Respiratory acidosis
Salt-losing nephritis
Syndrome of inappropriate antidiuretic hormone
Vomiting

notes

cholesterol

Type of test Blood

Normal findings

Adult/elderly: < 200 mg/dL or < 5.2 mmol/L (SI units)
Child: 120–200 mg/dL
Infant: 70–175 mg/dL
Newborn: 53–135 mg/dL

Test explanation and related physiology

Cholesterol is the main lipid associated with arteriosclerotic vascular disease. Nearly 75% of the cholesterol is bound to LDLs and 25% is bound to HDLs. Therefore cholesterol is the main component of LDLs and only a minimal component of HDLs and very low-density lipoproteins. LDLs are most directly associated with increased risk of coronary heart disease (CHD).

The purpose of cholesterol testing is to identify patients at risk for arteriosclerotic heart disease. Cholesterol testing is usually done as a part of *lipid profile* testing, which also evaluates lipoproteins (p. 462) and triglycerides (p. 737), because by itself cholesterol is not a totally accurate predictor of heart disease.

Because the liver is required to make cholesterol, low serum cholesterol levels are indicative of severe liver diseases. Furthermore, because our main source of cholesterol is our diet, malnutrition is also associated with low cholesterol levels. Certain illnesses can affect cholesterol levels. For example, patients with an acute myocardial infarction may have as much as a 50% reduction in cholesterol level for as many as 6 to 8 weeks.

The cholesterol-to-HDL ratio has been used to assess the risk of CHD (Table C3).

TABLE C3   Cholesterol-to-HDL ratio as an indicator of risk of coronary heart disease

	Ratio	
Risk	Male	Female
½ Average	3.4	3.3
Average	5	4.4
2 × Average	10	7
3 × Average	24	11

HDL, High-density lipoprotein.

Interfering factors
- Pregnancy is usually associated with elevated levels.
- Oophorectomy increases levels.

Procedure and patient care

C

- See inside front cover for Routine Blood Testing.
- Fasting: yes
- Blood tube commonly used: red
- PT Instruct the patient to fast 12 to 14 hours after eating a low-fat diet before testing. Only water is permitted.
- PT Inform the patient that dietary intake at least 2 weeks before testing will affect results.
- PT Tell the patient that no alcohol should be consumed 24 hours before the test.
- The fingerstick method is often used in mass screening.
- PT Instruct patients with high levels regarding a low-cholesterol diet, exercise, and appropriate body weight.

Abnormal findings

▲ **Increased levels**
Atherosclerosis
Biliary cirrhosis
Hypercholesterolemia
Hyperlipidemia
Hypothyroidism
Pregnancy
Stress

▼ **Decreased levels**
Cholesterol-lowering
  medication
Hemolytic anemia
Hyperthyroidism
Liver disease
Malabsorption
Malnutrition

notes

cholinesterase (CHS, Pseudocholinesterase [PChE], Cholinesterase RBC, Red blood cell cholinesterase, Acetylcholinesterase)

Type of test Blood

Normal findings

Serum cholinesterase: 8–18 units/mL or 8–18 kilo units/L
RBC cholinesterase: 5–10 units/mL or 5–10 kilo units/L
Dibucaine inhibition: 79%-84%

Test explanation and related physiology

This test is done to identify patients with pseudocholinesterase deficiency before anesthesia or to identify patients who may have been exposed to phosphate poisoning. Cholinesterases hydrolyze acetylcholine and other choline esters and thereby regulate nerve impulse transmission at the nerve synapse and neuromuscular junction. There are two types of cholinesterases: *acetylcholinesterase*, also known as *true cholinesterase*, and butyrylcholinesterase (pseudocholinesterase). Deficiencies in either of these enzymes can be acquired or congenital.

Because succinylcholine (the most commonly used muscle relaxant during anesthesia induction) is inactivated by pseudocholinesterase, people with an inherited pseudocholinesterase enzyme deficiency exhibit increased and/or prolonged effects of succinylcholine. Prolonged muscle paralysis and apnea will occur after anesthesia in these patients. This situation can be avoided by measuring serum cholinesterase activity in all patients with a family history of prolonged apnea after surgery.

Two tests are usually performed, one for the level of enzyme activity, and if enough activity exists, another test is performed for the dibucaine number. This number indicates the percent of inhibition of the enzyme when a standardized dose of dibucaine is added to the patient's serum. If total pseudocholinesterase is normal and dibucaine numbers are low, the presence of a nonfunctioning pseudocholinesterase variant is suspected, and the patient will be at risk for succinylcholine-induced prolonged paralysis. Genetic testing can also be performed to identify abnormal functioning cholinesterase genes.

A common form of acquired cholinesterase deficiency, either true or pseudocholinesterase, is caused by overexposure to pesticides, organophosphates, or nerve gas. Other factors that can reduce pseudocholinesterase activity and cause some prolonged paralysis with succinylcholine include liver disease, pregnancy, advanced age, renal failure, major burns, oral contraceptives, and echothiophate eye drops.

Increased cholinesterase activity, when found in the amniotic fluid, represents strong evidence for a *neural tube defect (NTD)*.

Interfering factors

• Pregnancy decreases test values.

Procedure and patient care

• See inside front cover for Routine Blood Testing.
• Fasting: no
• Blood tube commonly used: red
• It may be recommended to withhold medications that could alter test results for 12 to 24 hours before the test.

Abnormal findings

▲ **Increased serum levels**
Diabetes mellitus
Hyperlipidemia
Nephrosis

▼ **Decreased serum levels**
Hepatocellular disease
Malnutrition
Persons with congenital pseudocholinesterase enzyme deficiency
Poisoning from organophosphate insecticides

▲ **Increased RBC levels**
Reticulocytosis
Sickle cell disease

▼ **Decreased RBC levels**
Congenital cholinesterase deficiency
Poisoning from organophosphate insecticides

notes

chorionic villus sampling (CVS, Chorionic villus biopsy [CVB])

Type of test Cell analysis

Normal findings

No genetic or biochemical disorders

Test explanation and related physiology

CVS is performed on women whose unborn children may be at risk for life-threatening or significant life-altering genetic defects. This includes women who:

- Are older than age 35 years at the time of pregnancy
- Have had frequent spontaneous abortions
- Have had previous pregnancies with fetuses or infants with chromosomal or genetic defects (e.g., Down syndrome)
- Have a genetic defect themselves (e.g., hemoglobinopathies)

CVS can be performed between 8 and 12 weeks of gestation for the early detection of genetic and biochemical disorders. Because CVS detects congenital defects early, first-trimester therapeutic abortions can be performed if indicated.

For this study, a sample of chorionic villi from the chorion frondosum, which is the trophoblastic origin of the placenta, is obtained for analysis. These villi are present from 8 to 12 weeks on and reflect fetal chromosome, enzyme, and deoxyribonucleic acid content, thus permitting a much earlier diagnosis of prenatal problems than amniocentesis (p. 39), which cannot be done before 14 to 16 weeks. Furthermore, the cells derived by CVS are more easily grown in tissue culture for *karyotyping* (determination of chromosomal or genetic abnormalities). The cells obtained with amniocentesis take a longer time to grow in culture, further adding to the delay in obtaining results.

Potential complications

- Accidental abortion
- Bleeding
- Fetal limb deformities
- Infection

Procedure and patient care

Before

PT Explain the procedure to the patient.
- Be certain that the physician has obtained a signed consent.
PT Tell the patient that no food or fluid restrictions are necessary.

PT Encourage the patient to drink at least 1 to 2 glasses of fluid before testing.

PT Instruct the patient not to urinate for several hours before testing. A full bladder is an excellent reference point for pelvic ultrasound.

• Assess the vital signs of the mother and the fetal heart rate of the fetus before testing. These are baseline studies that should be repeated during and on completion of the test.

During

• Note the following procedural steps:
  1. The patient is placed in the lithotomy position.
  2. Samples of vaginal mucus may be obtained to rule out pre-procedural infections (e.g., *Chlamydia*).
  3. A cannula from the endoscope is inserted into the cervix and uterine cavity (Figure C2).
  4. Under ultrasound guidance, the cannula is rotated to the site of the developing placenta.

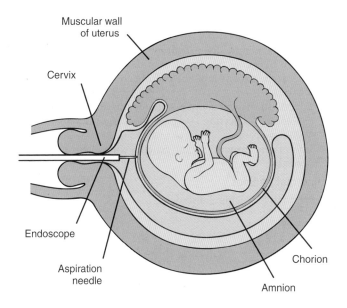

FIG. C2 Chorionic villus sampling. Diagram of an 8-week pregnancy showing endoscopic aspiration of extraplacental villi.

5. A syringe is attached, and suction is applied to obtain several samples of villi.
6. As many as three or more samples may be obtained to get sufficient tissue for accurate sampling.
7. If ultrasound indicates that the trophoblastic tissue is remote from the cervix, a transabdominal approach similar to that described for amniocentesis may be used.

- Note that this procedure is performed by an obstetrician in approximately 30 minutes.
- **PT** Inform the patient that discomfort associated with this test is similar to that of a Pap smear.

After

- Note that Rh-negative women (who have not been sensitized to Rh incompatibility) receive RhoGAM. This procedure may be contraindicated for women with known preexisting Rh sensitization.
- Monitor the vital signs and check for signs of bleeding.
- Schedule the patient for an ultrasound in 2 to 4 days to confirm the continued viability of the fetus.
- Assess the vaginal area for discharge and drainage; note the color and amount.
- **PT** Assess and educate the patient for signs of spontaneous abortion (e.g., cramps, bleeding).
- **PT** Inform the patient how she can obtain the results from her physician.
- **PT** Educate the patient about how to identify and report signs of endometrial infection (vaginal discharge, fever, crampy abdominal pain).
- **PT** Inform the patient about genetic counseling services if needed.

Abnormal findings

Genetic and biochemical disorders

notes

chromosome karyotype (Blood chromosome analysis, Chromosome studies, Cytogenetics, Karyotype)

Type of test Blood

Normal findings

Male: 44 autosomes + 1 X, 1 Y chromosome; karyotype: 46,XY
Female: 44 autosomes + 2 X chromosomes; karyotype: 46,XX

Test explanation and related physiology

This test is used to study an individual's chromosomal makeup to determine chromosomal defects associated with disease or the risk of developing disease. The term *karyotyping* refers to the arrangement and pairing of cell chromosomes in order from the largest to the smallest to analyze their number and structure. Variations in either can produce numerous developmental abnormalities and diseases. A normal karyotype of chromosomes consists of a pattern of 22 pairs of autosomal chromosomes and a pair of sex chromosomes (XY for the male and XX for the female). Chromosomal karyotype abnormalities can be congenital or acquired. These karyotype abnormalities can occur because of duplication, deletion, translocation, reciprocation, or genetic rearrangement.

Chromosomal karyotyping is useful in evaluating congenital anomalies, mental retardation, growth retardation, delayed puberty, infertility, hypogonadism, primary amenorrhea, ambiguous genitalia, chronic myelogenous leukemia, neoplasm, recurrent miscarriage, prenatal diagnosis of serious congenital diseases (especially in situations of advanced maternal age), Turner syndrome, Klinefelter syndrome, Down syndrome, and other suspected genetic disorders. The products of conception also can be studied to determine the cause of stillbirth or miscarriage.

Procedure and patient care

Before

PT Explain the procedure to the patient.

- Determine how the specimen will be collected. Obtain preparation guidelines from the laboratory if indicated.
- Many patients are fearful of the test results and require considerable emotional support.
- In some states, informed consent is required.

During

- Specimens for chromosome analysis can be obtained from numerous sources. Leukocytes from a peripheral venipuncture are most easily and most often used for this study.

- Bone marrow biopsies and surgical specimens also can be used sometimes as sources for analysis.
- During pregnancy, specimens can be collected by amniocentesis (p. 39) and chorionic villus sampling (p. 202).
- Fetal tissue or products of conception can be studied to determine the reason for loss of a pregnancy.
- Smears and stains of buccal mucosal cells are less costly but not as accurate as other tissue for karyotyping.

After

- Aftercare depends on how the specimen was collected.
- PT Inform the patient that test results generally will not be available for several months.
- If an abnormality is identified, often the entire family line must be tested. This can be exhaustive and expensive.
- PT If the test results show an abnormality, encourage the patient to verbalize his or her feelings. Provide emotional support.

Abnormal findings

Ambiguous genitalia
Chronic myelogenous leukemia
Congenital anomalies
Delayed puberty
Growth retardation
Hypogonadism
Infertility
Klinefelter syndrome
Mental retardation
Neoplasm
Primary amenorrhea
Recurrent miscarriage
Sickle cell anemia
Tay–Sachs disease
Trisomy 21 (Down syndrome)
Turner syndrome

notes

Clostridium difficile (C. diff, Clostridial toxin assay)

Type of test Stool

Normal findings

Negative (no *Clostridium* toxin identified)
No other infectious agent identified

Test explanation and related physiology

Clostridium difficile–associated disease (CDAD) bacterial infections usually affect the intestine (pseudomembranous colitis) and often occur in patients who are immunocompromised or taking broad-spectrum antibiotics (e.g., clindamycin, ampicillin, cephalosporins). The disease can be community acquired, and the severity can range from mild nuisance diarrhea to severe pseudomembranous colitis and bowel perforation.

The infection possibly results from depression of the normal flora of the bowel caused by the administration of antibiotics. The clostridial bacterium produces two toxins (A and B) that cause inflammation and necrosis of the colonic epithelium. Establishing a CDAD diagnosis is dependent on demonstrating the presence of toxin or toxigenic organism in stool samples.

Enzyme immunoassays (EIAs) can be used to detect either toxin A/B or glutamate dehydrogenase (GDH), an abundant enzyme whose presence is indicative of *C. difficile*. EIA, however, does not have high sensitivity and accuracy. *C. difficile* can be diagnosed by obtaining colonic-rectal tissue for this toxin. Stool cultures (p. 688) for *C. difficile* can be performed but are also labor intensive and take longer to get results.

A rapid detection of *C. difficile* toxin B gene (*tcdB*) in human liquid or soft stool specimens is available. This method rapidly provides a definitive diagnosis of *C. difficile*. Quickly reaching a definitive diagnosis allows CDAD patients to get the proper treatment without delay and reduces hospital stays for inpatients with CDAD. At the same time, they can be placed in isolation sooner to reduce transmission and prevent outbreaks.

Treatment of CDAD typically involves withdrawal of the associated antimicrobial(s) and orally administered and intraluminally active metronidazole, vancomycin, or fidaxomicin. Intravenous metronidazole may be used if an oral agent cannot be administered. In recent years, a more severe form of CDAD with increased morbidity and mortality has been recognized as being caused by an epidemic toxin-hyperproducing strain of *C. difficile* (NAP1 strain).

Procedure and patient care

Before

PT Explain the method of stool collection to the patient. Be matter of fact to avoid embarrassment for the patient.

PT Instruct the patient not to mix urine or toilet paper with the stool specimen.

• Handle the specimen carefully, as though it were capable of causing infection. Follow strict enteric precautions.

• Use soap and water instead of alcohol based hand sanitizers.

During

PT Instruct the patient to defecate into a clean container. A clean, dry bedpan or hat over the toilet or commode can be used. A rectal swab cannot be used because it collects inadequate amounts of stool. The stool cannot be retrieved from the toilet.

• Stool can be obtained from incontinence pads.

• The specimen can be obtained from a baby's diaper.

• A stool specimen also can be collected by proctoscopy.

• Place the specimen in a closed container and transport it to the laboratory to prevent deterioration of the toxin.

• If the specimen cannot be processed immediately, refrigerate it (depending on laboratory protocol).

After

• Maintain enteric isolation precautions on all patients until appropriate therapy is completed.

Abnormal findings

▲ **Increased levels**

Antibiotic-related pseudomembranous colitis
C. difficile colitis

notes

coagulating factors concentration (Coagulating factors, Blood-clotting factors)

Type of test Blood

Normal findings

Factor	Normal value (% of "normal")
II	80–120
V	50–150
VII	65–140
VIII	55–145
IX	60–140
X	45–155
XI	65–135
XII	50–150

Test explanation and related physiology

These tests measure the quantity of each specific factor thought to be responsible for suspected defects in hemostasis. Testing is available to measure the quantity of the factors listed in the normal findings section. When these factors exist in concentrations below their *minimal hemostatic levels*, clotting is impaired. Deficiencies of these factors may be a result of inherited genetic defects, acquired diseases, or drug therapy. Common medical conditions associated with abnormal factor concentrations are listed in Table C4.

The hemostasis and coagulation system is a homeostatic balance between factors encouraging clotting and those encouraging clot dissolution (Figure C3, p. 212). See Table C5, p. 213 for a list of factor names and routine coagulation test abnormalities associated with factor deficiency.

Fibrinogen (or factor I; p. 346), like many of the coagulation proteins, is considered an acute reactant protein and is elevated in many severe illnesses. It is also considered a risk factor for coronary heart disease and stroke.

Prothrombin is a vitamin K-dependent clotting factor. Its production in the liver requires vitamin K. This vitamin is fat soluble and is dependent on bile for absorption.

Factor VIII is actually a complex molecule with two components. The first component is related to hemophilia A and is involved in the hemostatic mechanism. The second component is von Willebrand factor and is related to von Willebrand disease. *Von Willebrand Disease gene (VWF gene)* detects pathogenic alterations within the *VWF* gene to delineate the underlying molecular defect in a patient

TABLE C4 **Conditions that may result in coagulation factor excess or deficiency**

Factor	Increased (excess)	Decreased (deficiency)
I (Fibrinogen)	Acute inflammatory reactions Trauma Coronary heart disease Cigarette smoking	Liver disease (hepatitis or cirrhosis) DIC Congenital deficiency
II (Prothrombin)	ND	Vitamin K deficiency Liver disease Congenital deficiency Warfarin ingestion
V (Proaccelerin)	ND	Liver disease DIC Fibrinolysis
VII (Proconvertin [stable factor])	ND	Congenital deficiency Vitamin K deficiency Liver disease Warfarin ingestion
VIII (Antihemophilic factor)	Acute inflammatory reactions Trauma or stress Pregnancy Birth control pills	Congenital deficiency (e.g., hemophilia A) DIC
von Willebrand factor	ND	Congenital deficiency (e.g., von Willebrand disease) Some myeloproliferative disorders
IX (Christmas factor)	ND	Congenital deficiency (e.g., hemophilia B) Liver disease Nephrotic syndrome Warfarin ingestion DIC Vitamin K deficiency

TABLE C4 Conditions that may result in coagulation factor excess or deficiency—cont'd

Factor	Increased (excess)	Decreased (deficiency)
X (Stuart factor)	ND	Congenital deficiency Liver disease Warfarin ingestion Vitamin K deficiency
XII (Hageman factor)	ND	Congenital deficiency Liver disease DIC

DIC, Disseminated intravascular coagulation; *ND,* there is no common disease state known to be associated with an excess of this factor.

with a laboratory diagnosis of von Willebrand disease (VWD). This second component is involved in platelet adhesion and aggregation.

Coagulation factor inhibitors arise in patients who are congenitally deficient in a specific factor in response to factor replacement therapy. They can also occur spontaneously without known cause or in response to a variety of medical conditions, including the postpartum state, immunologic disorders, certain antibiotic therapies, some malignancies, and old age.

In most cases, a factor deficiency can be diagnosed by identifying the mutated gene using next-generation sequencing (NGS). NGS is also helpful in identifying carrier status for close family members of an individual with a factor VII deficiency diagnosis.

Interfering factors
- Many of these proteins are heat sensitive, and levels are decreased if the specimen is kept at room temperature.
- Pregnancy or the use of contraceptive medication can increase levels of several of these factors, especially VIII and IX.
- Many of these protein coagulation factors are *acute reactant* proteins. Acute illness, stress, exercise, or inflammation can raise levels.

Procedure and patient care
- See inside front cover for Routine Blood Testing.
- Fasting: no
- Blood tube commonly used: blue

Abnormal findings
See Table C4

notes

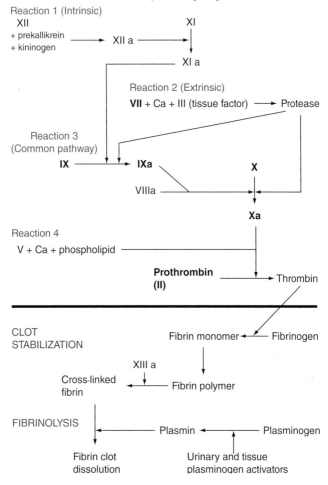

FIG. C3 Secondary hemostasis (fibrin clot formation) and fibrinolysis (fibrin clot dissolution). Primary hemostasis involves platelet plugging of the injured blood vessel. Secondary hemostasis, as described here, takes place most rapidly on the platelet surface after attachment to the fractured endothelium. Four different reactions result in the formation of fibrin. As seen beneath the dark line in the figure, the fibrin clot supports the platelet clump so that the clot does not get swept away by the tremendous shear forces of the fast-moving blood cells. Fibrinolysis follows formation of the fibrin clot in order to prevent complete occlusion of the injured blood vessel.

TABLE C5 List of minimum concentration of coagulation factors required for fibrin production[a]

Factor	Name	Quantitation of minimum hemostatic level (mg/dL)	Abnormal coagulation tests associated with deficiency	Blood components to provide specific factor
I	Fibrinogen	60–100	PT, APTT	C, FFP, FWB
II	Prothrombin	10–15	PT	P, WB, FFP, FWB
III	Tissue factor or thromboplastin	Not applicable	PT	
IV	Calcium	See calcium, p. 159		
V	Proaccelerin	5–10	PT, APTT	FFP, FWB
VII	Stable factor	5–20	PT	P, WB, FFP, FWB
VIII	Antihemophilic factor	30	APTT	C, FFP, VIII CONC
IX	Christmas factor	30	APTT	FFP, FWB
X	Stuart factor	8–10	PT, APTT	P, WB, FFP, FWB
XI	Plasma thromboplastin antecedent	25	APTT	P, WB, FFP, FWB
XII	Hageman factor	Yes	APTT	
XIII	Fibrin stabilizing factor	No		P, C, XIII CONC

[a]Recombinant factors are now available for factor VII, VIII, IX, and XIII. Concentrates are also now available for II, VII, IX, and XIII. APTT, Activated partial thromboplastin time; C, cryoprecipitate; FFP, fresh-frozen plasma; FWB, fresh whole blood (< 24 hours old); P, unfrozen banked plasma; PT, prothrombin time; VIII CONC, factor VIII concentrate; WB, banked whole blood; XIII CONC, factor XIII concentrate.

coagulation profile (Coagulation panel)

The coagulation panel is a screening test for abnormal blood clotting. It examines the factors most often associated with a bleeding problem. Abnormal test results can be followed up with other specific tests to confirm or rule out a diagnosis. These tests are listed below and discussed separately. For accuracy, check the normal values at the lab performing the test.

	Normal values
PT (prothrombin time)/INR (international normalized ratio) (p. 619)	11–12.5 seconds/0.8–1.1
APTT (activated partial thromboplastin time) (p. 557)	30–40 seconds
Platelet count (p. 577)	150,000–400,000/mm³

This screening profile does not address all causes of bleeding tendencies. Other tests to consider include fibrinogen (p. 346), D-dimer (p. 264), coagulation factors (p. 209), and disseminated intravascular coagulation (DIC) screening (p. 275).

Test results are often displayed as shown in Figure C4.

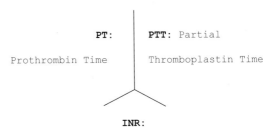

FIG. C4 Coagulation profile test.

cold agglutinins

Type of test Blood

Normal findings

No agglutination in titers $\leq 1:64$

Test explanation and related physiology

Cold agglutinins are antibodies (usually IgM) to erythrocytes. All individuals have circulating antibodies directed against RBCs, but their concentrations are often too low to trigger disease (titers < 1:64). In individuals with *cold agglutinin disease,* these antibodies are in much higher concentrations. At body temperatures of 28° C to 31° C, such as those encountered during winter months, these antibodies can cause a variety of symptoms, from chronic anemia because of intravascular hemolysis or extravascular sequestration of affected RBCs to acrocyanosis of the ears, fingers, or toes because of local blood stasis in the skin capillaries.

There are two forms of cold agglutinin disease: primary and secondary. The primary form has no precipitating cause. Secondary cold agglutinin disease is a result of an underlying condition, notably *Mycoplasma pneumoniae.* Other possible underlying conditions include influenza, mononucleosis, rheumatoid arthritis, lymphomas, HIV, Epstein–Barr virus, and cytomegalovirus. Temperature regulation is important for the performance of these tests. Under no circumstance should the cold agglutinin specimen be refrigerated.

The cold agglutinin screen is performed on all specimens first to identify most of those with titer values in the normal range. If the result is negative, no titration is required. If the result is positive, a titer with serial saline dilutions is performed.

Procedure and patient care

- See inside front cover for Routine Blood Testing.
- Fasting: no
- Blood tube commonly used: red

Abnormal findings

▲ **Increased levels**

Cirrhosis
Infectious mononucleosis
Influenza
Lymphoma
Multiple myeloma
Mycoplasma pneumoniae infection
Primary cold agglutinin disease
Rheumatoid arthritis
Scleroderma
Staphylococcemia
Systemic lupus erythematosus
Thymic tumor
Viral illness

notes

colonoscopy, sigmoidoscopy, proctoscopy, anoscopy

C

Type of test   Endoscopy

Normal findings

Normal anus, rectum, colon, and distal small bowel

Test explanation and related physiology

With fiberoptic colonoscopy, the entire colon from anus to cecum (and often a portion of terminal ileum) can be examined in most patients. *Anoscopy* refers to examination of the anus; *proctoscopy* to examination of the anus and rectum; and *sigmoidoscopy* to examination of the anus, rectum, and sigmoid colon. Sigmoidoscopy can be performed with a rigid ($\leq$ 25 cm from the anus) or flexible ($\leq$ 60 cm from the anus) sigmoidoscope.

Benign and malignant neoplasms, polyps, mucosal inflammation, ulceration, and sites of active hemorrhage can be visualized. Such diseases as cancer, polyps, ulcers, and arteriovenous (AV) malformations also can be visualized. Cancers, polyps, and inflammatory bowel diseases can be biopsied through the scope with cable-activated instruments; sites of active bleeding can be coagulated with the use of laser, electrocoagulation, and injection of sclerosing agents.

This test is recommended for patients who have Hemoccult-positive stools, abnormal sigmoidoscopy, lower GI tract bleeding, abdominal pain, or a change in bowel habits. Colonoscopy is also used for colorectal screening in asymptomatic patients without increased risks for cancer. The U.S. Preventive Services Task Force (USPSTF) recommends screening for colorectal cancer using high-sensitivity fecal occult blood testing, sigmoidoscopy, or colonoscopy beginning at age 45 years and continuing until age 75 years. For patients over 75 years, overall health and patient preference is considered. Virtual colonoscopy is now an option (p. 232).

Contraindications

- Patients whose medical condition is not stable
- Patients who are bleeding profusely from the rectum. The viewing lens will become covered with blood clots.
- Patients with a suspected perforation of the colon
- Patients with toxic megacolon. These patients may worsen with the test preparation.

- Patients with a recent colon anastomosis (within the past 14–21 days). The anastomosis may break down with significant insufflation of CO_2.

Potential complications

- Bowel perforation
- Persistent bleeding from a biopsy site
- Oversedation, resulting in respiratory depression

Interfering factors

- Poor bowel preparation may result in stool obstructing the lens and precluding adequate visualization of the colon.
- Active bleeding obstructs the lens system and precludes adequate visualization of the colon.

Procedure and patient care

Before

PT Explain the procedure to the patient.

PT Fully inform the patient about the risks of the procedure and obtain an informed consent.

PT Assure patients that they will be appropriately draped to avoid unnecessary embarrassment.

PT Instruct the patient on appropriate bowel preparation.

A typical preparation for *colonoscopy* may be as follows:

- *7 days before testing*
  - Aspirin or NSAIDs may be continued. But doctors must provide specific instructions for continuing blood thinners.
- *3 days before testing:*
  - Stop eating all nuts, seeds, and popcorn.
- *1 day before testing:*
  - Begin a clear liquid diet. Drink at least 8 glasses of water during the day to avoid dehydration.
  - At noon, take 3–4 Dulcolax tablets.
  - Mix the prescribed solution for bowel cleansing. Usually, this is a hypertonic polyethylene glycol with sodium - phosphate, picosulfate, or sulfate based solution.
  - Begin drinking the prescribied solution about 4–6 PM. Continue drinking one 8-oz glass every 15 minutes thereafter until the mixture is gone.
    - PT Instruct the patient to not drink anything colored red, orange, green, or blue because they may interrupt in interpretation and visualization of the intestines.

- A typical preparation for *sigmoidoscopy* is less severe and may be as follows:
  - Administer a Fleet enema in the morning of the test.
  - A light breakfast may be ingested.
- Oral tablets containing sodium sulfate, magnesium sulfate, or sodium phosphate diminish the volume required for bowel cleansing.

During

- Note the following procedural steps for a *colonoscopy*:
  1. IV access is obtained for anesthesia. Usually, Propofol is given.
  2. After a rectal examination indicates adequate bowel preparation, the patient is sedated.
  3. The patient is placed in the lateral decubitus position, and the colonoscope is placed into the rectum.
  4. Under direct visualization, the colonoscope is directed to the cecum. Often a significant amount of manipulation is required to obtain this position.
  5. As in all endoscopies, air is insufflated to distend the bowel for better visualization.
  6. Complete examination of the large bowel is carried out.
  7. Polypectomy, biopsy, and other endoscopic surgery is performed after appropriate visualization.
  8. When the laser or coagulator is used, the air is removed, and carbon dioxide is used as an insufflating agent to avoid explosion.
- Note the following procedural steps for a *sigmoidoscopy*:
  1. The patient is placed on the endoscopy table or bed in the left lateral decubitus position.
  2. Usually no sedation is required.
  3. The anus is mildly dilated with a well-lubricated finger.
  4. The rigid or flexible sigmoidoscope is placed into the rectum and advanced.
  5. Air is insufflated during the procedure to distend more fully the lower intestinal tract.
  6. The sigmoid, rectum, and anus are visualized.
  7. Biopsies can be obtained and polyps can be removed.

After

- PT Explain to the patient that air has been insufflated into the bowel. She or he may experience flatulence or gas pains.
- Examine the abdomen for evidence of colon perforation (abdominal distention, tenderness, fever, and chills).

- Monitor vital signs for a decrease in blood pressure and an increase in pulse as an indication of hemorrhage.
- Inspect the stool for gross blood.
- Notify the physician if the patient develops increased pain or significant GI bleeding.
- Allow the patient to eat when fully alert if no evidence of bowel perforation exists.
- PT Encourage the patient to drink a lot of fluids when intake is allowed. This will make up for the dehydration associated with the bowel preparation.
- PT Inform the patient that frequent, bloody bowel movements may indicate poor hemostasis after biopsy or polypectomy.
- PT Educate the patient to report abdominal bloating and inability to pass flatus, which may indicate colon obstruction if a neoplasm was identified.
- PT Assess the patient for and educate to report weakness and dizziness, which may indicate orthostasis and hypovolemia caused by dehydration.

Abnormal findings

Arteriovenous malformations
Colorectal cancer
Diverticulosis
Hemorrhoids
Inflammatory bowel disease (e.g., ulcerative or Crohn colitis)
Ischemic or postinflammatory strictures
Polyps
Tumors (benign or malignant)

notes

colorectal cancer tumor analysis (Microsatellite instability [MSI] testing, DNA mismatch repair [MMR] genetic testing, BRAF mutation analysis, Oncotype DX colon cancer assay)

Type of test Microscopic examination

Normal findings

Recurrence score < 10
No mismatch repair gene
No microsatellite instability

Test explanation and related physiology

The prognosis of patients with colorectal cancer (CRC) is primarily determined by the stage of the cancer. However, within each stage, the recurrence rate varies considerably. Colorectal tumor analysis/genomic testing can help determine prognosis within these large variations. This information can also be helpful in determining if additional therapy is helpful after surgery. Tumor analysis is used to indicate responsiveness to particular anti-cancer drugs. And finally, with the use of tumor molecular genetic analysis, genetic patterns can be determined and indicated whether a CRC is sporadic or familial (Lynch syndrome, etc.). This analysis is different than genetic testing for the identification of genetic alterations that cause familial CRC (p. 372). Furthermore, this analysis is somewhat different than the information provided by genomic testing of the particular genes of CRC tumor as described on p. 377. Here, these genes and the proteins whose synthesis they direct are discussed separately.

Deficiencies in DNA mismatch repair (MMR) gene function (because of either decreased gene expression or mutation) result in the accumulation of DNA alterations that can manifest as abnormal shortening or lengthening of microsatellite DNA sequences in the colon cancer cell. This causes microsatellite instability (MSI) and ultimately leads to the development of CRC. Patients with MMR-deficient (MMR-D) colon tumors have high MSI and have been shown to have significantly lower colon cancer recurrence risk. There are other MMR genes (MSH2, MSH6, and PMS2) that more rarely occur in CRC. Furthermore, hereditary colon cancers frequently are positive for MSI compared with sporadic colon cancers. Lynch syndrome (a hereditary form of colon cancer) can be suspected if the tumor is MSI positive.

Another important process in the development of CRC is chromosomal instability of the tumor cell. APC, TP53, KRAS, and NRAS are some of the mutations that occur in this pathway. KRAS and NRAS may indicate responsiveness to anti-EGFR therapy.

BRAF is another important tumor gene that is used to indicate the likelihood that a colon tumor is hereditary. The presence of a *BRAF* V600E mutation in a microsatellite unstable tumor indicates that the tumor is probably sporadic and not associated with hereditary nonpolyposis colorectal cancer (HNPCC).

BRAF is an important genetic mutation in other cancer cells such as melanoma, papillary thyroid cancer, hairy-cell leukemia, lung cancer, and other B-cell lymphomas. *BRAF* mutation may be associated with increased risk of recurrence, lymph node metastases, and advanced-stage cancer. Drugs that are BRAF inhibitors are specifically and successfully used on tumors that exhibit BRAF. Thus identifying *BRAF* mutations may be of critical therapeutic importance. *BRAF p.V600* mutations have shorter progression-free survival and overall survival. Other possible predictor markers that can be identified on the tumor include PIK3CA and TP53.

Procedure and patient care

Before

PT Inform the patient detection of these predictor markers may be performed on their colon cancer tissue.

PT Provide psychological and emotional support.

During

• The surgeon obtains tumor tissue.
• This tissue should be placed on ice or in formalin.
• Part of the tissue is used for routine histology. A portion of the paraffin block is sent to a reference laboratory.

After

PT Explain that results are usually available in 1 week.

Abnormal findings

Unfavorable test results indicating a high risk of cancer reoccurrence

notes

colposcopy

Type of test Endoscopy

Normal findings

Normal vagina and cervix

Test explanation and related physiology

Colposcopy provides an *in situ* microscope examination of the vagina and cervix with a *colposcope*, which is a microscope with a light source and a magnifying lens (Figure C5). With this procedure, tiny areas of dysplasia, carcinoma *in situ* (CIN), and invasive cancer that would be missed by the naked eye can be visualized, and biopsy specimens can be obtained. The study is performed on patients with abnormal vaginal epithelial patterns,

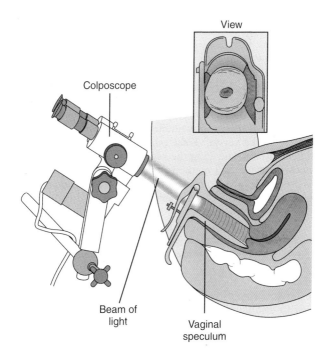

FIG. C5 Colposcopy. A colposcope is used to evaluate patients with an abnormal Pap smear and a grossly normal cervix.

cervical lesions, abnormal Pap smears, or positive HPV results and on those exposed to diethylstilbestrol *in utero*. This procedure is used to determine the need for cone biopsy.

It is important to realize that colposcopy is useful only in identifying a suspicious lesion. Definitive diagnosis requires biopsy of the tissue. One of the major advantages of this procedure is the capability of directing the biopsy to the area most likely to be truly representative of the lesion. A biopsy performed without colposcopy may not be representative of the lesion's pathology.

The patient will need to have diagnostic conization if

- Colposcopy and endocervical curettage do not explain the problem or match the cytologic findings of the Pap smear within one grade.
- The entire transformation zone is not seen.
- The lesion extends beyond the vision of the colposcope.

Endocervical curettage or brushings may accompany colposcopy to detect unknown lesions.

There are other promising methods to examine the cervix for neoplasm. *Cervicography* is a procedure in which the cervix is swabbed with an acetic acid solution to identify acetowhite changes in the cervix. A photograph of the cervix is taken with a special camera (Cerviscope) and is sent for imaging analysis for the presence of atypia or metaplasia, intraepithelial neoplasia, or cancer. *Speculoscopy* (PapSure) uses a chemiluminescent light to aid naked-eye or magnified visualization of acetowhite changes on the cervix. *Video colpography* (video colposcopy) has been used for imaging the vagina and cervix and has been proposed for use as a method of cervical cancer screening. In this procedure, a video camera is used to create computerized digital images of the cervix, vaginal fornices, and endocervical canal. Video colpography may be used in teaching, auditing, and screening of women with low-grade Pap smear abnormalities. *Spectroscopy* optical cervical imaging system is used as an adjunct to colposcopy to identify areas of the cervix with the highest likelihood of high-grade CIN on biopsy. Spectroscopy shines a light on the cervix and analyzes how different areas of the cervix respond to the light. The system produces a color map that distinguishes between healthy and potentially diseased tissue.

Finally, there are newer methods of gene identification using methylation markers and qualitative fluorescence *in situ* hybridization (FISH) methods to identify abnormal genes associated with early markers of neoplastic cervical disease.

Contraindications
- Patients with heavy menstrual flow

Interfering factors
- Failure to cleanse the cervix of foreign materials (e.g., creams, medications) may impair visualization.

Procedure and patient care

Before
PT Explain the procedure to the patient.
- Obtain informed consent if required by the institution.

During
- Note the following procedural steps:
  1. The patient is placed in the lithotomy position, and a vaginal speculum is used to expose the vagina and cervix.
  2. The cervix is cleansed with a 3% acetic acid solution to remove excess mucus and cellular debris. The acetic acid also accentuates the difference between normal and abnormal epithelial tissues.
  3. An aggressive ecto-endocervical Pap smear using curettage is then performed.
  4. The colposcope is focused on the cervix, which is then carefully examined.
  5. Usually the entire lesion can be outlined and the most atypical areas selected for biopsy specimen removal.
- Note that colposcopy is performed by a physician, nurse practitioner, or physician's assistant in approximately 5 to 10 minutes.
PT Tell the patient that some women complain of pressure pains from the vaginal speculum and that momentary discomfort may be felt if biopsy specimens are obtained.

After
PT Inform the patient that she may have vaginal bleeding if biopsy specimens were taken.
PT Instruct the patient to abstain from intercourse and to not insert anything (except a tampon) into the vagina until healing of a biopsy is confirmed.
PT Inform the patient about how to obtain test results.

Abnormal findings
Carcinoma *in situ*
Cervical lesions
Dysplasia
Invasive cancer

notes

complement assay (Total, C3 and C4 complement)

Type of test Blood

Normal findings

Total complement: 30–75 units/mL
C3: 75–175 mg/dL
C4: 22–45 units/mL

Test explanation and related physiology

Measurements of complement are used primarily to diagnose hereditary and acquired deficiencies of complement peptides and to monitor the activity of infectious or autoimmune diseases (e.g., systemic lupus erythematosus, nephritis, membranoproliferative nephritis, poststreptococcal nephritis).

Serum complement is a group of 31 proteins that act as enzymes, cofactors, inhibitors, and membrane-integrated proteins. These effect a cascade-like series of reactions that lead to the synthesis of a group of proteins that facilitate the immunologic and inflammatory responses.

Reduced complement levels can be congenital or acquired. As the complement system is activated, the complement components are consumed or used up. If the system is persistently or overly activated, serum levels can fall. The complement system is instigated by the presence of antibody–antigen complexes.

The total complement assay should be used as a screen for suspected complement-related diseases before ordering individual complement component assays. For a list of common diseases associated with complement abnormalities, see Table C6. Note, however, that this list is not complete.

Complement levels can also be measured in other bodily fluids such as pleural, pericardial, and synovial fluids. Low fluid complement levels are characteristic of effusions from patients with rheumatoid arthritis (despite elevated serum levels), systemic lupus erythematosus, and bacterial infections.

Procedure and patient care

- See inside front cover for Routine Blood Testing.
- Fasting: no
- Blood tube commonly used: red

TABLE C6   Diseases associated with complement deficiencies

Complement deficiency	Associated disease
C1q	Recurrent bacterial infection
C1r	Discoid lupus, glomerulonephritis
C1s	Systemic lupus
C1–INH	Hereditary angioedema
C1	Autoimmune diseases, hypogammaglobulinemia
C2	Lupus, glomerulonephritis, recurrent bacterial infections
C3	Recurrent bacterial infections
C4	Systemic lupus
C5	Systemic lupus, recurrent infections, *Neisseria* infection
C6	*Neisseria* infections
C7	Scleroderma, *Neisseria* infections, rheumatoid arthritis
C8	*Neisseria* infections
C9	*Neisseria* infections

Abnormal findings

▲ Increased levels
- Cancer
- Myocardial infarction (acute)
- Rheumatic fever (acute)
- Ulcerative colitis

▼ Decreased levels
- Anemia
- Autoimmune disease
- Cirrhosis
- Glomerulonephritis
- Hepatitis
- Lupus nephritis
- Malnutrition
- Protein malnutrition
- Renal transplant rejection
- Rheumatoid arthritis
- Serum sickness
- Severe sepsis
- Sjögren syndrome

notes

complete blood count and differential count (CBC and diff)

The CBC and differential count are a series of tests of the peripheral blood; they provide a tremendous amount of information about the hematologic system and many other organ systems. These tests are inexpensively, easily, and rapidly performed as a screening test. The CBC and differential count include automated measurement of the following studies, which are discussed separately:

RBC count (p. 631)
Hemoglobin (Hgb; p. 409)
Hematocrit (Hct; p. 406)
Blood smear (p. 128)
Platelet count (p. 577)
Platelet volume, mean (MPV) (p. 582)
RBC indices (p. 633)
    Mean corpuscular volume (MCV)
    Mean corpuscular hemoglobin (MCH)
    Mean corpuscular hemoglobin concentration (MCHC)
    Red blood cell distribution width (RDW)
WBC count and differential count (p. 809)
    Neutrophils (polymorphonuclear leukocytes or *polys*, segmented cells or *segs*, band cells, stab cells)
    Lymphocytes
    Monocytes
    Eosinophils
    Basophils

notes

comprehensive metabolic panel (CMP, Chem 12, Chemistry panel, SMA 12 (Sequential Multiple Analysis), SMA 20

The CMP is a broad screening tool used to evaluate organ function and to check for conditions such as liver disease, kidney disease, and diabetes. It is valuable for monitoring known conditions, such as hypertension, and for monitoring kidney- and liver-related side effects of medications. The CMP is often part of the blood workup for medical examinations or yearly physical examinations. Depending on the reason for the test, blood may be drawn after fasting or on a random basis. Abnormal test results can be followed up with other specific tests to rule out or confirm a suspected diagnosis. These tests are listed below and are discussed separately. Sample normal values are shown. For accuracy, use ranges from the lab performing the test.

	Normal values
Electrolytes	
Sodium (p. 676)	136–145 mEq/L
Potassium (p. 595)	3.5–5 mEq/L
Chloride (p. 196)	98–106 mEq/L
CO_2 (carbon dioxide, HCO_3; p. 167)	23–30 mEq/L
Calcium, total (p. 159)	9–10.5 mg/dL
Glucose	
Glucose (p. 386)	74–106 mg/dL
Kidney tests	
BUN (blood urea nitrogen; p. 134)	10–20 mg/dL
Creatine (p. 249)	0.5–1.1 mg/dL
Liver tests	
ALP (alkaline phosphatase; p. 23)	30–120 U/L
ALT (alanine aminotransferase; p. 16)	4–36 U/L
AST (aspartate aminotransferase; p. 105)	0–35 U/L
Albumin (p. 613)	3.5–5 g/dL
Total protein (p. 613)	6.4–8.3 g/dL
Bilirubin (p. 118)	
Total	0.3–1 mg/dL
Direct	0.1–0.3 mg/dL

Test results are often displayed as illustrated below in Figure C6.

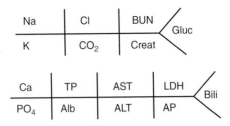

FIG. C6 Comprehensive metabolic panel.

C

computed tomography (CT scan abdomen, angiography, chest, extremity, head, heart, neck, spine)

Type of test X-ray with or without contrast

Normal findings

No evidence of abnormality

Test explanation and related physiology

CT scans can be performed on every region of the body for diagnostic, treatment planning, interventional procedures, or screening purposes. CT scans can detect traumatic injury, tumors, cysts, fluid collections, abscesses, infection, inflammation, perforation, bleeding, obstruction, emboli, thrombosis, aneurysms, vascular narrowing/occlusion, and calculi. Hundreds of individual images of an anatomic region can be obtained.

Helical CT scan (also called *spiral CT scan* or *volume-averaging CT scan*) can obtain images in a three-dimensional real-time display of the data that allows the interpreter to quickly visualize and analyze the data anatomically. *Multislice CT* scan or *multidetector CT scan* allows even more slices to be imaged in an even shorter period. The entire scan takes slightly more than a few minutes with a few breath holds. With thin slices and rapid accession, breathing and motion distortion are minimized producing more accurate images. *Fusion CT/positron emission tomography (PET) scans* are used to add anatomic information to the physiologic information obtained by a PET scan (p. 589). This allows the scan to locate pathology and to indicate whether it is benign or malignant. With computerized digital subtraction techniques, tissues obstructing anatomic areas are eliminated from views.

CT scans are commonly used in treatment planning for radiation therapy. The volume of radiation dose and its path can be determined to minimize side effects of radiation. CT scans may be repeated frequently to monitor the progress of any disease or to monitor the healing process. CT scan can be used to perform interventional procedures like image-directed biopsies of solid tumors or aspiration of fluid collections. CT scan has been expanded to the whole body to assist pathologists, coroners, and medical examiners to investigate cadavers for clues as to the cause of death. This is termed *virtual autopsy*.

CT scan may use a contrast agent. The contrast (usually an iodinated dye) may be injected into a vein or body cavity or given by mouth or by enema (usually barium or air). The contrast dye highlights specific areas and improves image quality. There are concerns for patients receiving iodinated IV contrast regarding allergic reaction, kidney injury, and lactic acidosis. See p. 231 regarding these concerns.

CT Scan of the Abdomen and Pelvis

The *CT scan of the abdomen/pelvis (abdominal CT)* is used to diagnose pathologic conditions of the abdominal and retroperitoneal organs. CT scans can be used as a guide to aspirate fluid from the abdomen or to guide biopsy needles. Catheters for draining intraabdominal abscesses can be placed with CT guidance as well. CT scans can be used to stage and monitor tumors before and after therapy. *Virtual colonoscopy* (*CT colonography*) uses a CT scanner and virtual reality software to look inside the colon without inserting a colonoscope (for conventional colonoscopy, see p. 217). *Virtual enteroscopy (CT enterography)* is used to examine the lumen of the small intestines. No sedation is required, and no discomfort is experienced. Patients need a cleansing bowel preparation before the test. Of course, polypectomy or biopsy cannot be performed with virtual testing. If abnormalities are found with virtual colonoscopy, conventional colonoscopy is needed.

CT urography or CT nephrotomography is designed to identify ureteral stones and can be performed with very little radiation exposure.

CT Angiography

Computerized tomography angiography (CTA) or CT angiography provides visualization of blood vessels. Major arteries and veins and even smaller vessels in a particular organ can be displayed after IV injection of contrast. CTA is commonly ordered for a variety of reasons, such as:

- CTA of the head and neck to detect cerebral aneurysm, carotid artery dissection, strokes, etc.
- CTA of the abdomen and pelvis for locating gastrointestinal bleeding, to detect mesenteric ischemia, renal artery stenosis, and hepatic vasculature for cancer-related resections. *Renal CTA* is used to demonstrate and evaluate each functional phase of urinary excretion. This is also called *dynamic CT scanning.*
- CTA of the chest to rule out pulmonary embolism, aortic dissection, and trauma
- CTA of the extremity to rule out arterial occlusion

- CTA of the coronary vessels. See below for CT scan of the heart for discussion on this topic.

CT Scan of the Chest

CT of the chest (chest CT) provides very accurate images of the heart, lungs, chest wall, pleura, esophagus, great vessels, and soft tissue. *Virtual bronchoscopy* and *virtual esophagoscopy* may increasingly be used in place of their endoscopic counterparts. *Low-dose CT (LDCT)* of the chest is used as a screening test for lung cancer. Adults aged 50–80 years who have a 20 pack-year smoking history and currently smoke or have quit within the past 15 years can benefit through early detection of lung cancer.

CT Scan of the Extremity

CT scan of the extremity is a study of the upper or lower extremities. Anatomic images of bones, muscle, soft tissue, and blood vessels are evaluated. It may evaluate swelling, pain, trauma, a mass, infection, or a questionable fracture in the extremity (shoulder, wrist, hands, fingers, hip, knee, ankle, or foot). These images are far more detailed than those done by conventional x-rays.

CT Scan of the Head

CT of the head provides examination of the cranial contents and soft tissues of the head. The CT scan is used in the differential diagnosis of intracranial neoplasms, cerebral infarctions, ventricular displacement or enlargement, cortical atrophy, cerebral aneurysms, intracranial hemorrhage and hematoma, and AV malformation. Information about the ventricular system is also evaluated. Multiple sclerosis and other degenerative abnormalities can be identified also. In most cases, CT scanning has eliminated the need for more invasive procedures, such as cerebral arteriography and pneumoencephalography. MRI brain scanning (p. 151) can provide more and different information in some instances and may be used in place of or in addition to CT scanning. However, CT scan of the head is more available in emergency situations than MRI.

CT Scan of the Heart

CT scan of the heart is used to help stratify patients according to risks of future cardiac events, to instigate preventive medicinal interventions (e.g., statin drugs), to monitor progression of coronary vascular disease, to evaluate chest pain, and to indicate the need for stress testing or coronary angiography. The entire heart can be scanned in

10 seconds with one breath hold. The scanner can allow routine cardiac gating that synchronizes the scanning with each heartbeat, thereby eliminating motion distortion.

Cardiac CT provides evaluation of the myocardium, cardiac chambers, cardiac valves, coronary arteries, and great vessels. Calcified atheromatous plaques can be seen and quantified (*calcium score* or *Agatston score*) with this study. Coronary calcium is a surrogate marker for coronary atherosclerotic plaque. Patients with Agatston scores above 400 have an increased incidence of coronary procedures (bypass, stent placement, angioplasty) and cardiac events (myocardial infarction and cardiac death) within 2 to 5 years after the test.

Coronary CT angiography (CCTA) can accurately visualize coronary artery lumen after IV injection of a contrast agent. This test is especially useful for patients who experience chest pain but have a low probability of coronary vascular disease. It can provide information regarding the patency of the coronary vessels. *Fractional flow reserve (FFR)* (i.e. measurement of the ratio between the maximum achievable blood flow in a diseased coronary artery and the theoretical maximum flow in a normal coronary artery) can determine the hemodynamic relevance of any changes.

CT Scan of the Neck

CT scan of the neck visualizes the soft tissue and organs of the neck, including the muscles, throat, tonsils, adenoids, airways, thyroid, parathyroids, and other glands. CT of the neck is very useful in the evaluation of penetrating trauma to the neck. Organ injury, vascular injury, and depth of penetration can be determined. Injury to the airway, esophagus, or soft tissue can be seen. Parathyroid tumors can be located to assist in surgical removal. Injury to and degenerative changes of the cervical spine can be evaluated.

CT Scan of the Spine

CT scan of the spine is used to evaluate spinal injuries, spinal anomalies, and tumors. It is also used to evaluate pain, trauma, masses, or questionable fractures in an area of the spine. These images are far more detailed than those done by conventional x-rays and can often diagnose injuries unseen on initial x-ray. Although the spine can be evaluated on other CT scans (e.g., neck, chest, abdomen and pelvis), protocols for CT of the spine improve the diagnostic accuracy of images.

CT is also preferred over magnetic resonance imaging (MRI) for evaluating hardware failure or lack of fusion in patients with indwelling orthopedic hardware from prior surgery. For evaluation of pain, *CT myelography* is performed only when MRI is not available or is contraindicated. However, if cord compression is suspected, CT myelography can be performed emergently.

Contraindications
- Patients who are allergic to iodinated contrast (if contrast is needed.)
- Patients who are pregnant, unless benefits outweigh risks
- Patients whose vital signs are unstable
- Patients who are very obese (usually > 400 lb.)

Potential complications
- Allergic reaction to iodinated contrast. See p. 516.
- Acute renal failure from dye infusion. (If risk outweighs benefit of testing). Adequate hydration before the infusion may reduce this likelihood.
- Lactic acidosis may occur in patients who are taking metformin and receiving iodine contrast.

Interfering factors
- Presence of metallic objects (e.g., hemostasis clips)
- Retained barium from previous studies
- Large amounts of fecal material or gas in the bowel

Procedure and patient care
Before
- PT Explain the procedure. The patient's cooperation is necessary because he or she must lie still during the procedure. See p. xviii for radiation exposure and risks.
- Assess the patient for allergies to iodinated contrast.
- PT Show the patient a pictures of the CT machine because some patients are claustrophobic.
- Keep the patient NPO (nothing by mouth) for at least 4 hours before the test if oral contrast is to be administered; however, this test can be performed on an emergency basis on patients who have recently eaten.
- Note that this procedure is usually performed by a radiologist in less than 30 minutes.
- PT Tell the patient that the discomforts associated with this study include lying still on a hard table and the peripheral venipuncture. Mild nausea is a common sensation when contrast is

used. An emesis basin should be readily available. Some patients may experience a metallic taste, flushing, and warmth during the contrast injection.

During

- Note the following procedural steps for CT scans:
  1. The patient is taken to the radiology department and placed on the CT scan table.
  2. The patient then is placed in an encircling body scanner (gantry). In a separate room, the technologist manipulates the CT scan table to change the level of the area that is scanned.
  3. Through audio communication, the patient is instructed to hold the breath at times of x-ray exposure.

After

PT Encourage the patient to drink fluids to avoid contrast-induced renal injury and to promote excretion of any intravenous dye.

PT Inform the patient that diarrhea may occur after ingestion of the non-barium oral contrast.

- Evaluate the patient for delayed reaction to contrast.

Abnormal findings

Appendicitis
Arthritis
Ascites
Bowel obstruction
Cancer
Cardiac valvular disease
Congenital abnormalities
Coronary vascular congenital
 anomalies
Cysts
Diverticulitis
Fractures
Gallstones
Hemoperitoneum
Hemorrhage
Hemothorax
Hernia
Infection/inflammation

Intestinal perforation
Joint trauma or dislocation
Ligamentous injury
Multiple sclerosis
Pleural effusion
Pneumonia
Pneumothorax
Pulmonary emboli
Rib fracture
Scarring
Soft tissue injury/infection
Trauma
Tumor
Ureteral obstruction
Urologic calculi
Vascular abnormalities
Ventricular displacement/
 enlargement

notes

Coombs test, direct (Direct antiglobulin test [DAT])

Type of test Blood

Normal findings

Negative; no agglutination

Test explanation and related physiology

   This test is performed to identify immune hemolysis (lysis of RBCs) or to investigate hemolytic transfusion reactions. Most of the antibodies to RBCs are directed against the ABO/Rh blood grouping antigens, such as those that occur in hemolytic anemia of the newborn or transfusion of incompatible blood. When a transfusion reaction occurs, the Coombs test can detect the patient's antibodies or complement components coating the transfused RBCs. Therefore the Coombs test is very helpful in evaluating suspected transfusion reactions.

   Non-blood grouping antigens can develop on the RBC membrane and stimulate formation of antibodies. Such drugs as levodopa or penicillin cause this. Also, in autoimmune diseases, antibodies not originally directed against the patient's RBCs can attach to the RBCs and cause hemolysis that is detected by the direct Coombs test. Frequently, the inciting factor for the production of these autoantibodies against RBCs is not associated with any identifiable disease, and the resulting hemolytic anemia is called *idiopathic*.

   The direct Coombs test demonstrates if the patient's RBCs have been attacked by antibodies in the patient's own bloodstream. Coombs serum is a solution containing antibodies to human globulin (antibodies). Coombs serum is mixed with the patient's RBCs. If the RBCs have antibodies on them, agglutination of the patient's RBCs will occur. The greater the quantity of antibodies against RBCs, the more clumping occurs. This test is read as *positive* with clumping on a scale of micropositive to +4. If the RBCs are not coated with autoantibodies against RBCs (immunoglobulins), agglutination will not occur; this is a *negative* test result.

Interfering factors

- Antiphospholipid antibodies (p. 568, anticardiolipin antibodies) can cause false-positive results.

Procedure and patient care

- See inside front cover for Routine Blood Testing.

- Fasting: no
- Blood tube commonly used: red or lavender
- Use venous blood from the umbilical cord to detect the presence of antibodies in the newborn

Abnormal findings

Autoimmune hemolytic anemia
Hemolytic disease of the newborn
Infectious mononucleosis
Lymphoma
Mycoplasmal infection
Systemic lupus erythematosus
Transfusion reaction

notes

C

Coombs test, indirect (Blood antibody screening, Indirect antiglobulin test [IAT])

Type of test Blood

Normal findings

Negative; no agglutination

Test explanation and related physiology

The indirect Coombs test detects circulating antibodies against RBCs. The major purpose of this test is to determine whether the patient has minor serum antibodies (other than the major ABO/Rh system) to RBCs that he or she is about to receive by blood transfusion. Therefore this test is the *screening* part of the *type and screen* routinely performed for blood compatibility testing (cross-matching in the blood bank).

Unlike the direct Coombs test that is performed on the patient's RBCs, this test is performed on the patient's serum. In this test, a small amount of the recipient's serum is added to donor RBCs containing known antigens on their surfaces. This is the first stage. In the second stage of the test, Coombs serum is added. If antibodies exist in the patient's serum, agglutination occurs. In blood transfusion screening, visible agglutination indicates that the recipient has antibodies to the donor's RBCs. If the recipient has no antibodies against the donor's RBCs, agglutination will not occur; transfusion should then proceed safely and without any transfusion reaction.

Procedure and patient care

- See inside front cover for Routine Blood Testing.
- Fasting: no
- Blood tube commonly used: red

Abnormal findings

Acquired immune hemolytic anemia
Hemolytic disease of the newborn
Incompatible cross-matched blood
Maternal anti-Rh antibodies
Presence of specific cold agglutinin antibody

notes

corticotropin-releasing hormone stimulation test (CRH stimulation test)

Type of test Blood

Normal findings

Increased response to CRH

Test explanation and related physiology

This test is used to differentiate Cushing disease (caused by an ACTH-producing pituitary adenoma) from Cushing syndrome, which has other adrenal causes. CRH and ACTH hormone secretion is part of a well-developed feedback mechanism dependent on the plasma cortisol levels. As plasma cortisol levels increase, CRH and ACTH secretion is suppressed; as cortisol levels decrease, CRH and ACTH secretion is stimulated. In patients with Cushing disease, ACTH and cortisol levels will increase with CRH administration. However, with less than a 50% increase in ACTH, or less than a 20% increase in cortisol, other adrenal causes of Cushing syndrome are suspected.

Procedure and patient care

Before

PT Explain the procedure to the patient

PT Instruct the patient to fast for at least 4 hours

• Monitor blood pressure and pulse throughout testing

• Establish intravenous (IV) access

• Draw the pretest blood before administration of CRH

• Blood tube commonly used: Lavender for ACTH, gold for cortisol

During

• Administer CRH 1 mcg/kg by IV, as ordered.

• Obtain ACTH and cortisol blood levels at 15, 30, 45, and 60 minutes after administration of CRH.

After

• Apply pressure or a pressure dressing to the venipuncture site.

Abnormal findings

Cushing disease

Cushing syndrome from adrenal-producing tumor

Cushing syndrome from an ectopic, ACTH-producing tumor

notes

cortisol, blood, urine, saliva (Hydrocortisone, Serum cortisol, Salivary cortisol, Total cortisol, Free cortisol)

Type of test Blood; urine; saliva

Normal findings

Serum

Free cortisol
    8 AM: 0.121–1.065 mcg/dL
Total cortisol:
    Adult/elderly
        8 AM: 5–23 mcg/dL or 138–635 nmol/L (SI units)
        4 PM: 3–13 mcg/dL or 83–359 nmol/L (SI units)
    Child 1–16 years
        8 AM: 3–21 mcg/dL
        4 PM: 3–10 mcg/dL
    Newborn: 1–24 mcg/dL

Urine (24-hour)

Adult/elderly: < 100 mcg/24 hr or < 276 nmol/day (SI units)
Adolescent: 5–55 mcg/24 hr
Child: 2–27 mcg/24 hr

Saliva

7 AM-9 AM: 100–750 ng/dL
3 PM-5 PM: < 401 ng/dL
11 PM-midnight: < 100 ng/dL

Test explanation and related physiology

The best method of evaluating adrenal activity is by directly measuring plasma cortisol levels. Normally, cortisol levels rise and fall during the day; this is called the diurnal variation. Cortisol levels are highest around 6 AM to 8 AM and gradually fall during the day, reaching their lowest point around midnight. High levels of cortisol indicate Cushing syndrome, and low levels of plasma cortisol are suggestive of Addison disease.

For this test, blood is usually collected at 8 AM and again at around 4 PM. The 4 PM value is anticipated to be one-third to two-thirds of the 8 AM value. Normal values may be transposed in individuals who have worked during the night and slept during the day for long periods of time.

The majority of cortisol circulates bound to corticosteroid-binding globulin (CBG) and albumin. Normally, less than 5% of circulating cortisol is free (unbound). Total cortisol includes measurements of free and bound cortisol. The measurement of late-night *salivary cortisol* is another effective test for Cushing syndrome.

Interfering factors
- Pregnancy is associated with increased levels.
- Physical and emotional stress can elevate cortisol levels.
- Variations in protein levels caused by renal or liver disease can affect free cortisol levels.

Procedure and patient care
Before
PT Explain the procedure to the patient to minimize anxiety.
- Assess the patient for signs of physical stress (e.g., infection).

During
Blood
- Collect a venous blood sample in a red-top or green-top tube in the morning after the patient has had a good night's sleep.
- Collect another blood sample at about 4 PM.

Saliva
1. Do not brush teeth before specimen collection.
2. Do not eat or drink for 15 minutes before specimen collection.
3. Collect the specimen between 11 PM and midnight and record the collection time.
4. Collect at least 1.5 mL of saliva in a Salivette as follows:
   a. Place swab directly into mouth by tipping container so that swab falls into mouth. Do not touch swab with fingers.
   b. Keep swab in mouth for approximately 2 minutes. Roll swab in mouth; do not chew swab.
   c. Place swab back into its container without touching and replace the cap.

Urine
PT Instruct the patient how to collect a 24-hour urine. See inside front cover for Routine Urine Testing.
- Keep the collection on ice and use a preservative.

After
- Apply pressure or a pressure dressing to the venipuncture site.

Abnormal findings
▲ **Increased levels**
Adrenal adenoma or carcinoma
Cushing syndrome
Ectopic ACTH-producing tumors
Hyperthyroidism
Obesity
Stress

▼ **Decreased levels**
Addison disease
Congenital adrenal hyperplasia
Hypopituitarism
Hypothyroidism
Liver disease

notes

C-peptide (Connecting peptide insulin, Insulin C-peptide, Proinsulin C-peptide)

Type of test Blood

Normal findings

Fasting: 0.78–1.89 ng/mL or 0.26–0.62 nmol/L (SI units)
1 hour after glucose load: 5–12 ng/mL

Test explanation and related physiology

In general, C-peptide levels correlate with insulin levels in the blood. The capacity of the pancreatic beta cells to secrete insulin can be evaluated by directly measuring either insulin or C-peptide. In most cases, direct measurement of insulin is more accurate. C-peptide levels, however, more accurately reflect islet cell function in the following situations:

- Patients with diabetes who are treated with exogenous insulin and who have antiinsulin antibodies.
- Patients who secretly administer insulin to themselves (factitious hypoglycemia). Insulin levels will be elevated. Direct insulin measurement in these patients tends to be high because the insulin measured is the self-administered exogenous insulin. But C-peptide levels in that same specimen will be low because exogenously administered insulin suppresses endogenous insulin (and C-peptide) production.
- Patients with diabetes who are taking insulin. This is done to see if the patient with diabetes is in remission and may not need exogenous insulin.
- Distinguishing type 1 from type 2 diabetes. This is particularly helpful in people who are newly diagnosed with diabetes. A person whose pancreas does not make any insulin (type 1 diabetes) has low levels of insulin and C-peptide. A person with type 2 diabetes has a normal or high level of C-peptide.

Furthermore, C-peptide is used in evaluating patients who are suspected of having an insulinoma. In patients with an autonomous secreting insulinoma, C-peptide levels are high. C-peptide can also be used to monitor treatment for insulinoma. A rise in C-peptide levels indicates a recurrence or progression of the insulinoma. In the same way, clinicians use C-peptide testing as an indicator of the adequacy of therapeutic surgical pancreatectomy in patients with pancreatic tumors. C-peptide can also be used to diagnose insulin resistance syndrome and to measure beta cell function after glucagon stimulation.

Interfering factors

- Because the majority of C-peptide is degraded in the kidney, renal failure can cause increased levels.

Procedure and patient care

- See inside front cover for Routine Blood Testing.
- Fasting: yes
- Blood tube commonly used: red

Abnormal findings

▲ **Increased levels**

Insulinoma
Pancreas transplant
Renal failure
Type 2 diabetes mellitus

▼ **Decreased levels**

Factitious hypoglycemia
Radical pancreatectomy
Type 1 diabetes mellitus

notes

C-reactive protein test (CRP, High-sensitivity C-reactive protein [hs-CRP], Ultra-sensitive CRP)

Type of test   Blood

Normal findings

< 1.0 mg/dL or < 10 mg/L (SI units)
   Cardiac risk:
     Low: < 1 mg/dL
     Average: 1–3 mg/dL
     High: > 3 mg/dL
hs-CRP: < 3 mg/L

Test explanation and related physiology

CRP is a nonspecific, acute-phase reactant used to diagnose bacterial infectious disease and inflammatory disorders, such as acute rheumatic fever and rheumatoid arthritis. CRP levels do not consistently rise with viral infections. CRP is a protein produced primarily by the liver during an acute inflammatory process and other diseases. A positive test result indicates the presence but not the cause of the disease. The synthesis of CRP is initiated by antigen–immune complexes, bacteria, fungi, and trauma.

The CRP test is a more sensitive and rapidly responding indicator than the erythrocyte sedimentation rate (ESR, p. 306). In an acute inflammatory change, CRP shows an earlier and more intense increase than ESR; with recovery, the disappearance of CRP precedes the return of ESR to normal.

The level of CRP correlates with peak levels of the muscle/brain (MB) isoenzyme of creatine kinase (p. 247), but CRP peaks occur 1 to 3 days later. Failure of CRP to normalize may indicate ongoing damage to the heart tissue. The level of CRP is a stronger predictor of cardiovascular events than the LDL cholesterol level. However, when used together with the lipid profile (in cholesterol, p. 462), it adds prognostic information to that conveyed by the Framingham risk score.

The development of an assay for *high-sensitivity CRP (hs-CRP)* has enabled accurate assays at even low levels. Because of the individual variability in hs-CRP, two separate measurements are required to classify a person's risk level. In patients with stable coronary disease or acute coronary syndromes, hs-CRP measurement may be useful as an independent marker for assessing the likelihood of harmful events, including death, myocardial infarction, or restenosis after percutaneous coronary intervention.

Interfering factors

- Elevated test results can occur in patients with hypertension, elevated body mass index, metabolic syndrome or diabetes mellitus, chronic infection (e.g., gingivitis, bronchitis), chronic inflammation (e.g., rheumatoid arthritis), and low HDL or high triglycerides.
- Cigarette smoking can cause increased levels.
- Decreased test levels can result from moderate alcohol consumption, weight loss, and increased activity/exercise.

Procedure and patient care

- See inside front cover for Routine Blood Testing.
- Fasting: verify with laboratory
- Blood tube commonly used: red

Abnormal findings

▲ **Increased levels**

Acute myocardial infarction
Acute rheumatic fever
Arthritis
Bacterial infection
Bacterial meningitis
Bone marrow transplant rejection
Crohn disease
Kidney transplant rejection
Malignant disease
Postoperative wound infection
Pulmonary infarction
Reiter syndrome
Soft tissue trauma
Systemic lupus erythematosus
Tissue infarction or damage
Tuberculosis
Urinary tract infection
Vasculitis syndrome

notes

creatine kinase (CK, Creatine phosphokinase [CPK])

Type of test Blood

Normal findings

(Varies according to lab and patient statistics)
Total CK: 20–200 U/L

Test explanation and related physiology

Creatine kinase (CK) is an enzyme most commonly used to diagnose and follow muscle disease or injury. Age, gender, race, and physical activity can affect CK. It occurs in three isoenzyme forms (CK-MM, CK-MB, and CK-BB). Skeletal muscle has the highest concentration of CK (> 99% is CK-MM form) of any tissue. Cardiac tissue has the highest concentration of CK-MB, and brain tissue has the highest concentration of CK-BB.

Rhabdomyolysis is a syndrome characterized by muscle necrosis and the release of CK into circulation (mainly CK-MM). CK levels are typically over five times the normal value range, and muscle pain and myoglobinuria may be present. The severity of illness ranges from asymptomatic elevations in serum muscle enzymes to life-threatening disease.

CK-MB for the assessment of acute myocardial infarction (AMI) has largely been replaced by troponins (p. 741). The clinical application of CK-BB is limited. Levels are elevated with injury or disease to either the brain or lungs.

Interfering factors

- IM injections may cause elevated CPK levels.
- Strenuous exercise and recent surgery may cause increases.
- Early pregnancy may cause decreased levels.

Procedure and patient care

- See inside front cover for Routine Blood Testing.
- Fasting: no
- Blood tube commonly used: red or green
- **PT** Discuss with the patient the need and reason for frequent venipuncture in diagnosing myocardial infarction.
- Avoid IM injections, which may falsely elevate the total CK.
- Record the exact time and date of venipuncture.

Abnormal findings

▲ **Increased levels of total CK**
Disease or injury affecting the heart, skeletal muscle, or brain

▲ **Increased levels of CK-BB**
Adenocarcinoma (especially breast and lung)
Disease affecting the central nervous system
Pulmonary infarction

▲ **Increased levels of CK-MB**
Acute myocardial infarction and cardiac ischemia
Cardiac arrhythmias, defibrillation or cardioversion
Cardiac surgery
Extreme exercise
Inflammatory myopathy
Muscular dystrophy

▲ **Increased levels of CK-MM**
Drug-induced myopathies
Electromyography
Exercise
Hypokalemia and hyponatremia
Hypothyroidism
IM injections
Malignant hyperthermia
Muscular dystrophy
Myositis
Neuroleptic malignant syndrome
Recent surgery
Rhabdomyolysis
Seizures and electroconvulsive therapy
Trauma and crush injuries

notes

creatinine, blood (Serum creatinine)

Type of test Blood

Normal findings

Adult:

   Male: 0.6–1.2 mg/dL or 53–106 μmol/L (SI units)
   Female: 0.5–1.1 mg/dL or 44–97 μmol/L (SI units)

Elderly: decrease in muscle mass may cause decreased values

Adolescent: 0.5–1 mg/dL

Child: 0.3–0.7 mg/dL

Infant: 0.2–0.4 mg/dL

Newborn: 0.3–1.2 mg/dL

Possible critical values

> 4 mg/dL (indicates serious impairment in renal function)

Test explanation and related physiology

This test measures the amount of creatinine in the blood. Creatinine is a catabolic product of CPK, which is used in skeletal muscle contraction. The daily production of creatine, and subsequently creatinine, depends on muscle mass, which fluctuates very little. Creatinine, as with BUN (p. 134), is excreted entirely by the kidneys and therefore is directly proportional to renal excretory function. Besides dehydration, only such renal disorders as glomerulonephritis, pyelonephritis, acute tubular necrosis, and urinary obstruction will cause abnormal elevations in creatinine.

The serum creatinine test, as with BUN, is used to diagnose impaired renal function. The creatinine test is used as an approximation of *glomerular filtration rate (GFR)*. The serum creatinine level has much the same significance as the BUN level but tends to rise later. Therefore elevations in creatinine suggest chronicity of the disease process. In general, a doubling of creatinine suggests a 50% reduction in GFR. The creatinine level is interpreted in conjunction with the BUN test. These tests are referred to as *renal function studies*. The BUN/creatinine ratio is a good measurement of kidney and liver function. The normal adult range is 6 to 25, with 15.5 being the optimal adult value for this ratio.

Although serum creatinine is the most commonly used biochemical parameter to estimate GFR in routine practice, there are some shortcomings. Such factors as muscle mass and protein intake can influence serum creatinine, leading to an inaccurate estimation of GFR. On the other hand, *cystatin C*, a protein that is produced at a constant rate by all nucleated cells, is probably a better indicator of GFR. Because of its constant rate of production, its serum concentration is determined only by glomerular filtration. Its level is not influenced by those factors that affect creatinine and BUN.

Cystatin C is a protein that is widely made and distributed throughout the body and exists in plasma. Since it is formed at a constant rate and freely filtered by the healthy kidney, cystatin C is a good marker of renal function. Serum concentrations of cystatin C are almost totally dependent on glomerular filtration rate (GFR). Cystatin C has not been shown to be affected by factors such as muscle mass and nutrition, factors that have been demonstrated to affect creatinine values. In addition, a rise in creatinine does not become evident until the GFR has fallen by approximately 50%. A small reduction in GFR causes a rise in the concentration of cystatin C. Cystatin C is often used as a confirmatory test for the diagnosis of chronic kidney disease (CKD) in patients with a decreased GFR as estimated from creatinine. Increased levels of cystatin C are associated with risk of death and several types of cardiovascular disease. For women, the average reference interval is 0.52 to 0.9 mg/L with a mean of 0.71 mg/L. For men, the average reference interval is 0.56 to 0.98 mg/L with a mean of 0.77 mg/L.

Procedure and patient care

- See inside front cover for Routine Blood Testing.
- Fasting: no
- Blood tube commonly used: red
- For pediatric patients, blood is drawn from a heel stick.

Abnormal findings

▲ **Increased levels**
  Acromegaly
  Acute tubular necrosis
  Diabetic nephropathy
  Gigantism
  Glomerulonephritis
  Nephritis
  Pyelonephritis
  Reduced renal blood flow
    (e.g., shock, dehydration,
    congestive heart failure,
    atherosclerosis)
  Rhabdomyolysis
  Urinary tract obstruction

▼ **Decreased levels**
  Decreased muscle mass
    (e.g., muscular dystrophy,
    myasthenia gravis)
  Debilitation

notes

creatinine clearance (CC, Estimated glomerular filtration rate [eGFR])

Type of test Urine (24-hour); blood

Normal findings

Adult (< 40 years)
>Male: 107–139 mL/min or 1.78–2.32 mL/s (SI units)
>Female: 87–107 mL/min or 1.45–1.78 mL/s (SI units)

Newborn: 40–65 mL/min

Values decrease 6.5 mL/min/decade of life because of decline in GFR.

eGFR: > 60 mL/min/1.73 m^2

Test explanation and related physiology

Creatinine is a catabolic product of creatine phosphate. Creatinine is entirely excreted by the kidneys and therefore is directly proportional to the glomerular filtration rate (GFR; i.e., the number of milliliters filtered by all the nephrons in the kidneys per minute). The creatinine clearance (CC) is a measure of the GFR.

The CC depends on the amount of blood present to be filtered and the ability of the nephron to act as a filter. The amount of blood present for filtration is decreased in renal artery atherosclerosis, dehydration, or shock. The ability of the nephron to act as a filter is decreased by such diseases as glomerulonephritis, acute tubular necrosis, and most other primary renal diseases.

When one kidney becomes diseased, the opposite kidney, if normal, has the ability to compensate by increasing its filtration rate. Therefore with unilateral kidney disease or nephrectomy, a decrease in CC is not expected if the other kidney is normal.

Several nonrenal factors may influence CC. With each decade of age, the CC decreases 6.5 mL/min because of a decrease in the GFR. Urine collections are timed, and incomplete collections will falsely decrease CC. Muscle mass varies among people. Decreased muscle mass will give lower CC values.

The CC test requires a 24-hour urine collection and a serum creatinine level. However, 24-hour urine collections are too time-consuming and expensive for routine clinical use. The GFR can be estimated *(eGFR)* using the Modification of Diet in Renal Disease (MDRD) Study equation. This is an equation that uses the serum creatinine, age, and numbers that vary depending on sex and ethnicity to calculate the GFR with very good accuracy. GFR can also be measured by using Cystatin C instead of Creatinine. See page 251.

The eGFR calculation can be programmed into most laboratory information systems. As a result, chronic renal disease is being recognized more frequently in its early stages. The eGFR can also be used to calculate medication dosage in patients with decreased renal function.

Table C7 shows population estimates for mean (average) eGFR by age. There is no difference between races or sexes when eGFRs are expressed per meter squared body surface area. For diagnostic purposes, most laboratories report eGFR values above 60 as greater than 60 mL/min/1.73 m², not as an exact number.

Interfering factors

- Exercise may cause increased creatinine values.
- Incomplete urine collection may give a falsely lowered value.
- Pregnancy increases CC.
- A diet high in meat can transiently elevate CC.
- The eGFR may be inaccurate in extremes of age and in patients with obesity, severe malnutrition, paraplegia, quadriplegia, or pregnancy.

Procedure and patient care

- See inside front cover for Routine Urine Testing.
- PT Note that some laboratories instruct the patient to avoid cooked meat, tea, coffee, or drugs on the day of the test.
- Make sure a venous blood sample is drawn in a red-top tube during the 24-hour urine collection.

TABLE C7   Mean estimated glomerular filtration rates (eGFRs)

Age (years)	Mean eGFR (mL/min/1.73 m²)
20–29	116
30–39	107
40–49	99
50–59	93
60–69	85
70+	75

Abnormal findings

▲ **Increased levels**
Exercise
High cardiac output syndromes
Pregnancy

▼ **Decreased levels**
Conditions causing decreased GFR (e.g., congestive heart failure, cirrhosis with ascites, shock, dehydration)
Impaired kidney function (e.g., renal artery atherosclerosis, glomerulonephritis, acute tubular necrosis)

notes

cryoglobulin

Type of test   Blood

Normal findings

No cryoglobulins detected

Test explanation and related physiology

Cryoglobulins are abnormal globulin protein complexes that exist in the blood of patients with various diseases. These proteins precipitate reversibly at low temperatures and redissolve with rewarming. They can precipitate in the blood vessels of the fingers when exposed to cold temperatures. This precipitation causes sludging of the blood in those blood vessels. These patients may have symptoms of purpura, arthralgia, or Raynaud phenomenon.

Type I (monoclonal) cryoglobulinemia is associated with monoclonal gammopathy of undetermined significance, macroglobulinemia, or multiple myeloma. Type II (mixed, two or more immunoglobulins of which one is monoclonal) cryoglobulinemia is associated with autoimmune disorders, such as systemic lupus erythematosus, rheumatoid arthritis, and Sjögren syndrome. Type III (polyclonal) cryoglobulinemia is associated with the same disease spectrum as type II cryoglobulinemia.

Procedure and patient care

- See inside front cover for Routine Blood Testing.
- Fasting: verify with laboratory
- Blood tube commonly used: red
- PT Inform the patient that an 8-hour fast may be required.
- PT If cryoglobulins are found to be present, warn the patient to avoid cold temperatures and contact with cold objects to minimize Raynaud symptoms.

Abnormal findings

Acute and chronic infections (e.g., infectious mononucleosis, endocarditis, poststreptococcal glomerulonephritis)

Connective tissue disease (e.g., lupus erythematosus, Sjögren syndrome, rheumatoid arthritis)

Liver disease (e.g., hepatitis, cirrhosis)

Lymphoid malignancies (e.g., multiple myeloma, leukemia, Waldenström macroglobulinemia, lymphoma)

notes

culture and sensitivity (C&S)

Type of test Microscopic examination

Normal findings

Negative

Test explanation and related physiology

Cultures are obtained to determine the presence of pathogens in patients with suspected wound infections.

All cultures should be performed before antibiotic therapy is initiated. Otherwise, the antibiotic may interrupt the growth of the organism in the laboratory. All forms of bacteria are grossly classified by Gram stain: gram positive (blue staining) or gram negative (red staining). Knowledge of the shape of the organism (e.g., spheric, rod shaped) also may be helpful in identification of the infecting organism. With the use of molecular technologies, organisms can be rapidly identified.

Usually 48 to 72 hours is required for growth and identification of the organism. Cultures may be repeated after appropriate antibiotic therapy to assess for complete resolution of the infection. The *sensitivity* of a bacterium to antibiotics can be determined by adding small antibiotic infused discs to the culture to identify bacterial growth inhibition. The amount of inhibition can be quantitated and provide an accurate list of appropriate antibiotics to which the bacteria will be sensitive. Here, again, molecular laboratory technology has allowed sensitivity testing to be available in 2 hours.

Procedure and patient care

Before

PT Explain the procedure to the patient. Here we describe the procedure for a culture of a wound.

During

- Aseptically place a sterile cotton swab into the pus of the patient's wound and then place the swab into a sterile, covered test tube. (Culturing specimens from the skin edge is much less accurate than culturing the suppurative material.)
- If an anaerobic organism is suspected, obtain an anaerobic culture tube from the microbiology laboratory.
- If wound cultures are to be obtained on a patient requiring wound irrigation, obtain the culture before the wound is irrigated.

- If any antibiotic ointment or solution has been previously applied, remove it with sterile water or saline before obtaining the culture.
- Indicate on the laboratory slip any medications the patient may be taking that could affect test results.

C

After

- Transport the specimen to the laboratory immediately after testing.
- Notify the physician of any positive results so that appropriate antibiotic therapy can be initiated.

Abnormal findings

Infection

notes

cystography (Cystogram, Cystourethrography, Voiding cystography, Voiding cystourethrography [VCUG])

Type of test X-ray with contrast

Normal findings

Normal bladder structure and function

Test explanation and related physiology

Filling the bladder with radiopaque contrast material provides visualization of the bladder for radiographic study. Either fluoroscopic or x-ray images demonstrate bladder filling and collapse after emptying. Filling defects or shadows within the bladder indicate primary bladder tumors. Extrinsic compression or distortion of the bladder is seen with pelvic tumor (e.g., rectal, cervical) or hematoma (secondary to pelvic bone fractures). Extravasation of the dye is seen with traumatic rupture, perforation, and fistula of the bladder. Vesicoureteral reflux (abnormal backflow of urine from bladder to ureters), which can cause persistent or recurrent pyelonephritis, also may be demonstrated during cystography.

Contraindications

• Patients with urethral or bladder infection or injury

Procedure and patient care

Before

PT Explain the procedure to the patient. See p. xviii for radiation exposure and risks.

• Obtain informed consent if required by the institution.

• Give clear liquids for breakfast on the morning of the test.

PT Assure the patient that he or she will be draped to prevent unnecessary exposure.

• Insert a Foley catheter if ordered.

During

• Note the following procedural steps:
    1. The patient is taken to the radiology department and placed in a supine or lithotomy position.
    2. Unless the catheter is already present, one is placed.
    3. Through the catheter, approximately 300 mL of air or radiopaque dye (much less for children) is injected into the bladder.
    4. The catheter is clamped.

   5. X-ray images are taken.
   6. If the patient is able to void, the catheter is removed, and
      the patient is asked to urinate while images are taken of the
      bladder and urethra (voiding cystourethrogram).
- Note that a radiologist performs the study in approximately
  15 to 30 minutes.
PT Tell the patient that this test is moderately uncomfortable if
  bladder catheterization is required.

After
- Assess the patient for signs of urinary tract infection.
PT Encourage the patient to drink fluids to eliminate the dye and
  to prevent accumulation of bacteria.

Abnormal findings

Bladder trauma
Bladder tumor
Hematoma
Pelvic tumor
Vesicoureteral reflux

notes

Type of test Endoscopy

Normal findings

Normal structure and function of the urethra, bladder, ureters, and prostate (in males)

Test explanation and related physiology

Cystoscopy provides direct visualization of the urethra and bladder through the transurethral insertion of a cystoscope into the bladder (Figure C7). Cystoscopy is used *diagnostically* to allow

- Direct inspection and biopsy of the prostate, bladder, and urethra
- Collection of a separate urine specimen directly from each kidney by the placement of ureteral catheters

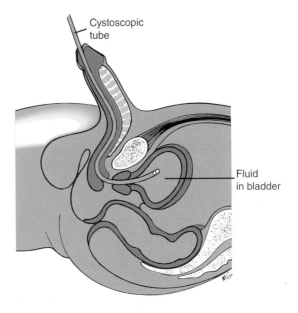

FIG. C7 Cystoscopic examination of the male bladder. The cystoscope is passed through the urethra into the bladder. Although shown here as a flexible scope, usually the scope is rigid. Through the scope, fluid is instilled to maintain bladder distention.

- Measurement of bladder capacity and determination of ureteral reflux
- Identification of bladder and ureteral calculi
- Placement of ureteral catheters (Figure C8) for retrograde pyelography (p. 629)
- Identification of the source of hematuria

Cystoscopy is used *therapeutically* to provide

- Resection of small, superficial bladder tumors
- Removal of foreign bodies and stones
- Dilation of the urethra and ureters
- Placement of stents to drain urine from the renal pelvis
- Coagulation of bleeding areas
- Implantation of radium seeds into a tumor
- Resection of hypertrophied or malignant prostate gland overgrowth
- Placement of ureteral stents during pelvic surgery

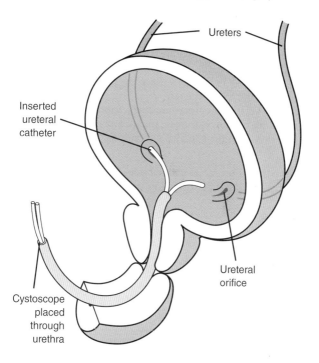

FIG. C8 Ureteral catheterization through the cystoscope. Note the ureteral catheter inserted into the right orifice. The left ureteral catheter is ready to be inserted.

Transendoscopic instruments (e.g., forceps, scissors, needles, electrodes) are used when appropriate.

Potential complications
- Perforation of the bladder
- Sepsis caused by bacteria from infected urine
- Hematuria
- Urinary retention

Procedure and patient care

Before
PT Explain the procedure to the patient.
- Ensure that an informed consent is obtained.
- If enemas are ordered to clear the bowel, assist the patient as needed.
PT Encourage the patient to drink fluids several hours before the procedure to maintain a continuous flow of urine for collection and to prevent multiplication of bacteria.
- If the procedure will be done with the patient under local anesthesia, allow a liquid breakfast.
- If the procedure will be performed under general anesthesia, follow routine precautions. Keep the patient NPO after midnight on the day of the test.
- Administer the preprocedure medications as ordered before the study. Sedatives decrease the spasm of the bladder sphincter, decreasing the patient's discomfort.

During
- Note the following procedural steps:
  1. Cystoscopy is performed in the operating room or in the urologist's office.
  2. The patient is placed in the lithotomy position with his or her feet in stirrups.
  3. The external genitalia are cleansed with an antiseptic.
  4. A local anesthetic is instilled into the urethra if general anesthesia has not been used.
  5. The cystoscope is inserted, and the desired diagnostic or therapeutic studies are performed.
PT Tell the patient that he or she will have the desire to void as the cystoscope passes the bladder neck.
PT When local anesthesia is used, inform the patient of the associated discomfort (more than with urethral catheterization).

After
- Assess the patient's ability to void for at least 24 hours after the procedure. Urinary retention may be secondary to edema caused by instrumentation.
- PT Instruct the patient to note the urine color. Pink-tinged urine is common. The presence of bright red blood or clots should be reported to the physician.
- PT Encourage increased intake of fluids. A dilute urine decreases dysuria. Fluids also maintain a constant flow of urine to prevent stasis and the accumulation of bacteria in the bladder.
- Monitor the patient's vital signs for a decrease in blood pressure and an increase in pulse as an indication of hemorrhage.
- Observe for signs and symptoms of sepsis (elevated temperature, flush, chills, decreased blood pressure, increased pulse).
- PT Note that antibiotics are occasionally ordered before and after the procedure to reduce the incidence of bacteremia that may result from instrumentation.
- PT Instruct the patient to watch for fever, shaking chills, or prolonged dysuria as possible signs of a urinary tract infection.
- PT Encourage the patient to use cathartics, especially after cystoscopic surgery. Increases in intraabdominal pressure caused by constipation may initiate urologic bleeding.
- If postprocedure irrigation is ordered, use an isotonic solution containing mannitol, glycine, or sorbitol to prevent fluid overhydration in the event any of the irrigation is absorbed through opened venous sinuses in the bladder.
- PT If a catheter is left in after the procedure, provide catheter care instructions.

Abnormal findings

Inflammation of the bladder and urethra
Lower urologic tract tumor
Prostate cancer
Prostatic hypertrophy
Prostatitis
Stones in the ureter or bladder
Urethral or ureteral stricture
Vesical neck contracture

notes

cytokines (interleukins)

Type of test Blood

Normal findings

Vary by laboratory and technique

Test explanation and related physiology

Cytokines were renamed as *interleukins* and were numbered by the sequence of discovery. Interleukins, in general, are made up of leukocytes. Lymphokines and monokines are made up of lymphocytes and monocytes, respectively. Other cytokines include *interferon* and *growth factors.*

Some cytokines are produced at increased levels in certain disease states and therefore become markers for disease extent, progression, and response to therapy. They can act as tumor markers in cancers associated with elevated cytokines. *Human interferon inducible protein 10* is an accurate predictor of multiple organ failure.

Clinically, cytokine assays may have the following uses:

- Measurement of AIDS progression
- Measurement of progression of inflammatory diseases
- Tumor markers (e.g., breast cancer, lymphoma, and leukemia)
- Determination of disease risk
- Determination of treatment of disease
- Determination of immune function and response
- Monitoring of patients receiving cytokine therapy or anticytokine therapy
- Determination of degree of inflammation caused by COVID-19

Usually, cytokine testing is performed on serum. However, joint fluid is often tested in the evaluation of the patient with arthritis. Likewise, if inflammatory encephalitis or meningitis is considered, cerebrospinal fluid may be the specimen.

Interfering factors

- Cells can still produce cytokines after specimen collection. It is best to freeze the specimen.

Procedure and patient care

- See inside front cover for Routine Blood Testing.
- Fasting: no
- Blood tube commonly used: red

Abnormal findings

AIDS   Various malignancies
Inflammatory disease

notes

cytolethal distending toxin B (CdtB) and antivinculin antibodies

C

Type of test Blood
Normal findings
1–2.5 titers
Test explanation and related physiology
With no clear pathophysiology, irritable bowel syndrome (IBS) is currently identified through a diagnosis of exclusion. The Rome IV criteria are used to diagnose IBS. These criteria include the following: symptoms of recurrent abdominal pain or discomfort with a marked change in bowel habit for at least 6 months, symptoms on at least 3 days for at least 3 months, and two or more of the following pain descriptions:
- Pain relieved by a bowel movement
- Pain onset linked to a change in frequency of stool
- Pain onset linked to a change in appearance of stool

Patients undergo extensive testing to rule out inflammatory bowel disease (IBD), and maldigestion (such as celiac disease). Diarrhea-predominant irritable bowel syndrome (D-IBS) can be precipitated by acute gastroenteritis. Anti-CdtB and antivinculin antibodies may occur after an acute bout of gastroenteritis. Persistent elevation of these antibodies is predictive of D-IBS rather than IBD or celiac disease.

Procedure and patient care
- See inside front cover for Routine Blood Testing.
- Fasting: no
- Blood tube commonly used: A central laboratory testing kit
- Obtain a list of foods ingested in the last 48 hours.
- Assess severity of symptoms and the hydrational status of the patient with diarrhea.

Abnormal findings
Acute gastroenteritis
Diarrhea-predominate irritable bowel syndrome

notes

D-dimer (Fragment D-dimer, Fibrin degradation product [FDP], Fibrin split products)

Type of test Blood

Normal findings

< 500 μg/ or ≤ 0.5 mg/L Fibrinogen Equivalent Untis (FEU)

Test explanation and related physiology

D-dimer is a fibrin degradation fragment that is made through lysis of crosslinked (D-dimerized) fibrin. As plasmin acts on the fibrin polymer clot, fibrin degradation products (FDPs) and D-dimer are produced. The D-dimer assay provides a highly specific measurement of the amount of fibrin degradation that occurs. Normal plasma does not have detectable amounts of fragment D-dimer. For discussion of other fibrin degradation products, see thrombosis indicators (p. 714).

This test provides a simple and confirmatory test for intravascular thrombosis such as disseminated intravascular coagulation (DIC), deep vein thrombosis (DVT), pulmonary embolism (PE), sickle cell anemia, and thrombosis of malignancy. D-dimer is used as an effective screening test for DVT. If the D-dimer test is negative, it is unlikely that significant DVT or pulmonary embolism exists.

D-dimer levels increase with age. As a result, the clinical usefulness of the test, the proportion of the patients with a D-dimer level lower than the predetermined cutoff value (500 μg/L for most available commercial assays) and in whom the diagnosis of PE may be ruled out by the test, is reduced. The *optimal age-adjusted D-dimer* cutoff has been redefined as patient's age multiplied by 5 to 10 in patients 50 years or older.

When combining D-dimer with testing for *soluble fibrin monomers*, diagnosis of thrombosis may be more sensitive. The D-dimer test, however, is often positive in patients who are already hospitalized.

Finally, the D-dimer test can be used to determine the duration of anticoagulation therapy in patients with DVT. Patients with an abnormal D-dimer level 1 month after the discontinuation of anticoagulant therapy have a significant incidence of recurrent DVT. This incidence can be reduced by restarting anticoagulation therapy.

Interfering factors

- D-dimer level may be decreased in lipemic patients.
- The presence of rheumatoid factor at a level > 50 IU/mL may lead to increased D-dimer levels.

Procedure and patient care

- See inside front cover for Routine Blood Testing.
- Fasting: no
- Blood tube commonly used: blue
- Remember that if the patient is receiving anticoagulants or has coagulopathies, the bleeding time will be increased.

Abnormal findings

▲ **Increased levels**

Arterial thromboembolism

Deep vein thrombosis

Disseminated intravascular coagulation

During thrombolytic or defibrination therapy with tissue plasminogen activator

Fibrinolysis

Malignancy

Pregnancy

Pulmonary embolism

Sickle cell anemia with or without vasoocclusive crisis

Surgery

notes

delta-aminolevulinic acid (Aminolevulinic acid [ALA], d-ALA)

Type of test Urine (24-hour)

Normal findings

1.5–7.5 mg/24 hr or 11–57 μmol/24 hr (SI units)

Possible critical values

> 20 mg/24 hr

Test explanation and related physiology

As the basic precursor for the porphyrins (p. 587), d-ALA is needed for the normal production of porphobilinogen, which ultimately leads to heme synthesis in erythroid cells. Heme is used in the synthesis of hemoglobin. Genetic disorders (porphyria) are associated with a lack of a particular enzyme vital to heme metabolism. These disorders are characterized by an accumulation of porphyrin products in the liver or red blood cells. Acute intermittent porphyria (AIP) is the most common form of the liver porphyrias.

In lead intoxication, heme synthesis is similarly diminished by the inhibition of ALA dehydrase. This enzyme assists in the conversion of ALA to porphobilinogen. As a result of lead poisoning, ALA accumulates in the blood and urine.

Procedure and patient care

- See inside front cover for Routine Urine Testing.
- Keep the urine in a light-resistant container with a preservative.
- If the patient has a Foley catheter in place, cover the drainage bag to prevent exposure to light.

Abnormal findings

▲ **Increased levels**

  Chronic alcoholic disorders
  Diabetic ketoacidosis
  Lead intoxication
  Porphyria

notes

dental x-ray (Dental radiography)

Type of test X-ray

Normal findings

No evidence of dental caries (tooth decay/cavity), tumor, tooth impaction, or congenital abnormalities

Test explanation and related physiology

Dental x-rays can be taken intraorally and extraorally. They give a high level of detail of the tooth, bone, and supporting tissues of the mouth. These x-rays allow dentists to:
- Find cavities.
- Look at the tooth roots.
- Check the health of the bony area around the tooth.
- Determine periodontal disease.
- See the status of developing teeth and impacted teeth.
- Keep track of growth and development.
- Examine the relationships between teeth and jaws.
- Examine the bones of the face.

Interfering factors
- Earrings can obstruct radiographic visualization.

Procedure and patient care

Before
- PT Explain the procedure to the patient. See p. xviii for a discussion of radiation exposure and risk.
- PT Instruct the patient that he or she will need to keep still while the x-ray image is being taken (about 1 second).
- PT Tell the patient that no fasting or sedation is required.

During
- Note that this test is routinely performed by a dental hygienist within several minutes.
- PT Tell the patient that no discomfort is associated with this test.

After
- PT Explain the radiographic interpretation to the patient.

Abnormal findings

Bone or jaw tumors, resorption, infection
Dental caries
Dental malformation and growth
Periodontal or endodontal disease
Tooth injury

notes

dexamethasone suppression test (DST, Prolonged/rapid DST, Cortisol suppression test, ACTH suppression test)

Type of test Blood; urine (24-hour)

Normal findings

Prolonged method

Low dose: > 50% reduction of plasma cortisol
High dose: > 50% reduction of plasma cortisol
Urinary free cortisol: < 20 mcg/24 hr (< 50 nmol/24 hr)

Rapid (overnight) method

Normal: plasma cortisol levels suppressed to < 2 mcg/dL

Test explanation and related physiology

The DST is based on pituitary adrenocorticotropic hormone (ACTH) secretion being dependent on the plasma cortisol feedback mechanism. As plasma cortisol levels increase, ACTH secretion is suppressed; as cortisol levels decrease, ACTH secretion is stimulated. Dexamethasone is a synthetic steroid (similar to cortisol) that normally should suppress ACTH secretion. Under normal circumstances, administration of dexamethasone results in reduced stimulation to the adrenal glands and ultimately a drop of 50% or more in plasma cortisol and 17-OCHS levels. In general, blood testing is more easily obtained and is equally accurate and reliable as urine testing, especially in low-dose DST. This important feedback system does not function properly in patients with hypercortisol states.

When elevated cortisol levels caused by an ACTH-producing pituitary tumor lead to bilateral adrenal hyperplasia (Cushing disease), the pituitary gland is reset upward and responds only to high plasma levels of dexamethasone. There is no response to low-dose dexamethasone. In Cushing syndrome caused by adrenal adenoma or cancer (which acts autonomously), cortisol secretion continues despite a suppression in ACTH even at high doses of dexamethasone. Likewise, when Cushing syndrome is caused by an ectopic ACTH-producing tumor (e.g., lung cancer), that tumor is also considered autonomous and will continue to secrete ACTH despite high-dose suppression with dexamethasone. ACTH and plasma cortisol levels are measured during this test. Dexamethasone levels may also be measured to ensure adequacy of suppressive doses administered.

When hypercortisol is caused by:
- *Bilateral adrenal hyperplasia (Cushing disease)*
  - Low dose: no change

- ○ High dose: > 50% reduction of plasma cortisol and ACTH is elevated
- *Adrenal adenoma or carcinoma (primary hypercortisolism)*
  - ○ Low dose: no change
  - ○ High dose: no change
  - ○ ACTH is undetectable or low
- *Ectopic ACTH-producing tumor*
  - ○ Low dose: no change
  - ○ High dose: no change
  - ○ ACTH is normal to elevated

The DST may also identify depressed persons likely to respond to electroconvulsive therapy or antidepressants rather than to psychological or social interventions. ACTH production will not be fully suppressed after administration of low-dose dexamethasone in these patients.

The *prolonged* DST (high-dose DST—usually 8 mg of dexamethasone) can be performed over a 2-day period on an outpatient basis. The *rapid* DST (low dose—1 mg of dexamethasone) is easily and quickly performed and is used primarily as a screening test to diagnose Cushing syndrome. It is less accurate and informative than the prolonged DST, but when its results are normal, the diagnosis of Cushing syndrome can be safely excluded. The high-dose DST is used if the results of the low-dose DST are equivocal. Corticotropin-releasing hormone can be added to dexamethasone to increase the accuracy of this test in order to differentiate Cushing syndrome from "pseudo-Cushing states." In pseudo-Cushing, one would expect elevations of ACTH and cortisol levels.

Interfering factors

- Physical and emotional stress can elevate ACTH release.

Procedure and patient care

Before

PT Explain the procedure (prolonged or rapid test) to the patient.
- Check with the lab to see if fasting is needed.

During

- There are several documented methods of performing this test by varying the dose and duration of testing.

Prolonged test
- Obtain a baseline 24-hour urine collection for urinary free cortisol (p. 241). See inside front cover for Routine Urine Testing.
- Collect blood for determination of baseline plasma cortisol levels, if indicated.

- Collect 24-hour urine specimens daily over a 2-day period. Because 2 continuous days of urine collections are needed, no urine specimens are discarded except for the first voided specimen on day 1, after which the collection begins.
- On days 1 and 2, administer a low dose of dexamethasone by mouth every 6 hours for 48 hours.
- Administer the dexamethasone with milk or an antacid to prevent gastric irritation.
- Note that creatinine is measured in all the 24-hour urine collections to demonstrate their accuracy and adequacy.
- Keep the urine specimens refrigerated or on ice during the collection period.

Rapid test
- Give the patient a low dose of dexamethasone by mouth at bedtime.
- Administer the dexamethasone with milk or an antacid.
- Attempt to ensure a good night's sleep. However, use sedative-hypnotic drugs only if absolutely necessary.
- At 8 AM the next morning, draw fasting blood for determination of plasma cortisol level before the patient arises.
- If no cortisol suppression occurs after the dose of dexamethasone, administer a higher dose at bedtime and obtain a cortisol level as described previously. This is referred to as the *overnight dexamethasone suppression test*. Patients with adrenal hyperplasia will suppress. Patients with adrenal or ectopic tumors will not suppress.

After
- Assess the patient for steroid-induced side effects by monitoring glucose levels and potassium levels.

Abnormal findings

Adrenal adenoma or carcinoma
Bilateral adrenal hyperplasia
Cushing disease
Cushing syndrome
Ectopic ACTH-producing tumors
Hyperthyroidism
Mental depression

notes

D

diabetes mellitus autoantibody panel (diabetes-associated autoantibodies, Insulin autoantibody [IAA], Islet cell antibody [ICA], Glutamic acid decarboxylase antibody [GAD Ab])

Type of test   Blood

Normal findings

< 1:4 titer; no antibody detected

Test explanation and related physiology

Type 1 diabetes mellitus (DM) is insulin-dependent (IDDM). This disease is an *organ-specific* form of autoimmune disease that results in destruction of the pancreatic islet cells and their products. These antibodies are used to differentiate type I DM from type II non-insulin-dependent DM. Nearly 90% of people with type 1 DM have one or more of these autoantibodies at the time of their diagnosis. People with type 2 DM have low or negative titers. Determining which type of diabetes a patient has is critical in providing the proper care and treatment. However, a rise in childhood obesity has made distinguishing between type 1 and type 2 diabetes increasingly more challenging. Maturity-onset diabetes of the young (MODY) type 3 is important to identify so that treatment can be most appropriately provided.

These antibodies often appear years before the onset of symptoms. The panel is useful to screen relatives of IDDM patients who are at risk of developing the disease. *GAD Ab* provide confirmatory evidence. The presence of these antibodies identifies which woman with gestational diabetes will eventually require insulin permanently.

Because identifying the type of diabetes can be complex, DNA molecular testing for *NF1A* (MODY3), *GCK* (MODY2), *HNF4A* (MODY1), and *HNF1B* (MODY5) is valuable. Defects in these genes are a cause of MODY.

The presence of insulin antibodies is diagnostic of factitious hypoglycemia from surreptitious administration of insulin (see C-peptide, p. 243). This antibody panel is also used in surveillance of patients who have received pancreatic islet cell transplantation. Finally, these antibodies can be used to identify late onset type 1 diabetes in those patients previously thought to have type 2 diabetes.

Procedure and patient care

- See inside front cover for Routine Blood Testing.
- Fasting: no
- Blood tube commonly used: red or serum separator

Abnormal findings

▲ **Increased levels**

Allergies to insulin
Factitious hypoglycemia
Insulin-dependent diabetes mellitus
Insulin resistance

notes

2,3-diphosphoglycerate (2,3-DPG in erythrocytes)

Type of test Blood

Normal findings

12.3 ± 1.87 µmol/g of hemoglobin or 0.79 ± 0.12 mol/mol hemoglobin (SI units)

4.2 ± 0.64 µmol/mL of erythrocytes or 4.2 ± 0.64 mmol/L erythrocytes (SI units)

(Levels are lower in newborns and even lower in premature infants.)

Test explanation and related physiology

This test is used in the evaluation of nonspherocytic hemolytic anemia. 2,3-DPG is a byproduct of the glycolytic respiratory pathway of the red blood cell (RBC). A congenital enzyme deficiency in this vital pathway alters the RBC shape and survival significantly. Anemia is the result. Another result of the enzyme deficiency is reduced synthesis of 2,3-DPG.

Usually, 2,3-DPG levels increase in response to anemia or hypoxic conditions (e.g., obstructive lung disease, congenital cyanotic heart disease, after vigorous exercise). Increases in 2,3-DPG decrease the oxygen binding to hemoglobin so that oxygen is more easily released to the tissues when needed (lower arterial PO_2). Levels of 2,3-DPG are decreased as a result of inherited genetic defects. This genetic defect parallels that of sickle cell anemia and hemoglobin C diseases.

Interfering factors

- Vigorous exercise may cause increased levels.
- High altitudes may increase levels.
- Banked blood has decreased amounts of 2,3-DPG.
- Acidosis decreases levels.

Procedure and patient care

- See inside front cover for Routine Blood Testing.
- Fasting: no
- Blood tube commonly used: red

Abnormal findings

▲ **Increased levels**

Adjustment to higher
altitudes

Anemia

Chronic renal failure

Cystic fibrosis

Hyperthyroidism

Hypoxic heart (e.g.,
cyanotic heart disease)
or lung (e.g., chronic
obstructive pulmonary
disease) diseases

Pyruvate kinase deficiency

▼ **Decreased levels**

Acidosis

Polycythemia

Post–massive blood
transfusion

Respiratory distress
syndrome

2,3-DPG mutase
deficiency

2,3-DPG phosphatase
deficiency

notes

disseminated intravascular coagulation screening (DIC screening)

D

Type of test Blood

Normal findings

No evidence of DIC

Test explanation and related physiology

This is a group of tests used to detect disseminated intravascular coagulation (DIC). Many pathologic conditions can instigate or are associated with DIC. The more common ones include bacterial septicemia, amniotic fluid embolism, retention of a dead fetus, malignant neoplasia, liver cirrhosis, extensive surgery (especially on the liver), post–extracorporeal heart bypass, extensive trauma, severe burns, and transfusion reactions.

In DIC, the entire clotting mechanism is inappropriately triggered. This results in significant systemic or localized intravascular formation of fibrin clots. The consequences of this futile clotting are blood vessel occlusion and excessive bleeding caused by consumption of the platelets and clotting factors that have been used in intravascular clotting. The fibrinolytic system is also activated to break down the clot formation and the fibrin involved in the intravascular coagulation. This fibrinolysis results in the formation of fibrin degradation products (FDPs), which by themselves act as anticoagulants; these FDPs serve only to enhance the bleeding tendency (Figure D1). See thrombosis indicators, p. 714.

When a patient with a bleeding tendency is suspected of having DIC, a series of readily performed laboratory tests should be conducted (Table D1. These tests are discussed separately in this book.)

Abnormal findings

Disseminated intravascular coagulation

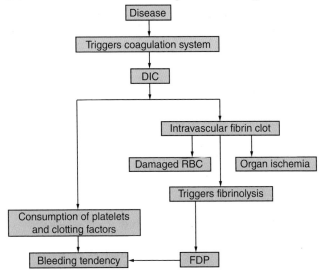

FIG. D1 Pathology of disseminated intravascular coagulation (DIC) may result in bleeding tendency, organ ischemia, and hemolytic anemia. *FDP,* Fibrin degradation product; *RBC,* red blood cell.

TABLE D1   Disseminated intravascular coagulation screening tests

Test	Result
Blood smear (p. 128)	Evidence of microangiopathic hemolytic anemia (schistocytes and helmet cells)
Coagulating factors (p. 209)	Decreased factors I, II, V, VIII, X, and XIII (more commonly used for diagnosis rather than for screening)
D-dimer (p. 264)	Increased
Fibrin degradation products (p. 714)	Increased
Fibrinogen (p. 346)	Decreased
Fibrinopeptide A (p. 714)	Increased
Partial thromboplastin time (p. 557)	Prolonged
Platelet count (p. 577)	Decreased
Prothrombin fragment (p. 714)	Increased
Prothrombin time (p. 619)	Prolonged

drug monitoring (Therapeutic drug monitoring [TDM], Drug sensitivity genotyping)

Type of test Blood

Normal findings

See Table D2.

Test explanation and related physiology

TDM entails measuring blood drug levels to determine effective drug dosages and to prevent toxicity. Drug monitoring is helpful in patients who take other medicines that may affect drug levels or act in a synergistic or antagonistic manner with the drug to be tested. There are some medicines (e.g., antiarrhythmics, bronchodilators, antibiotics, anticonvulsants, cardiotonics) that have a very narrow therapeutic margin (i.e., the difference between therapeutic and toxic drug levels is small).

Table D2 lists the therapeutic and toxic ranges for the average patient for some commonly tested drug levels. This list is far from complete. These ranges may not apply to all patients because clinical response is influenced by many factors.

Blood is routinely used for TDM because results indicate what is presently going on with the drug at any one particular time. Urine drug levels reflect the presence of the drug over the previous several days.

Blood samples can be taken at the drug's *peak level* (highest concentration) or at the *trough level* (lowest concentration). Peak levels are useful when testing for toxicity, and trough levels are useful for demonstrating a satisfactory therapeutic level. Trough levels are often referred to as residual levels. The time when the sample should be drawn after the last dose of the medication varies according to whether a peak or trough level is requested and according to the half-life of the drug (the time required for the body to decrease the drug blood level by 50%). If peak levels are higher than the therapeutic range, toxicity may be experienced. If trough levels are lower than the therapeutic range, drug therapy is inadequate.

Pharmacogenetics (genotyping for drug monitoring)

TDM is used to alter the dosage of medications to maximize efficacy and minimize side effects. There are several factors that affect efficacy and toxicity: patient compliance, patient age and size, access to adequate care, optimal dosing, and drug pharmacology issues (e.g., absorption, elimination, and drug interactions). Drugs undergo metabolism by enzyme systems to activate

TABLE D2 Drug monitoring data

Drug	Use	Therapeutic level[a]	Toxic level[a]
Acetaminophen	Analgesic, antipyretic	Depends on use	> 25 mcg/mL
Aminophylline	Bronchodilator	10–20 mcg/mL	> 20 mcg/mL
Digoxin	Cardiac glycoside	0.8–2 ng/mL	> 2.4 ng/mL
Gentamicin	Antibiotic	5–10 mcg/mL	> 12 mcg/mL
Lidocaine	Antiarrhythmic	1.5–5 mcg/mL	> 5 mcg/mL
Lithium	Manic episodes of bipolar psychosis	0.8–1.2 mEq/L	> 2 mEq/L
Methotrexate	Antitumor agent	0.1–1 μmol/24 hr	> 10 μmol/24 hr
Phenobarbital	Anticonvulsant	10–30 mcg/mL	> 40 mcg/mL
Phenytoin	Anticonvulsant	10–20 mcg/mL	> 30 mcg/mL
Propranolol	Antiarrhythmic	50–100 ng/mL	> 150 ng/mL
Salicylate	Antipyretic, antiinflammatory, analgesic	100–250 mcg/mL	> 300 mcg/mL
Theophylline	Bronchodilator	10–20 mcg/mL	> 20 mcg/mL
Tobramycin	Antibiotic	5–10 mcg/mL	> 12 mcg/mL
Valproic acid	Anticonvulsant	50–100 mcg/mL	> 100 mcg/mL
Vancomycin	Antibiotic	Peak: 20–40 mcg/mL Trough: 5–15 mcg/mL	> 40 mcg/mL

[a] Levels vary according to the institution performing the test.

a bound (proactive) drug or to deactivate an active drug. The effectiveness of these enzyme systems of metabolism are determined by the genetic makeup of the patient. Based on the results of genotyping, a phenotype is predicted for a gene. Assessment of multiple genes (gene panels) may assist the clinician with personalized drug recommendations, avoidance of adverse drug reactions, and optimization of drug treatment.

Using the cytochromes as an example, four categories of drug metabolizers can be identified through genotype testing:

- Poor metabolizers (PMs)
- Intermediate metabolizers (IMs)
- Extensive metabolizers (EMs)
- Ultrarapid metabolizers (UMs)

Overall, whereas PMs and, to a lesser extent, IMs are prone to exaggerated side effects from active drugs, normal doses of the same drugs tend to be ineffectual for UMs. If a proactive drug is administered and must be hydrolyzed to its active form, PMs will not benefit from normal doses, but UMs will experience drug benefit from even small doses.

The cytochrome P450 (CYP450) system is a major family of drug-metabolizing enzymes. Several CYP450 enzymes are involved in the metabolism of a significant proportion of drugs. Drugs affected by cytochrome metabolism include medications used for allergy, pain, inflammatory, cardiovascular, cancer, viral, neurologic, mental diseases, and prostate diseases. Other medications using the cytochrome system for metabolism are anticoagulants, newer anti-platelets, immunosuppressives, antacids, and sedative hypnotics. A commonly used proprietary genetic test called *Genesight Psychotropic Test* provides testing of the cytochrome p450 system used in the metabolism of antidepression medications. Use of this test provides the prescriber with the patient's ability to metabolize a particular antidepressive medication. Armed with this information, a medication can be provided that has the least side effects and the greatest efficacy.

Thiopurine methyltransferase (TPMT) and Nudix hydrolase (NUDT15) are other examples of metabolic enzyme systems that are specifically used in the metabolism of thiopurine drugs (e.g., azathioprine, 6-mercaptopurine [6MP], and 6-thioguanine).

Pharmacogenetics allows physicians to consider genetic information from patients in selecting medications and dosages of medications for a variety of common conditions (e.g., cardiac disease, psychiatric disease, and cancer).

Biologic drug monitoring assays measure both drug concentration and anti-drug antibodies to improve clinical outcomes and to characterize patients who may have diminished response to therapy. This testing is available for a host of new biologic drugs and for the metabolites of many long-provided medications.

Procedure and patient care

Before

PT Explain the procedure to the patient.

PT Tell the patient that no food or fluid restrictions are needed,

- For patients suspected of having symptoms of drug toxicity, the best time to draw the blood specimen is when the symptoms are occurring.
- If there is a concern regarding whether an adequate dose of the drug is achieved, it is best to obtain trough levels.

During

- Collect a venous blood sample in a tube designated by the laboratory. Peak levels are usually obtained 1 to 2 hours after oral intake, approximately 1 hour after intramuscular (IM) administration, or approximately 30 minutes after intravenous (IV) administration. Residual (trough) levels are usually obtained shortly before (0–15 minutes) the next scheduled dose. Consult with the pharmacy for specific times.

After

- Apply pressure or a pressure dressing to the venipuncture site.
- Promptly send the specimen to the laboratory.

Abnormal findings

Nontherapeutic levels of drugs
Toxic levels of drugs

notes

echocardiography (Cardiac echo, Heart sonogram, Transthoracic echocardiography [TTE]), Transesophageal echocardiography (TEE))

Type of test Ultrasound

Normal findings

Normal position, size, and movement of the cardiac valves and heart muscle wall

Normal directional flow of blood within the heart chambers

Test explanation and related physiology

Echocardiography is a noninvasive ultrasound procedure used to evaluate the structure and function of the heart. Echocardiography is also used in *cardiac stress testing*. During an exercise or chemical cardiac stress test, ischemic muscle areas are evident as hypokinetic areas within the myocardium. Echocardiography is used frequency in emergent and urgent evaluations of patients with chest pains.

The most useful application of the color flow imaging is in determining the direction and turbulence of blood flow across regurgitant or narrowed valves. Doppler color flow imaging also may be helpful in assessing proper functioning of prosthetic valves.

Echocardiography is also used in the diagnosis of a pericardial effusion, valvular heart disease (e.g., mitral valve prolapse, stenosis, regurgitation), subaortic stenosis, myocardial wall abnormalities (e.g., cardiomyopathy), infarction, and aneurysm. Cardiac tumors (e.g., myxomas) are easily diagnosed with ultrasound. Atrial and ventricular septal defects and other congenital heart diseases are also recognized by ultrasound. Finally, postinfarction mural thrombi are readily apparent with this testing.

Echocardiography can be performed with use of a probe passed into the lower esophagus. This is referred to as *transesophageal echocardiography* or *TEE*. TEE sees the heart from a retrocardiac vantage point, avoiding interference with the ultrasound by the interposed subcutaneous tissue, bony thorax, and lungs (Figure E1). TEE is especially helpful in patients who are obese or have large lung-air spaces. This test is used in addition to TTE:
- To monitor high-risk patients during surgery
- To better visualize the heart valves
- To differentiate intracardiac from extracardiac masses and tumors
- To better visualize the atrial septum (for atrial septal defects)
- To diagnose thoracic aortic dissection
- To better detect valvular vegetation indicative of endocarditis
- To determine cardiac sources of arterial embolism
- To detect coronary artery disease and ischemia

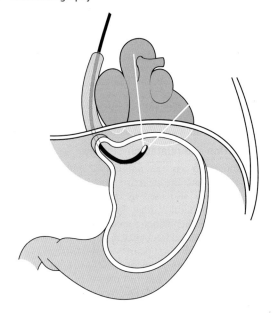

FIG. E1 Transesophageal echocardiography. The diagram illustrates the location of the transesophageal endoscope in the esophagus.

Emergent use of TEE during surgery is sometimes called "rescue TEE." In this case, it is used to diagnose causes of hemodynamic instability or cardiopulmonary arrest. Contrast echocardiography is a technique for improving echocardiographic resolution by the use of an injectable agent such as lipid or air bubbles. It enhances endocardial borders and provides real-time assessment of intracardiac blood flow (right to left shunts).

Contraindications

- Patients who are uncooperative
- Patients with known upper esophageal pathology
- Patients with Zenker diverticulum

Interfering factors

- Chronic obstructive pulmonary disease (COPD)

    Patients who have severe COPD have a significant amount of air space between the heart and the chest cavity. Air space does not conduct ultrasound waves well.
- Obesity

    In obese patients, the space between the heart and the transducer is greatly enlarged; therefore accuracy of the test is decreased.

Procedure and patient care

Before

PT Explain the test and assure the patient that this is painless.

PT For TEE
- Instruct the patient to fast for 4 to 6 hours before the test.
- Tell the patient to remove all oral prostheses.
- Obtain IV access.

During
- Note the following procedural steps for echocardiography:
  1. The patient is placed in the supine position.
  2. Electrocardiographic (ECG) leads are placed (p. 284).
  3. A gel, which allows better transmission of sound waves, is placed on the chest wall under the transducer.
  4. Ultrasound is directed to the heart, and appropriate tracings are obtained.
- Note the steps for TEE:
  1. The pharynx is anesthetized with a local topical agent to depress the gag reflex.
  2. IV sedation is commonly provided.
  3. The patient is placed in the left lateral decubitus position.
  4. The transducer is advanced into position behind the heart.
- Note that this procedure usually takes approximately 45 minutes and is performed by an ultrasound technician in a darkened room within the cardiac or radiology department.

After
- Remove the gel from the patient's chest wall and the esophageal tranducer.
- PT Inform the patient that the physician must interpret the study and that the results will be available in a few hours.

Abnormal findings

Endocarditis
Mitral valve prolapse
Myxoma
Pericardial effusion
Poor ventricular muscle motion
Septal defects
Valvular regurgitation
Valvular stenosis
Ventricular hypertrophy
Ventricular or atrial mural thrombi

notes

electrocardiography (Electrocardiogram [ECG, EKG])

Type of test Electrodiagnostic

Normal findings

Normal rhythm, wave deflections, and heart rate (60–100 beats/min)

Test explanation and related physiology

The ECG is a graphic representation of the electrical impulses that the heart generates during the cardiac cycle. The monitoring electrodes detect the electrical activity of the heart from a variety of spatial perspectives. There are six limb leads (combination of electrodes on the extremities) and six chest leads (corresponding to six sites on the chest) (Figure E2).

The normal ECG pattern is composed of waves arbitrarily designated by the letters *P*, *Q*, *R*, *S*, *T*, and *U*. The significance of the waves and time intervals is as follows (Figure E3):

- *P wave*. This represents atrial electrical depolarization associated with atrial contraction.
- *PR interval*. This represents the time required for the impulse to travel from the SA node to the atrioventricular (AV) node.
- *QRS complex*. This represents ventricular electrical depolarization associated with ventricular contraction.
- *ST segment*. This represents the period between the completion of depolarization and the beginning of repolarization of the ventricular muscle. This segment may be elevated or depressed in transient muscle ischemia (e.g., angina) or in muscle injury (e.g., the early stages of myocardial infarction).
- *T wave*. This represents ventricular repolarization (i.e., return to the resting state).
- *U wave*. This deflection follows the T wave and is usually quite small. It represents repolarization of the Purkinje nerve fibers within the ventricles.

The ECG is used primarily to identify abnormal heart rhythms and to diagnose acute coronary occlusive disease, conduction defects, and ventricular hypertrophy.

Interfering factors

- Inaccurate placement of the electrodes
- Electrolyte imbalances
- Poor contact between the skin and the electrodes
- Movement or muscle twitching during the test

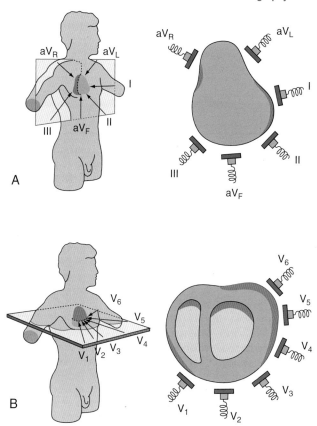

FIG. E2 Planes of reference. **A**, The frontal plane. **B**, The horizontal plane.

Procedure and patient care

Before

PT Explain the procedure to the patient.

PT Tell the patient that no food or fluid restriction is necessary.

PT Assure the patient that the flow of electric current is *from* the patient. He or she will feel nothing during this procedure.

• Expose only the patient's chest upper arms, and lower legs. Keep the abdomen and thighs adequately covered.

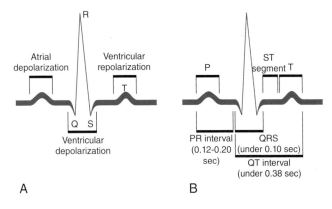

FIG. E3 Electrocardiography. **A,** Normal electrocardiographic (ECG) deflections during depolarization and repolarization of the atria and ventricles. **B,** Principal ECG intervals between P, QRS, and T waves.

During
- Note the following procedural steps:
    1. The skin areas designated for electrode placement are prepared by using alcohol swabs or sandpaper to remove skin oil or debris. Sometimes the skin is shaved if the patient has a large amount of hair.
    2. Pads with special gel are applied to ensure electrical conduction between the skin and the electrodes.
    3. Electrodes are applied to the four extremities.
    4. The chest leads are applied as follows:
        V_1: in the fourth intercostal space (4ICS) at the right sternal border
        V_2: in 4ICS at the left sternal border
        V_3: midway between V_2 and V_4
        V_4: in 5ICS at the midclavicular line
        V_5: at the left anterior axillary line at the level of V_4 horizontally
        V_6: at the left midaxillary line on the level of V_4 horizontally
- Note that cardiac technicians, nurses, or physicians perform this procedure in less than 5 minutes at the bedside or in the cardiology clinic.

E

After

- Remove the electrodes from the patient's skin and wipe off the electrode gel.
- Indicate on the ECG strip or request slip if the patient was experiencing chest pain during the study. The pain may be correlated with an arrhythmia on the ECG.

Abnormal findings

Acute myocardial infarction
Cardiac arrhythmias
Conduction defects
Cor pulmonale
Electrolyte imbalance
Myocardial ischemia
Old myocardial infarction
Pericarditis
Pulmonary embolus
Ventricular hypertrophy
Wolff-Parkinson-White syndrome

notes

electroencephalography (Electroencephalogram [EEG])

Type of test Electrodiagnostic

Normal findings

Normal frequency, amplitude, and characteristics of brain waves

Test explanation and related physiology

The EEG is a graphic recording of the electrical activity of the brain. EEG electrodes are placed on the scalp over multiple areas of the brain to detect the focus of seizure activity. Because this study determines the overall activity of the brain, it can be used to evaluate drug intoxication and to determine cerebral death in comatose patients. The EEG also can be used to monitor cerebral blood flow during carotid endarterectomy.

Electrocorticography (ECoG) is a form of EEG performed during craniotomy. The same information can be obtained by a noninvasive brain imaging technique called *magnetoencephalography (MEG)*. MEG is also used in localizing important adjacent cortical areas for surgical planning in patients with intractable epilepsy.

Interfering factors

- Drinks containing caffeine (e.g., coffee, tea, cocoa, cola) interfere with test results.
- Body and eye movements during the test can cause changes in brain wave patterns.
- Drugs that may affect test results include sedatives.

Procedure and patient care

Before

PT Explain the procedure to the patient.

PT Assure the patient that this test cannot read the mind or detect senility.

PT Assure the patient that the flow of electrical activity is *from* the patient. He or she will not feel anything.

PT Instruct the patient to wash his or her hair the night before the test. No oils, sprays, or lotion should be used.

- Check to see if the physician wants to discontinue any medications before the study. Sedatives should be avoided.

PT Instruct the patient if sleeping time should be shortened the night before the test. Adults may not be allowed to sleep more than 4 or 5 hours and children not more than 5 to 7 hours if a sleep EEG will be done.

During
- Note the following procedural steps:
    1. The EEG is usually performed in a specially constructed room that is shielded from outside disturbances.
    2. The patient is placed in a supine position on a bed or reclining in a chair.
    3. Sixteen or more electrodes are applied to the scalp with electrode paste in a uniform pattern.
    4. The technician observes the patient during the EEG recording for movements that could alter results.
- In addition, an EEG may be recorded during hyperventilation, photostimulation, or sleep.
- Note that this study is performed by an EEG technician in approximately 45 minutes to 2 hours.

After
- Help the patient remove the electrode paste.

Abnormal findings

Alzheimer disease
Brain abscess
Brain tumor
Cerebral death
Cerebral infarct
Encephalitis
Head injury
Intracranial hemorrhage
Narcolepsy
Seizure disorders (e.g., epilepsy)

notes

electromyography (EMG)

Type of test Electrodiagnostic

Normal findings

No evidence of neuromuscular abnormalities

Test explanation and related physiology

EMG is used to detect primary muscular disorders, along with muscular abnormalities caused by other system diseases (e.g., nerve dysfunction, sarcoidosis, paraneoplastic syndrome). Spontaneous muscle movement such as spasm, fibrillation, and fasciculation can be detected during EMG. When evident, these waveforms indicate injury or disease of the nerve or muscle being evaluated. A decrease in the number of muscle fibers able to contract is typically observed with peripheral nerve damage. This study is usually done in conjunction with nerve conduction studies (p. 292) and may also be called *electromyoneurography*.

EMG is particularly helpful in evaluating the pelvic muscles (*EMG of the pelvis*) because they cannot be evaluated on physical exam. Placement of electrodes around the anus/perineum provides neuromuscular functional evaluation of the pelvic muscles, urinary, or anal sphincter. It is performed most often in patients who have urinary or fecal incontinence. Change in the muscle activity before and during voiding is also observed.

Interfering factors

- Thick subcutaneous fat.
- Patients with excessive pain.

Procedure and patient care

Before

PT Explain the procedure to the patient.

PT Tell the patient that fasting is not usually required; however, some facilities may restrict stimulants (coffee, tea, cocoa, cola, cigarettes) for 2 to 3 hours before the test.

- If serum enzyme tests are ordered, the specimen should be drawn before EMG or 5 to 10 days after the test because the EMG may cause misleading elevations of these enzymes.
- Premedication or sedation is usually avoided because of the need for patient cooperation.

During
- Note the following procedural steps:
  1. This study is usually done in an EMG laboratory.
  2. The patient's position depends on the muscle being studied.
  3. A sticky patch electrode is applied to the skin overlying the muscle to be evaluated.
  4. A reference patch electrode is placed nearby on the skin surface.
  5. The patient is asked to keep the muscle at rest.
  6. Electrical activity of the muscle is displayed on a monitor to which the electrodes are attached. The electrical waves are observed during voluntary contraction and relaxation.
- Note that the EMG is performed by a physical therapist, physiatrist, or neurologist in approximately 20 minutes.

After

Abnormal findings

Acetylcholine blockers (e.g., curare, snake venom)
Amyotrophic lateral sclerosis
Guillain–Barré syndrome
Multiple sclerosis
Muscle denervation
Muscle spasm
Muscular dystrophy
Myasthenia gravis
Myopathy
Peripheral nerve injury, entrapment, or compression
Polymyositis
Spinal cord injury or disease
Traumatic injury

notes

electroneurography (ENG, Nerve conduction studies)

Type of test Electrodiagnostic

Normal findings

No evidence of peripheral nerve injury or disease

Test explanation and related physiology

Nerve conduction studies (NCS) evaluate the integrity of the nerves and allow for the detection and location of peripheral nerve injury or disease. By initiating an electrical impulse at one site (proximal when evaluating motor nerves or distal when evaluating sensory nerves) of a nerve and recording the time required for that impulse to travel to a second site (opposite above) of the same nerve, the conduction velocity of an impulse in that nerve can be determined. This study is usually done in conjunction with EMG (p. 290) and also may be called *electromyoneurography*.

Because conduction velocity may require contraction of a muscle as an indication of an impulse arriving at the recording electrode, significant primary muscular disorders may cause a falsely slow nerve conduction velocity. This "muscular" variable is eliminated if one evaluates the suspected pathologic muscle group before performing NCS. This muscular factor is evaluated by measuring distal latency (i.e., the time required for stimulation of the nerve to cause muscular contraction). As the distal latency is calculated, the motor NCS is performed normally by stimulating the nerve bundle. Conduction velocity can then be determined by the following equation:

$$\frac{\text{Conduction velocity}}{\text{(in meters per second)}} = \frac{\text{Distance (in meters)}}{\text{Total latency} - \text{Distal latency}}$$

Interfering factors

- Patients in severe pain may have false results.

Procedure and patient care

Before

PT Explain the procedure to the patient. Allay any fears.

- Obtain informed consent if required by the institution.

PT Tell the patient that no fasting or sedation is usually required.

During

- Note the following procedural steps:
  1. This test can be performed in a nerve conduction laboratory or at the patient's bedside.
  2. The patient's position depends on the area of suspected peripheral nerve injury or disease.
  3. A recording electrode is placed on the skin overlying a muscle innervated solely by the relevant nerve or overlying the nerve itself. All skin-to-electrode connections are ensured by using electrical gel.
  4. A reference electrode is placed nearby.
  5. The nerve is stimulated by a shock-emitting device at an adjacent location.
  6. The time between nerve impulse and muscular contraction (distal latency) is measured in milliseconds.
  7. The nerve is similarly stimulated at a location proximal to the area of suspected injury or disease.
  8. The time required for the impulse to travel from the site of initiation to muscle contraction (total latency) is recorded in milliseconds.
  9. The distance between the site of stimulation and the recording electrode is measured in centimeters.
  10. Conduction velocity is converted to meters per second and is computed as in the previous equation.
- Note that this test takes approximately 40 minutes and is performed by a physiatrist or a neurologist.
- **PT** Tell the patient that this test may be uncomfortable because a mild shock is required for nerve impulse stimulation.

After

- Remove the electrode gel from the patient's skin.

Abnormal findings

Carpal tunnel syndrome
Diabetic neuropathy
Guillain–Barré syndrome
Herniated disc disease
Myasthenia gravis
Peripheral nerve injury or disease
Poliomyelitis

notes

electronystagmography (Electrooculography)

Type of test   Electrodiagnostic

Normal findings

Normal nystagmus response
Normal oculovestibular reflex

Test explanation and related physiology

Electronystagmography is used to evaluate nystagmus (involuntary rapid eye movement) and the muscles controlling eye movement. By measuring changes in the electrical field around the eye, this study can make a permanent recording of eye movement at rest, with a change in head position, and in response to various stimuli. The test delineates the presence or absence of nystagmus, which is caused by the initiation of the oculovestibular reflex. Nystagmus should occur when initiated by positional, visual, or caloric stimuli. Unlike caloric studies (p. 162), in which nystagmus is usually determined visually, electronystagmography electrically records the direction, velocity, and degree of nystagmus.

If nystagmus does not occur with stimulation, the vestibular cochlear apparatus, cerebral cortex (temporal lobe), auditory nerve, or brainstem is abnormal. Tumors, infection, ischemia, and degeneration can cause such abnormalities. When put together with the entire clinical picture, the pattern of nystagmus helps in the differentiation between central and peripheral vertigo.

This study also may help evaluate unilateral hearing loss and vertigo. Unilateral hearing loss may be caused by middle ear problems or nerve injury. If the patient experiences nystagmus with stimulation, the auditory nerve is working and hearing loss can be blamed on the middle ear.

Contraindications

- Patients with perforated eardrums, who should not have water irrigation
- Patients with pacemakers

Interfering factors

- Blinking of the eyes can alter test results.

Procedure and patient care

Before

PT Explain the procedure to the patient.
PT Instruct the patient not to apply facial makeup before the test because electrodes will be taped to the skin around the eyes.

PT Instruct the patient not to eat solid food before the test to reduce the likelihood of vomiting.

PT Instruct the patient not to drink caffeine or alcoholic beverages for approximately 24 to 48 hours (as ordered).

• Check with the physician regarding withholding any medications that could interfere with the test results.

During

• Note the following procedural steps:
    1. This procedure is usually performed in a darkened room with the patient seated or lying down.
    2. If there is any wax in the ear, it is removed.
    3. Electrodes are taped to the skin around the eyes.
    4. Various procedures are used to stimulate nystagmus such as pendulum tracking, changing head position, changing gaze position, and caloric tests.
    5. Several recordings are made with the patient at rest and to demonstrate patient response to various procedures (e.g., blowing air into the ear, irrigating the ear with water).
    6. Nystagmus response is compared with the expected ranges, and the results are recorded as normal, borderline, or abnormal.

• Note that this procedure is performed by a physician or audiologist in approximately 1 hour.

PT Tell the patient that nausea and vomiting may occur.

After

• Consider prescribing bed rest until nausea, vertigo, or weakness subsides.

Abnormal findings

Auditory nerve damage
Brainstem lesions
Cerebellum lesions
Congenital disorder
Demyelinating disease
Vestibular system lesions

notes

electrophysiologic study (EPS, Cardiac mapping)

Type of test Electrodiagnostic; manometric

Normal findings

Normal conduction intervals, refractive periods, and recovery times

Tilt-table testing

< 20 mm Hg decrease in systolic blood pressure
< 10 mm Hg increase in diastolic blood pressure
Heart rate increase should be less than 10 beats/min.

Test explanation and related physiology

In this invasive procedure, multiple electrode catheters are fluoroscopically placed through a peripheral vein and into the right atrium and/or ventricle or, less often, through an artery into the left atrium and/or ventricle. With close cardiac monitoring, the electrode catheters are used to pace the heart and potentially induce arrhythmias. Defects in the heart conduction system can then be identified; arrhythmias that are otherwise not apparent also can be induced, identified, and treated. The effectiveness of antiarrhythmic drugs can be assessed.

EPS can also be therapeutic. With the use of radiofrequency, sites with documented low thresholds for inducing arrhythmias can be obliterated to stop the arrhythmias.

The *tilt-table test* is sometimes performed with an EPS cardiac study and is a provocative test used to diagnose vasopressor syncope syndrome. Patients with this syndrome usually demonstrate symptomatic hypotension and syncope within a few to 30 minutes of being tilted upright by approximately 60 to 80 degrees. The tilt-table test is often used to assess the efficacy of prophylactic pacing in some patients with vasopressor syncope. It is also used to evaluate the influence of posture with some forms of tachyarrhythmias. Normally, a minimal drop in systolic blood pressure, rise in diastolic blood pressure, and increase in heart rate occur in the tilted position.

Contraindications

- Patients with acute myocardial infarction

Potential complications

- Cardiac arrhythmias
- Perforation of the myocardium
- Catheter-induced embolic cerebrovascular accident (CVA; stroke) or myocardial infarction

- Peripheral vascular problems
- Hemorrhage
- Phlebitis at the venipuncture site

Interfering factors

- Patients with dehydration or hypovolemia demonstrate similar changes in blood pressure and heart rate with tilt-table testing. This is especially true in elderly patients.

E

Procedure and patient care

Before

PT Instruct the patient to fast for 6 to 8 hours before the procedure. Usually fluids are permitted until 3 hours before.
- Obtain an informed consent from the patient.
PT Encourage the patient to verbalize any fears.
- Prepare the catheter insertion site as directed.
- Obtain peripheral IV access for the administration of drugs.
- Inquire as to whether the patient has had excessive fluid loss (diarrhea or vomiting) in the previous 24 hours.
- Record the use of antihypertensive or diuretic medicines.

During

- Note the following procedural steps:

Electrophysiologic study

1. In the cardiac catheterization laboratory, the patient has ECG leads attached.
2. The catheter insertion site, usually the femoral vein, is prepared and draped in a sterile manner.
3. Under fluoroscopic guidance, the catheter is passed to the atrium and ventricle.
4. Baseline surface intracardiac ECGs are recorded.
5. Various parts of the cardiac electroconduction system are stimulated by atrial or ventricular pacing.
6. Mapping of the electroconduction system is performed.
7. Arrhythmias are identified.
8. Drugs may be administered to assess their efficacy in preventing EPS-induced arrhythmias.
9. Because dangerous arrhythmias can be prolonged, cardioversion must be immediately available.
10. The patient is also constantly engaged in light conversation to assess mental status and consciousness.

Tilt-table test

1. The patient lies supine on a horizontal tilt table.
2. Obtain the patient's blood pressure and pulse as baseline values before tilting is carried out.

3. Monitor these vital signs during the procedure.
4. Question the patient as to the presence of symptoms of dizziness and lightheadedness.
5. The table is progressively tilted 60 to 80 degrees while the patient is being monitored. Alternatively, the patient is asked to sit or stand.

PT Tell the patient that he or she may experience palpitations, lightheadedness, or dizziness when arrhythmias are induced. For most patients, this is an anxiety-producing experience.

After

- Keep the patient on bed rest for about 6 to 8 hours. Limit straining and heavy lifting for 24 hours.
- Evaluate the access site for swelling and bleeding.
- Monitor the patient's vital signs for at least 2 to 4 hours for hypotension and arrhythmias.
- Continue cardiac monitoring to identify arrhythmias.
- Cover the area with sterile dressings if the electrical catheter is left in place for subsequent studies.

Abnormal findings

Atrioventricular node defects and heart blocks
Cardiac arrhythmias
Electroconduction defects
Inducible arrhythmias (e.g., ventricular tachycardia and Wolff-Parkinson-White syndrome)
SA node defects (e.g., sick sinus syndrome)
Vasomotor syncope syndrome

notes

endometrial biopsy

Type of test   Microscopic examination of tissue

Normal findings

No pathologic conditions
Presence of a secretory-type endometrium 3 to 5 days before
   normal menses

E

Test explanation and related physiology

   An endometrial biopsy can determine whether ovulation has
occurred. A biopsy specimen taken 3 to 5 days before normal
menses should demonstrate a *secretory-type* endometrium on
histologic examination if ovulation and corpus luteum formation have occurred. If not, only a preovulatory *proliferative-type*
endometrium will be seen.
   This test can determine whether a woman has adequate ovarian estrogen and progesterone levels. Another major use of endometrial biopsy is to diagnose endometrial cancer, tuberculosis,
polyps, or inflammatory conditions and to evaluate dysfunctional
uterine bleeding.

Contraindications

- Patients with infections (e.g., trichomonal, candidal, or suspected gonococcal) of the cervix or vagina
- Patients in whom the cervix cannot be visualized (e.g.,
  because of previous surgery)
- Patients who are or may be pregnant because the procedure
  may induce labor or abortion

Potential complications

- Perforation of the uterus
- Uterine bleeding
- Interference with early pregnancy
- Infection

Procedure and patient care

Before

PT Explain the procedure to the patient.
- Ensure that written and informed consent is obtained.
PT Tell the patient that neither fasting nor sedation is usually
   required.

During

- Note the following procedural steps:
  1. The patient is placed in the lithotomy position, and a pelvic examination is performed to determine the position of the uterus.
  2. The cervix is exposed and cleansed.
  3. A biopsy instrument is inserted into the uterus, and specimens are obtained from the anterior, posterior, and lateral walls. This can be performed as part of a dilation and curettage or hysteroscopy (p. 435).
  4. The specimens are placed in a solution containing 10% formalin solution and sent to pathology.
- Note that this procedure is performed by an obstetrician/gynecologist in approximately 10 to 30 minutes.
- **PT** Tell the patient that this procedure may cause momentary discomfort (menstrual-type cramping).

After

- Assess the patient's vital signs at regular intervals. Any temperature elevation should be reported to the physician because this procedure may activate pelvic inflammatory disease.
- **PT** Advise the patient to wear a pad because some vaginal bleeding is to be expected. Tell the patient to call her physician if there is excessive bleeding (> 1 pad per hour).
- **PT** Inform the patient that douching and intercourse are not permitted for 72 hours after the biopsy.
- **PT** Instruct the patient to rest during the next 24 hours and to avoid heavy lifting to prevent uterine hemorrhage.

Abnormal findings

Anovulation
Inflammatory condition
Polyps
Tuberculosis
Tumor

notes

endoscopic retrograde cholangiopancreatography (ERCP)

E

Type of test Endoscopy

Normal findings

Normal size of biliary and pancreatic ducts
No obstruction or filling defects in the biliary or pancreatic ducts

Test explanation and related physiology

With the use of a fiberoptic endoscope, ERCP provides radiographic visualization of the biliary and pancreatic ducts. This is especially useful in patients with jaundice. Stones, benign strictures, cysts, ampullary stenosis, anatomic variations, and malignant tumors can be identified.

Incision of the papillary muscle in the ampulla of Vater can be performed through the scope at the time of ERCP. This incision widens the distal common duct so that common bile duct gallstones can be removed. Stents can be placed through narrowed bile ducts with the use of ERCP, and the bile of jaundiced patients can be internally drained. Pieces of tissue and brushings of the common bile duct can be obtained by ERCP for pathologic review and genomic testing.

Percutaneous transhepatic cholangiography (PTHC) is another method of bile duct visualization through a percutaneous catheter placed into the bile duct.

Magnetic resonance imaging cholangiopancreatography (p. 490) is a noninvasive test that can provide information similar to ERCP. However, interventional procedures such as papillotomy cannot be performed with this testing method.

Contraindications

- Patients who are uncooperative. Cannulation of the ampulla of Vater requires that the patient lie very still.
- Patients whose ampulla of Vater is not accessible endoscopically because of previous upper gastrointestinal (GI) surgery
- Patients with esophageal diverticula. The scope can fall into a diverticulum and perforate its wall.
- Patients with known acute pancreatitis

Potential complications

- Perforation of the esophagus, stomach, or duodenum
- Gram-negative sepsis. This results from introducing bacteria through the biliary system and into the blood.

- Pancreatitis resulting from pressure of the contrast injection
- Aspiration of gastric contents into the lungs
- Respiratory arrest as a result of oversedation

Interfering factors

- Barium in the abdomen as a result of a previous upper GI series or barium enema x-ray study precludes adequate visualization of the biliary and pancreatic ducts.

Procedure and patient care

Before

PT Explain the procedure to the patient. See p. xviii for radiation exposure and risks.
- Obtain informed consent from the patient.
- Keep the patient NPO as of midnight the day of the test.
- Administer appropriate premedication if ordered.

During

- Note the following procedural steps:
  1. After sedation, the pharynx is sprayed with a local anesthetic to inactivate the gag reflex.
  2. A fiberoptic duodenoscope is inserted through the oral pharynx and passed through the esophagus and stomach and then into the duodenum.
  3. A small catheter is passed through the ampulla of Vater and into the common bile or pancreatic ducts.
  4. Radiographic contrast is injected, and x-ray images are taken.
- Note that the test usually takes approximately 1 hour and is performed by a physician trained in endoscopy. The x-ray images are interpreted by a radiologist.
- Tell the patient that no discomfort is associated with the dye injection but that minimal gagging may occur during the initial introduction of the scope into the oral pharynx.

After

- Do not allow the patient to eat or drink until the gag reflex returns. Encourage light eating for the next 12 to 24 hours.
- Observe the patient closely for development of abdominal pain, nausea, and vomiting. This may herald the onset of ERCP-induced pancreatitis or gastroduodenal perforation.
- Observe safety precautions until the effects of the sedatives have worn off.
PT Instruct the patient to notify the physician immediately of fever or shaking chills. This may indicate possible cholangitis.

Abnormal findings

Anatomic biliary or pancreatic duct variations
Biliary sclerosis
Cancer of the duodenum or ampulla of Vater
Chronic pancreatitis
Cysts of the common bile duct
Pseudocyst of the pancreatic duct
Sclerosing cholangitis
Tumor, strictures, or gallstones of the common bile duct
Tumor, strictures, or inflammation of the pancreatic duct

notes

E

erythrocyte fragility (Osmotic fragility [OF], Red blood cell fragility)

Type of test   Blood

Normal findings

Hemolysis begins at 0.5% NaCl.
Hemolysis complete at 0.3% NaCl.

Test explanation and related physiology

The osmotic fragility (OF) test is used to determine the concentration of solute inside the cell by subjecting it to salt solutions of different concentrations. When intravascular hemolysis is identified, OF is used to determine whether the RBCs have increased fragility (tend to burst open when exposed to a higher concentrated NaCl solution) or decreased fragility (tend to burst open in lower concentrated, and thus more hypotonic, NaCl solution).

This test is performed to detect hereditary spherocytosis and thalassemia when intravascular hemolysis is identified. Round cells (spherocytes) have increased OF compared with normal indented RBCs. In hereditary spherocytosis, there is abnormal morphology because of a lack of spectrin, a key RBC cytoskeletal membrane protein. This produces membrane instability, which forces the cell to the smallest volume—that of a sphere. This common disorder is associated with intravascular hemolysis. This is shown by increased osmotic fragility. Thalassemia, on the other hand, is associated with thinner leptocytes whose OF is decreased.

Interfering factors

- Acute hemolysis. The osmotically labile cells are already hemolyzed and therefore are not found in the blood specimen.

Procedure and patient care

- See inside front cover for Routine Blood Testing.
- Fasting: no
- Blood tube commonly used: green

Abnormal findings

▲ **Increased erythrocyte fragility**

Acquired hemolytic anemia

Hemolytic disease of the newborn

Hereditary spherocytosis

Malaria

Pyruvate kinase deficiency

▼ **Decreased erythrocyte fragility**

Hemoglobinopathies (C and S disease)

Iron deficiency anemia

Reticulocytosis

Thalassemia

E

notes

erythrocyte sedimentation rate (ESR, Sed rate test)

Type of test Blood

Normal findings

Westergren method

Male: ≤15 mm/hr
Female: ≤ 20 mm/hr
Elderly: up to 40 mm/hr
Child: ≤ 10 mm/hr
Newborn: 0–2 mm/hr

Test explanation and related physiology

ESR is a measurement of the rate with which the RBCs settle in saline or plasma over a specified time period. It is nonspecific and therefore not diagnostic for any particular organ disease or injury. Because acute and chronic infection, inflammation (collagen-vascular diseases), advanced neoplasm, and tissue necrosis or infarction increase the protein (mainly fibrinogen) content of plasma, RBCs have a tendency to stack up on one another, increasing their weight and causing them to descend faster. Therefore in these diseases, the ESR is increased. ESR is considered an *acute-phase* or a *reactant* protein (i.e., it occurs as a reaction to acute illnesses).

The test can be used to detect occult disease. Many physicians use the ESR test in this way for routine patient evaluation for vague symptoms. Other physicians regard this test as so nonspecific that it is useless as a routine study. The ESR test occasionally can be helpful in differentiating disease entities or complaints.

The ESR is a fairly reliable indicator of the course of disease and can be used to monitor disease therapy, especially for inflammatory autoimmune diseases (e.g., temporal arteritis or polymyalgia rheumatica). In general, as the disease worsens, the ESR increases; as the disease improves, the ESR decreases. If the results of the ESR are equivocal or inconsistent with clinical impressions, the C-reactive protein test (p. 245) is often performed.

Interfering factors

- Artificially low results can occur when the collected specimen is allowed to stand longer than 3 hours before the testing.
- Pregnancy (second and third trimesters) can cause elevations.
- Menstruation can cause elevated levels.
- Polycythemia is associated with decreased ESR.

Procedure and patient care

- See inside front cover for Routine Blood Testing.
- Fasting: no
- Blood tube commonly used: lavender (verify with laboratory)

Abnormal findings

▲ **Increased levels**

Bacterial infection
Chronic renal failure
Hyperfibrinogenemia
Inflammatory diseases
Macroglobulinemia
Malignant diseases
Necrotic tissue diseases
Severe anemias (e.g., iron
   deficiency or B_{12} deficiency)

▼ **Decreased levels**

Hypofibrinogenemia
Polycythemia vera
Sickle cell anemia
Spherocytosis

E

notes

erythropoietin (EPO)

Type of test Blood

Normal findings

5–35 IU/L

Test explanation and related physiology

EPO is a hormone produced by the kidney. In response to decreased oxygen, the production of EPO is increased. EPO stimulates the bone marrow to increase RBC production. This improves oxygenation in the kidney, and the stimulus for EPO is reduced. This feedback mechanism is very sensitive to minimal persistent changes in oxygen levels. In patients with normal renal function, EPO levels are inversely proportional to the hemoglobin concentration.

As a hormone, EPO is often administered to patients who experience anemia as a result of chemotherapy. Occasionally athletes, in order to improve oxygen-carrying capacity and thereby improve performance, abuse this hormone.

EPO testing is performed to assist in the differential diagnosis of patients with anemia or polycythemia. EPO is elevated in patients who have low hemoglobin due to failure of marrow production or with increased RBC destruction (iron-deficiency or hemolytic anemia, respectively). However, patients with anemia caused by renal diseases (or bilateral nephrectomy) do not have elevated EPO levels. The renal cells are damaged by disease. EPO levels fall and these patients develop anemia.

Patients who have polycythemia as an appropriate response to chronic hypoxemia have elevated EPO levels. Yet patients who have malignant marrow causes of polycythemia vera may have reduced EPO levels. Some renal cell or adrenal carcinomas can produce elevated EPO levels.

Interfering factors

- Pregnancy is associated with elevated EPO levels.
- The use of transfused blood decreases EPO levels.

Procedure and patient care

- See inside front cover for Routine Blood Testing.
- Fasting: no
- Blood tube commonly used: red or gel separator

Abnormal findings

▲ **Increased levels**
Adrenal carcinoma
AIDS
Chemotherapy
Hemolytic anemia
Iron-deficiency anemia
Megaloblastic anemia
Myelodysplastic syndrome
Pheochromocytoma
Renal cell carcinoma

▼ **Decreased levels**
Polycythemia vera
Renal diseases
Renal failure

E

notes

esophageal function studies (Esophageal manometry, Esophageal motility studies)

Type of test Manometric

Normal findings

Lower esophageal sphincter pressure: 10–20 mm Hg
Swallowing pattern: normal peristaltic waves
Acid reflux: negative
Acid clearing: < 10 swallows
Bernstein test: negative

Test explanation and related physiology

Esophageal function studies may include:

- Determination of the *lower esophageal sphincter (LES)* pressure (manometry)
- Graphic recording of esophageal swallowing waves or *swallowing pattern* (manometry)
- Detection of reflux of gastric acid back into the esophagus (acid reflux)
- Detection of the ability of the esophagus to clear acid (acid clearing)
- An attempt to reproduce symptoms of heartburn (Bernstein test)

Manometry studies

Two manometry studies are used in assessing esophageal function: measurement of LES pressure and graphic recording of swallowing waves. The LES is a sphincter muscle that acts as a valve to prevent reflux of gastric acid into the esophagus. Free reflux of gastric acid occurs when sphincter pressures are low. This occurs in adults with gastroesophageal reflux; in children, it is called chalasia (incompetent LES).

With increased sphincter pressure, as found in patients with achalasia (failure of the LES to relax normally with swallowing) and diffuse esophageal spasms, food cannot pass from the esophagus into the stomach.

Acid reflux with pH probe

Acid reflux is the primary component of gastroesophageal reflux. Patients with an incompetent LES will regurgitate gastric acid into the esophagus. This then causes a drop in the esophageal pH during *esophageal pH monitoring*.

For this test, a small pH probe is passed into the esophagus as the patient swallows. The catheter is connected to a recorder that registers acid reflux and marks meals, sleep, and symptoms. The recorder is worn on a belt or over the shoulder for 24 to 48 hours. A newer, *wireless pH probe* uses a capsule and makes pH monitoring easier.

The use of *esophageal electrical impedance studies (EEI)* records the contractions of the esophagus, with normal being a progressive wave from the top to the bottom of the esophagus when drinking.

Acid clearing

Patients with normal esophageal function can completely clear hydrochloric acid from the esophagus in less than 10 swallows. Patients with decreased esophageal motility require a greater number of swallows to clear the acid.

Bernstein test (acid perfusion)

The Bernstein test is simply an attempt to reproduce the symptoms of gastroesophageal reflux. If the patient has pain with the instillation of hydrochloric acid into the esophagus, the test result is positive and proves that the patient's symptoms are caused by reflux esophagitis. If the patient has no discomfort, a cause other than esophageal reflux must be found.

Potential complications

• Aspiration of gastric contents

Interfering factors

• Eating shortly before the test may affect results.

Procedure and patient care

Before

PT Explain the procedure to the patient. Inform the patient that some medications may be stopped up to 7 days before testing.

PT Instruct the patient not to eat or drink anything for at least 8 hours before the test.

PT Allay any fears and allow the patient to verbalize concerns.

During

• Note the following procedural steps:
  1. These studies are performed in the endoscopy laboratory.
  2. The fasting, unsedated patient is asked to swallow a thin pressure recording tube or a thin pH probe after the nasopharynx is anesthestized topically.
  3. Pressures and pH are recorded per testing protocol.

- Note that these tests are performed by an esophageal technician in approximately 30 minutes.

PT Tell the patient that, except for some initial gagging when swallowing the tubes, these tests are not uncomfortable.

After

PT Inform the patient that it is not unusual to have a mild sore throat after placement of the tubes.

Abnormal findings

Achalasia
Chalasia
Diffuse esophageal spasm
Gastroesophageal reflux
Presbyesophagus
Reflux esophagitis

notes

esophagogastroduodenoscopy (EGD, Upper gastrointestinal [UGI] endoscopy, Gastroscopy)

Type of test   Endoscopy

Normal findings

Normal esophagus, stomach, and duodenum

Test explanation and related physiology

Endoscopy enables direct visualization of the upper GI tract by means of a long, flexible, fiberoptic-lighted scope. The esophagus, stomach, and duodenum are examined for tumors, varices, mucosal inflammations, hiatal hernias, polyps, ulcers, and obstructions. It is used to evaluate patients with dysphagia, weight loss, early satiety, upper abdominal pain, ulcer symptoms, or dyspepsia. It is also used to detect esophageal varices in cirrhotic patients. Suspicious barium swallow or upper GI x-ray findings can be corroborated by EGD.

With upper GI endoscopy, one can also visualize and perform a biopsy of tissue in most of the small intestinal tract. This procedure is referred to as *enteroscopy*. Abnormalities of the small intestine such as arteriovenous (AV) malformations, tumors, enteropathies (e.g., celiac disease), and ulcerations can be diagnosed with enteroscopy.

Capsule endoscopy (or *wireless capsule endoscopy*) uses a capsule containing a miniature camera that records images of the entire digestive tract, particularly the small intestine. The capsule is swallowed with water. The most common reason for doing capsule endoscopy is to search for a cause of bleeding from the small intestine. It may also be useful for detecting polyps, inflammatory bowel disease (Crohn disease), ulcers, and tumors of the small intestine.

An endoscopist often can control active GI bleeding by electrocoagulation, laser coagulation, or the injection of sclerosing agents (e.g., alcohol for esophageal varices). Also, with the endoscope, benign and malignant strictures can be dilated to reestablish patency of the upper GI tract. Biliary, esophageal, and duodenal stents and percutaneous gastrostomy can be placed with the use of EGD.

Contraindications

- Patients with severe upper GI bleeding. The viewing lens will become covered with blood clots.
- Patients with esophageal diverticula. The scope can easily fall into the diverticulum and perforate the wall of the esophagus.

- Patients with suspected perforation. The perforation can be worsened by the insufflation of pressurized air into the GI tract.
- Patients who have had recent GI surgery. The anastomosis may not be able to withstand the pressure of the required air insufflation.

Potential complications
- Perforation of the esophagus, stomach, or duodenum
- Bleeding from a biopsy site or scope trauma
- Pulmonary aspiration of gastric contents
- Oversedation from medication administered during the test
- Hypotension induced by the sedative medication

Interfering factors
- Food in the stomach
- Excessive GI bleeding

Procedure and patient care
Before
- PT Explain the procedure to the patient. See p. xviii for radiation exposure and risks.
- Obtain informed consent.
- PT Instruct the patient to abstain from eating for 8 to 10 hours before the test.
- PT Reassure the patient that this test is not painful but may be mildly uncomfortable. Tell the patient that the throat will be anesthetized with a spray to depress the gag reflex.
- PT Encourage the patient to verbalize fears. Provide support.
- Remove the patient's dentures and eyewear before testing.
- PT Remind the patient that he or she will not be able to speak during the test but that respiration will not be affected.
- PT Instruct the patient not to bite down on the endoscope.
- PT Instruct the patient as to appropriate oral hygiene because the tube will be passed through the mouth.
- If *capsule endoscopy* is to be performed, apply the recording mechanism to the patient's abdomen and waist.

During
- Note the following procedural steps for routine endoscopy:
  1. The patient is placed on the endoscopy table in the left lateral decubitus position.
  2. The throat is topically anesthetized with viscous lidocaine or another anesthetic spray.
  3. The patient is usually sedated with Propofol. This minimizes anxiety and allows the patient to experience a light sleep.

4. The endoscope is gently passed through the mouth and finally into the esophagus.

5. Air is insufflated to distend the upper GI tract for adequate visualization.

6. The esophagus, stomach, and duodenum are evaluated.

7. During enteroscopy, the upper small bowel is visualized and a biopsy is performed if needed.

8. Biopsy or any endoscopic intervention is performed with direct visualization.

9. On completion of direct inspection and surgery, the excess air and GI secretions are aspirated through the scope.

• Note that the test is performed in the endoscopy laboratory by a physician trained in GI endoscopy and takes approximately 20 to 30 minutes.

PT Instruct the patient that eating is allowed about 2 to 4 hours after swallowing the capsule for capsule endoscopy.

PT For *capsule endoscopy*, instruct the patient to return to the physician's office in 6 to 10 hours to return the recording device and have all recording wires removed.

PT For *capsule endoscopy*, instruct the patient that he or she can continue regular activities throughout the examination and will not feel any sensations resulting from the capsule's passage.

After

PT Inform the patient that he or she may have hoarseness or a sore throat after the test. A soothing mouthwash may help.

• Withhold any fluids until the patient is alert and the swallowing reflex returns to normal, usually in 2 to 4 hours.

• Observe the patient's vital signs. Evaluate the patient for bleeding, fever, abdominal pain, dyspnea, or dysphagia.

• Observe safety precautions until the effects of the sedatives have worn off.

PT Inform the patient that it is normal to have some bloating, belching, and flatulence after the procedure.

PT Inform the patient that the sedation may cause some retrograde and antegrade amnesia for a few hours.

PT For *capsule endoscopy*, instruct the patient that there is no need to retrieve the capsule or camera from the stool.

Abnormal findings

Esophageal diverticula
Esophagitis, gastritis, duodenitis
Extrinsic compression by a cyst or tumor outside the upper
   GI tract
Gastroesophageal varices
Helicobacter pylori infection
Hiatal hernia
Peptic stricture and subsequent scarring
Peptic ulcer
Source of upper GI bleeding
Tumor (benign or malignant) of the esophagus, stomach, or
   duodenum

notes

estrogen fractions (Estriol excretion, Estradiol, Estrone)

Type of test Urine (24-hour); blood

Normal findings

	Serum	Urine mcg/24 hours
Estradiol		
Adult male	10–50 pg/mL	0–6
Adult female		
Follicular phase	20–350 pg/mL	0–13
Midcycle peak	150–750 pg/mL	4–14
Luteal phase	30–450 pg/mL	4–10
Postmenopause	≤ 20 pg/mL	0–4
Child < 10 years old	< 15 pg/mL	0–6
Estriol		
Male or child < 10 years old	N/A	1–11
Female, adult		
Follicular phase	N/A	0–14
Ovulatory phase	N/A	13–54
Luteal phase	N/A	8–60
Postmenopausal	N/A	0–11
Female, pregnant		
1st trimester	< 38 ng/mL	0–800
2nd trimester	38–140 ng/mL	800–12,000
3rd trimester	31–460 ng/mL	5000–12,000
Total estrogen		
Male or child < 10 years old	N/A	4–25
Female, nonpregnant	N/A	4–60
Female, pregnant		
1st trimester	N/A	0–800
2nd trimester	N/A	800–5000
3rd trimester	N/A	5000–50,000

Possible critical values

Values 40% lower than the average of two previous values demand immediate evaluation of fetal well-being during pregnancy.

Test explanation and related physiology

There are three major estrogens. Estradiol (E_2), the most potent estrogen, is produced predominantly in the ovary. This hormone is measured most often to evaluate menstrual and fertility problems, menopausal status, sexual maturity, gynecomastia, feminization syndromes, or as a tumor marker for patients with certain ovarian tumors.

Estrone (E_1) is also secreted by the ovary and is the major circulating estrogen after menopause.

Estriol (E_3) is the major estrogen in the pregnant female. Serial urine and blood studies for E_3 excretion provide objective means of assessing placental function and fetal normality in high-risk pregnancies. Unfortunately, only severe placental distress will decrease urinary E_3 sufficiently to reliably predict fetoplacental stress. Furthermore, plasma and urinary E_3 levels are normally associated with significant daily variation, which may confuse serial results. Most clinicians use nonstress fetal monitoring (p. 336) to indicate fetoplacental health.

Interfering factors

- Recent administration of radioisotopes may alter test results.
- Glycosuria and urinary tract infections can increase urine E_3 levels.

Procedure and patient care

- See inside front cover for Routine Blood Testing.
- Fasting: no
- Blood tube commonly used: red
- See inside front cover for Routine Urine Testing for spot urine.

Abnormal findings

▲ **Increased levels**
Adrenal tumor
Feminization syndromes
Hepatic cirrhosis
Hepatic necrosis
Hyperthyroidism
Normal pregnancy
Ovarian tumor
Precocious puberty
Testicular tumor

▼ **Decreased levels**
Anorexia nervosa
Failing pregnancy
Hypopituitarism
Menopause
Primary and secondary
  hypogonadism
Stein-Leventhal syndrome
Turner syndrome

notes

estrogen receptor assay (ER assay, ERA, Estradiol receptor)

Type of test Microscopic examination

Normal findings

Immunohistochemistry
Negative: < 5% of the cells stain for receptors
Positive: > 5% of the cells stain for receptors
Reverse-transcriptase polymerase chain reaction (RT-PCR)
Negative: < 6.5 units
Positive: > 6.5 units

Test explanation and related physiology

The ER assay is useful in determining the prognosis and treatment of breast cancer. The assay is used to determine whether a tumor is likely to respond to endocrine therapy. Tumors with a positive ER assay are more than twice as likely to respond to endocrine therapy than ER-negative tumors.

Interfering factors

- Delay in tissue fixation or too long in fixative solution may cause deterioration of receptor proteins.

Procedure and patient care

Before
PT Explain the procedure to the patient.
PT Instruct the patient to discontinue hormones before breast biopsy is performed. Verify with the physician.

During
- The surgeon obtains tumor tissue.
- Part of the tissue is used for routine histology. A portion of the paraffin block or a slide containing cancer is used for immunohistochemistry (IHC) staining.

After
- Results are usually available in 1 week.

Abnormal findings

Not applicable

notes

ethanol (Ethyl alcohol, Blood alcohol, Blood EtOH)

Type of test Blood; urine; gastric; breath

Normal findings

Blood: 0–50 mg/dL, or 0%-0.05%

Possible critical values

Blood: > 300 mg/dL

Test explanation and related physiology

This test is usually performed to evaluate alcohol-impaired driving or alcohol overdose. Proper collection, handling, and storage of blood alcohol are important for medicolegal cases involving sobriety. Legal testing must be done by specially trained people and must have a strict chain of custody (a paper trail that records sample movement and handling).

Samples tested for legal purposes may include blood, breath, urine, or saliva. Blood is the specimen of choice. Blood is taken from a peripheral vein in living patients and from the aorta in cadavers. Results are given as mg/dL, g/100 mL, or a percentage. Each represents the same amount of alcohol. Blood alcohol concentrations (BACs) greater than 80 mg/dL (0.08%) may cause flushing, slowing of reflexes, and impaired visual activity. Depression of the central nervous system occurs with BACs over 0.1%, and fatalities are reported with levels greater than 0.4%. Persons with BACs less than 0.05% are not considered under the influence of alcohol. Levels greater than 0.05% are considered in most states to be illegal for the operation of motor vehicles and as definite evidence of intoxication.

For legal purposes, when outside of a laboratory or hospital, taking a blood sample for later analysis in the laboratory is not practical or efficient. Breath testing is the most common test performed on automobile drivers. It uses the tail end sample of breath from deep in the lungs and uses a conversion factor to estimate the amount of alcohol in the blood. Blood alcohol testing may be ordered to confirm or refute findings. Alcohol that a person drinks shows up in the breath because it gets absorbed from the intestinal tract into the bloodstream. The alcohol is not metabolized on first pass through the liver. As the blood goes through the lungs, some of the volatile alcohol moves across the alveolar membranes and is exhaled.

Urine testing may also be performed as an alternative to blood. Usually, a patient collects and discards a urine sample and then collects a second sample 20 to 30 minutes later. Saliva alcohol testing is not as widely used but may be used as an alternate screening test. Alcohol stays in the saliva for 6 to 12 hours. Finally, hair testing is used but represents a more chronic use of alcohol.

Interfering factors

- Elevated blood ketones (as with diabetic ketoacidosis) can cause false elevations of blood and breath test results.
- Bacteria in the urine of diabetic patients with glucosuria can metabolize the glucose to alcohol.
- Alcohols other than ethanol (e.g., isopropyl [rubbing alcohol] or methanol [grain alcohol]) will cause positive results.
- **PT** The use of alcohol-based mouthwash or cough syrup may cause false positives on a breath test.

Procedure and patient care

- See inside front cover for Routine Blood Testing.
- Fasting: no
- Blood tube commonly used: gray or red
- Follow the institution's chain-of-custody protocol.
- Follow the agency's protocol regarding specimen collection.
- Use a povidone-iodine wipe instead of an alcohol wipe for cleansing the venipuncture site.
- If a gastric or urine specimen is indicated, approximately 20 to 50 mL of fluid is necessary.
- Breath analyzers are taken at the end of expiration after a deep inspiration.
- The exact time of specimen collection should be indicated.

Abnormal findings

Alcohol intoxication or overdose

notes

evoked potential studies (EP studies, Evoked brain potentials, Evoked responses)

Type of test Electrodiagnostic

Normal findings

No neural conduction delay

Test explanation and related physiology

EP studies are indicated for patients who are suspected of having a sensory deficit but are unable to or cannot reliably indicate recognition of a stimulus. These may include infants, comatose patients, or patients with an inability to communicate. These tests are also used to evaluate specific areas of the cortex that receive incoming stimuli from the eyes, ears, and lower or upper extremity sensory nerves. They are used to monitor natural progression or treatment of deteriorating neurologic diseases.

EP studies focus on changes and responses in brain waves that are evoked from stimulation of a sensory pathway. The EP study measures minute voltage changes produced in response to a specific stimulus such as a light pattern, a click, or a shock.

Evoked potential studies measure and assess the entire sensory pathway from the peripheral sensory organ all the way to the brain cortex. Clinical abnormalities are usually detected by an increase in *latency,* which refers to the delay between the stimulus and the wave response. The sensory stimulus chosen depends on which sensory system is suspected of being pathologic (e.g., questionable blindness, deafness, or numbness) and the area of the brain in which pathology is suspected (auditory stimuli check the brainstem and temporal lobes of the brain; visual stimuli test the optic nerve, central neural visual pathway, and occipital parts of the brain; and somatosensory stimuli check the peripheral nerves, spinal cord, and parietal lobe of the brain).

Visual-evoked responses (VERs) are usually stimulated by a strobe light flash, reversible checkerboard pattern, or retinal stimuli. Most patients with multiple sclerosis show abnormal latencies of VERs, a phenomenon attributed to demyelination of nerve fibers. In addition, patients with other neurologic disorders (e.g., Parkinson disease) show an abnormal latency of VERs. The degree of latency seems to correlate with the severity of the disease. Abnormal results also may be seen in patients with lesions of the optic nerve, optic tract, visual left, and the eye itself. Absence of binocularity, which is a neurologic developmental disorder in infants, can be detected and evaluated by VERs. Eyesight problems or blindness can be detected in infants through VERs or *electroretinography*. This test can also be used during eye surgery to provide a warning of possible damage to the optic nerve.

Auditory brainstem-evoked potentials (ABEPs) or brainstem auditory revoked responses (BAER) are used to evaluate the central auditory pathways of the brainstem. Either ear can be evoked to detect lesions in the brainstem. One of the most successful applications of ABEPs has been screening newborns and other infants for hearing disorders. ABEPs also have great therapeutic implications in the early detection of posterior fossa brain tumors.

Somatosensory-evoked responses (SERs) are usually stimulated by sensory stimulus to an area of the body. The time is then measured for the current of the stimulus to travel along the nerve to the cortex of the brain. SERs are used to evaluate patients with spinal cord injuries and to monitor spinal cord functioning during spinal surgery. They are also used to monitor treatment of diseases, to evaluate the location and extent of areas of brain dysfunction after head injury, and to pinpoint tumors at an early stage.

One of the main benefits of EPs is their objectivity because voluntary patient response is not needed. This objectivity makes EPs useful with nonverbal and uncooperative patients. It permits the distinction of organic from psychogenic problems.

Procedure and patient care

Before

PT Explain the procedure to the patient.

PT Instruct the patient to shampoo his or her hair before the test.

PT Tell the patient that no fasting or sedation is required.

During

- Note that the position of the electrode depends on the type of EP study to be done:
  1. *VERs* are measured using electrodes placed on the scalp along the vertex and cortex lobes. Stimulation occurs by using a strobe light, checkerboard pattern, or retinal stimuli.
  2. *ABEPs* are stimulated with clicking noises or tone bursts delivered via earphones. The responses are detected by electrodes placed along the vertex and on each earlobe.
  3. *SERs* are stimulated using electrical stimuli applied to nerves at the wrist (medial nerve) or knee (peroneal nerve). The response is detected by electrodes placed over the sensory cortex of the opposite hemisphere on the scalp.

- Note that this study is performed by a physician or technician in less than 30 minutes.
- **PT** Tell the patient that little or no discomfort is associated with this study.

After

- If gel was used for the adherence of the electrodes, remove it.

Abnormal findings

Prolonged latency for VER

Absence of binocularity
Blindness
Demyelinating diseases (e.g., multiple sclerosis)
Occipital lobe tumor or CVA
Ocular disease or injury
Optic nerve damage
Optic tract disease
Parkinson disease
Visual field defects

Prolonged latency for ABEP

Auditory nerve damage
Cerebrovascular accident
Deafness
Demyelinating diseases (e.g., multiple sclerosis)
Tumor (e.g., acoustic neuroma)

Abnormal latency for SER

Cervical disc disease
Parietal cortical tumor or CVA
Peripheral nerve injury, transection, or disease
Spinal cord demyelinating diseases
Spinal cord injury

notes

factor V leiden (FVL, Leiden factor V, Mutation analysis)

Type of test Blood

Normal findings

Negative for factor V Leiden

Test explanation and related physiology

Factor V is an important factor in reaction 4 (common pathway) of normal hemostasis (p. 212). The term *factor V Leiden* (FVL) refers to an inherited abnormal form of the gene for factor V. The endogenous anticoagulant protein C (p. 617) is normally able to break down factor V at one of these cleavage sites. However, protein C cannot inactivate this same cleavage site on FVL. Therefore FVL is inactivated at a rate slower than that of normal factor V and persists longer in the circulation. This results in increased thrombin generation and a hypercoagulable state reflected by elevated levels of prothrombin fragment F1 + 2 and other activated coagulation markers. This test is used to diagnose FVL-associated thrombophilia.

Individuals *heterozygous* for the FVL mutation have a slightly increased risk for venous thrombosis. *Homozygous* individuals have a much greater thrombotic risk (e.g., deep vein thrombosis [DVT], arterial thrombosis, or pulmonary embolism).

Individuals who are candidates for FVL testing include patients who

- experienced a thrombotic event without any predisposing factors
- have a strong family history of thrombotic events
- experienced a thrombotic event before 30 years of age
- experienced DVT during pregnancy or while taking birth control pills
- had venous thrombosis at unusual sites (e.g., cerebral, mesenteric, portal, and hepatic veins)
- experienced an arterial clot

Testing for FVL is sometimes preceded by a coagulation screening test called the *activated protein C (APC) resistance test*. This test identifies resistance of factor V to APC. If APC resistance is identified, the patient then may choose to undergo mutation testing by DNA analysis of the *F5* gene, which encodes the factor V protein. This testing should be accompanied by professional genetic counseling for the patient and family members.

Procedure and patient care

- See inside front cover for Routine Blood Testing.
- Fasting: no
- Blood tube commonly used: purple
- If the patient is having FVL mutation analysis, anticoagulants will not interfere with testing.
- As an alternative, genetic testing can be done on the patient's cells obtained by a smear of the oral surface of the cheek.
- Remember: if the patient is receiving anticoagulants, the bleeding time will be increased.

Abnormal findings

Activated protein C resistance

Factor V Leiden genetic mutation (homozygous or heterozygous)

notes

febrile antibodies (Febrile agglutinins)

Type of test Blood

Normal findings

Titers $\leq 1{:}80$

Test explanation and related physiology

Febrile antibodies are used to support the diagnosis and monitoring of infectious diseases (e.g., salmonellosis, rickettsial diseases, brucellosis, and tularemia). Neoplastic diseases, such as leukemias and lymphomas, are also associated with febrile agglutinins. Appropriate antibiotic treatment of the infectious agent is associated with a drop in the titer activity of febrile antibodies.

Procedure and patient care

- See inside front cover for Routine Blood Testing.
- Fasting: no
- Blood tube commonly used: red

Abnormal findings

▲ **Increased febrile antibodies**
   Brucellosis
   Lymphoma
   Rickettsial disease
   Salmonellosis infection
   Systemic lupus erythematosus
   Tularemia leukemia

notes

fecal calprotectin

Type of test Stool

Normal findings

≤ 50 mcg/g
Borderline: 50.1–120 mcg/g
Abnormal: ≥ 120.1 mcg/g

Test explanation and related physiology

Calprotectin comprises a majority of soluble protein content in the cytosol of neutrophils. Elevated fecal calprotectin indicates the migration of neutrophils to the intestinal mucosa that occurs during inflammation. This test is used to identify patients with inflammation of the intestines (e.g., celiac disease) and particularly inflammatory bowel diseases (e.g., Crohn disease and ulcerative colitis).

The test is helpful as an ancillary diagnostic test for inflammatory bowel diseases and is a biomarker for treatment assessment. The level of calprotectin in stool correlates significantly with endoscopic colonic inflammation in both ulcerative colitis and Crohn disease and fecal lactoferrin.

Procedure and patient care

Before

PT Explain the procedure to the patient.
PT Tell the patient that no fasting is needed.

During

- Collect a fresh random stool specimen.
- The specimen must be frozen within 18 hours of collection.
- Collect separate specimens when multiple tests are ordered.
- Note that specimens cannot be collected from a diaper.

Abnormal findings

▲ **Increased levels**
Antineutrophil cytoplasmic antibody
Celiac disease
Crohn disease
Infectious colitis
Necrotizing enterocolitis
Ulcerative colitis

notes

fecal fat (Fat absorption, Quantitative stool fat determination)

Type of test Stool

Normal findings

Fat: 2–6 g/24 hr or 7–21 mmol/day (SI units)
Retention coefficient: ≥ 95%

Test explanation and related physiology

This qualitative or quantitative test is performed to confirm the diagnosis of steatorrhea. Steatorrhea occurs when fat content in the stool is high. It is suspected when the patient has large, greasy, and foul-smelling stools. Determining an abnormally high fecal fat content confirms the diagnosis. Short-gut syndrome and any condition that may cause malabsorption (e.g., sprue, Crohn disease, Whipple disease) or maldigestion (e.g., bile duct obstruction, pancreatic duct obstruction secondary to tumor or gallstones) are also associated with increased fecal fat.

The total output of fecal fat can be tested on a random stool specimen but is more accurate when total 24-, 48-, or 72-hour collection is carried out. Abnormal results from a random specimen should be confirmed by submission of a timed collection. Test values for random fecal fat collections are reported in terms of percent fat.

Procedure and patient care

Before

PT Explain the procedure to the patient.

PT Instruct the patient to abstain from alcohol ingestion for 3 days before testing.

PT Tell the patient to avoid enemas and laxatives.

PT Give the patient instructions regarding the appropriate diet (a diet diary may be requested by the laboratory):

• For adults, usually 100 g of fat per day is suggested for 3 days before and during the collection period.

• Children, and especially infants, cannot ingest 100 g of fat. Therefore a *fat retention coefficient* is determined by measuring the difference between ingested fat and fecal fat and then expressing that difference (the amount of fat retained) as a percentage of the ingested fat:

$$\frac{\text{Ingested fat} - \text{Fecal fat}}{\text{Ingested fat}} \times 100\% = \text{Fat retention coefficient}$$

- Note that the normal fat retention coefficient is 95% or greater. A low value indicates steatorrhea.
- PT Instruct the patient to defecate in a dry, clean container.
- PT Tell the patient not to urinate in the stool container.
- PT Inform the patient to collect diarrheal stools.
- PT Instruct the patient that toilet paper should not be placed in the stool container.
- PT Tell the patient not to take any laxatives or enemas during this test because they will interfere with intestinal motility and alter test results.

During

- Collect each stool specimen and send immediately to the laboratory during the 24- to 72-hour testing period. Label each specimen and include the time and date of collection.
- If the specimen is collected at home, give the patient a stool container to keep in the freezer.

After

- Inform the patient that a normal diet can be resumed.

Abnormal findings

▲ **Increased levels**

Cystic fibrosis

Malabsorption secondary to sprue, celiac disease, Whipple disease, Crohn disease, or radiation enteritis

Maldigestion secondary to obstruction of the pancreaticobiliary tree (e.g., cancer, stricture, gallstones)

Short-gut syndrome secondary to surgical resection, surgical bypass, or congenital anomaly

notes

ferritin

Type of test Blood

Normal findings

Male: 12–300 ng/mL or 12–300 mcg/L (SI units)
Female: 10–150 ng/mL or 10–150 mcg/L (SI units)
Levels may be lower in the elderly
Children
  6 months-15 years: 7–142 ng/mL
  2–5 months: 50–200 ng/mL
  ≤ 1 month: 200–600 ng/mL
  Newborn: 25–200 ng/mL

Test explanation and related physiology

The serum ferritin study is a good indicator of available iron stores in the body. Ferritin, the major iron storage protein, is normally present in the serum in concentrations directly related to iron storage.

Decreases in ferritin levels indicate a decrease in iron storage associated with iron deficiency anemia. A ferritin level less than 10 ng/100 mL is diagnostic of iron deficiency anemia. Increased levels are a sign of iron excess, as seen in hemochromatosis, hemosiderosis, iron poisoning, or recent blood transfusions. Increased ferritin is also noted in patients with megaloblastic anemia, hemolytic anemia, and chronic hepatitis. Furthermore, ferritin is factitiously elevated in patients with chronic disease states, such as neoplasm, alcoholism, uremia, collagen diseases, or chronic liver diseases.

A limitation of this study is that ferritin levels also can act as an acute-phase reactant protein and may be elevated in conditions not reflecting iron stores (e.g., acute inflammatory diseases, infections, metastatic cancer, lymphomas).

Interfering factors

- Recent transfusions and recent ingestion of a meal with high iron content may cause elevated ferritin levels.
- Hemolytic diseases may be associated with an artificially high iron content.
- Disorders of excessive iron storage (e.g., hemochromatosis, hemosiderosis) are associated with high ferritin levels.
- Iron-deficient menstruating women may have decreased ferritin levels.

- Acute and chronic inflammatory conditions and Gaucher disease can falsely increase ferritin levels.

Procedure and patient care

- See inside front cover for Routine Blood Testing.
- Fasting: no
- Blood tube commonly used: red

Abnormal findings

▲ **Increased levels**

Advanced cancers
Alcoholic or inflammatory
  hepatocellular disease
Chronic illnesses (e.g.,
  leukemias, cirrhosis,
  chronic hepatitis)
Collagen vascular diseases
Congenital and acquired
  sideroblastic anemias
Hemochromatosis
Hemolytic anemia
Hemophagocytic syndromes
Hemosiderosis
Inflammatory disease
Megaloblastic anemia

▼ **Decreased levels**

Hemodialysis
Iron-deficiency anemia
Severe protein deficiency

notes

fetal biophysical profile (Biophysical profile [BPP])

Type of test   Ultrasound; fetal activity study

Normal findings

Score of 8–10 points

Possible critical values

Score of less than 4 points may necessitate immediate delivery.

Test explanation and related physiology

The BPP is a method of evaluating fetal status during the antepartal period based on five variables originating within the fetus: fetal heart rate (FHR), fetal breathing movement, gross fetal movements, fetal muscle tone, and amniotic fluid volume. FHR reactivity is measured by the nonstress test (NST) (p. 336); the other four parameters are measured by ultrasound scanning. BPP is often done to assess fetal well-being in the face of a nonreactive NST.

The major premise behind the BPP is that variable assessments of fetal biophysical activity are more reliable than an examination of a single parameter (e.g., FHR). Indications for this test include such factors as postdate pregnancy, maternal hypertension, diabetes mellitus, vaginal bleeding, maternal Rh sensitization, maternal history of stillbirth, and premature rupture of membranes.

The five parameters are briefly described here. Each parameter is scored and contributes either a 2 or a 0 to the score. Therefore 10 is the perfect score, and 0 is the lowest score. Gestational age influences these results. For example, fetal breathing movements are the latest parameter to develop.

- *FHR reactivity*. This is measured and interpreted in the same way as the nonstress test. The FHR is considered reactive when there are movement-associated FHR accelerations of at least 15 beats/min above baseline and 15 seconds in duration over a 20-minute period. A score of 2 is given for reactivity; a score of 0 indicates that the FHR is nonreactive.
- *Fetal breathing movements*. This parameter is assessed based on the assumption that fetal breathing movements indicate fetal well-being and their absence may indicate hypoxemia. To earn a score of 2, the fetus must have at least one episode of fetal breathing lasting at least 30 seconds within a 30-minute observation. Absence of this breathing pattern is scored a 0 on the BPP. It is important to note that fetal breathing

movements increase during the second and third hours after maternal meals and at night. Fetal breathing movements may decrease in such conditions as hypoxemia, hypoglycemia, nicotine use, and alcohol ingestion.

- *Fetal body movements.* Fetal activity is a reflection of neurologic integrity and function. The presence of at least three discrete episodes of fetal movements within a 30-minute observation period is given a score of 2. A score of 0 is given with two or fewer fetal movements in this time period. Fetal activity is greatest 1 to 3 hours after the mother has consumed a meal.

- *Fetal tone.* In the uterus, the fetus is normally in a position of flexion. However, the fetus also stretches, rolls, and moves in the uterus. The arms, legs, trunk, and head may be flexed and extended. A score of 2 is earned when there is at least one episode of active extension with return to flexion. An example of this is the opening and closing of a hand. A score of 0 is given for slow extension with a return to only partial flexion, fetal movement not followed by return to flexion, limbs or spine in extension, and an open fetal hand.

- *Amniotic fluid volume.* Oligohydramnios (too little amniotic fluid) has been associated with fetal anomalies, intrauterine growth retardation, and postterm pregnancy. A score of 2 is given for this parameter when there is at least one pocket of amniotic fluid that measures 2 cm in two perpendicular planes. A score of 0 indicates either that fluid is absent in most areas of the uterine cavity or that the largest pocket measures 1 cm or less in the vertical axis.

A score of 8 or 10 with a normal amount of amniotic fluid indicates a healthy fetus. A score of 8 with oligohydramnios or a score of 4 to 6 is equivocal. An equivocal test result is interpreted as possibly abnormal. A score of 0 or 2 is abnormal and indicates the need for assessment of immediate delivery.

Modifications can be made to the BPP. Some physicians omit the nonstress test if the ultrasound parameters are normal. Some physicians have added placental grading as a sixth parameter.

Another measure of fetal well-being is the *amniotic fluid index (AFI).* Ultrasound is used to measure the largest collection of amniotic fluid in each of the four quadrants within the uterus. The numbers are added together, and the sum is the AFI. The normal range for the AFI is 8 to 18 cm. The sum is plotted on a graph in which the age of gestation also is taken into account. If the AFI is less than the 2.4 percentile, oligohydramnios is present. If AFI exceeds the 97th percentile, polyhydramnios exists.

An abnormally low AFI observed in antepartum testing is associated with an increased risk of intrauterine growth restriction and overall adverse perinatal outcome. The percentile value seems to be a better indicator than an absolute fluid volume. Oligohydramnios is associated with placental failure, fetal gastrointestinal problems, or fetal renal problems. Polyhydramnios is associated with maternal diabetes or fetal upper GI malformation or obstruction.

Doppler ultrasound evaluations of the placenta and the *umbilical artery velocity* can recognize alterations in umbilical artery flow and direction that may indicate fetal stress or illness.

Interfering factors

• If no eye movement or respiratory movement is noted, the fetus may be sleeping. Testing is then extended.

Procedure and patient care

Before
PT Explain the procedure to the patient.
PT Inform the patient that no fasting is required.
PT Explain that stimulants and sedatives can impact test results.

During
• FHR reactivity is measured and interpreted from a nonstress test.
• Fetal breathing movements, fetal body movements, fetal tone, and amniotic fluid volume are determined by ultrasound imaging (see obstetric ultrasonography, p. 754).

After
• If the test results are abnormal or equivocal, support the patient in the next phase of the fetal evaluation process.

Abnormal findings

Congenital anomalies
Fetal asphyxia/death/stress
Intrauterine growth retardation
Oligohydramnios
Postterm pregnancy

notes

fetal nonstress test (Non stress test [NST], Fetal activity determination, Fetal stress test, Contraction stress test [CST], Oxytocin challenge test [OCT])

Type of test Electrodiagnostic

Normal findings

Negative

Test explanation and related physiology

The NST is a method of evaluating the viability of a fetus. It documents the function of the placenta in its ability to supply adequate blood to the fetus. The NST can be used to evaluate any high-risk pregnancy in which fetal well-being may be threatened. The NST is a noninvasive study that monitors acceleration of the FHR in response to fetal movement. Healthy babies will react with an increased heart rate during times of movement, and the heart rate will decrease at rest. When oxygen levels are low, the fetus may not react. Fetal activity may be spontaneous, induced by uterine contraction, or induced by external manipulation. Fetal response is characterized as reactive or nonreactive. This test a reliable indication of fetal viability and negates the need for the contraction stress test.

If NST detects a nonreactive fetus within 40 minutes, the patient is a candidate for the CST. An NST is routinely performed before the CST to avoid the complications associated with oxytocin administration. The CST, frequently called the oxytocin challenge test (OCT), is also used in the assessment of high-risk pregnancy.

For CST, a temporary stress in the form of uterine contractions is applied to the fetus after the IV administration of oxytocin. The reaction of the FHR to the contractions is assessed by an external fetal heart monitor. If the placental reserve is adequate, the maternal–fetal oxygen transfer is not significantly compromised during the contractions and the FHR remains normal (a negative test result). Late FHR decelerations following contractions indicates the placental reserve is inadequate. Although this test can be performed reliably at 32 weeks of gestation, it usually is done after 34 weeks.

Contraindications

- Patient pregnant with multiple fetuses (e.g., twins) because the myometrium is under greater tension and is more likely to be stimulated to premature labor
- Patient with a prematurely ruptured membrane, because labor may be stimulated by the CST

- Patient with placenta previa because vaginal delivery may be induced
- Patient with abruptio placentae because the placenta may separate from the uterus as a result of uterine contractions
- Patient with a previous hysterotomy because the strong uterine contractions may cause uterine rupture
- Patient with pregnancy of less than 32 weeks because early delivery may be induced by the procedure

Potential complications

- Premature labor

Interfering factors

- Hypotension may cause false-positive results.

Procedure and patient care

Before

PT Explain the procedure to the patient.
- Obtain informed consent for the procedure.
PT Teach the patient breathing and relaxation techniques.
- Record the patient's blood pressure and FHR before the test as baseline values.
- If the CST is performed on an elective basis, the patient may be kept nothing by mouth (NPO) in case labor occurs.

During

- Note the following procedural steps:
  1. Monitor vital signs every 10 minutes.
  2. Place an external fetal monitor over the patient's abdomen to record the fetal heart tones.
  3. Monitor baseline FHR and uterine activity for 20 minutes.
  4. If uterine contractions are detected during NST, withhold oxytocin and monitor the response of the fetal heart tone to spontaneous uterine contractions.
  5. If no spontaneous uterine contractions occur, administer oxytocin by intravenous (IV) infusion pump.
- Note that the CST is performed safely on an outpatient basis in the labor and delivery unit, where qualified nurses and necessary equipment are available. The test is performed by a nurse with a physician available.
- Note that the duration of this study is approximately 2 hours.
PT Tell the patient that the discomfort associated with the CST may consist of mild labor contractions. Usually, breathing exercises are sufficient to control any discomfort. Administer analgesics if needed.

After

- Monitor the patient's blood pressure and FHR.
- Discontinue the IV line and assess the site for bleeding.

Abnormal findings

Fetoplacental inadequacy

notes

fetal fibronectin (fFN, Fibronectin)

Type of test Fluid analysis

Normal findings

Negative: $\leq 0.05\,\text{mcg/mL}$

Test explanation and related physiology

Fibronectin may help with implantation of the fertilized egg into the uterine lining. Normally, fibronectin cannot be identified in vaginal secretions after 22 weeks of pregnancy. However, concentrations are very high in the amniotic fluid. If fibronectin is identified in vaginal secretions after 24 weeks, the patient is at high risk for preterm delivery (i.e., before 37 weeks of gestation). The use of fFN is limited to symptomatic women with contractions whose membranes are intact and who have cervical dilation of less than 3 cm.

Procedure and patient care

Before

PT Explain the procedure to the patient.

PT Tell the patient that no fasting is required.

• Determine whether the patient has had a cervical examination or intercourse within the past 24 hours. Results may be inaccurate.

During

• Note the following procedural steps:
  1. The patient is placed in the lithotomy position.
  2. A vaginal speculum is inserted to expose the cervix.
  3. Vaginal secretions are collected from the posterior vagina and paracervical area using a swab from a kit.
  4. The container with appropriate medium is labeled with the patient's name, age, and estimated date of confinement.

PT Tell the patient that no discomfort, except for insertion of the speculum, is associated with this procedure.

• Note that this procedure is performed by a physician or other licensed health care provider in several minutes.

After

PT Tell the patient that results will be available the same or next day.

PT Educate the patient about the signs of preterm labor.

Abnormal findings

High risk for preterm premature delivery

notes

fetal hemoglobin (Kleihauer–Betke)

Type of test Blood

Normal findings

< 1% of red blood cells (RBCs)

Test explanation and related physiology

Fetal hemoglobin may be present in the mother's blood because of fetal–maternal hemorrhage (FMH), which causes leakage of fetal cells into the maternal circulation. When large volumes of fetal blood are lost in this way, neonatal outcomes can be serious and potentially fatal.

Leakage of fetal RBCs results from a breach in the integrity of the placental circulation. As pregnancy continues, more women will show evidence of fetal RBCs in their circulation; by term, about 50% will have detectable fetal cells.

Risk factors correlated with the increasing risk of massive FMH include maternal trauma, placental abruption, placental tumors, third-trimester amniocentesis, fetal hydrops, pale fetal organs, antecedent sinusoidal fetal heart tracing, and twinning. Having one or more of these features should be an indication for fetal hemoglobin testing.

This test is often performed on women who have delivered a stillborn baby to see if FMH was a potential cause of fetal death.

Interfering factors

- Any maternal condition that involves persistence of fetal hemoglobin will cause a false positive.
- If the blood is drawn after C-section, a false positive could occur.

Procedure and patient care

- See inside front cover for Routine Blood Testing.
- Fasting: no
- Blood tube commonly used: red

Abnormal findings

Fetal–maternal hemorrhage
Hereditary persistence of fetal hemoglobin
Intrachorionic thrombi

notes

fetal scalp blood pH

Type of test Blood

Normal findings

pH: 7.25–7.35
O_2 saturation: 30%-50%
Po_2: 18–22 mm Hg
Pco_2: 40–50 mm Hg
Base excess: 0 to -10 mEq/L

Test explanation and related physiology

Measurement of fetal scalp blood pH provides valuable information on fetal acid–base status. This test is useful clinically for diagnosing fetal distress. The pH normally ranges from 7.25 to 7.35 during labor; a mild decline within the normal range is noted with contractions and as labor progresses.

Fetal hypoxia causes anaerobic glycolysis, resulting in excess production of lactic acid. This causes an increase in hydrogen ion concentration (acidosis) and a decrease in pH. Acidosis reflects the effect of hypoxia on cellular metabolism. A high correlation exists between low pH levels and low Apgar scores.

Fetal oxygen saturation monitoring (FSpo₂) also is available to assist the monitoring of fetal well-being during delivery. After membranes are ruptured, and if the baby is in vertex position with good cervical dilatation, a specialized probe can be placed on the temple or cheek of the fetus for FSpo₂ monitoring. The normal oxygen saturation for a baby in the womb receiving oxygenated blood from the placenta is usually between 30% and 70%.

Contraindications

- Patients with premature membrane rupture
- Patients with active cervical infection

Potential complications

- Continued bleeding from the puncture site
- Hematoma
- Ecchymosis
- Infection

Procedure and patient care

Before

PT Explain the procedure to the patient.
- Obtain informed consent for this procedure.
PT Tell the patient that no fasting or sedation is required.

During

- Note the following procedural steps for fetal scalp pH:
  1. Amnioscopy is performed with the mother in the lithotomy position.
  2. The cervix is dilated, and the endoscope (amnioscope) is introduced into the cervical canal.
  3. The fetal scalp is cleansed with an antiseptic and dried with a sterile cotton ball.
  4. A small amount of petroleum jelly is applied to the fetal scalp to cause droplets of fetal blood to bead.
  5. After the skin on the scalp is pierced with a small metal blade, beaded droplets of blood are collected in long, heparinized capillary tubes.
  6. The tube is sealed with wax and placed on ice to retard cellular respiration, which can alter the pH.
  7. The physician performing the procedure applies firm pressure to the puncture site to retard bleeding.
  8. Scalp blood sampling can be repeated as necessary.
- Note that this study is performed by a physician in approximately 10 to 15 minutes.
- **PT** Tell the patient that she may be uncomfortable during the cervical dilation.

After

- **PT** Inform the patient that she may have vaginal discomfort and menstrual-type cramping.

After delivery

- Assess the newborn and document the puncture site(s).
- Cleanse the fetal scalp puncture site with an antiseptic solution and apply an antibiotic ointment.

Abnormal findings

Fetal distress

notes

fetoscopy

Type of test Endoscopy

Normal findings

No fetal distress

Test explanation and related physiology

Fetoscopy is an endoscopic procedure that allows direct visualization of the fetus via the insertion of a tiny, telescope-like instrument through the abdominal wall and into the uterine cavity (Figure F1). Direct visualization may lead to the diagnosis of a severe malformation (e.g., a neural tube defect). During the procedure, fetal blood samples to detect congenital blood disorders (e.g., hemophilia, sickle cell anemia) can be drawn from a blood vessel in the umbilical cord for biochemical analysis. Fetal skin biopsies also can be done to detect primary skin disorders.

Fetoscopy is performed at approximately 18 weeks of gestation. At this time, the vessels of the placental surface are of adequate size, and the fetal parts are readily identifiable. A therapeutic abortion would not be as hazardous at this time as it would be if it were done later in the pregnancy.

Fetoscopy provides access for surgeons to perform minimally invasive surgical procedures on the fetus that are caused by congenital birth defects. For example, central nervous system (CNS) shunts can be inserted.

Potential complications

- Amnionitis
- Amniotic fluid leak
- Intrauterine fetal death
- Premature delivery
- Spontaneous abortion

Procedure and patient care

Before

PT Explain the procedure to the patient.
- Obtain informed consent.
- Assess the FHR to serve as a baseline value.
- Administer fentanyl, if ordered, before the test because it crosses the placenta and quiets the fetus. This prevents excessive fetal movement, which would make the procedure more difficult.

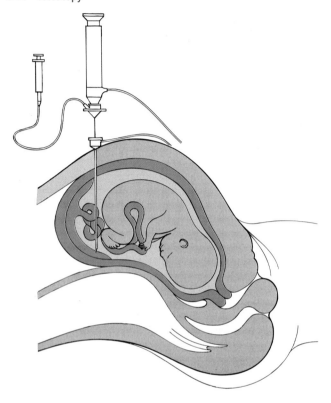

FIG. F1 Fetoscopy for fetal blood sampling.

During
- Note the following procedural steps:
  1. The woman is placed in the supine position on an examining table.
  2. The abdominal wall is anesthetized locally.
  3. Ultrasonography is done to locate the fetus and placenta.
  4. The endoscope is inserted.
  5. Biopsies and blood samples may be obtained.
- Note that this procedure is performed by a physician in 1 to 2 hours.
- PT Tell the patient that the only discomfort associated with this study is the injection of the local anesthetic.

After

- Assess the FHR and compare with the baseline value to detect any side effects related to the procedure.
- Monitor the mother and fetus carefully for alterations in blood pressure, pulse, uterine activity, and fetal activity; vaginal bleeding; and loss of amniotic fluid.
- Administer RhoGAM to mothers who are Rh negative unless the fetal blood is found to be Rh negative.
- Note that a repeat ultrasound is usually performed the day after the procedure to confirm the adequacy of the amniotic fluid and fetal viability.
- If ordered, administer antibiotics prophylactically after the test to prevent amnionitis.
- PT Instruct the mother to avoid strenuous activity for 1 to 2 weeks after the procedure.
- PT Advise the mother to report any pain, bleeding, amniotic fluid loss, or fever.

Abnormal findings

Congenital blood disorders (e.g., hemophilia, sickle cell anemia)
Developmental defects (e.g., neural tube defects)
Primary skin disorders

notes

fibrinogen (Factor I, Quantitative fibrinogen)

Type of test Blood

Normal findings

Adult: 200–400 mg/dL or 2–4 g/L (SI units)
Newborn: 125–300 mg/dL
Levels may be increased in the elderly

Possible critical values

< 100 mg/dL

Test explanation and related physiology

Fibrinogen is essential to the blood-clotting mechanism. It is part of the common pathway in the coagulation system. (See discussion of coagulating factors, p. 209). Fibrinogen, which is produced by the liver, is also an acute-phase protein reactant. It rises sharply during instances of tissue inflammation or necrosis. High levels of fibrinogen have been associated with an increased risk of coronary heart disease, stroke, myocardial infarction, and peripheral arterial disease.

Fibrinogen is used primarily to aid in the diagnosis of suspected bleeding disorders. This testing is used to detect increased or decreased fibrinogen concentration of acquired or congenital origin. It is also used for monitoring the severity and treatment of disseminated intravascular coagulation and fibrinolysis.

Reduced levels of fibrinogen can be seen in patients with liver disease, malnourished states, and consumptive coagulopathies (e.g., disseminated intravascular coagulation). Large-volume blood transfusions are also associated with low levels of fibrinogen because banked blood does not contain fibrinogen. Reduced levels of fibrinogen will cause a prolonged prothrombin time and partial thromboplastin time.

Interfering factors

- Blood transfusions within the past month.
- Diets rich in omega-3 and omega-6 fatty acids reduce levels.

Procedure and patient care

- See inside front cover for Routine Blood Testing.
- Fasting: no
- Blood tube commonly used: blue

Abrmal findings

▲ **Increased levels**
Acute infection (e.g., pneumonia)
Acute inflammatory reactions (e.g., rheumatoid arthritis, glomerulonephritis)
Cerebrovascular accident
Cigarette smoking
Coronary heart disease
Myocardial infarction
Peripheral arterial disease
Pregnancy
Trauma

▼ **Decreased levels**
Advanced carcinoma
Congenital afibrinogenemia
Consumptive coagulopathy
Fibrinolysins
Hemophagocytic lymphohistiocytosis
Large-volume blood transfusion
Liver disease (e.g., hepatitis, cirrhosis)
Malnutrition

notes

F

fluorescein angiography (FA, Ocular photography)

Type of test Other

Normal findings

Normal retinal and choroidal vasculature

Test explanation and related physiology

With the use of fluorescein angiography, the patency and integrity of the retinal circulation can be determined. This test involves injection of sodium fluorescein into the systemic circulation followed by timed-interval photographs performed with a fundus camera. The timed images are then reviewed for specific patterns indicative of disease states. This test is performed to diagnose disease affecting the posterior eye, including the retina, choroid, and optic nerve. The test is often repeated at intervals to monitor treatment or disease progression.

Pathologic changes are recognized by the detection of either hyperfluorescence or hypofluorescence.

Potential complications

- Allergic reactions. Allergies to fluorescein dye are rare. If they occur, they may cause a skin rash and itching.

Procedure and patient care

Before

PT Explain the procedure to the patient.
- Obtain an informed consent.
PT Reinforce the need for the patient to remain still during the few seconds after fluorescein injection.
- Obtain an ocular history of cataracts, prior retinal surgery, and other diseases that may inhibit photography.
PT Instruct the patient to remove any ocular lenses.
PT Inform the patient that there are no dietary restrictions.
- Note that pupil dilatation can improve access to the posterior eye. If ordered, administer appropriate mydriatic medications. Note, however, that these medications are contraindicated for patients with glaucoma because they may dangerously increase ocular pressures.

During

- Note the following procedural steps:
  1. The patient is positioned in the fundus camera with the chin on the bar.

2. The patient is told to pick a spot in the far distance and to concentrate on that spot during the examination.
3. Intravenous access is obtained.
4. Fluorescein dye is injected with the assistance of an autoinjector.
5. Photographs are taken by the ophthalmologist at timed intervals.
- The test is performed and interpreted by an ophthalmologist, usually in the office setting. Results are available in less than 30 minutes.

After

- Remove the intravenous access device and apply pressure to the venipuncture site.
- PT Inform the patient that fluorescein dye is excreted by the kidneys and to expect very yellow urine for the next 24 hours.

Abnormal findings

▲ **Increased levels**
Detached retina
Diabetic retinopathy
Inflammation
Papilledema
Retinitis pigmentosa
Trauma
Tumor

▼ **Decreased levels**
Diabetes
Edema
Hemorrhage
Prior photocoagulation
  therapy
Radiation to the eye
Vascular disease

Focused Assessment with Sonography for Trauma (FAST)

Type of test Ultrasound

Normal findings

No sign of abdominal or thoracic trauma

Test explanation and related physiology

The Focused Assessment with Sonography for Trauma (FAST) is a series of ultrasound views typically performed at the bedside as part of an initial evaluation of trauma patients to detect abnormal free fluid in the chest and abdomen. The extended FAST examination (E-FAST) adds views to evaluate for pneumothorax. The presence of abnormal free fluid appears as a hypoechoic or anechoic (dark gray or black) collection on ultrasound. This fluid is presumed to be blood, although it may represent urine in cases of pelvic trauma. If any view reveals an anechoic collection, the FAST examination is considered positive. If all views are free of abnormal fluid, it is a negative FAST examination. If any view cannot be adequately assessed, the study is indeterminate.

The standard evaluation includes ultrasound views in the following four serial locations so as to identify the most life-threatening injuries first.

1. *Pericardial:* The ultrasound probe is often placed in the subxiphoid area to obtain a subcostal view of all four cardiac chambers and the pericardium. This area is assessed for pericardial fluid and signs of tamponade.
2. *Right flank:* The ultrasound probe evaluates the pleural space, the subphrenic space, the hepatorenal space (Morison's pouch), and the inferior pole of the right kidney. Morison's pouch is one of the first sites to demonstrate abnormal fluid collection representing intraabdominal injury.
3. *Left flank:* The ultrasound evaluates the pleural space, the subphrenic space, the perisplenic space, and the inferior pole of the left kidney.
4. *Pelvic:* The ultrasound probe is placed just above the symphysis pubis to look for fluid collections behind the bladder in males and behind the uterus in females.

A fifth thoracic view is used as part of the E-FAST examination to rule out pneumothorax. This is done by viewing the normal sliding of the pleura using either the gray-scale B-mode,

M-mode, or Doppler ultrasound. In addition, the lung is evaluated for the normal presence of "comet tails" that extend perpendicular from the surface to the deeper portion of the lung.

The limitation of the FAST examination is that a number of injuries are not detectable by ultrasound, such as diaphragm tears, bowel perforations, and abdominal injuries that do not produce free fluid in amounts detectable by ultrasound (generally >200 mL).

Contraindications

- Patients who require immediate surgery because there should be no delay for ultrasound

Interfering factors

- Severe obesity makes it more difficult.
- Chronic obstructive pulmonary disease results in hyperinflated lungs and reduces the accuracy of cardiac images.
- Women of reproductive age often have a trace amount of free pelvic fluid associated with ovulation.

Procedure and patient care

Before
PT Explain the procedure to the patient.
PT Tell the patient that no discomfort is expected.

During
- Note the following procedural steps:
  1. The patient is placed in the supine position.
  2. A gel lubricant is applied to the patient's skin to enhance sound wave transmission and reception.
  3. A transducer is placed over the skin.
  4. Images are made of the space being studied.
- The test can be completed within a few minutes and interpreted immediately at the bedside.

After
- Remove the gel from the patient's skin.
PT Explain findings and follow up to the patient.

Abnormal findings

Cardiac tamponade
Hemopericardium
Hemothorax
Intraperitoneal free fluid
Pneumothorax

notes

folic acid (Folate)

Type of test Blood

Normal findings

Serum: 5–25 ng/mL or 11–57 nmol/L (SI units)
RBC folate: 360–1400 nmol/L

Test explanation and related physiology

Folic acid (folate), one of the B vitamins, is necessary for normal function of RBCs and white blood cells (WBCs). It is needed for the adequate synthesis of certain purines and pyrimidines, which are precursors for DNA. Blood folate levels require normal absorption by the intestinal tract.

Tissue folate is best tested by determining the content of folate in RBCs. A low RBC folate can mean either that there is tissue folate depletion because of folate deficiency, which requires folate therapy, or that the patient has primary vitamin B_{12} (p. 805) deficiency, which blocks the ability of cells to take up folate. In the latter case, the proper therapy would be with vitamin B_{12} rather than with folic acid.

Folic acid blood levels are performed to assess folate availability in pregnancy, to evaluate hemolytic disorders, and to detect anemia caused by folic acid deficiency (in which the RBCs are abnormally large, causing a megaloblastic anemia). These RBCs have a shortened life span and impaired oxygen-carrying capacity. If folic acid blood levels are low, RBC folate is measured.

Folate deficiency is present in about 33% of pregnant women; many people with alcoholism; and patients with a variety of malabsorption syndromes, including celiac disease, sprue, Crohn disease, and jejunal/ileal bypass procedure. Folate binds to aluminum hydroxide. Patients with a chronic use of antacids or H_2-receptor antagonists and with diets marginal in folate may experience low folate levels.

Elevated serum levels of folic acid may be seen in patients with pernicious anemia because vitamin B_{12} is needed to allow incorporation of folate into tissue cells. The folic acid tests are often done in conjunction with tests for vitamin B_{12} levels.

Interfering factors

- A falsely normal result may occur in a folate-deficient patient who has received a blood transfusion.

Procedure and patient care

- See inside front cover for Routine Blood Testing.
- Fasting: verify with laboratory
- Blood tube commonly used: red
- Some laboratories prefer an 8-hour fast.
- PT Instruct the patient not to consume alcoholic beverages before the test.
- Draw the specimen before starting folate therapy.

Abnormal findings

▲ **Increased levels**

Pernicious anemia
Recent blood transfusions
Vegetarianism

▼ **Decreased levels**

Alcoholism
Anorexia nervosa
Folic acid deficiency anemia
Hemolytic anemia
Malabsorption syndrome
  (e.g., sprue, celiac disease)
Malignancy
Malnutrition
Pregnancy

notes

> **fungal testing** (Antifungal antibodies; Beta-D-glucan,(1,3)-
> β-D-glucan, Fungitell, Fungal culture, Fungal antigen assay, Fungal PCR
> testing)

Type of test Blood, microscopic examination

Normal findings

No antibodies detected
β-D-glucan:

Negative	< 60 pg/mL
Indeterminate	60–79 pg/mL
Positive	≥ 80 pg/mL

Culture: no growth in 24 days
Gram stain: no fungus seen

Test explanation and related physiology

Few fungal diseases can be diagnosed clinically; many are diagnosed by isolating and identifying the infecting fungus in the clinical laboratory. Fungal infections can be superficial, subcutaneous, or systemic (deep). The systemic fungal infections (mycoses) are the most important, for which serologic antibody testing is performed. In general, mycoses are caused by the inhalation of airborne fungal spores. In the United States, the most serious fungal infections are coccidioidomycosis, blastomycosis, histoplasmosis, and paracoccidioidomycosis. These infections start out as primary pulmonary infections. *Aspergillus, Candida,* and *Cryptococcus* systemic infections usually affect only those with compromised immunity.

Fungal antibody testing is not highly reliable. In general, this testing is used for screening for antibodies to dimorphic fungi (*Blastomyces, Coccidioides, Histoplasma* spp.) and the antigen of *Cryptococcus neoformans* during acute infection. Antibodies are present in only about 70% to 80% of infected patients. When positive, they merely indicate that the person has an active or has had a recent fungal infection. These antibodies can be identified in the blood or cerebrospinal fluid (CSF). Antibodies can be tested singularly or as a fungal panel.

(1,3)-β-D-glucan is used to support the diagnosis of invasive fungal disease (IFD) in at-risk patients. Normally, serum contains low levels of (1,3)-β-D-glucan, presumably from yeasts present in the alimentary and GI tract. D-glucan becomes elevated well in advance of conventional clinical signs and symptoms of IFD. As opportunistic infections, IFDs are common among patients with

hematologic malignancies or AIDS. They account for a growing number of nosocomial infections, particularly among organ transplant recipients and other patients receiving immunosuppressive treatments. $(1,3)$-β-D-glucan is produced by most invasive fungal organisms. *Blastomyces* and *Cryptococcus* produce very low levels of $(1,3)$-β-D-glucan. Mucoromycetes do not produce $(1,3)$-β-D-glucan. It is important to note that negative results do not exclude fungal etiology, especially in the early stages of infection.

Correlation of the patient clinical condition with culture results is necessary. Fungus can be cultured from blood, body fluids, CSF, fresh tissue, bronchopulmonary secretions, or swabs of the ear, nose, and throat or from urine. Accurate fungal culture is labor intensive and requires a highly experienced laboratory. Results are not available quickly.

Interfering factors

- False-positive results can occur if a patient's intestinal tract is colonized with *Candida* spp.
- False-positive results occur in patients on hemodialysis using cellulose membranes.
- False-negative results occur in serum that is hemolyzed, icteric, lipemic, or turbid.

Procedure and patient care

- See inside front cover for Routine Blood Testing.
- Fasting: no
- Blood tube commonly used: red or serum separator
- Indicate on the laboratory request the particular antibody or panel of antibodies that are to be tested.
- Because some patients with fungal infection may be immunocompromised, instruct them to check for signs of infection at the venipuncture site.

Abnormal findings

▲ Increased levels

Acute fungal infection

Previous systemic exposure to fungal disease

notes

galectin-3 (GAL-3)

Type of test Blood

Normal findings

≤ 22.1 ng/mL

Test explanation and related physiology

Heart failure progresses primarily by dilatation of the ventricular cardiac chamber through remodeling in fibrosis as a response to cardiac injury and/or overload. Galectin-3 (GAL-3) is a biomarker that appears to be actively involved in both the inflammatory and fibrotic pathways involved in remodeling. GAL-3 is a carbohydrate-binding lectin whose expression is associated with inflammatory cells, including macrophages, neutrophils, and mast cells. GAL-3 has been linked to cardiac remodeling in the setting of heart failure and a variety of other cardiac insults. Elevated levels are associated with increased risk of mortality.

Interfering factors

- Hemolysis increases GAL-3 levels.
- Heterophile antibodies (p. 797) increase GAL-3 levels.

Procedure and patient care

- See inside front cover for Routine Blood Testing.
- Fasting: no
- Blood tube commonly used: lavender

Abnormal findings

▲ Increased levels

Congestive heart failure

notes

gallbladder nuclear scanning (Hepatobiliary scintigraphy, Cholescintigraphy, DISIDA scanning, HIDA scanning)

Type of test Nuclear scan

Normal findings

Gallbladder, common bile duct, and duodenum are visualized within 60 minutes after radionuclide injection. (This confirms patency of the cystic and common bile ducts.)

Test explanation and related physiology

Through the use of iminodiacetic acid analogs (IDAs) labeled with technetium-99 m (^{99m}Tc), the biliary tract can be evaluated in a safe, accurate, and noninvasive manner.

Failure to visualize the gallbladder 60 to 120 minutes after injection of the radionuclide dye is virtually diagnostic of an obstruction of the cystic duct (acute cholecystitis). Delayed filling of the gallbladder is associated with chronic or acalculous cholecystitis. The identification of the radionuclide in the biliary tree, but not in the bowel, is diagnostic of common bile duct obstruction.

Gallbladder function can be numerically determined by calculating the capability of the gallbladder to eject its contents after the injection of a cholecystokinetic drug. It is believed that an ejection fraction lower than 35% indicates chronic cholecystitis or functional obstruction of the cystic duct.

Occasionally, morphine sulfate is given intravenously during nuclear scanning. The morphine causes increased ampullary contraction. This reproduces the patient's symptoms of biliary colic and forces the bile containing the radionuclide into the gallbladder, shortening the expected time of visualization of the gallbladder.

Contraindications

• Patients who are pregnant because of the risk of fetal damage

Interfering factors

• If the patient has not eaten for more than 24 hours, the radionuclide may not fill the gallbladder. This would produce a false-positive result.

Procedure and patient care

Before

PT Explain the procedure to the patient. See p. xviii for radiation exposure and risks.

PT Assure the patient that he or she will not be exposed to large amounts of radioactivity.

PT Instruct the patient to fast for at least 2 to 4 hours before the test. This fasting is preferable but not mandatory.

During

- Note the following procedural steps:
  1. After IV administration of a ^{99m}Tc-labeled IDA analog (e.g., mebrofenin, disofenin), the right upper quadrant of the abdomen is scanned.
  2. Serial images are obtained over 1 hour.
  3. Subsequent images can be obtained at 15- to 30-minute intervals.
  4. If the gallbladder, common bile duct, or duodenum is not visualized within 60 minutes after injection, delayed images are obtained up to 4 hours later.
  5. When an *ejection fraction* is to be determined, the patient is given a fatty meal or cholecystokinin to evaluate emptying of the gallbladder. The gallbladder is continually scanned to measure the percentage of isotope ejected.
- Note that a radiologist performs this study in 1 to 4 hours in the nuclear medicine department.

PT Tell the patient that the only discomfort associated with this procedure is the intravenous (IV) injection of radionuclide.

After

- Obtain a meal for the patient if indicated.

Abnormal findings

Acalculous cholecystitis
Acute cholecystitis
Chronic cholecystitis
Common bile duct obstruction secondary to gallstones, tumor, or stricture
Cystic duct syndrome

notes

gallium scan

Type of test Nuclear scan

Normal findings

Diffuse, low level of gallium uptake, especially in the liver and spleen

No increased gallium uptake within the body

Test explanation and related physiology

A gallium scan of the total body may be performed 24, 48, and 72 hours after an IV injection of radioactive gallium. Most commonly, a single scan is performed 2 to 4 days after the gallium injection. Gallium is a radionuclide that is concentrated by areas of inflammation and infection, abscesses, and benign and malignant tumors. Lymphomas are particularly gallium avid. Other tumors that can be detected by a gallium scan include sarcomas, hepatomas, and carcinomas of the gastrointestinal (GI) tract, kidney, uterus, stomach, and testicle.

This test is useful in detecting metastatic tumor. However, to a large degree, positron emission tomography (PET) scans (p. 589) have replaced gallium scans for the identification of malignancy. The gallium scan is useful in demonstrating a source of infection in patients with a fever of unknown origin. Gallium can be used to identify noninfectious inflammation within the body in patients who have an elevated sedimentation rate. PET scans are more commonly used to identify areas of acute infection.

Another method of scanning is called *single-photon emission computed tomography (SPECT) imaging.* This provides a more detailed image.

Contraindications

- Patients who are pregnant unless benefits outweigh risks

Interfering factors

- Recent barium studies will interfere with visualization of gallium within the abdomen.

Procedure and patient care

Before

PT Explain the procedure to the patient. See p. xviii for radiation exposure and risks.

- If ordered, administer a cathartic or enema to the patient to minimize increased gallium uptake in the bowel.

During
- Note the following procedural steps:
  1. The unsedated patient is injected with gallium.
  2. A total-body scan may be performed 4 to 6 hours later by slowly passing a radionuclide detector over the body.
  3. Additional scans are usually taken 24, 48, and 72 hours later.
  4. During the scanning process, the patient is placed in the supine position and occasionally in the lateral position.
- Note that a nuclear medicine technologist performs each scan in approximately 30 to 60 minutes. Repeated scanning is required. Repeated injections are not necessary.
- PT Inform the patient that test results are interpreted by a nuclear medicine physician and are usually available 72 hours after the injection.

After
- PT Assure the patient that only tracer doses of radioisotopes have been used and that no precautions against radioactive exposure to others are necessary.

Abnormal findings

Abscess
Infection
Noninfectious inflammation
Tumor

notes

gamma-glutamyl transpeptidase (GGTP, γ-GTP, Gamma-glutamyl transferase [GGT])

Type of test Blood

Normal findings

Male and female age 45 years and older: 8–38 units/L or 8–38 international units/L (SI units)

Female younger than age 45 years: 5–27 units/L or 5–27 international units/L (SI units)

Elderly: slightly higher than adult level

Child: similar to adult level

Newborn: five times higher than adult level

Test explanation and related physiology

This test is used to detect liver cell dysfunction, and it very accurately indicates even the slightest degree of cholestasis. This is the most sensitive liver enzyme in detecting biliary obstruction, cholangitis, or cholecystitis. As with leucine aminopeptidase and 5-nucleotidase (pp. 459 and 528), the elevation of GGTP generally parallels that of alkaline phosphatase; however, GGTP is more sensitive. GGTP is not increased in bone diseases as is alkaline phosphatase. A normal GGTP level with an elevated alkaline phosphatase level implies skeletal disease. Elevated GGTP and alkaline phosphatase levels imply hepatobiliary disease. Another important clinical aspect of GGTP is that it can detect chronic alcohol ingestion. Therefore it is very useful in the screening and evaluation of patients with alcoholism. GGTP is elevated in approximately 75% of patients who chronically drink alcohol.

Why this enzyme is elevated after an acute myocardial infarction is not clear. The elevation usually occurs 1 to 2 weeks after infarction.

Interfering factors

• Values may be decreased in late pregnancy.

Procedure and patient care

• See inside front cover for Routine Blood Testing.
• Fasting: yes
• Blood tube commonly used: red
• Patients with liver dysfunction often have prolonged clotting times.

Abnormal findings

▲ **Increased levels**

Alcohol ingestion
Cancer of the pancreas
Cholestasis
Cirrhosis
Cytomegalovirus infections
Epstein-Barr virus (infectious mononucleosis)
Hepatic necrosis
Hepatic tumor or metastasis
Hepatitis
Hepatotoxic drugs
Jaundice
Myocardial infarction
Pancreatitis
Reye syndrome

notes

gastric emptying scan

Type of test Nuclear scan

Normal findings

Normal values are determined by type and quantity of radiolabeled ingested food.

Time	Lower normal limits (%)	Upper normal limits (%)
0 minutes		
30 minutes	70	
1 hour	30	90
2 hours		60
3 hours		30
4 hours		10

Values lower than normal represent abnormally fast gastric emptying. Values higher than upper limits represent delayed gastric emptying.

Test explanation and related physiology

In this study, the patient ingests a solid or liquid "test meal" containing a radionuclide such as technetium (Tc). The stomach is then scanned until gastric emptying is complete. This study is used to assess the stomach's ability to empty solids or liquids and to evaluate disorders that may cause a delay in gastric emptying, such as obstruction (caused by peptic ulcers or gastric malignancies) and gastroparesis. This scan is also useful in determining the rate of gastric emptying. This is helpful in the diagnosis of gastric retention secondary to gastroparesis or gastric obstruction. It is helpful in evaluating patients who have postcibal nausea, vomiting, bloating, early satiety, belching, or abdominal pain.

Contraindications

• Patients who are pregnant or lactating, unless the benefits outweigh the risk of fetal or newborn injury

Procedure and patient care

Before

PT Explain the procedure to the patient. See p. xviii for radiation exposure and risks.

PT Instruct the patient to keep on nothing by mouth (NPO) status after midnight on the day of the test.

PT Tell the patient that smoking is prohibited on the day of examination because tobacco can inhibit gastric emptying.

During

- Note the following procedural steps:
  1. In the nuclear medicine department, the patient is asked to ingest a test meal. In the *solid-emptying* study, the patient eats scrambled egg whites containing Tc. In the *liquid-emptying* study, the patient drinks orange juice or water containing ^{99m}Tc diethylenetriamine pentaacetic acid (DTPA) or indium-111 DTPA.
  2. After ingestion of the test meal, the patient is imaged by a gamma camera that records gastric images. Images are obtained for 2 minutes every 30 to 60 minutes until gastric emptying is complete. This may take several hours, although each particular timed scan takes a few minutes.
  3. With the use of computer calculations of timed images, the rate of gastric emptying can be determined.

After

PT Assure the patient that no radiation precautions need to be taken since only a small dose of nuclear material was given.

Abnormal findings

Gastric obstruction caused by gastric ulcer or cancer
Gastroparesis
Nonfunctioning GI anastomosis

gastrin

Type of test Blood

Normal findings

Adult: 0–180 pg/mL or 0–180 ng/L (SI units)
   Levels are higher in elderly patients.
Child: 0–125 pg/mL

Test explanation and related physiology

Zollinger-Ellison (ZE) syndrome (gastrin-producing pancreatic tumor) and G-cell hyperplasia (overfunctioning of G cells in the distal stomach) are associated with high serum gastrin levels. Patients with these tumors have aggressive peptic ulcer disease. Unlike a patient with routine peptic ulcers, a patient with ZE syndrome or G-cell hyperplasia has a high incidence of complicated and recurrent peptic ulcers. It is important to identify this latter group of patients to institute more appropriate, aggressive medical and surgical therapy. The serum gastrin level is normal in patients with routine peptic ulcer and greatly elevated in patients with ZE syndrome or G-cell hyperplasia.

It is important to note that patients who are taking antacid peptic ulcer medicines or have had peptic ulcer surgery or have atrophic gastritis will have a high serum gastrin level. However, levels usually are not as high as in patients with ZE syndrome or G-cell hyperplasia.

Not all patients with ZE syndrome exhibit increased levels of serum gastrin. Some may have *top normal* gastrin levels, which makes these patients difficult to differentiate from patients with routine peptic ulcer disease. ZE syndrome or G-cell hyperplasia can be diagnosed in these top normal patients by *gastrin stimulation tests* with the use of calcium or secretin. Patients with these diseases have greatly increased serum gastrin levels associated with the infusion of these drugs.

Interfering factors

- Peptic ulcer surgery creates a persistent alkaline environment, which is the strongest stimulant to gastrin.
- Ingestion of high-protein food can result in an increase in serum gastrin two to five times the normal level.

Procedure and patient care

- See inside front cover for Routine Blood Testing.
- Fasting: yes
- Blood tube commonly used: red
- PT Tell the patient to avoid alcohol for at least 24 hours.
- For the *calcium infusion test,* administer calcium gluconate intravenously. A preinfusion serum gastrin level is then compared with specimens taken every 30 minutes for 4 hours.
- For the *secretin test,* administer secretin intravenously over 1 minute. Preinjection and postinjection serum gastrin levels are taken at 2, 5, 10, 15, and 20 minutes after injection.

Abnormal findings

▲ **Increased levels**
  Atrophic gastritis
  Chronic renal failure
  G-cell hyperplasia
  Gastric carcinoma
  Pernicious anemia
  Pyloric obstruction or gastric outlet obstruction
  Retained antrum after gastric surgery
  Zollinger-Ellison syndrome

notes

gastroesophageal reflux scan (GE reflux scan, Aspiration scan)

Type of test Nuclear scan

Normal findings
No evidence of GE reflux

Test explanation and related physiology

GE reflux scans are used to evaluate patients with symptoms of heartburn, regurgitation, vomiting, and dysphagia. They are also used to evaluate the medical or surgical treatment of patients with GE reflux. *Aspiration scans* may be used to detect aspiration of gastric contents into the lungs.

G

Contraindications
- Patients who cannot tolerate abdominal compression
- Patients who are pregnant or lactating unless the benefits outweigh the risks

Procedure and patient care

Before
- PT Explain the procedure to the patient. See p. xviii for radiation exposure and risks.
- PT Assure the patient that no pain is associated with this test.
- PT Instruct the patient not to eat anything after midnight.

During
- Note the following procedural steps:

GE reflux scan
1. The patient is placed in the supine position and asked to swallow a tracer cocktail (e.g., orange juice, diluted hydrochloric acid, and ^{99m}Tc colloid).
2. Images are taken of the patient's esophageal area.
3. The patient is asked to assume other positions to determine whether GE reflux occurs and, if so, in what position.
4. A large abdominal binder that contains an air-inflatable cuff is placed on the patient's abdomen. This is insufflated to increase abdominal pressure.
5. Images are again taken to detect GE reflux.

Aspiration scans
- Delayed images are made over the lung fields 24 hours after injection of technetium to detect esophagotracheal aspiration.
- Note that this procedure is performed in the nuclear medicine department in approximately 30 minutes.

PT Remind the patient that no discomfort is associated with this test.

• For infants being evaluated for achalasia, note that the tracer is added to the feeding or formula. Nuclear tracer films are then taken over the next hour, with 24-hour delayed films as needed.

After

PT Assure the patient that he or she has ingested only a small dose of nuclear material. No radiation precautions need to be taken against the patient or his or her bodily secretions.

Abnormal findings

GE reflux
Pulmonary aspiration

notes

genetic testing (Breast cancer [*BRCA*] and ovarian cancer, Colon cancer, Cardiovascular disease, Tay–Sachs disease, Cystic fibrosis, Melanoma, Hemochromatosis, Thyroid cancer, Paternity [parentage analysis], Forensic genetic testing)

Type of test Blood; miscellaneous

Normal findings

No genetic mutation

Test explanation and related physiology

Genetic testing is used to identify a predisposition to disease, to establish the presence of a disease, to establish or refute paternity, or to provide forensic evidence used in criminal investigations. Prenatal and newborn genetic tests are discussed on pp. 501 and 523.

Predictive tests for defective genes known to be associated with certain diseases are now commonly used in screening people who have certain phenotypes and family histories compatible with a genetic mutation. Genetic testing is done in addition to a family history (pedigree). In this section, we discuss commonly performed genetic tests. There are many more familial diseases that can be predicted by genetic testing (see Table G1).

There are now direct-to-consumer (DTC) genetic testing kits that provide predictability about some diseases, allergies, body habitus, hair / eye color, and even paternity. There are potential risks and drawbacks to the use of DTC testing. Most DTC genetic tests look for only the major variants associated with a particular disease and do not test for minor harmful variants, causing a false sense of security for the patient who receives a "negative result." Furthermore, interpretation of the genetic tests can be difficult and should be provided by a knowledgeable health care provider in order to avoid unneeded anxiety or false reassurance and to assist in making important decisions about preventative care.

Breast cancer and ovarian cancer genetic testing

Inherited mutations in *BRCA* (BReast CAncer) genes indicate an increased susceptibility for development of breast cancer. The two genes in which mutations are most commonly seen are *BRCA1* and *BRCA2*. More than half of women who inherit mutations will develop breast cancer by the age of 50 years, compared with fewer than 2% of women without the genetic defect

TABLE G1   Genetic susceptibility syndromes

Organ affected	Familial cancer susceptibility syndromes
Breast and Gynecologic	Cowden
	Fanconi Anemia
	Li-Fraumeni
	Peutz-Jeghers
Endocrine and Neuroendocrine Neoplasias	Carney-Stratakis
	Hyperparathyroidism
	Medullary Thyroid Cancer
	Pheochromocytoma
Renal Cell Cancer	Birt-Hogg
	Von Hippel-Lindau
Skin Cancer	Bloom
	Brooke-Spiegler
	Dyskeratosis Congenita
	Epidermodysplasia Verruciformis,
	Epidermolysis Bullosa
	Muir-Torre
	Multiple Familial Trichoepithelioma
	Oculocutaneous Albinism
	Werner
	Xeroderma Pigmentosum
	PTEN Hamartoma Tumor

(Table G2). Also, see Table G3 for Interpretation of *BRCA* results.

The *BRCA* genes also confer an increased susceptibility for ovarian cancer. In the normal population, fewer than 2% of women develop ovarian cancer by age 70 years. Of women with mutations of the *BRCA1* gene, 44% develop ovarian cancer by that age. Ovarian cancer is less commonly associated with the *BRCA2* gene (20%). Furthermore, a woman with a *BRCA* mutation who has already had breast cancer has a 65% chance of developing a contralateral breast cancer in her lifetime (compared with < 15% of women without the genetic defect). A woman with breast cancer and a *BRCA* genetic defect has a 10 times greater risk of developing ovarian cancer as a second primary cancer compared with similar women without the mutated form of the gene.

TABLE G2 Who should be tested for *BRCA* mutations?

Patient with breast cancer	Family history (with at least one characteristic)
Diagnosed at ≤50 years of age	• No other family history
Diagnosed with 2 primary breast cancers	
Triple negative breast cancer at ≤60 years of age	
Breast cancer at any age	• One relative ≤50 years of age with breast cancer
Diagnosed at any age	• One relative with ovarian cancer at any age
	• Two relatives with breast cancer at any age
	• Two relatives with pancreatic or prostate cancer
	• Personal history of ovarian cancer
	• Ashkenazi Jewish heritage
	• First- or second-degree relative with *BRCA* mutation
	• Close relative with male breast cancer
Male breast cancer at any age	• Family history not needed.
No personal history of breast cancer	Male breast cancer in a close relative

G

TABLE G3 Interpretation of BRCA genetic testing results

Result	Risk of breast cancer
Positive for a deleterious mutation	Increased risk
Genetic variant; suspected deleterious	Uncertain increased risk
Genetic variant; favor polymorphism	Normal risk
Genetic variant; uncertain significance	Uncertain risk
No deleterious mutation	Normal risk

These mutations have an autosomal dominant inheritance pattern, indicating that women who inherit just one genetic defect can develop the phenotypic cancers. Men with *BRCA* genetic mutations are at an increased risk for the development of breast, prostate, pancreas, and colon cancer. In addition, they can pass the mutation to their daughters. Because BRCA is an autosomal dominant gene, 50% of the children are at risk.

Colon cancer genetic testing

There are multiple forms of colon cancer strongly associated with family history. These genetic defects are inherited in an autosomal dominant fashion and are important for genome mismatch repair.

The most common form is familial adenomatous polyposis (FAP). The patient presents with over one hundred polyps in his or her colon—one or more of which may degenerate into cancer. FAP is caused by a genetic mutation in the 5q 21–22 (APC) gene on chromosome 5. These genes encode tumor suppression proteins.

Hereditary nonpolyposis colorectal cancer (HNPCC) syndrome is also known as Lynch syndrome. These patients are more difficult to recognize because they may have few polyps. HNPCC is associated most often with mutations (defective DNA mismatch repair) of MLH1, MLH2, and MSH6.

Tay–Sachs disease genetic testing

Tay–Sachs disease is characterized by the onset of severe mental and developmental retardation in the first few months of life. Affected children become totally debilitated by 2 to 5 years of age and die by ages 5 to 8 years. Another form of the same disease is late-onset *Tay–Sachs* or chronic GM2, also known as gangliosidosis. The basic defect in affected patients is a mutation in the hexosaminidase A gene, which is on chromosome 15. This gene is responsible for the synthesis of hexosaminidase (HEX), an enzyme that normally breaks down a fatty substance called GM2 gangliosides. Ashkenazi (Eastern European) Jews and non-Jewish French Canadians, particularly those in the Cajun population in Louisiana, are affected most. This gene is inherited as an autosomal recessive gene. Carriers have one affected gene. Affected individuals have both defective genes. A *carrier couple* has a 25% chance of having a child affected with the disease.

HEX A protein testing (p. 414) has been extremely effective for identification of carriers and affected individuals. Both the test for the protein and that for the gene mutation are performed on a blood sample or during amniocentesis (p. 39).

Cystic fibrosis genetic testing

Cystic fibrosis (CF) is caused by a mutation in the cystic fibrosis transmembrane conductance regulator (*CFTR*) gene located on chromosome 7. A mutation in this gene alters the cell's ability to regulate sodium, postassium, and chloride transport.

There are more than 1000 mutations and 200 polymorphisms of the CFTR gene. Gene mutation analysis is utilized for carrier identification, prenatal diagnosis in at-risk pregnancies, and newborn screening programs for CF.

CF is an autosomal recessive disease. A carrier has one mutated *CFTR* gene. The person affected by CF has mutations on both copies of *CFTR*. Genetic testing is now used to identify both carriers of CF and neonates with the disease, as well as to detect fetal disease during pregnancy. The sweat test (p. 698) is a more accurate method to diagnose the disease in affected children. The use of genetic testing for CF is often limited to those with a family history of CF, partners of CF patients, and pregnant couples with a family history of CF. Genetic testing can be performed on blood samples or on samples taken during chorionic villus sampling (CVS, p. 202) or during amniocentesis (p. 39).

Melanoma genetic testing

There are two melanoma susceptibility genes:
- The tumor suppressor gene *CDKN2A* encoding the p16 protein on chromosome 9 p21
- The *CDK4* gene on chromosome 12 q13

The p16 genetic mutation is by far the most common form of hereditary melanoma. Characteristics of familial melanoma include frequent multiple primary melanomas, early age of onset of first melanoma, and frequently the presence of atypical or dysplastic nevi (moles). Family members with the following characteristics may consider testing for p16 genetic mutations:
- Multiple diagnoses of primary melanoma
- Two or more family members with melanoma
- Melanoma and pancreatic cancer
- Melanoma and a family history of multiple atypical nevi
- Relatives of a patient with a p16 genetic mutation

The average age at diagnosis is 35 years for those with a mutation in p16 versus 57 years in the general population.

Hemochromatosis genetic testing

The diagnosis of hemochromatosis is traditionally made by using serum iron studies. When hereditary hemochromatosis

(HH) is suspected, mutation analysis of the *hemochromatosis-associated HFE genes* (*C282Y* and *H63D*) is done. HH is an iron overload disorder that is considered to be the most common inherited disease in whites; it affects 1 in 500 individuals. Increased intestinal iron absorption and intracellular iron accumulation lead to progressive damage of the liver, heart, pancreas, joints, reproductive organs, and endocrine glands.

Patients with symptoms and early biochemical signs of iron overload consistent with HH should be tested. Relatives of individuals with HH should also be studied. Serum iron markers are monitored at more frequent intervals if an HFE mutation is detected. Early initiation of phlebotomy therapy reduces the hemochromatosis-related symptoms and organ damage.

Hereditary transthyretin cardiac amyloidosis (hATTR-CA)

Amyloidosis is a generic term used to describe the deposition of misfolded proteins causing impairment of organ and tissue function. The two most common forms of amyloidosis are immunoglobulin light chain amyloidosis (AL) and transthyretin amyloidosis (ATTR). The accepted nomenclature for the different forms of amyloidosis is "A" for amyloid followed by the abbreviation of the precursor protein. For example, in *ATTR amyloidosis, transthyretin (TTR)* is the precursor protein that forms amyloid fibrils, and in AL, the precursor protein is a monoclonal immunoglobulin light chain. Transthyretin amyloidosis can occur either due to a mutation in the transthyretin gene that is inherited in an autosomal dominant fashion or due to age-related protein misfolding. The current nomenclature guidelines also recommend that familial forms of ATTR now be called hereditary ATTR (hATTR). Patients may receive genetic testing, via saliva or blood, for known or likely pathogenic TTR variants. Direct-to-consumer testing can be initiated by the patient.

Thyroid cancer genetic testing

Genetic testing for RET germline mutations has shown 100% sensitivity and specificity for identifying those at risk for developing inherited medullary thyroid cancer (multiple endocrine neoplasia [MEN] 2A, MEN 2B, or familial medullary thyroid carcinoma [FMTC]).

Use of the genetic assay allows earlier and more definitive identification and clinical management of those with a risk for FMTC. FMTC is surgically curable if detected before it has spread to regional lymph nodes. Thus there is an emphasis on early detection and intervention.

Cardiac genetic testing

Mutations in sarcomeric genes cause early onset cardiac channelopathies and cardiomyopathies. These are rare but potentially lethal heart conditions that include long QT syndrome (LQTS), catecholaminergic polymorphic ventricular tachycardia (CPVT), hypertrophic cardiomyopathy (HCM), arrhythmogenic right ventricular cardiomyopathy, and dilated cardiomyopathy (DCM).

Limited genetic testing for familial hypercholesterolemia (FH) looks for inherited genetic changes in three different genes (LDLR, APOB, and PCSK9) known to cause FH. In affected people, medical intervention can be more aggressively pursued.

Gastric cancer genetic testing

Hereditary diffuse gastric cancer (HDGC) is an autosomal dominant cancer predisposition syndrome predominantly caused by loss-of-function germline variants in the tumor suppressor CDH1. CDH1 encodes for E-cadherin. Nearly 90% of patients who have an aberrant CDH1 gene have evidence of signet ring carcinoma of the stomach on subsequent gastrectomy.

Paternity genetic testing (parentage analysis)

DNA testing is the most accurate form of testing to prove or exclude paternity when the identity of the biological father of a child is in doubt. By comparing DNA variants in the mother and child, it is possible to determine variants that the child inherited from the biological mother. Thus any remaining DNA variation must have come from the biological father. If the DNA from the tested man is found to contain these paternal characteristics, then the probability of paternity can be determined. Testing is more than 99% accurate. Testing can be done on a mouth swab or blood. Results are usually available in 1 to 3 weeks.

Many parents are given misinformation at the time of twin births as to whether the twins are identical or fraternal. DNA samples from siblings can be analyzed to indicate whether twins are identical or fraternal with an accuracy of greater than 99%.

There are times, particularly in circumstances of rape, when early pregnancy paternity identification is desired. *Noninvasive prenatal paternity testing* can now be performed accurately by extracting and amplifying fetal chromosome alleles from maternal blood.

Forensic genetic testing

Forensic DNA testing is used with increasing frequency in today's courtrooms because of its accuracy. Furthermore, DNA testing can be so conclusive that it often motivates plea bargaining and thereby reduces court time. It can quickly establish guilt or innocence beyond a reasonable doubt. Because DNA does not change and deteriorates very slowly even after death, testing can be performed on any body part, cadaver, or live person. Specimens considered adequate for DNA testing include blood, teeth, semen, saliva, bone, nails, skin scrapings, and hair.

Contraindications

• Patients who are not emotionally able to deal with the results

Procedure and patient care

Before

PT Explain the procedure to the patient.

PT Tell the patient that no fasting is required.

PT Tell the patient the time it will take to have the results back.

PT Inform the patient of the high costs of genetic testing and that it may not be covered by all medical insurance plans.

During

• Obtain the specimen in a manner provided by the specialized testing laboratory.
  ○ **Blood:** A venous blood sample is collected in a lavender-top tube. Cord blood can be used for infants.
  ○ **Buccal swab:** A cotton swab is placed between the lower cheek and gums. It is twisted and then placed on a special paper or in a special container.
  ○ **Amniotic fluid:** At least 20 mL of fluid is preferred.
  ○ **CVS:** 10 mg of cleaned villi as prescribed by the laboratory.
  ○ **Product of conception:** 10 mg of placental tissue are preserved in a sterile medium.
  ○ **Other body parts:** As much tissue as is available is tested.

After

• Apply pressure or a dressing to the venipuncture site.
• Make sure that the patient has an appointment scheduled for obtaining the results.
• Ensure counseling after results are obtained.

Abnormal findings

Affected state
Genetic carrier state

notes

genomic cancer testing (Oncotype DX, Genotyping, Genomics)

Type of test Microscopic examination

Normal findings

Low risk genomic score

Test explanation and related physiology

Genomic testing of cancers is a multigene assay that provides an assessment of the likelihood of the presence of a particular cancer or the risk for distant or local cancer recurrence. It can also assess the benefit of therapy in newly diagnosed cancer patients. In cancer treatment, the evaluation of the likelihood of distant recurrence is usually based on multiple pathologic factors, such as nodal status, tumor size, tumor grade, targeted receptors, and other pathologic findings. However, these factors may not be adequate to sufficiently quantify the recurrence risk to provide significant insight into the risks and benefits of therapy.

Genomic testing is designed to provide additional quantitative data regarding the patient's tumor biology to assist in clinical decision making regarding the use of anticancer therapies. By providing answers to key questions about the aggressiveness of and appropriate treatment for early-stage cancer, these practice-changing tests can help select the right treatment at the right time in each individual case. Genomic testing can help patients and their physicians optimize their cancer care and outcomes, enabling many patients to avoid unnecessary procedures and therapies. For example, a genomic test performed on the patient's tumor after part or all of the tumor has been excised can provide a risk score. If the patient's tumor genomics indicate a "low risk score," she or he has only a slight chance of the tumor acting aggressively and will only derive minimal or no benefit from aggressive anticancer therapy. Patients with tumor genomics indicating a "high risk" score may have a significant chance of the tumor acting aggressively and can experience considerable benefit from anticancer therapy.

At present, genomic testing is available for assessing cancers of the breast, bladder, lung, thyroid, prostate, and colon; lymphomas; and hematologic malignancies. Genomic testing is also being used to treat chronic benign diseases. This, along with molecular testing, offers the promise of very extensive information regarding pathogenesis, prognosis, and treatment options for benign and malignant diseases.

Our use of genomic testing as it relates to cancer care refers to identifying particular panels of numerous genes of a tumor that statistically have been shown to provide more accurate prognostic and therapeutic data. Information gained from genomic testing is quite different from the information derived from other genetic testing, which identifies a gene causing a specific disease in a patient. For the sake of clarity, we have chosen to discuss genetic testing separately (p. 369). Furthermore, genomic testing is different from other tumor markers determined by other molecular laboratory methods and may provide similar information regarding prognosis and treatment of cancer.

Bladder cancer genomics

This genomic assay is able to provide an assessment of bladder tumor aggressiveness. It is able to separate less aggressive bladder cancer from the more aggressive muscle invasive bladder cancer. The test is also able to predict the response and survival outcome to neoadjuvant chemotherapy.

Another bladder cancer-related genomic assay is performed on urine. This test is designed to help rule out the presence of bladder (or any urothelial) cancer at an early stage. It is particularly appropriate for low-risk patients with hematuria. This is also a noninvasive and accurate method of performing bladder cancer surveillance because of its ability to detect early recurrence of bladder cancer. A "low risk" score would indicate no evidence of a new or recurrent urothelial cancer. The *Cx Bladder* is an example of a genomic test for bladder cancer.

Breast cancer genomic testing

The test is intended for use in all newly diagnosed patients with early-stage (stage I, II or IIIa), invasive breast cancer who have node-negative or node-positive (1–3), estrogen receptor-positive (ER+), HER2-negative disease. The Oncotype DX rtPCR assay provides a recurrence score between 0 and 100. A low score means the cancer has a lower chance of returning and therefore the patient has a lower chance of benefiting from chemotherapy. A high score means the cancer has a higher chance of recurring, and the patient has a higher chance of benefiting from chemotherapy.

A second genomic test is available for noninvasive breast cancer to determine which women with this type of cancer are at high risk of having their cancer return, either as ductal carcinoma in situ (DCIS) or as an invasive carcinoma. The *Oncotype DX* breast cancer test for patients with DCIS provides an individualized prediction of the 10-year risk of local recurrence (either

DCIS or invasive carcinoma). This diagnostic test helps guide treatment decision regarding extent of surgery, hormone therapy, and radiation therapy. *MammaPrint* and *Mammostrat* are other examples of genomic tests for breast cancer.

Hyperactive signaling in the PI3K pathway has been implicated in processes that contribute to the progression of breast and colon cancer. *PIK3CA* (phosphatidylinositol 3-kinase, catalytic, alpha polypeptide) mutations may lead to hyperactivation of PI3K increasing cellular growth, transformation, adhesion, apoptosis, survival, and motility. A mutation in this gene is associated with a more aggressively acting breast or colon cancer. PIK3CA mutation can be detected using samples from the primary breast or metastatic cancer. It can also be detected in the plasma.

Colon cancer genomic testing

The genomic colon cancer test is used to predict recurrence risk in patients with stage II and stage III colon cancer to provide an individualized approach to treatment planning. Based on a recurrence risk score, a better-informed decision can be made about whether chemotherapy is needed following surgery (stage II) or whether oxaliplatin should be added to the chemotherapy regimen after surgery (stage III). In this way, the test may help some patients avoid the complications of treatments they do not need, while directing others to the therapy that is most likely to benefit them.

Additionally, some genomic testing provides microsatellite instability (MSI) gene and mismatch repair (MMR) gene testing to detect the protein expression of MSI and the 2 MMR genes (MLH1 and MSH2) (see colo-rectal cancer tumor analysis, p. 221). Used in conjunction with the *Colon Recurrence Score* test, MMR status offers deeper insight into the risk of recurrence. Approximately 15% of stage II colon cancer patients with MMR-deficient (MMR-D) tumors have a lower risk of recurrence.

Furthermore, genomic testing and molecular testing can be used to identify particular cancer markers (see cancer tumor marker, p. 164) to indicate associative inherited syndromes, such as FAP and HNPCC (Lynch syndrome).

Lung cancer genomic testing

Subsets of lung cancers can be defined by the presence of mutations that may occur in oncogenes (see cancer markers, p. 164). These mutations may be found in adenocarcinoma, squamous cell carcinoma (SCC), and large cell carcinoma. There are targeted drugs that can inhibit the tumor development of these proteins and thereby inhibit tumor growth. Most significantly, the therapeutic importance of genes that encode pharmacologically targetable *tyrosine kinases* involved in growth factor receptor signaling, *epidermal growth factor receptor (EGFR)*, and *anaplastic lymphoma kinase (ALK)* has changed the way these cancers are diagnosed and treated.

Lymphoma and hematologic cancer genomics

A major challenge in diagnosing hematologic and solid tumor cancers is the high degree of heterogeneity of the tumor cells. Mutations that have critical clinical implications regarding diagnosis and treatment may only be present in very low levels, making detection of these mutations difficult. Genomic testing can identify mutations that can provide insight into prognosis by providing a comprehensive view of the tumor's genomic profile. Particular testing panels have been developed for follicular and B cell lymphomas and for other non-Hodgkin lymphomas and leukemias.

Prostate cancer genomic testing

Genomic testing for prostate cancer was developed to help men with early-stage prostate cancer make the most informed treatment decision (specifically, aggressive therapy versus close surveillance). Men with genomic scores that are "low risk" have only a 3% chance that their disease will become life threatening and therefore may choose no treatment. Those with "high risk" scores would benefit from immediate surgery or radiation therapy. Genomic prostate tests build on traditional clinical and pathologic factors to provide additional, clinically relevant insight into the underlying tumor biology. The result is a more precise and accurate assessment of risk, which helps more men avoid the lifelong complications associated with treatments they do not need, while directing aggressive therapy to men who require immediate treatment. Decipher, Prolaris, and ProMark are examples of genomic tests for prostate cancer.

Thyroid cancer genomic testing

Thyroid cancer genomics can identify a benign gene expression signature in thyroid nodules that are identified as "indeterminate" on needle aspiration biopsy of the thyroid. In these cases, diagnostic thyroidectomy would not be required. This testing can also guide treatment decision when a "suspicious for malignancy" result is obtained. A thyroid nodule is most commonly evaluated for the possibility of malignancy by ultrasound (p. 761), thyroid scanning (p. 720), thyroid hormone testing (p. 716), and thyroid aspiration (p. 718). Genomic testing can be used on the aspirate (see thyroid fine needle biopsy, p. 718) of indeterminate nodules and classify them as either benign (< 5% risk for malignancy) or suspicious (> 50% risk for malignancy). With a benign score, observation or ultrasound follow-up could be recommended *in lieu* of thyroid surgery, avoiding unnecessary surgery. With a suspicious score, thyroid surgery is recommended.

Furthermore, if a thyroid aspirate is suspicious for cancer, genomic testing can also identify genes that can classify the tumor as medullary thyroid cancer (MTC). If positive, more aggressive lymph node surgery may be indicated. Thyroid genomics of a suspicious aspirate could also identify the V600E *BRAF* mutation indicating the presence of a papillary thyroid cancer (PTC) and encourage more extensive planned surgery. The presence of the *BRAF* gene mutation may be a prognostic marker of aggressive papillary thyroid cancer and is significantly associated with recurrence, lymph node metastases, extrathyroidal extension, and advanced stage in papillary thyroid cancer. Mutated *BRAF* is virtually absent in follicular, Hurthle cell, medullary carcinomas, and in benign thyroid tumors. The *Afirma gene expressive classifier (GEC)* is an example of genomic test for thyroid cancer.

Procedure and patient care
Before
- PT Explain the significance of the prognostic data available for the patient's tumor.
- PT Explain the benefits of genomics in helping make appropriate decisions regarding the use of adjuvant chemotherapy.
- Provide the patient with emotional support.
- Ensure that insurance will cover this expensive testing.

During
- The pathologist will send paraffin-embedded tumor tissue to the centralized laboratory.
- Results will be available in about 1 to 3 weeks.
- For bladder cancer identification, a urine specimen is provided.

After
- PT Provide education and support to patients as they evaluate their results.

Abnormal findings
Aggressive versus nonaggressive cancer
High likelihood of benefit for aggressive anticancer treatment
High risk for the presence of cancer or recurrence

notes

gliadin, endomysial, and tissue transglutaminase antibodies (Celiac serology, Deamidated gliadin peptide [DGP], Endomysial antibody [EMA], Tissue transglutaminase [tTG])

Type of test Blood
Normal findings

	Age	Normal
Gliadin IgA/IgG	0–2 years	< 20 EU
	3 years and older	< 25 EU
Endomysial IgA	All	Negative
Tissue transglutaminase IgA	All	< 20 EU

Test explanation and related physiology

Gliadin and gluten are proteins found in wheat and wheat products. Patients with celiac disease cannot tolerate ingestion of these proteins or any products containing wheat. When an affected patient ingests wheat-containing foods, gluten and gliadin build up in the intestinal mucosa. These gliadin and gluten proteins (and their metabolites) cause direct mucosal damage.

Furthermore, IgA immunoglobulins (antigliadin, antiendomysial, and antitissue transglutaminase [tTG-ab]) are made, appearing in the gut mucosa and in the serum of severely affected patients. The identification of these antibodies in the blood of patients with malabsorption is helpful in supporting the diagnosis of celiac sprue or dermatitis herpetiformis. However, a definitive diagnosis of celiac disease can be made only when a patient with malabsorption is found to have the pathologic intestinal lesions characteristic of celiac disease. Also, the patient's symptoms must be improved with a gluten-free diet. Both are needed for the diagnosis. Because of the high specificity of IgA endomysial antibodies for celiac disease, the test may obviate the need for multiple small bowel biopsies to verify the diagnosis.

In patients with known celiac disease, these antibodies can be used to monitor disease status and dietary compliance. Furthermore, these antibodies identify successful treatment because they will become negative in patients on a gluten-free diet.

When celiac disease is suspected but the patient does not improve with gluten-free diet, one should consider the possibility of autoimmune enteropathy (AIE). In these patients, serology should include testing for *antienterocyte and/or antigoblet cell antibodies*.

Interfering factors

- Other GI diseases (e.g., Crohn disease, colitis, and severe lactose intolerance) can cause elevated gliadin antibodies.

Procedure and patient care

- See inside front cover for Routine Blood Testing.
- Fasting: no
- Blood tube commonly used: red
- Obtain a list of foods eaten in the last 48 hours.
- Assess how many malabsorption symptoms the patient has been experiencing in the last few weeks.

Abnormal findings

Celiac disease
Celiac sprue
Dermatitis herpetiformis

notes

glucagon

Type of test Blood

Normal findings

50–100 pg/mL or 50–100 ng/L (SI units)

Test explanation and related physiology

Glucagon is a hormone secreted by the alpha cells of the pancreatic islets of Langerhans. It is secreted in response to hypoglycemia and increases the blood glucose. As serum glucose levels rise in the blood, glucagon is inhibited by a negative feedback mechanism.

Elevated glucagon levels may indicate the diagnosis of a *glucagonoma* (i.e., an alpha islet cell neoplasm). Glucagon deficiency occurs with extensive pancreatic resection or with burned-out pancreatitis. Arginine is a potent stimulator of glucagon. If glucagon levels fail to rise even with arginine infusion, a diagnosis of glucagon deficiency as a result of pancreatic insufficiency is confirmed.

In an insulin-dependent patient with diabetes, glucagon stimulation caused by hypoglycemia does not occur. To differentiate the causes of glucagon insufficiency between pancreatic insufficiency and diabetes, *arginine stimulation* is performed. Patients with diabetes will have an exaggerated elevation of glucagon with arginine. In pancreatic insufficiency, glucagon is not stimulated with arginine. Furthermore, in patients with diabetes, hypoglycemia fails to stimulate glucagon release as would occur in a nondiabetic person.

Because glucagon is thought to be metabolized by the kidneys, renal failure is associated with high glucagon and, as a result, high glucose levels. When rejection of a transplanted kidney occurs, one of the first signs of rejection may be increased serum glucagon levels.

Interfering factors

• Levels may be elevated after prolonged fasting or moderate to severe exercise.

Procedure and patient care

• See inside front cover for Routine Blood Testing.
• Fasting: yes
• Blood tube commonly used: lavender

Abnormal findings

▲ **Increased levels**
Acromegaly
Acute pancreatitis
Chronic renal failure
Diabetes mellitus
Familial hyperglucagonemia
Glucagonoma
Hyperlipidemia
Pheochromocytoma
Severe stress including
  infection, burns, surgery,
  and acute hypoglycemia

▼ **Decreased levels**
Cancer of the pancreas
Chronic pancreatitis
Cystic fibrosis
Diabetes mellitus
Idiopathic glucagon
  deficiency
Postpancreatectomy

notes

glucose measurements (Blood sugar; Fasting blood sugar;
Diabetic control index; Glucose, blood; Glucose, postprandial;
2-hour Postprandial glucose [2-hour PPG]; 1-hour Glucose screen;
Glycosylated hemoglobin [GHb, GHB, Hb A1c], Glycohemoglobin

Type of test Blood

Normal findings

Glucose

Cord: 45–96 mg/dL or 2.5–5.3 mmol/L (SI units)
Premature infant: 20–60 mg/dL or 1.1–3.3 mmol/L
Neonate: 30–60 mg/dL or 1.7–3.3 mmol/L
Infant: 40–90 mg/dL or 2.2–5 mmol/L
Child < 2 years: 60–100 mg/dL or 3.3–5.5 mmol/L
Child > 2 years to adult:

    Fasting: 70–110 mg/dL or < 6.1 mmol/L (Fasting is defined
      as no caloric intake for at least 8 hours.)

    Casual: ≤ 200 mg/dL (< 11.1 mmol/L) (Casual is defined
      as any time of day regardless of food intake.)

Elderly:

    60–90 years: 82–115 mg/dL or 4.6–6.4 mmol/L
    > 90 years: 75–121 mg/dL or 4.2–6.7 mmol/L

Possible critical values

Adult: < 54 and > 400 mg/dL
Infant: < 40 mg/dL
Newborn: < 30 and > 300 mg/dL

2-Hour PPG

0–50 years: < 140 mg/dL or < 7.8 mmol/L (SI units)
50–60 years: < 150 mg/dL
60 years and older: < 160 mg/dL

1-hour glucose screen for gestational diabetes

< 140 mg/dL

Glycosylated hemoglobin

Nondiabetic adult or child: 4% to 5.9%
Good diabetic control: < 7%
Fair diabetic control: 8% to 9%
Poor diabetic control: > 9%

Test explanation and related physiology

    In general, glucose measurements are used to diagnose and
monitor *diabetes mellitus* and its treatment. Serum blood sugar
can be measured directly in the laboratory with a blood sample.

More easily, glucose levels can be obtained from a fingerstick using a glucose meter. Blood glucose can be continuously monitored with the use of a continuous glucose monitor (CGM). If diabetes is suspected by elevated fasting blood levels, glycosylated hemoglobin or glucose tolerance tests can be performed.

Glucose results are affected by dietary intake. Blood sugar should peak at about an hour after ingesting a meal (1-hour postprandial glucose) and then slowly return to normal baseline levels at 2 hours (2-hour postprandial glucose). In patients with diabetes, the glucose level is still elevated 2 hours after the meal. The PPG is an easily performed screening test for diabetes mellitus. The 1-hour glucose screen is used to detect gestational diabetes mellitus after a 50- to 100-g oral glucose load *(Sullivan test)*.

Glycosylated hemoglobin (GHB or HbA_{1c}) is used to diagnose and monitor diabetes. HbA_{1c} measures of the amount of hemoglobin A_{1c} in a red blood cell. Because HbA_{1c} strongly binds glucose over its 120-day lifespan, high levels of glucose over the last 120 days cause HbA_{1c} to be elevated. Therefore, HbA_{1c} reflects the average blood sugar level for the 100 to 120 days prior to testing. Another advantage of HbA_{1c} is that it is not affected by short-term variations (e.g., food intake, exercise, stress, hypoglycemic agents). HbA_{1c} is helpful in differentiating short-term hyperglycemia in patients whose glucose is elevated because of a recent physical stress (e.g., myocardial infarction) from those who have diabetes.

Glycated proteins are another measurement of glucose. Because the turnover rate of proteins is much faster than hemoglobin, the measurement of serum glycated proteins (e.g., *glycated albumin* or *glycated fructosamine*) provides more recent information about glucose levels. Glycated proteins reflect an average blood glucose level of the past 15 to 20 days.

By a relatively simple calculation, GHb can be accurately correlated with the *estimated average glucose (eAG)*, which is the average glucose level throughout the day. This has been very helpful for diabetics and health care professionals in determining and evaluating daily glucose goals. See Table G4.

Glucose can be directly measured in the urine when the level exceeds the ability of the kidneys to reabsorb the glucose. See p. 386.

Interfering factors

- Many forms of stress (e.g., general anesthesia, surgery, myocardial infarction, shock, strenuous exercise, burns) can cause transient increased serum glucose levels.

TABLE G4 Correlation between glycosylated hemoglobin and estimated average glucose (diabetes.org)

A_{1c} (%)	eAG (mg/dL)	Interpretation
4	68	Nondiabetic range
5	97	Nondiabetic range
6	125	Nondiabetic range
7	154	ADA target
8	183	Action suggested

- Many pregnant women experience some degree of glucose intolerance. If significant, it is called gestational diabetes.
- Some IV fluids contain dextrose, which is quickly converted to glucose. Therefore, patients receiving IV fluids may have increased glucose levels.
- If the patient is not able to eat the entire test meal or vomits some or all the meal, levels will be falsely decreased.
- Hemoglobinopathies can affect results because the quantity of hemoglobin A (and, as a result, HbA1) varies considerably.
- Abnormally low levels of proteins may falsely indicate normal glycated protein levels despite high glucose levels.
- Falsely elevated values occur when the RBC life span is lengthened (e.g., after splenectomy).

Procedure and patient care

- See inside front cover for Routine Blood Testing.
- Fasting: yes (for fasting blood glucose)
- Blood tube commonly used: red or gray
- PT For *fasting blood sugar*, instruct the patient to fast for 8 hours. Water is permitted.
- PT To prevent starvation, which may artificially raise the glucose levels, tell the patient not to fast much longer than 8 hours.
- Withhold insulin or oral hypoglycemics until after blood is obtained.
- PT For the *2-hour PPG*, instruct the patient to eat the entire meal (with at least 75 g of carbohydrates) and then not to eat anything else until the blood is drawn.
- PT For the *1-hour glucose screen* for GDM, instruct the patient to consume the 50-g oral glucose load and then not to eat anything until the blood is drawn

PT   Instruct the patient not to smoke during the testing. Smoking may increase glucose levels.

Abnormal findings

▲ **Increased levels (hyperglycemia) and HbA$_{1c}$**

Acromegaly
Acute pancreatitis
Acute stress response
Chronic renal failure
Corticosteroid therapy
Cushing syndrome
Diabetes mellitus
Diuretic therapy
Glucagonoma
Pheochromocytoma

▼ **Decreased level (hypoglycemia)**

Addison disease
Extensive liver disease
Hypopituitarism
Hypothyroidism
Insulinoma
Insulin overdose
Starvation

▼ **Decreased levels of HbA$_{1c}$**

Chronic blood loss
Chronic renal failure
Hemolytic anemia

G

notes

glucose-6-phosphate dehydrogenase (G-6-PD screen, G-6-PD quantification, Glucose-6-phosphate dehydrogenase [G-6-PD] deficiency DNA sequencing)

Type of test Blood

Normal findings

Negative (quantification)
12.1 ± 2 IU/g of hemoglobin
146–376 units/trillion RBC
G-6-PD sequencing: no mutation noted

Test explanation and related physiology

This test is used to identify G-6-PD deficiency in patients who have developed hemolysis after taking certain oxidizing drugs. It is especially useful in males of certain ethnic populations who are susceptible to this genetic defect.

G-6-PD is an enzyme used in glucose metabolism. G-6-PD deficiency causes precipitation of oxidized hemoglobin. This may result in hemolysis of variable severity. This disease is a sex-linked, recessive trait carried on the X chromosome. The full effect of this genetic defect is not seen if the normal gene is present on a second X chromosome to oppose the genetic defect. In males, there is no second X gene and the genetic defect is unopposed. Affected males inherit this abnormal gene from their mothers, who are usually asymptomatic. In these males, the disease is most severe. G-6-PD activity is higher in premature infants than in term infants. In the United States, G-6-PD deficiency is found mainly in African Americans. Also, those of Mediterranean descent (Italians, Greeks, Sephardic Jews) are at risk for the genetic defect.

With the administration of an oxidizing drug, hemolysis can start as early as the first day and usually by the fourth day. The most common oxidizing drugs known to precipitate hemolysis and anemia in G-6-PD deficiency are noted in Box G1.

BOX G1   Medications that can precipitate G-6-PD deficiency

- Antibiotics, such as quinolones, nitrofurantoin
- Antimalarial medicines, such as quinine
- Aspirin (high doses)
- Nonsteroidal antiinflammatory drugs (NSAIDs)
- Quinidine
- Sulfa drugs

Acute bacterial or viral infections or acidosis can also precipitate a hemolytic process in these patients.

There are several different testing methods available for G-6-PD deficiency screening and testing. G-6-PD enzyme assay direct quantitation is most definitive. The Beutler test is a semiquantitative rapid fluorescent spot test. *Glucose-6-phosphate dehydrogenase* (G-6-PD) *deficiency DNA sequencing* by polymerase chain reaction/sequencing can most accurately make the diagnosis of this disease. As in all genetic diseases, pretesting counseling and informed consent are recommended. A number of rapid point-of-care diagnostic tests for determining G-6-PD deficiency status exist. Screening tests are particularly helpful in malaria-endemic areas for permitting safe use of primaquine, which can provoke hemolysis in persons with G-6-PD deficiency.

Procedure and patient care

- See inside front cover for Routine Blood Testing.
- Fasting: no
- Blood tube commonly used: lavender or green
- PT If the test indicates a G-6-PD deficiency, give the patient a list of drugs that may precipitate hemolysis. Instruct patients with the Mediterranean type of this disease not to eat fava beans. Teach patients to read labels on any over-the-counter (OTC) drugs for the presence of agents (e.g., aspirin) that may cause hemolytic anemia.

Abnormal findings

▼ **Decreased levels**
  G-6-PD deficiency

notes

glucose tolerance test (GTT, Oral glucose tolerance test [OGTT])

Type of test Blood; urine

Normal findings

Plasma test

Fasting: < 110 mg/dL or < 6.1 mmol/L (SI units)
1 hour: < 180 mg/dL or < 10 mmol/L
2 hours: < 140 mg/dL or < 7.8 mmol/L

Urine test

Negative

Test explanation and related physiology

The GTT is used when diabetes is suspected. It is also suggested for the following:

- Patients with a family history of diabetes
- Patients who are markedly obese
- Patients with a history of recurrent infections
- Patients with delayed healing of wounds
- Women who have a history of delivering large babies, still-births, or neonatal births
- Patients who have transient glycosuria or hyperglycemia during pregnancy or after myocardial infarction, surgery, or stress

In the GTT, the patient's ability to tolerate a standard oral glucose load is evaluated by obtaining plasma and urine specimens for glucose level determinations before glucose administration and then at 1 hour and 2 hours afterward. Normally, there is a rapid insulin response to the ingestion of a large oral glucose load. This response peaks in 30 to 60 minutes and returns to normal in about 3 hours. Patients with an appropriate insulin response are able to tolerate the glucose load quite easily, with only a minimal and transient rise in plasma glucose levels within 1 to 2 hours after ingestion.

Patients with diabetes will not be able to tolerate this load. As a result, their serum glucose levels will be greatly elevated from 1 to 5 hours (Figure G1). It is important to note that intestinal absorption may vary among individuals. For this reason, some centers prefer the glucose load to be administered intravenously.

Pregnant women who have not previously had an abnormal GTT should be tested between 24 and 28 weeks of gestation. Generally, a fasting glucose, 2-hour postprandial glucose during a 75-g OGTT, and A1C are equally appropriate for diagnostic

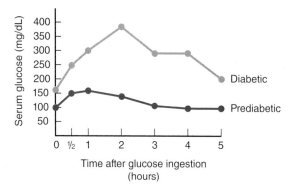

FIG. G1 Glucose tolerance test curve for a diabetic and a prediabetic patient.

screening. The OGTT is being used less often because of its inconvenience.

Contraindications

- Patients with serious concurrent infections or endocrine disorders because glucose intolerance will be observed

Potential complications

- Dizziness, tremors, anxiety, sweating, euphoria, or fainting during testing. If these symptoms occur, a blood specimen is obtained.

Interfering factors

- Smoking during the testing period stimulates glucose production because of the nicotine.
- Stress (e.g., from surgery, infection) can increase levels.
- Exercise during the testing can affect glucose levels.
- Fasting before GTT can cause glucose intolerance.

Procedure and patient care

Before

PT Explain the procedure to the patient.

PT Instruct the patient to fast for 12 hours before the test.

PT Instruct the patient to discontinue drugs (including tobacco) that could interfere with the test results.

- Obtain the patient's weight to determine the appropriate glucose loading dose (especially in children).

During
- Obtain fasting blood and urine specimens.
- Administer the prescribed oral glucose.
- Give pediatric patients a dose based on body weight.
- PT Tell the patient that he or she cannot eat anything until the test is completed. However, encourage the patient to drink water.
- PT Inform the patient that tobacco, coffee, and tea are not allowed because they cause physiologic stimulation.
- Collect a venous blood sample in a gray-top tube at 30 minutes and at hourly periods. Collect urine specimens at hourly periods.
- Assess the patient for such reactions as dizziness, sweating, weakness, and giddiness. (These are usually transient.)
- For the IV GTT, administer the glucose load intravenously over 3 to 4 minutes.

After
- Send all specimens promptly to the laboratory.
- Allow the patient to eat and drink normally.
- Apply pressure to the venipuncture site.

Abnormal findings

Acromegaly
Acute pancreatitis
Acute stress response
Chronic renal failure
Corticosteroid therapy
Cushing syndrome
Diabetes mellitus
Diuretic therapy
Glucagonoma
Myxedema
Pheochromocytoma
Postgastrectomy
Somogyi response to hypoglycemia

notes

growth hormone (GH, Human growth hormone [HGH], Somatotropin hormone [SH])

Type of test Blood

Normal findings

Men: < 5 ng/mL (mcg/L [SI units])
Women: < 10 ng/mL (mcg/L [SI units])
Children:

    1 year male: 0–6 ng/mL (mcg/L [SI units])
    1 year female: 0–10 ng/mL (mcg/L [SI units])
    1–12 months: 2–10 ng/mL (mcg/L [SI units])
    1 week: 2–27 ng/mL (mcg/L [SI units])
    Newborn: 5–23 ng/mL (mcg/L [SI units])

Test explanation and related physiology

This test is used to identify GH deficiency in adolescents who have short stature, delayed sexual maturity, or other growth deficiencies. It is also used to document the diagnosis of GH excess in patients with gigantism or acromegalia. GH is used to identify and follow patients with ectopic GH production by neoplasm. Finally, it is often used as a screening test for pituitary hypofunction or hyperfunction.

Because GH release is episodic, a random measurement of GH is unreliable to predict GH deficiency in adolescents. Measurement of free insulin-like growth factor (IGF) 1 and IGF BP 3 (see insulin-like growth factor, p. 442) is preferred in cases of short stature.

GH, or somatotropin, is secreted by the acidophilic cells in the anterior pituitary gland. It plays a central role in modulating growth from birth until the end of puberty. GH exerts its effects on many tissues through a group of peptides called *somatomedins*. The most commonly tested somatomedin is somatomedin C (also known as IGF-1), which is produced by the liver and has its major effect on cartilage.

If GH secretion is insufficient during childhood, limited growth and dwarfism may result. Also, a delay in sexual maturity may be a result in adolescents with reduced GH levels. Conversely, overproduction of GH during childhood results in gigantism, with the person sometimes reaching nearly 7 to 8 feet in height. An excess of GH during adulthood (after closure of long bone end plates) results in acromegaly, which is characterized by an increase in bone thickness and width but no increase in height.

Normal GH levels overlap significantly with deficient levels. Low GH levels may indicate deficiency or may be normal for certain individuals at certain times of the day. To negate time variables in GH testing, GH can be drawn 60 to 90 minutes after deep sleep has occurred. Levels increase during sleep. Also, strenuous exercise can be performed for 30 minutes in an effort to stimulate GH production.

To negate the common variations in GH secretion, screening for *IGF-1* or *somatomedin C* provides a more accurate reflection of the mean plasma concentration of GH. These proteins are not affected by the time of day or food intake like GH is. A *GH stimulation test* (p. 398) can be performed to evaluate the body's ability to produce GH. *Growth hormone suppression testing* is used to identify gigantism in children or acromegaly in the adult. The most commonly used suppression test is the oral glucose tolerance test (p. 392).

Interfering factors

- Random measurements of GH are not adequate determinants of GH deficiency because hormone secretion is episodic.
- GH secretion is increased by stress, exercise, and low blood glucose levels.

Procedure and patient care

Before

PT Explain the procedure to the patient.
- The patient should not be emotionally or physically stressed because this can increase GH levels.
- It is preferred that the patient be fasting and well rested. Water is permitted.
- For *GH suppression testing*, the patient is kept NPO after midnight.

During

Growth hormone test
- Collect a venous blood sample in a red-top tube.
- Because approximately two-thirds of the total release of GH occurs during sleep, GH secretion also can be measured during hospitalization by obtaining blood samples when the patient is sleeping.

Growth hormone suppression test
- Obtain peripheral venous access with normal saline solution.
- Obtain baseline GH and glucose levels as described previously.
- Administer the prescribed dose of glucose over 5 minutes.

- Obtain GH and glucose levels at 10, 60, and 120 minutes after glucose ingestion.

After

- Indicate the patient's fasting status and the time the blood is collected. Include the patient's recent activity (e.g., sleeping, walking, eating).
- Send the blood to the laboratory immediately after collection.

Abnormal findings

▲ **Increased levels**
   Acromegaly
   Anorexia nervosa
   Deep-sleep state
   Diabetes mellitus
   Exercise
   Gigantism
   Hypoglycemia
   Major surgery
   Starvation
   Stress

▼ **Decreased levels**
   Dwarfism
   Failure to thrive
   GH deficiency
   Hyperglycemia
   Pituitary insufficiency

notes

growth hormone stimulation test (GH provocation test, Insulin tolerance test [ITT], Arginine test, Glucagon Stimulation test)

Type of test Blood

Normal findings

GH levels > 10 ng/mL or > 10 mcg/L (SI units)
IGF-1 > 80 ng/mL

Test explanation and related physiology

Because GH (see previous test) secretion is episodic, a random measurement of plasma GH is not adequate to make a diagnosis of GH deficiency. IGF-1 screening (p. 442) followed by GH stimulation is indicated for children and adults suspected of GH deficiency. To diagnose GH deficiency, GH stimulation tests are sometimes needed. One of the most reliable GH stimulators is insulin-induced hypoglycemia, in which the blood glucose declines to less than 40 mg/dL. Other GH stimulants include vigorous exercise and drugs (e.g., arginine, clonidine, glucagon, levodopa). Glucagon is more widely used for GH stimulation, especially if there are safety concerns with insulin-induced hypoglycemia.

This test can also evaluate the entire hypothalamic–pituitary–adrenal endocrine pathway. Induced hypoglycemia is a potent stressor that strongly instigates ACTH and cortisol besides growth hormone.

Usually a *double-stimulated test* is performed using an arginine infusion followed by insulin-induced hypoglycemia. A GH concentration of more than 10 mcg/L after stimulation effectively excludes the diagnosis of GH deficiency. Hypothyroidism should be excluded before GH stimulation testing.

Contraindications

- Patients with epilepsy
- Patients with cerebrovascular disease
- Patients with myocardial infarction
- Patients with low basal plasma cortisol levels

Potential complications

- Hypoglycemia so significant and severe as to cause ketosis, acidosis, and shock; with close observation, this is unlikely

Procedure and patient care

Before

PT Explain the procedure to the patient and, if appropriate, to the parents.

PT Instruct the patient to remain NPO after midnight on the morning of the test. Water is permitted.

• Ensure that a syringe of 50% glucose solution is readily available in the event of severe hypoglycemia.

During

• Note the following procedural steps:
   1. A saline lock IV line is inserted for the administration of medications and for the withdrawal of blood samples.
   2. Baseline blood levels are obtained for GH, glucose, and cortisol.
   3. Venous samples for GH are obtained at 15, 30, 45, 60, 90, and 120 minutes after injection of arginine, insulin, or glucagon. Redosing may be required if glucose does not decrease by 30 minutes.
   4. Blood glucose levels can also be monitored with a glucometer. The blood sugar should drop to less than 40 mg/dL for effective measurement of GH reserve.

• Monitor the patient for signs of hypoglycemia, postural hypotension, somnolence, diaphoresis, and nervousness. Ice chips are often given during the test for patient comfort.

• This procedure is usually performed by a nurse with a physician in proximity.

• This test takes approximately 2 hours to perform.

PT Tell the patient that the minor discomfort associated with this test results from the insertion of the IV line and the hypoglycemic response induced by the insulin injection.

After

• Observe the venipuncture site for bleeding.

• Send the blood to the laboratory immediately after collection.

• Give the patient cookies and punch or an IV glucose infusion.

PT Inform the patient and family that results may not be available for approximately 7 days.

Abnormal findings

Growth hormone deficiency
Pituitary deficiency

notes

haptoglobin

Type of test Blood

Normal findings

Adult: 50–220 mg/dL or 0.5–2.2 g/L (SI units)
Newborn: 0–10 mg/dL or 0–0.1 g/L (SI units)

Possible critical values

< 40 mg/dL

Test explanation and related physiology

The serum haptoglobin test is used to detect intravascular destruction (lysis) of red blood cells (RBCs), also called *hemolysis*. Haptoglobins are produced by the liver and are powerful, free hemoglobin (Hgb)-binding proteins. In hemolytic anemias the released Hgb is quickly bound to haptoglobin, and the new complex is quickly catabolized. This results in a diminished amount of free haptoglobin in the serum; this decrease cannot be quickly compensated for by normal liver production. As a result, the patient demonstrates a transient, reduced level of haptoglobin in the serum. Megaloblastic anemias can reduce the haptoglobin level because of increased destruction of megaloblastic RBC precursors in the bone marrow.

Haptoglobins are also decreased in patients with primary liver disease not associated with hemolytic anemias. This occurs because the diseased liver is unable to produce these glycoproteins. Hematoma can reduce haptoglobin levels by the absorption of Hgb into the blood and binding with haptoglobin.

Elevated haptoglobin concentrations are found in many inflammatory diseases and can be used as a nonspecific acute-phase protein in much the same way as a sedimentation rate test is used (p. 306).

Interfering factors

- A slight decrease in haptoglobin levels is noted in pregnancy.
- Ongoing infection can cause falsely elevated test results.

Procedure and patient care

- See inside front cover for Routine Blood Testing.
- Fasting: no
- Blood tube commonly used: red

Abnormal findings

▲ **Increased levels**
Acute rheumatic disease
Biliary obstruction
Collagen vascular disease
Infection
Myocardial infarction
Neoplasia
Nephritis
Peptic ulcer
Pyelonephritis
Tissue destruction
Ulcerative colitis

▼ **Decreased levels**
Hematoma
Hemolytic anemia
Hemolytic disease of the
  newborn
Megaloblastic anemia
Primary liver disease not
  associated with hemolytic
  anemia
Prosthetic heart valves
Severe malnutrition
Systemic lupus
  erythematosus
Tissue hemorrhage
Transfusion reactions

notes

H

Heinz body preparation

Type of test Blood

Normal findings

No Heinz bodies detected

Test explanation and related physiology

Heinz bodies are water-insoluble precipitates of oxidated–denatured Hgb that form within RBCs. They occur as a result of exposure to oxidative chemicals and drugs. Mutations of Hgb, thalassemias, and defects in the Hgb reductive defense system against oxidation lead to an enhanced tendency toward oxidative hemolysis. The diagnosis of these problems can be suspected by the detection of Heinz bodies in RBCs.

Heinz bodies are often associated with hemolytic anemias and the presence of spherocytosis.

Procedure and patient care

- See inside front cover for Routine Blood Testing.
- Fasting: no
- Blood tube commonly used: lavender, pink, or green

Abnormal findings

▲ **Increased levels**

Heinz body hemolytic anemia
RBC enzymopathies (e.g., G6PD)
Thalassemia
Unstable hemoglobinopathies (e.g., Hb Gun Hill)

notes

H

Helicobacter pylori testing (Anti–*Helicobacter pylori* antibody, *Campylobacter*-like organism [CLO] test, *H. pylori* stool antigen, Urea Breath Test [UBT])

Type of test Blood, microscopic examination of antral or duodenal biopsy specimen, breath test, stool

Normal findings

Blood test

IgM	IgG
≤ 30 U/mL (negative)	< 0.75 (negative)
30.01–39.99 U/mL (equivocal)	0.75–0.99 (equivocal)
≥ 40 U/mL (positive)	≥ 1 (positive)

Breath test

No evidence of *H. pylori*

Stool test

No evidence of *H. pylori*

Test explanation and related physiology

H. pylori, a bacterium found in the mucus overlying the gastric mucosa and in the mucosa (cells that line the stomach), is a risk factor for gastric and duodenal ulcers, chronic gastritis, or even ulcerative esophagitis. There are several methods of detecting the presence of this organism. The organism can be cultured from a specimen of mucus obtained through a gastroscope (p. 313). The organism can also be detected on a gastric mucosal biopsy (from the antrum and greater curvature of the corpus). This is very accurate. The gold standard for diagnosis of *H. pylori* disease is identifying the infected tissue by Gram, silver, Giemsa, or acridine orange stains.

It often takes several weeks before the results from cultures are available. It is preferable to start treatment before that time on a patient with symptomatic or active ulcer disease. For that reason, *rapid urease testing* for *H. pylori* was developed. *H. pylori* can break down large quantities of urea because of its ability to produce great amounts of an enzyme called urease. In the *CLO test,* a small piece of gastric mucosa (obtained through gastroscopy) is placed onto a specialized testing gel containing urea and a pH indicator. If *H. pylori* organisms are present in the gastric mucosa, the urease (made by the *H. pylori*) will break down to urea to ammonia and change the colors of the test material.

A *breath test* is also available for the detection of *H. pylori*. In the *Urea Breath Test*, radioactive carbon (^{13}C) labeled urea is administered orally. The urea, if *H. pylori* is present, will be converted to $^{13}CO_2$ (where the carbon is radiolabeled). The $^{13}CO_2$ is then taken up by the capillaries in the stomach wall and delivered to the lungs. There the $^{13}CO_2$ is exhaled.

Although *H. pylori* does not survive in the stool, anti–*H. pylori* antibody can detect the presence of *H. pylori* antigen in a fresh stool specimen. Negative results indicate the absence of detectable antigen but do not eliminate the possibility of infection because of *H. pylori*.

Serologic testing is a noninvasive way of screening and diagnosing *H. pylori* infection. It is also used as a supportive diagnostic in which no preparation or abstinence from antacids is required. The IgG anti–*H. pylori* antibody is most commonly used. It becomes elevated 2 months after infection and stays elevated for more than 1 year after treatment. The IgA anti–*H. pylori* antibody, like IgG, becomes elevated 2 months after infection but decreases 3 to 4 weeks after treatment. The IgM anti–*H. pylori* antibody is the first to become elevated (about 3–4 weeks after infection) and is not detected 2 to 3 months after treatment. Serologic testing is often used several months after treatment to document cure of *H. pylori* infection. Serologic testing is also used to corroborate the findings of other *H. pylori* testing methods.

Quantitative polymerase chain reaction (PCR) testing on gastric biopsies can be used to detect low bacterial loads and to detect genetic mutations associated with therapeutic antimicrobial resistance.

Contraindications

- Patients who are pregnant or are children
- The breath tests use radioactive carbon to which children should not be exposed.

Interfering factors

- *H. pylori* can be transmitted by contaminated endoscopic equipment during endoscopic procedures.

Procedure and patient care

Before

PT Explain the procedure to the patient.

PT Tell the patient that no fasting is required for the blood test.

- If a biopsy or culture will be obtained by endoscopy, see discussion of esophagogastroduodenoscopy (EGD, p. 313).

- If culture is to be performed, be sure that the patient has not had any antibiotic, antacid, or bismuth treatment for 5 to 14 days before the endoscopy.

During
- Collect a venous blood sample according to the protocol of the laboratory performing the test.
- A gastric or duodenal biopsy can be obtained by endoscopy.
- For the breath test, a dose of radioactive ^{14}C or nonradioactive ^{13}C urea is given by mouth.

After
- Apply pressure to the venipuncture site.
- If endoscopy was used to obtain a culture, see procedure for EGD. The specimen should be transported to the laboratory within 30 minutes after collection.

H

Abnormal findings

▲ **Increased levels**
   Acute and chronic gastritis
   Duodenal ulcer
   Gastric carcinoma
   Gastric ulcer

notes

hematocrit (Hct, Packed red blood cell volume, Packed cell volume [PCV])

Type of test Blood

Normal findings

Male: 42%–52% or 0.42–0.52 volume fraction (SI units)
Female: 37%–47% or 0.37–0.47 volume fraction (SI units)
Pregnant female: > 33%
Elderly: values may be slightly decreased
Children (%)
  6–18 years: 32–44
  1–6 years: 30–40
  6 months-1 year: 29–43
  2–6 months: 35–50
  2–8 weeks: 39–59
  Newborn: 44–64

Possible critical values

< 21% or > 60%

Test explanation and related physiology

The Hct is a measure of the percentage of the total blood volume that is made up by the RBCs. The height of the RBC column is measured after centrifugation. It is compared with the height of the column of the total whole blood (Figure H1). The ratio of the height of the RBC column compared with the original total blood column is multiplied by 100%. This is the Hct value. It is routinely performed as part of a complete blood count. The Hct closely reflects the Hgb and RBC values. The Hct in percentage points usually is approximately three times the Hgb concentration in grams per deciliter when RBCs are of normal size and contain normal amounts of Hgb.

Abnormal values indicate the same pathologic states as abnormal RBC counts and Hgb concentrations (see next test). Decreased levels indicate anemia (reduced number of RBCs). Increased levels can indicate erythrocytosis. Like other RBC values, the Hct can be altered by many factors, such as hydration status and RBC morphology.

Interfering factors

- Abnormalities in RBC size may alter Hct values.
- Extremely elevated white blood cell counts may affect values.
- Hemodilution and dehydration may affect the Hct level.

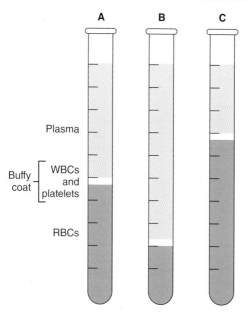

FIG. H1 Tubes showing hematocrit levels of normal blood, blood with evidence of anemia, and blood with evidence of polycythemia. Note the buffy coat located between the packed red blood cells (RBCs) and the plasma. **A,** Normal percentage of RBCs. **B,** Anemia (low percentage of RBCs). **C,** Polycythemia (high percentage of RBCs). *WBC,* White blood cell.

- Pregnancy usually causes slightly decreased values because of hemodilution.
- Living in high altitudes causes increased values.
- Values may not be reliable immediately after hemorrhage.

Procedure and patient care

- See inside front cover for Routine Blood Testing.
- Fasting: no
- Blood tube commonly used: lavender

Abnormal findings

▲ **Increased levels**

Burns
Chronic obstructive
  pulmonary disease
Congenital heart disease
Eclampsia
Erythrocytosis
Polycythemia vera
Severe dehydration

▼ **Decreased levels**

Anemia
Bone marrow failure
Cirrhosis
Dietary deficiency
Hemoglobinopathy
Hemolytic reaction
Hemorrhage
Hodgkin disease
Hyperthyroidism
Leukemia
Lymphoma
Multiple myeloma
Normal pregnancy
Prosthetic valves
Renal disease
Rheumatoid arthritis

notes

hemoglobin (Hb, Hgb)

Type of test   Blood

Normal findings

Male: 14–18 g/dL or 8.7–11.2 mmol/L (SI units)
Female: 12–16 g/dL or 7.4–9.9 mmol/L (SI units)
Pregnant female: > 11 g/dL
Elderly: values are slightly decreased
Children:

    6–18 years: 10–15.5 g/dL
    1–6 years: 9.5–14 g/dL
    6 months-1 year: 9.5–14 g/dL
    2–6 months: 10–17 g/dL
    0–2 weeks: 12–20 g/dL
    Newborn: 14–24 g/dL

Possible critical values

< 7 g/dL or > 20 g/dL

H

Test explanation and related physiology

The Hgb concentration is a measure of the total amount of Hgb in the peripheral blood, which reflects the number of RBCs in the blood. The test is normally performed as part of a complete blood count.

The Hct in percentage points usually is approximately three times the Hgb concentration in grams per deciliter when RBCs are of normal size and contain normal amounts of Hgb. Abnormal values indicate the same pathologic states as abnormal RBC counts and Hct concentrations (see previous test). Decreased levels indicate anemia (reduced number of RBCs). Increased levels can indicate erythrocytosis. In addition, however, changes in plasma volume are more accurately reflected by the Hgb concentration. Hemoglobinopathies, such as sickle cell disease and Hgb C disease, are also associated with reduced Hgb levels.

Interfering factors

- Slight Hgb decreases occurs normally during pregnancy because of the expanded blood volume.
- Living in high-altitude areas causes high Hgb values.
- Heavy smokers have higher levels than nonsmokers.

Procedure and patient care

- See inside front cover for Routine Blood Testing.
- Fasting: no
- Blood tube commonly used: lavender

Abnormal findings

▲ **Increased levels**

Chronic obstructive
  pulmonary disease
Congenital heart disease
Congestive heart failure
Dehydration
Hemoconcentration of the
  blood
High altitudes
Polycythemia vera
Severe burns

▼ **Decreased levels**

Anemia
Chronic hemorrhage
Hemoglobinopathies
Hemolysis
Hemorrhage
Kidney disease
Lymphoma
Neoplasia
Nutritional deficiency
Sarcoidosis
Splenomegaly
Systemic lupus
  erythematosus

notes

hemoglobin electrophoresis (Hgb electrophoresis)

Type of test Blood

Normal findings

Adult/elderly: percentage of total Hgb

Hgb A$_1$: 95%–98%

Hgb A$_2$: 2%–3%

Hgb F: 0.8%–2%

Hgb S: 0%

Hgb C: 0%

Hgb E: 0%

Hgb H: 0%

Children: Hgb F

> 6 months: 1%–2%

< 6 months: < 8%

Newborn: 50%–80%

Test explanation and related physiology

Hgb electrophoresis is a test that identifies and quantifies normal and abnormal forms of Hgb (hemoglobinopathies). Although many different forms of Hgb have been described, the more common types are A$_1$, A$_2$, F, S, E, and C. Each major Hgb type is electrically charged to varying degrees. Each electrophoretic band can be quantitated as a percentage of the total Hgb.

The form *Hgb A$_1$* constitutes the major component of Hgb in the normal RBC. *Hgb A$_2$* is only a minor component (2%–3%) of the normal Hgb total. *Hgb F* is the major Hgb component in a fetus but normally exists in only minimal quantities in a normal adult. Levels of Hgb F greater than 2% in patients older than age 3 years are considered abnormal. Hgb F is able to transport oxygen when only small amounts of oxygen are available (as in fetal life). In patients requiring compensation for prolonged chronic hypoxia (as in congenital cardiac abnormalities), Hgb F may be found in increased levels to assist in the transport of the available oxygen.

Hgb S and *Hgb C* are abnormal forms of Hgb that occur predominantly in African Americans. Hgb E occurs predominantly in Southeast Asians. The Hgb contents of some common disorders affecting Hgb, as determined by electrophoresis, are indicated in Table H1. Hgb E is produced less efficiently by RBC precursors; if there is an increased Hgb E content in the RBCs, those cells will have a low mean corpuscular volume (MCV, p. 633).

TABLE H1   Hemoglobin (Hgb) contents of some common hemoglobinopathies

	Hgb A₁	Hgb A₂	Hgb F	Hgb S	Hgb H	Hgb C	Hgb E
	$Hgb\ A_1$	$Hgb\ A_2$	Hgb F	Hgb S	Hgb H	Hgb C	Hgb E
				Percentage range			
Sickle cell disease	0	2–3	2	95–98	0	0	0
Sickle cell trait	50–65	2–3	2	35–45	0	0	0
Hgb C disease	0	2–3	2	0	0	90–100	0
Three gene deletion α-thalassemia (Hgb H disease)	65–90	0.3–1.5	0.6–4.5	0	0–30	0	0
β-Thalassemia major	0	0–15	85–100	0	0	0	0
β-Thalassemia trait	50–85	4–8	1–5	0	0	0	0
Hgb E disease	0	0	0	0	0	0	100

Quantification of abnormal Hgb proteins provides a method of monitoring treatments.

Interfering factors

- Blood transfusions within the previous 12 weeks.
- Glycosylated Hgb can blur the peak of Hgb F and cause falsely low levels of Hgb F.

Procedure and patient care

- See inside front cover for Routine Blood Testing.
- Fasting: no
- Blood tube commonly used: lavender

Abnormal findings

Hgb C disease
Hgb E disease
Hgb H disease
Sickle cell disease
Sickle cell trait
Thalassemia major
Thalassemia minor

notes

hexosaminidase (Hexosaminidase A, Hex A, Total hexosaminidase, Hexosaminidase A and B)

Type of test Blood

Normal findings

Hexosaminidase A: 7.5–9.8 units/L (SI units)
Total hexosaminidase: 9.9–15.9 units/L (SI units)
(Check with the laboratory because of the variety of testing methods.)

Test explanation and related physiology

Tay–Sachs disease (TSD) is a *lysosomal storage disease* (LSD), which, in infancy and early childhood, is characterized by loss of motor skills. Major categories of LSD include mucopolysaccharidoses, oligosaccharidoses, neuronal ceroid lipofuscinoses, and sphingolipidoses.

TSD, like other LSDs, is usually a result of a mutation in an autosomal recessive gene. This gene encodes the synthesis of an enzyme called hexosaminidase. Without this enzyme, lysosomes of GM2 accumulate, particularly in the CNS.

Two clinically important isoenzymes of hexosaminidase have been detected in the serum: hexosaminidase A (hex A, made up of 1 alpha subunit and 1 beta subunit) and hexosaminidase B (hex B, made up of 2 beta subunits). Any genetic mutation that affects the alpha unit will cause a deficiency of hexosaminidase A, resulting in TSD. A mutation that affects the beta unit will cause a deficiency in hex A and B. Sandhoff disease, an uncommon variant of TSD, occurs with deficiency of both of these enzymes.

Hex A has been found to be abnormally low in carriers, whereas hex B is high. Therefore testing for total hexosaminidase is not useful. A carrier has a 25% chance of having a child with TSD if the other biological parent is also a carrier. In communities in which the Ashkenazi Jewish population is high, hex A screening has been very effective for identifying carriers. Furthermore, hex A is used to diagnose TSD in infants, young children, and adults.

Interfering factors

- Hemolysis of the blood sample can cause inaccurate results.
- Pregnancy can cause markedly increased values. For this reason, blood tests are not done during pregnancy.

Procedure and patient care

- See inside front cover for Routine Blood Testing.
- Fasting: no
- Blood tube commonly used: red
- **PT** Emphasize the importance of this test to Jewish couples of Eastern European ancestry who plan to have children. Explain that both must carry the defective gene to transmit TSD to their offspring.
- Professional genetic counseling should be provided to every person considering undergoing this test.
- Check with the laboratory regarding withholding oral contraceptives.
- Note that pregnant women can be evaluated by amniocentesis (p. 39) or chorionic villus biopsy (p. 202).
- Note that infants may have blood obtained by heel sticks. Neonates often have blood drawn through the umbilical cord.

Abnormal findings

▼ **Decreased hexosaminidase A**
Tay–Sachs disease

▼ **Decreased hexosaminidase A and B**
Sandhoff disease

notes

HIV drug resistance testing (HIV genotype)

Type of test Blood

Normal findings

No resistant HIV

Test explanation and related physiology

There are several factors that affect the success of HIV antiviral medications, including patient compliance, access to adequate care, optimal dosing, and drug pharmacology issues. Another significant factor that determines a patient's response to antiviral HIV drugs is the percentage of an HIV viral population that is resistant to the drugs that are administered. HIV genotyping is able to detect changes in the viral genome that are associated with drug resistance and is particularly able to predict HIV-1 resistance to protease and reverse-transcriptase inhibitor antiretroviral drugs.

HIV genotyping is particularly useful when failure of the most active antiviral therapy is suspected. HIV genotyping can also be performed in conjunction with *HIV drug sensitivity testing.* HIV sensitivity testing estimates the ability of a cloned copy of the patient's virus to replicate in a cell culture in the presence of a particular antiviral drug. This same testing can help determine the amount of drug needed to inhibit viral replication.

More recently, using *next-generation sequencing (NGS)* to detect drug-resistance mutations in HIV-1 342 drug-resistance mutations have been identified.

Interfering factors

- If the plasma HIV-1 RNA viral load is less than 1000 copies per mL of plasma, genotyping may be inaccurate.

Procedure and patient care

- See inside front cover for Routine Blood Testing.
- Fasting: no
- Blood tube commonly used: lavender or pink

Abnormal findings

Drug resistance

notes

HIV RNA quantification (HIV viral load)

Type of test Blood

Normal findings

Undetected

Test explanation and related physiology

Quantification of HIV RNA in the blood of patients infected with HIV can be used after immunoassay tests (p. 417) are positive. Quantification is also helpful when confirmatory tests are indeterminate or cannot be accurately interpreted. Direct viral testing is helpful in differentiating newborn HIV infection from passive transmission of HIV antibodies from an HIV-infective mother. Finally, HIV RNA quantification testing determines HIV viral load. Determining viral load is used:

- to establish a baseline viral load before initiating therapy
- to identify HIV-1 drug resistance while on therapy
- to identify noncompliance with anti–HIV-1 drug therapy
- to monitor HIV-1 disease progression
- to recommend the initiation of antiretroviral treatment (Table H2)
- to indicate the course of the disease
- as a determinant of patient survival (Table H3)

HIV viral load is most accurately determined by quantifying the amount of genetic material of the virus in the blood. In general, it is recommended to determine the baseline viral load by obtaining two measurements 2 to 4 weeks apart after HIV infection. Monitoring may continue with testing every 3 to 4 months in conjunction with CD4 counts. Both tests provide data used to determine when to start antiviral treatment. The viral load test can be repeated every 4 to 6 weeks after starting or changing antiviral therapy. It is important to recognize that a *nondetectable* result does not mean that no virus is left in the blood after treatment; it means that the viral load has fallen below the limit of detection by the test. A significant rise of viral load should warrant re-evaluation of therapy.

Interfering factors

- Incorrect handling and processing of the specimen can cause inconsistent results.
- Recent vaccinations may affect viral levels.
- Concurrent infections can cause inconsistent results.
- Variable compliance to therapy may alter test results.

TABLE H2 Recommendations for antiretroviral therapy based on viral load and CD4 count

CD 4 count ($\times 10^5$/L)	HIV RNA viral load, copies/mL		
	< 5000	5000–30,000	> 30,000
< 350	Recommend therapy	Recommend therapy	Recommend therapy
350–500	Consider therapy	Recommend therapy	Recommend therapy
> 500	Defer therapy	Consider therapy	Recommend therapy
Symptomatic		Recommend therapy	Recommend therapy

TABLE H3 Using the viral load to predict disease course

	HIV RNA viral load (copies/mL)				
	< 500	501–3000	3001–10,000	10,001–30,000	> 30,000
Developing AIDS (%)	5.4	16.6	31.7	55.2	80
Dying of AIDS (%)	0.9	6.3	18.1	34.9	69.5

Procedure and patient care

- See inside front cover for Routine Blood Testing.
- Fasting: no
- Blood tube commonly used: lavender
- Specimens are often sent to a central laboratory.
- PT Instruct the patient to observe the venipuncture site for infection. Patients with AIDS are immunocompromised and susceptible to infection.
- PT Encourage the patient to discuss his or her concerns regarding the prognostic information from test results.
- Do not give test results over the phone. Increasing viral load results can have devastating consequences.
- Because test results vary according to the laboratory test method, it is important to use the same laboratory method for monitoring the course of the disease.
- Viral loads are usually repeated after starting or changing antiviral therapy.

Abnormal findings

HIV infection

notes

Holter monitoring

Type of test Electrodiagnostic

Normal findings

Normal sinus rhythm

Test explanation and related physiology

Holter monitoring is a continuous recording of the electrical activity of the heart. This can be performed for periods of up to 72 hours. With this technique, an electrocardiogram (ECG) is recorded continuously on magnetic tape during unrestricted activity, rest, and sleep (Figure H2). The Holter monitor is equipped with a clock that permits accurate time monitoring on the ECG tape. The patient is asked to carry a diary and to record daily activities as well as any cardiac symptoms that may develop during the period of monitoring.

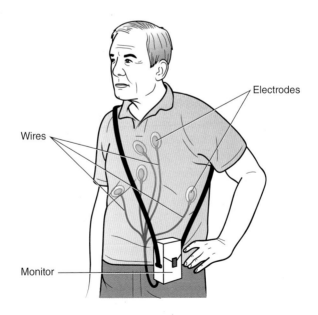

FIG. H2 Electrical activity of the heart is recorded on a Holter monitor.

Most units are equipped with an *event marker.* This is a button the patient can push when such symptoms as chest pain, syncope, or palpitations are experienced.

The Holter monitor is used primarily to identify suspected cardiac rhythm disturbances and to correlate these disturbances with symptoms (e.g., dizziness, syncope, palpitations, or chest pain). The monitor is also used to assess pacemaker function and the effectiveness of antiarrhythmic medications.

After completion of the determined time period, the Holter monitor is removed from the patient. The ECG tracing is usually interpreted by computer, which can detect any significant, abnormal waveform patterns that occurred during the testing.

Implantable loop recorders (ILRs) are used when long-term monitoring is required. These recorders are implanted subcutaneously via a small incision. ILRs can record ECG tracings continuously or only when purposefully activated by the patient. The ILR can be automatically activated by a predefined arrhythmia that will trigger device recording. If nothing irregular happens, then the information is subsequently erased. But if an arrhythmia does occur, the device locks it in and saves it to memory. ILRs can provide a diagnosis in many patients with unexplained syncope or presyncope.

Contraindications

- Patients who are unable to cooperate with maintaining the lead placement from the monitor to the body
- Patients who are unable to maintain an accurate diary of significant activities or events

Interfering factors

- Interruption in the electrode contact with the skin

Procedure and patient care

Before

PT Explain the procedure to the patient.

PT Instruct the patient about care of the Holter monitor. If it gets wet (from bathing or swimming), it will be damaged.

PT Inform the patient about the necessity of ensuring good contact between the electrodes and the skin.

PT Teach the patient how to maintain an accurate diary. Stress the need to record significant symptoms, such as palpitations, skipped beats, dizziness, syncope or chest pain.

PT Instruct the patient to note in the diary if any interruption in Holter monitoring occurs.

PT Assure the patient that the electrical flow is coming from the patient and that he or she will not experience any electrical stimulation from the machine.

PT Tell the patient to minimize the use of electrical devices (e.g., electric toothbrushes, shavers) that may cause artificial changes in the ECG tracing.

During

- Prepare the sites for electrode placement with alcohol. (This is usually done in the cardiology department by a technologist.)
- Place the gel and electrodes at the appropriate sites. Usually, the chest and abdomen are the most appropriate locations for limb-lead electrode placement. The precordial leads also may be placed.

PT Encourage the patient to call if he or she has any difficulties.

After

- Gently remove the tape and other paraphernalia securing the electrodes.
- Wipe the patient clean of electrode gel.

PT Inform the patient when the Holter monitoring interpretation will be available.

Abnormal findings

Cardiac arrhythmia
Ischemic changes

notes

homocysteine (Hcy)

Type of test Blood

Normal findings

4–14 µmol/L
(Levels may increase with age.)

Test explanation and related physiology

Elevated blood levels of homocysteine may act as an independent risk factor for ischemic heart disease, cerebrovascular disease, peripheral arterial disease, and venous thrombosis. Homocysteine appears to promote the progression of atherosclerosis by causing endothelial damage, promoting low-density lipoprotein (LDL) deposition, and promoting vascular smooth muscle growth.

Dietary deficiency of vitamins B_6, B_{12}, or folate is the most common cause of elevated homocysteine. These vitamins are essential for the enzymatic metabolism of homocysteine to methionine (a protein). Homocysteine levels are elevated in patients with megaloblastic anemia. Some practitioners recommend homocysteine testing in patients with known poor nutritional status (alcoholics, drug abusers) and the elderly. Homocysteine is elevated in children with inborn errors of methionine metabolism.

Both fasting and postmethionine loading levels of homocysteine can be measured. When blood levels are elevated, urine homocysteine levels are also increased.

Contraindications

- Patients whose creatinine levels exceed 1.5 mg/dL are not candidates for methionine loading.

Interfering factors

- Patients with renal impairment have elevated levels of homocysteine because of poor excretion of the protein.
- Men usually have higher levels of homocysteine than women. Most likely, this is because of higher creatinine values and greater muscle mass. Values also increase with age.
- Smoking is associated with increased homocysteine levels.

Procedure and patient care

- See inside front cover for Routine Blood Testing.
- Fasting: yes (10–12 hours)
- Blood tube commonly used: purple, green, or blue

- For *methionine loading*, the patient ingests approximately 100 mg/kg of methionine after fasting for 10 to 12 hours. A blood sample is obtained. Repeat blood samples are collected at 2, 4, 8, 12, and 24 hours to compare levels of B vitamins and amino acids in the plasma.

Abnormal findings

▲ **Increased levels**

Cardiovascular disease

Cerebrovascular disease

Cystinuria

Folate deficiency

Peripheral vascular disease

Vitamin B_6 or B_{12} deficiency

notes

human chorionic gonadotropin (hCG, Pregnancy tests, hCG beta subunit)

Type of test   Blood; urine

Normal findings

- Negative: < 5 IU/L
- Indeterminate: 5–25 IU/L
- Positive: > 25 IU/L
- Males and nonpregnant females: < 2 IU/L

Test explanation and related physiology

All pregnancy tests are based on the detection of human chorionic gonadotropin (hCG). hCG appears in the blood and urine of pregnant women within days after conception.

hCG is made up of alpha and beta subunits. The beta subunit is specific for hCG.

Very small levels of hCG can be detected and pregnancy can be determined 3 to 7 days after conception. There is no crossover reactivity with other non-hCG glycoprotein hormones. Results can be confirmed with a repeat test in 72 hours. Values in pregnancy should double every 3 days for the first 6 weeks. When an embryo is first large enough to be visible on transvaginal ultrasonography (p. 755), the patient generally will have hCG concentrations between 1000 and 2000 IU/L. If the hCG value is high and gestational contents are not visible in the uterus, an ectopic pregnancy is suggested.

There are qualitative serum and urine hCG assays and quantitative serum hCG assays (Table H4). In the home setting, the urine is applied to a testing apparatus, and the color change is compared with a standard. If the color matches that standard, pregnancy is present. Other test kits use the development of a line or plus symbol that may appear indicating pregnancy. These tests take only a few minutes to perform and to obtain results. They are best if performed a few days after a missed menses. However, results can be positive on the day of an expected menses.

TABLE H4   Recommended uses for hCG testing

Test name	Recommended use
Qualitative beta hCG	Rapid pregnancy test
Quantitative hCG	More accurate pregnancy test
	Used to monitor high-risk pregnancy
Quantitative hCG (tumor marker)	Monitor patients with hCG-secreting tumors

Concentrations of hCG level off around week 20, significantly above prepregnancy levels. After delivery, miscarriage, or pregnancy termination, hCG falls until prepregnancy levels are reached.

Normally, hCG is not present in nonpregnant women. In a very small number of women, hCG exists in minute levels. The presence of hCG does not necessarily indicate a normal pregnancy. Ectopic pregnancy, hydatidiform mole of the uterus, recent abortion, and choriocarcinoma can all produce hCG. However, hCG levels in ectopic pregnancy typically fail to double appropriately, and decreased levels eventually result relative to the values expected in normal intrauterine pregnancies of similar gestational age. hCG is also an effective cancer tumor marker, see page 164.

Interfering factors

- Tests performed too early in the pregnancy, before a significant hCG level exists, may cause false-negative results.
- Hematuria and proteinuria may cause false-positive results.
- Hemolysis of blood may interfere with test results.
- Urine pregnancy tests can vary according to the dilution of the urine. hCG levels may not be detectable in dilute urine but may be detectable in concentrated urine.

Procedure and patient care

Before

PT Explain the procedure to the patient.
- If a urine specimen will be collected, give the patient a urine container the evening before so that she can provide a first-voided morning specimen. This specimen generally contains the greatest concentration of hCG.

During

- Collect the first-voided urine specimen for urine testing.
- Collect a venous blood sample in a red-top tube.

After

- Apply pressure to the venipuncture site.

Abnormal findings

▲ **Increased levels**
Choriocarcinoma of the uterus, testes, or ovaries
Ectopic pregnancy
Hydatidiform mole of the uterus
Pregnancy
Tumor

▼ **Decreased levels**
Ectopic pregnancy
Fetal death
Spontaneous abortion

notes

human lymphocyte antigen B27 (HLA-B27 antigen, Human leukocyte A antigen, White blood cell antigens, Histocompatibility leukocyte A antigen)

Type of test   Blood

Normal findings

Negative

Test explanation and related physiology

The HLA antigens exist on the surface of white blood cells and on the surface of all nucleated cells in other tissues. The presence or absence of these antigens is determined genetically. Each gene controls the presence or absence of HLA A, B, C, or D.

The HLA system is used to assist in the diagnosis of certain diseases. For example, HLA-B27 is present in 80% of patients with Reiter syndrome. When a patient has recurrent and multiple arthritic complaints, the presence of HLA-B27 supports the diagnosis of Reiter syndrome. Other HLA–disease associations are mentioned below in abnormal findings.

The HLA system of antigens has been used to indicate tissue compatibility in transplantation. Because HLA antigens are genetically determined, they can also be used to resolve *paternity investigations.*

Procedure and patient care

- See inside front cover for Routine Blood Testing.
- Fasting: no
- Blood tube commonly used: verify with laboratory

Abnormal findings

▲ **Increased levels (HLA-B27 antigens present)**

Ankylosing spondylitis
Anterior uveitis
Celiac disease or gluten enteropathy
Chronic active hepatitis
Dermatitis herpetiformis
Graves disease
Hemochromatosis
Juvenile diabetes
Myasthenia gravis
Multiple sclerosis
Psoriasis
Reiter syndrome
Rheumatoid arthritis
Yersinia enterocolitica arthritis

notes

human placental lactogen (hPL, Human chorionic somatomammotropin [HCS])

Type of test Blood
Normal findings

Weeks of pregnancy	hPL concentration (mg/L = mcg/mL)
≤ 20	0.05–1
≤ 22	1.5–3
≤ 26	2.5–5
≤ 30	4–6.5
≤ 34	5–8
≤ 38	5.5–9.5
≤ 42	5–7

Test explanation and related physiology

The human placenta produces hPL, which maintains pregnancy. Serum levels of hPL rise very early in normal pregnancy and continue to increase until a plateau is reached at about the 35th week after conception. Assays for maternal serum levels of hPL are useful in monitoring placental function. Measurements of hPL also are used in pregnancies complicated by hypertension, proteinuria, edema, postmaturity, placental insufficiency, or possible miscarriage.

A decreased serum concentration of hPL is pathognomonic for a malfunction of the placenta, which may cause intrauterine growth retardation, intrauterine death of the fetus, or imminent miscarriage. Pregnant women with hypertonia also show low serum concentrations of hPL. Because of the short biological half-life of hPL in serum, the determination of hPL gives a very accurate representation of placental function.

Increased serum concentrations of hPL are found in women with diabetes mellitus and, because of the higher placental mass, in multiple pregnancies. In contrast to estriol, the hPL concentration depends only on the placental mass and not on fetal function. The simultaneous determination of hPL and estriol can be helpful in the differential evaluation of placental function.

Procedure and patient care
- See inside front cover for Routine Blood Testing.
- Fasting: no
- Blood tube commonly used: red
- Indicate the date of the patient's last menstrual period on the laboratory slip.

PT Explain the possibility that serial testing is often required.

Abnormal findings

▲ **Increased levels**
Diabetes
Intact molar pregnancy
Multiple pregnancies
Placental-site trophoblastic tumor
Rh incompatibility

▼ **Decreased levels**
Choriocarcinoma
Hydatidiform mole
Placental insufficiency
Preeclampsia
Toxemia

notes

17-hydroxycorticosteroids (17-OCHS)

Type of test   Urine (24-hour)

Normal findings

Adult

    Male: 3–10 mg/24 hr or 8.3–27.6 µmol/day (SI units)

    Female: 2–8 mg/24 hr or 5.2–22.1 µmol/day (SI units)

Elderly: values slightly lower than that of an adult

Children

    8–12 years: < 4.5 mg/24 hr

    < 8 years: < 1.5 mg/24 hr

Test explanation and related physiology

Elevated levels of 17-OCHS are seen in patients with hyperfunctioning of the adrenal gland (Cushing syndrome), whether this condition is caused by a pituitary or adrenal tumor, bilateral adrenal hyperplasia, or ectopic tumors producing adrenocorticotropic hormone (ACTH). Low levels of 17-OCHS are seen in patients who have a hypofunctioning adrenal gland (Addison disease) as a result of destruction of the adrenals (by hemorrhage, infarction, metastatic tumor, or autoimmunity), surgical removal of an adrenal gland, congenital enzyme deficiency, hypopituitarism, or adrenal suppression after prolonged exogenous steroid ingestion.

Interfering factors

• Emotional and physical stress (e.g., infection) and licorice ingestion may cause increased adrenal activity.

Procedure and patient care

• See inside front cover for Routine Urine Testing.
• Note that some drugs may be withheld several days before the urine collection. Check with the physician.

Abnormal findings

▲ **Increased levels**

    Adrenal adenoma or
       carcinoma

    Cushing syndrome

    Ectopic ACTH-producing
       tumors

    Hyperthyroidism

    Obesity

▼ **Decreased levels**

    Addison disease

    Adrenal hyperplasia
       (adrenogenital syndrome)

    Adrenal suppression from
       steroid therapy

    Hypopituitarism

    Hypothyroidism

notes

5-hydroxyindoleacetic acid (5-HIAA)

Type of test   Urine (24-hour)

Normal findings

2–8 mg/24 hr or 10–40 µmol/day (SI units)
Female levels lower than male levels

Test explanation and related physiology

Quantitative analysis of urine levels of 5-HIAA is used to detect and follow the clinical course of patients with carcinoid tumors. Carcinoid tumors are serotonin-secreting tumors that may grow in the appendix, intestine, lung, or any tissue derived from the neuroectoderm. These tumors contain *argentaffin-staining (enteroendocrine)* cells, which produce serotonin and other powerful neurohormones that are metabolized by the liver to 5-HIAA and excreted in the urine. These powerful neurohormones are responsible for the clinical presentation of carcinoid syndrome (bronchospasm, flushing, diarrhea).

Procedure and patient care

- See inside front cover for Routine Urine Testing for 24-hour collection.
- PT Instruct the patient to refrain from eating foods containing serotonin (e.g., plums, pineapples, bananas, eggplant) for several days before and during testing.
- Keep the specimen on ice or in a refrigerator during the 24-hour collection. A preservative is needed.

Abnormal findings

▲ **Increased levels**
  Carcinoid tumors
  Cystic fibrosis
  Intestinal malabsorption
  Noncarcinoid illness

▼ **Decreased levels**
  Mental depression
  Migraine headaches

notes

21-hydroxylase antibodies

Type of test   Blood

Normal findings

< 1 U/mL

Test explanation and related physiology

Chronic primary adrenal insufficiency (Addison disease) is most commonly caused by the insidious autoimmune destruction of the adrenal cortex and is characterized by the presence of adrenal cortex autoantibodies in the serum. It can occur sporadically or in combination with other autoimmune endocrine diseases. This antibody may precipitate this disease. Measurement of this antibody is used in the investigation of causes of adrenal insufficiency.

Procedure and patient care

- See inside front cover for Routine Blood Testing.
- Fasting: no
- Blood tube commonly used: red

Abnormal findings

▲ Increased levels

Autoimmune adrenal insufficiency
Autoimmune polyglandular syndrome

notes

hysterosalpingography (Uterotubography, Uterosalpingography, Hysterogram)

Type of test X-ray with contrast

Normal findings

Patent fallopian tubes
No defects in uterine cavity

Test explanation and related physiology

This test is part of the workup for infertility. The results can indicate patency or obstruction of the fallopian tubes. It can also investigate repeated miscarriage from uterine problems, such as fibroids. In hysterosalpingography, the uterine cavity and fallopian tubes are visualized radiographically after the injection of contrast material through the cervix. Uterine tumors, intrauterine adhesions, and developmental anomalies can be seen. Tubal obstruction caused by internal scarring, tumor, or kinking also can be detected. A possible therapeutic effect of this test is that passage of dye through the tubes may clear mucous plugs, straighten kinked tubes, or break up adhesions. This test also may be used to document adequacy of surgical tubal ligation.

Contraindications

- Patients with infections of the vagina, cervix, or fallopian tubes, because there is risk of extending the infection
- Patients with suspected pregnancy, because contrast material might induce abortion

Potential complications

- Infection of the endometrium (endometritis)
- Infection of the fallopian tubes (salpingitis)
- Uterine perforation

Procedure and patient care

Before

PT Explain the procedure to the patient. See p. xviii for radiation exposure and risks.
- Determine pregnancy status of the patient.
- Administer sedatives or antispasmodics, if ordered.
PT Tell the patient that no food or fluid restrictions are needed.

During

- Note the following procedural steps:
  1. After voiding, the patient is placed on the fluoroscopy table in the lithotomy position.

2. With a speculum in the vagina, contrast material is injected through the cervix. The dye fills the entire upper genital tract (uterus and tubes).

3. Fluoroscopy is performed, and x-ray images are taken.

- Note that this procedure is performed by a physician in approximately 15 to 30 minutes.

PT Tell the patient that she may feel occasional transient menstrual-type cramping and that she may have shoulder pain caused by subphrenic irritation from the dye as it leaks into the peritoneal cavity.

After

PT Inform the patient that a vaginal discharge (sometimes bloody) may be present for 1 to 2 days after the test.

PT Instruct the patient to report signs and symptoms of infection (e.g., fever, increased pulse rate, pain).

Abnormal findings

Developmental anomaly (e.g., uterus bicornis) of the uterus
Extrauterine pregnancy
Intrauterine adhesions or polyps
Obstruction, kinking, or twisting of the fallopian tubes
Tumor of the fallopian tubes
Uterine fistula
Uterine tumor (e.g., leiomyoma, cancer) or polyps

notes

hysteroscopy

Type of test Endoscopy

Normal findings

Normal structure and function of the uterus

Test explanation and related physiology

Hysteroscopy is an endoscopic procedure that provides direct visualization of the uterine cavity by inserting a hysteroscope (a thin, telescope-like instrument) through the vagina and cervix and into the uterus (Figure H3). Hysteroscopy can be used to identify the cause of abnormal uterine bleeding, infertility, and

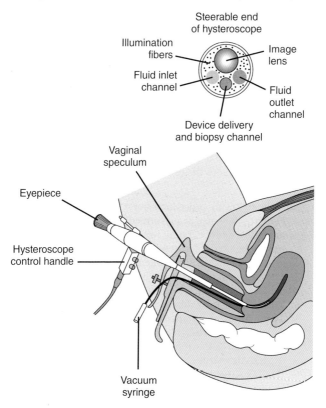

FIG. H3 Hysteroscopy.

repeated miscarriages. It is also used to identify, evaluate, and perform biopsies of uterine adhesions (Asherman syndrome), polyps, cancer, fibroids, and to detect displaced intrauterine devices (IUDs).

In addition to diagnosing and evaluating uterine problems, hysteroscopy can correct uterine problems. For example, uterine adhesions and small fibroids can be removed through the hysteroscope, thus avoiding open abdominal surgery. Hysteroscopy can also be used to perform endometrial ablation, which destroys the uterine lining to treat some cases of heavy dysfunctional uterine bleeding.

Contraindications

- Patients with pelvic inflammatory disease
- Patients with vaginal discharge

Potential complications

- Uterine perforation
- Infection

Procedure and patient care

Before

- **PT** Explain the procedure to the patient.
- Obtain informed consent for this procedure.
- Assess the pregnancy status of the patient.
- **PT** Instruct the patient to be NPO (nothing by mouth) for at least 8 hours before the test.

During

- Note the following procedural steps:
  1. Hysteroscopy may be performed in the operating room or the doctor's office. Local, regional, general, or no anesthesia may be used. (The type of anesthesia depends on other procedures that may be done at the same time.)
  2. The patient is placed in the lithotomy position. The vaginal area is cleansed with an antiseptic solution.
  3. The cervix may be dilated before this procedure.
  4. The hysteroscope is inserted through the vagina and cervix and into the uterus.
  5. A liquid or gas is released through the hysteroscope to expand the uterus for better visualization.
  6. If minor surgery is to be performed, small instruments will be inserted through the hysteroscope.

7. For more detailed or complicated procedures, a laparoscope may be used to concurrently view the outside of the uterus.

• Note that hysteroscopy is performed by a physician in approximately 30 minutes.

After

PT Tell the patient that it is normal to have slight vaginal bleeding and cramps for a day or two after the procedure.

PT Inform the patient that signs of fever, severe abdominal pain, or heavy vaginal discharge or bleeding should be reported to her physician.

Abnormal findings

Asherman syndrome
Displaced IUD
Endometrial cancer, polyps, or hyperplasia
Septate uterus
Uterine fibroids

H

notes

immunoglobulin quantification

Type of test Blood

Normal findings

Results vary by age and methods.

IgG (mg/dL)
>   Adults: 565–1765
>   Children: 250–1600

IgA (mg/dL)
>   Adults: 85–385
>   Children: 1–350

IgM (mg/dL)
>   Adults: 55–375
>   Children: 20–200

IgD and IgE
>   Minimal

Test explanation and related physiology

This test is used to detect and monitor the course of hypersensitivity diseases, immune deficiencies, autoimmune diseases, chronic infections, and intrauterine fetal infections.

Antibodies are made up of gamma globulin protein and are called *immunoglobulins*. There are many classes of immunoglobulins. *Immunoglobulin G (IgG)* constitutes approximately 75% of the serum immunoglobulins. *IgA* constitutes approximately 15% of the immunoglobulins in the body and is present primarily in secretions of the respiratory and gastrointestinal tracts, in saliva, in colostrum, and in tears. IgA is also present to a smaller degree in the blood. *IgM* is primarily responsible for ABO blood grouping and rheumatoid factor; it is also involved in the immunologic reaction to many infections. *IgE* often mediates an allergic response and is measured to detect allergic diseases. *IgD*, which constitutes the smallest part of the immunoglobulins, is rarely evaluated or detected.

Increased serum immunoglobulin concentrations occur because of polyclonal or oligoclonal immunoglobulin proliferation in hepatic disease, connective tissue diseases, and acute and chronic infections. Elevation of immunoglobulins may occur in monoclonal gammopathies (e.g., multiple myeloma, primary systemic amyloidosis, and monoclonal gammopathies of undetermined significance). Decreased immunoglobulin levels are found in patients with acquired or congenital immune deficiencies. It can be used to monitor therapy and recurrence. Testing can determine the type of connective tissue disease, its severity, its clinical course, and its response to therapy.

Procedure and patient care

- See inside front cover for Routine Blood Testing.
- Fasting: no
- Blood tube commonly used: red
- Indicate if the patient has received any vaccinations or immunizations in the past 6 months.

Abnormal findings

▲ **Increased IgA levels**
Chronic infections
Chronic liver diseases
(e.g., primary biliary
cirrhosis)
Inflammatory bowel disease

▼ **Decreased IgA levels**
Ataxia or telangiectasia
Congenital deficiency
Hypoproteinemia (e.g.,
nephrotic syndrome
or protein-losing
enteropathies)
Immunosuppressive drugs
(e.g., steroids, dextran)

▲ **Increased IgG levels**
Autoimmune diseases (e.g.,
rheumatoid arthritis,
Sjögren disease, systemic
lupus erythematosus)
Chronic granulomatous
infections (e.g.,
tuberculosis, Wegener
granulomatosis,
sarcoidosis)
Chronic liver disease
Hyperimmunization
reactions
Intrauterine devices
Multiple myeloma
(monoclonal IgG type)

▼ **Decreased IgG levels**
Agammaglobulinemia
AIDS
Drug immunosuppression
(e.g., steroids, dextran)
Hypoproteinemia (e.g.,
nephrotic syndrome,
protein-losing
enteropathies)
Leukemia
Non-IgG multiple myeloma
Wiskott-Aldrich syndrome

440 immunoglobulin quantification

▲ **Increased IgM levels**

Acute infections
Autoimmune diseases
(e.g., systemic lupus
erythematosus, rheumatoid
arthritis)
Chronic infections (e.g.,
hepatitis, mononucleosis,
sarcoidosis)
Chronic liver disorders (e.g.,
biliary cirrhosis)
Waldenström
macroglobulinemia

▼ **Decreased IgM levels**

Agammaglobulinemia
AIDS
Drug immunosuppression
(e.g., steroids, dextran)
Hypoproteinemia (e.g.,
nephrotic syndrome,
protein-losing
enteropathies)
IgG or IgA multiple
myeloma
Leukemia

▲ **Increased IgE levels**

Allergic infections (e.g.,
aspergillosis or parasites)
Allergy reactions (e.g., hay
fever, asthma, eczema,
anaphylaxis)

▼ **Decreased IgE levels**

Agammaglobulinemia

notes

insulin assay

Type of test Blood

Normal findings

6–26 µU/mL or 43–186 pmol/L (SI units)
Newborn: 3–20 µU/mL

Possible critical values

> 30 µU/mL

Test explanation and related physiology

Insulin assay is used to diagnose insulinoma (tumor of the islets of Langerhans). It is also used in the evaluation of patients with fasting hypoglycemia. Also see C-peptide, p. 243.

Some investigators believe that measuring the ratio of the blood sugar and insulin on the same specimen obtained during the oral glucose tolerance test (GTT; p. 392) is more reliable than measuring insulin levels alone. Combined with the oral GTT, the insulin assay can show characteristic curves.

Type 2 diabetes (adult onset) is characterized by an excess of insulin production in response to GTT. This hyperresponse of insulin may precede hyperglycemia by many years, allowing the patient time and opportunity to take action to reduce the incidence of outright diabetes through diet management and lifestyle changes.

Procedure and patient care

- See inside front cover for Routine Blood Testing.
- Fasting: yes
- Blood tube commonly used: red

Abnormal findings

▲ Increased levels
Acromegaly
Cushing syndrome
Fructose or galactose
  intolerance
Insulinoma
Obesity

▼ Decreased levels
Diabetes mellitus
Hypopituitarism

notes

insulin-like growth factor (IGF-1, Somatomedin C, Insulin-like growth factor binding proteins [IGF BP])

Type of test Blood

Normal findings

Adults: 42–110 ng/mL
Children:

Age (yr)	Girls (ng/mL)	Boys (ng/mL)
0–8	5–128	2–118
9–10	24–158	15–148
11–13	65–226	55–216
14–15	124–242	114–232
16–17	94–231	84–211
18–19	66–186	56–177

Test explanation and related physiology

Growth hormone (GH) exerts its effects on many tissues through a group of peptides called *somatomedins*. The most commonly tested somatomedins are insulin-like growth factor 1 (IGF-1) and IGF-3. Measurement of free IGF-1 and IGF binding protein (BP) 3 is preferred to GH measurements in cases of short stature in early adolescence. IGF is the test of choice in identifying and monitoring treatment of acromegaly.

To diminish the common variations in GH secretion, screening for IGF-1 provides a more accurate reflection of the mean plasma concentration of GH. Somatomedins are not affected (as GH is) by the time of day, food intake, or exercise because they circulate bound to proteins that are durable or long-lasting. Normally there is a large increase during the pubertal growth spurt.

Levels of IGF-1 depend on levels of GH. As a result, IGF-1 levels are low when GH levels are deficient. (See GH, p. 395.) Nonpituitary causes of reduced IGF-1 levels include malnutrition, severe chronic illnesses, severe liver disease, hypothyroidism, renal failure, inflammatory bowel disease, and Laron dwarfism.

Pediatricians commonly use *IGF BPs* to even further diminish the influence of the variables affecting GH and somatomedin levels. Specifically, IGF BP 2 and IGF BP 3 are the most commonly measured. However, if GH deficiency is strongly suspected yet documentation using GH or somatomedins is questionable, IGF BP determinations are helpful. IGF BP 3 is less age-dependent and is the most accurate (97% sensitivity and specificity). These proteins help to evaluate GH deficiencies and GH-resistant syndromes (e.g., Laron dwarfism). Finally, these binding proteins are very useful in predicting responses to therapeutic exogenous GH administration.

Procedure and patient care

- See inside front cover for Routine Blood Testing.
- Fasting: yes
- Blood tube commonly used: lavender or red

Abnormal findings

▲ **Increased levels**

Acromegaly
Gigantism
Hyperpituitarism
Obesity
Precocious puberty
Pregnancy

▼ **Decreased levels**

Cirrhosis of the liver
Delayed puberty
GH deficiency/resistance
Hypopituitarism
Inactive GH
Laron dwarfism
Nutritional deficiency
Pituitary tumor
Resistance to somatomedins

notes

intrinsic factor antibody (IF ab)

Type of test Blood

Normal findings

Negative

Test explanation and related physiology

IF ab is used to diagnose pernicious anemia (PA). PA is a vitamin B_{12} deficiency and is a megaloblastic anemia. It is a disease of the stomach in which secretion of IF is severely reduced or absent, resulting in malabsorption of vitamin B_{12}. PA appears to be an autoimmune process.

More than half of adult patients have IF abs. There are two types of this antibody. Type I, blocking antibody, is more common and prevents the binding of vitamin B_{12} and IF. Type II binding antibody is less specific for PA and affects the binding of IF in the ileum. The blocking antibody is extremely specific for PA and is more sensitive than the binding antibody. In the context of a low or borderline B_{12} result, in which other clinical and hematologic findings are compatible with a diagnosis of B_{12} deficiency, the presence of IF blocking antibody can be taken as confirmation of this diagnosis and, at the same time, as an indication of its cause. A negative result, on the other hand, cannot rule out the possibility of PA because blocking antibody is not demonstrable in nearly 50% of all patients with this disorder.

Interfering factors

- Levels are *decreased* if an injection of vitamin B_{12} is administered within 48 hours of testing.

Procedure and patient care

- See inside front cover for Routine Blood Testing.
- Fasting: no
- Blood tube commonly used: red

Abnormal findings

▲ **Increased levels**

Pernicious anemia

notes

iron level and total iron-binding capacity (Fe and TIBC, Transferrin saturation, Transferrin)

Type of test Blood

Normal findings

Iron

Male: 80–180 mcg/dL or 14–32 μmol/L (SI units)
Female: 60–160 mcg/dL or 11–29 μmol/L (SI units)
Results may be decreased in the elderly
Child: 50–120 mcg/dL
Newborn: 100–250 mcg/dL

TIBC

250–460 mcg/dL or 45–82 μmol/L (SI units)

Transferrin

Adult male: 215–365 mg/dL or 2.15–3.65 g/L (SI units)
Adult female: 250–380 mg/dL or 2.5–3.8 g/L (SI units)
Child: 203–360 mg/dL
Newborn: 130–275 mg/dL

Transferrin saturation

Male: 20%-50%
Female: 15%-50%

Test explanation and related physiology

Serum iron

Abnormal levels of iron are characteristic of many diseases, including iron deficiency anemia and hemochromatosis. Seventy percent of iron in the body is found in the hemoglobin of red blood cells (RBCs). The other 30% is stored iron in the form of *ferritin* (p. 331) and hemosiderin. Iron is supplied by the diet. Iron is bound to a globulin protein called *transferrin*. When iron stores are low, transferrin levels increase. Transferrin is low when there is too much iron. Usually about one-third of the transferrin is used to transport iron. Because of this, the blood serum has considerable extra iron-binding capacity, which is the *unsaturated iron-binding capacity (UIBC)*. The TIBC equals UIBC plus the serum iron measurement. The serum iron determination is a measurement of the quantity of iron bound to transferrin.

Iron-deficiency anemia is a result of reduced serum iron. Iron-deficiency anemia has many causes, including the following:

- Insufficient iron intake

- Inadequate gut absorption
- Increased requirements (e.g., in growing children)
- Loss of blood (e.g., menstruation, bleeding peptic ulcer)

Iron deficiency results in decreased production of hemoglobin, which in turn results in small, pale (microcytic, hypochromic) RBCs.

Acute iron poisoning is characterized by a serum iron level that exceeds the TIBC. Chronic iron overload or poisoning is called *hemochromatosis* or *hemosiderosis*. Excess iron is usually deposited in the brain, liver, and heart and causes severe dysfunction of these organs.

Total iron-binding capacity and transferrin

TIBC is a measurement of all proteins available for binding mobile iron. Transferrin represents the largest quantity of iron-binding proteins. Therefore TIBC is an indirect yet accurate measurement of transferrin. Ferritin is not included in TIBC because it binds only stored iron. TIBC is increased in 70% of patients with iron deficiency.

Transferrin is a *negative* acute-phase reactant protein. That is, in various acute inflammatory reactions, transferrin levels diminish. Transferrin also is diminished in the face of chronic illnesses, such as malignancy, collagen vascular diseases, or liver diseases.

TIBC varies minimally according to iron intake and is more of a reflection of liver function (transferrin is produced by the liver) and nutrition than of iron metabolism.

Soluble transferrin receptor (sTfR), also called *circulating transferrin receptor* or *serum transferrin receptor*, is a circulating protein derived from cleavage of the membrane transferrin receptor on bone marrow erythroid precursor cells. Its concentration in serum is directly proportional to RBC synthesis and inversely proportional to tissue iron availability.

Total iron-binding capacity and transferrin saturation

The percentage of transferrin and other mobile iron-binding proteins saturated with iron is calculated by dividing the serum iron level by the TIBC:

$$TS(\%) = \frac{\text{Serum iron level}}{\text{TIBC}} \times 100\%$$

TS is decreased to less than 15% in patients with iron-deficiency anemia. It is increased in patients with hemolytic, sideroblastic, or megaloblastic anemias. TS is also increased in patients with iron overload or poisoning. Increased intake or absorption of iron (as in hemochromatosis) leads to elevated iron levels. In such cases, TIBC is unchanged; as a result, the percentage of TS is very high. UIBC has been proposed as an inexpensive alternative to transferrin saturation.

Chronic illness is characterized by a low serum iron level, decreased TIBC, and normal TS. Pregnancy is marked by high levels of protein, including transferrin. Because iron requirements are high, it is not unusual to find low serum iron levels, high TIBC, and a low percentage of TS in late pregnancy.

Contraindications
• Patients with hemolytic diseases, because they may have an artificially high iron content

Interfering factors
• Recent blood transfusions.
• Recent ingestion of a meal containing high iron content.
• Hemolytic diseases may be associated with an artificially high iron content.

Procedure and patient care
• See inside front cover for Routine Blood Testing.
• Fasting: yes (12 hours)
• Blood tube commonly used: red
• Avoid hemolysis, because the iron contained in the RBCs will pour out into the serum.

Abnormal findings

▲ **Increased serum iron levels**
Hemochromatosis
Hemolytic anemia
Hemosiderosis
Hepatic necrosis
Hepatitis
Iron poisoning
Lead toxicity
Massive blood transfusion

▼ **Decreased serum iron levels**
Chronic blood loss
  (e.g., gastrointestinal)
Chronic menstruation
Chronic hematuria
Inadequate iron absorption
Insufficient dietary iron
Iron deficiency anemia
Neoplasia
Pregnancy (late)

▲ **Increased TIBC or transferrin levels**
Iron deficiency anemia
Oral contraceptives
Polycythemia vera
Pregnancy (late)

▼ **Decreased TIBC or transferrin levels**
Cirrhosis
Hemolytic anemia
Hypoproteinemia
Inflammatory diseases
Pernicious anemia
Sickle cell anemia

▲ **Increased TS or TIBC saturation**

Acute iron overdose
Hemochromatosis
Hemolytic anemia
Hemosiderosis

▼ **Decreased TS or TIBC saturation**

Chronic illnesses (e.g., malignancy)
Iron deficiency anemia

notes

ischemia-modified albumin (IMA)

Type of test Blood

Normal findings

< 85 IU/mL

Test explanation and related physiology

When albumin is exposed to an ischemic environment, its N terminal is altered; this causes an alteration of the albumin called *ischemia-modified albumin (IMA)*. This has become particularly helpful in identifying cardiac ischemia in patients with chest pain. When combined with troponins (p. 741), myoglobin (p. 518), and electrocardiography, the diagnosis of an ischemic cardiac event can be corroborated or ruled out. IMA is produced continually during the period of ischemia. Blood levels rise within 10 minutes of the initiation of the ischemic event and stay elevated for 6 hours after ischemia has resolved.

IMA may also be elevated in patients with pulmonary embolus or acute stroke. False positives can occur in other clinical circumstances, such as advanced cancers, acute infections, and end-stage renal or liver disease.

Procedure and patient care

- See inside front cover for Routine Blood Testing.
- Fasting: no
- Blood tube commonly used: yellow
- This test is usually done after the initial onset of chest pain, then 12 hours later, and then daily testing for 3 to 5 days.

Abnormal findings

▲ Increased levels

Brain ischemia

Myocardial ischemia

Pulmonary ischemia

notes

kidney stone analysis (Urinary stone analysis, Renal calculus analysis)

Type of test Urine

Normal findings

All urinary stones are pathologic.

Test explanation and related physiology

Kidney stone analysis is performed to identify the chemical composition of a kidney stone. This can guide treatment and help prevent more stones from forming (Box K1). Eighty percent of patients with kidney stones have a history of recurrent stone formation. Treatment can be done by altering urine pH and by adjusting dietary intake of fluids, electrolytes, and protein.

Analysis is done on a kidney stone that has been passed in the urine or removed from the urinary tract during surgery.

In general, the following patterns are often treated as follows:

- Hyperuricuria and predominately uric acid stones are treated by alkalinizing the urine to increase uric acid solubility.
- Hypercalciuria and predominately hydroxyapatite stones are treated by acidifying the urine to increase calcium solubility.
- Hyperoxaluria and calcium oxalate stones are treated by increasing daily fluid intake and by possibly reducing daily calcium intake. This type of stone represents 80% of kidney stones found.
- Magnesium ammonium phosphate (struvite) stones are caused by infection and are prevented by treatment of the urinary tract infection.
- Cystine stones are rare and caused by hereditary cystinuria. They are treated by increasing fluid intake, by restricting sodium and protein intake, and by alkalinizing the urine.

Interfering factors

- Tape used to attach a stone to paper may affect the ability to accurately identify the composition of the stone.

BOX K1 Evaluating the patient with kidney stones

- Focused history to determine predisposing factors
- Radiographic diagnostic testing to identify the stone
- Stone analysis
- Laboratory testing for metabolic evaluation
- Monitoring for new stones

Procedure and patient care

Before
- PT Explain the procedure to the patient. Tell the patient that a stone could look like a grain of sand or a small piece of gravel.
- PT Explain that there are no dietary restrictions for this test.
- PT Provide and explain the use of the urine strainer.

During
- PT Instruct the patient to urinate into the strainer provided.
- PT If a stone is found, tell the patient to allow it to air dry at room temperature for 24 hours on a tissue or towel before placing it into a clean, dry container.

After
- Transport the specimen to the laboratory promptly.
- PT Encourage fluids.

Abnormal findings

Kidney stones

K

notes

lactic acid (Lactate)

Type of test Blood

Normal findings

Venous blood: 5–20 mg/dL or 0.6–2.2 mmol/L (SI units)
Arterial blood: 3–7 mg/dL or 0.3–0.8 mmol/L (SI units)

Test explanation and related physiology

Under conditions of normal oxygen availability to tissues, glucose is metabolized to CO_2 and H_2O for energy. When oxygen to the tissues is diminished, anaerobic metabolism of glucose occurs, and lactate (lactic acid) is formed instead of CO_2 and H_2O. To compound the problem of lactic acid buildup, when the liver is hypoxic, it fails to clear the lactic acid. Lactic acid levels accumulate, causing lactic acidosis (LA). Lactic acid blood levels are used to document the presence of tissue hypoxia, determine the degree of hypoxia, and monitor the effect of therapy. Levels increase when strenuous exercise or conditions such as heart failure, sepsis, or shock lower the flow of blood and oxygen in the body.

Procedure and patient care

- See inside front cover for Routine Blood Testing.
- Fasting: no
- Blood tube commonly used: red
- **PT** Instruct the patient to avoid making a fist before and while blood is being withdrawn. This can increase levels.
- Avoid the use of a tourniquet if possible.

Abnormal findings

▲ Increased levels

Carbon monoxide poisoning
Diabetes mellitus (nonketotic)
Genetic errors of metabolism
Liver disease
Sepsis
Shock
Strenuous exercise
Tissue ischemia

notes

lactic dehydrogenase (LDH, Lactate dehydrogenase)

Type of test Blood

Normal findings

Total

Adult/elderly: 100–190 units/L at 37° C (lactate → pyruvate) or 100–190 units/L (SI units)

Child: 60–170 units/L (30° C)

Infant: 100–250 units/L

Newborn: 160–450 units/L

Isoenzymes

Adult/elderly:

    LDH-1: 17%-27%

    LDH-2: 27%-37%

    LDH-3: 18%-25%

    LDH-4: 3%-8%

    LDH-5: 0%-5%

Test explanation and related physiology

The LDH test is a measure of total LDH. There are actually five separate fractions (isoenzymes) that make up the total LDH. In general, isoenzyme LDH-1 comes mainly from the heart; LDH-2 comes primarily from the reticuloendothelial system; LDH-3 comes from the lungs and other tissues; LDH-4 comes from the kidney, placenta, and pancreas; and LDH-5 comes mainly from the liver and striated muscle. In normal persons, LDH-2 makes up the greatest percentage of total LDH.

LDH is also measured in other body fluids. Elevated urine levels of total LDH indicate neoplasm or injury to the urologic system. When the LDH in an effusion (pleural, cardiac, or peritoneal) is more than 60% of the serum total LDH, the effusion is said to be an *exudate* and not a transudate.

Interfering factors

- Strenuous exercise may cause elevations.
- Hemolysis of blood will cause false-positive LDH levels.

Procedure and patient care

- See inside front cover for Routine Blood Testing.
- Fasting: no
- Blood tube commonly used: red

Abnormal findings

▲ **Increased values**

Advanced solid tumor malignancies
Diffuse disease or injury (e.g., heatstroke)
Hepatic disease (e.g., hepatitis, active cirrhosis, neoplasm)
Intestinal ischemia and infarction
Lymphoma and other reticuloendothelial system tumors
Myocardial infarction
Pancreatitis
Pulmonary disease (e.g., embolism, infarction, pneumonia)
Red blood cell disease
Renal parenchymal disease (e.g., infarction,
   glomerulonephritis, acute tubular necrosis)
Skeletal muscle disease and injury (e.g., muscular trauma)
Testicular tumors (seminoma or dysgerminomas)

notes

lactoferrin

Type of test Stool

Normal findings

None detected

Test explanation and related physiology

Lactoferrin is a glycoprotein expressed by activated neutrophils. The detection of lactoferrin in a fecal sample therefore serves as a surrogate marker for inflammatory white blood cells (WBCs) in the intestinal tract. Lactoferrin assay has allowed the identification of inflammatory cells in the stool without the use of microscopy.

Detection of fecal lactoferrin allows for the differentiation of inflammatory and noninflammatory intestinal disorders in patients with diarrhea. Usually the test is used as a diagnostic aid to help identify patients with active inflammatory bowel disease (e.g., Crohn disease or ulcerative colitis) and to rule out those with active irritable bowel syndrome, which is noninflammatory. Lactoferrin is also present in patients with bacterial enteritis (e.g., *Shigella* spp., *Salmonella* spp., *Campylobacter jejuni,* and *Clostridium difficile*). Diarrhea caused by viruses and most parasites is not associated with elevated lactoferrin levels.

Interfering factors

- Breastfeeding can affect test results in breastfed infants.

Procedure and patient care

Before

PT Explain the procedure to the patient.

PT Instruct the patient not to mix urine or toilet paper with the specimen.

During

- Stool is collected in a clean bedpan.
- Place at least 5 g of stool in a clean specimen container.

After

- Observe appropriate contamination precautions.
- Transfer the specimen to the laboratory immediately.

Abnormal findings

Bacterial enteritis

Crohn disease

Ulcerative colitis

notes

lactose tolerance test (Hydrogen breath test)

Type of test   Blood

Normal findings

Blood: Adult/elderly: rise in plasma glucose levels > 20 mg/dL
   No abdominal cramps or diarrhea
Breath: < 50 ppm hydrogen increase over baseline

Test explanation and related physiology

This test is performed to detect lactose intolerance, intestinal malabsorption, maldigestion, or bacterial overgrowth in the small intestine. Because lactose-intolerant patients have an absence of lactase, any lactose (the common sugar in dairy products) ingested will not be digested in the small bowel. Thus the colon is flooded with a high lactose load. Although all adults have some degree of lactase reduction, severe lactose intolerance can occur in patients with inflammatory bowel disease, short-gut syndrome, and other malabsorption syndromes. Lactase deficiency can be congenital and become apparent in newborns. These infants present with vomiting, diarrhea, malabsorption, and failure to thrive.

In this test, the patient is given an oral lactose load. If lactase is not present in sufficient quantities, lactose is not metabolized to glucose and galactose. Plasma levels of glucose do not rise as expected.

There is a breath-test portion of this diagnostic test in which exhaled air is analyzed for hydrogen content. This is called the *lactose breath test* (or *hydrogen breath test*). The bacteria in the colon produce hydrogen when exposed to unabsorbed food, particularly the lactose load that was not absorbed in the small intestine. Large amounts of hydrogen may also be produced when the colonic bacteria move back into the small intestine, a condition called *bacterial overgrowth of the small bowel.* In this instance the overgrowth bacteria are exposed to the lactose load that has not had a chance to completely traverse the small intestine to be fully digested and absorbed. Large amounts of the hydrogen produced by the bacteria are absorbed into the blood flowing through the wall of the small intestine and colon. This hydrogen-containing blood travels to the lungs, where the hydrogen is released and exhaled in the breath in measurable quantities.

More recently, lactose (and other disaccharidases) deficiency can be detected by identifying the disaccharidase in the tissue of the colon, obtained by colonoscopy. Maltase, palatinase, and sucrase deficiencies can also be evaluated with this technique.

Interfering factors
- Enterogenous steatorrhea
- Ethnicity has a major effect on primary lactose deficiency.
- Patients with diabetes may have glucose levels that exceed 20 mg/dL despite lactase insufficiency.

Procedure and patient care

Before
PT Explain the procedure to the patient. Inform the patient that four blood samples will be needed.

PT Instruct the patient to fast for 12 hours before testing.

PT Instruct the patient to avoid strenuous exercise for 8 hours before testing because exercise may factitiously affect the blood glucose level.

PT Inform the patient that smoking is prohibited for approximately 8 hours before testing because smoking can increase the blood glucose level.

During
- Collect a venous blood sample in a gray-top tube.
- Provide a specified dose of lactose for the patient.
- Note that pediatric doses of lactose are based on weight.
- Collect three more blood samples at 30, 60, and 120 minutes after the ingestion of lactose.

PT Tell the patient that the only discomfort is the venipuncture; however, patients with lactase deficiency may have symptoms of lactose intolerance (e.g., cramps and diarrhea).

- If the breath test is being done, the exhaled air is evaluated for hydrogen content before ingestion of lactose and every 15 minutes thereafter. Hydrogen levels are recorded.

After
- Apply pressure to the venipuncture site.
- Note that patients with abnormal test results may receive a monosaccharide tolerance test (e.g., glucose or galactose tolerance test).

Abnormal findings

▼ **Decreased levels**

Intestinal malabsorption or maldigestion

Lactase insufficiency

Small bowel overgrowth of bacteria

notes

Legionnaires' disease antibody test

Type of test Blood

Normal findings

Legionella PCR: negative

Test explanation and related physiology

Legionnaires' disease was originally described as a fulminating pneumonia caused by *Legionella pneumophila*. *PCR testing for Legionella* DNA is the preferred test for the diagnosis of this disease. PCR can be performed on nearly any sample type and detects all clinically important *Legionella* species and serotypes. The best sample for a patient with pneumonia is a lower respiratory sputum or transbronchial aspirate.

The *Legionella urinary antigen test* is a commonly used alternative test for Legionnaires' disease especially if sputum cannot be obtained. *Legionella* antigens can be detected in urine as early as 1 day after symptom onset and persist for days to weeks.

Culture on special media is considered the gold standard for diagnosis of *Legionella* infections. Culture can be performed on nearly any sample type and results are typically obtained in approximately 3 to 5 days.

Sputum samples require prompt processing because *Legionella* bacteria do not survive for prolonged periods in respiratory secretions.

Procedure and patient care

- See inside front cover for Routine Blood Testing.
- Fasting: no
- Blood tube commonly used: red
- For culture: Obtain sputum as described in sputum culture (p. 682).

Abnormal findings

▲ **Increased levels**

Legionnaires' disease

leucine aminopeptidase (LAP)

Type of test Blood; urine (24-hour)

Normal findings

Blood

Male: 80–200 units/mL or 19.2–48 units/L (SI units)
Female: 75–185 units/mL or 18–44.4 units/L (SI units)

Urine

2–18 units/24 hr

Test explanation and related physiology

LAP is an intracellular enzyme that exists in the hepatobiliary system and, to a much smaller degree, in the pancreas and small intestine. LAP is mainly used in diagnosing liver disorders and in the differential diagnosis of increased levels of alkaline phosphatase (ALP; p. 23). LAP levels tend to parallel ALP levels in hepatic disease. LAP is a sensitive indicator of cholestasis; however, unlike ALP, LAP remains normal in bone disease.

Interfering factors

• Pregnancy may cause increased values.

Procedure and patient care

• See inside front cover for Routine Blood Testing.
• Fasting: no
• Blood tube commonly used: red
• If a urine sample is needed, see inside front cover for Routine Urine Testing.

Abnormal findings

▲ Increased levels

Cholestasis
Cirrhosis
Gallstones
Hepatic necrosis, ischemia, tumor
Hepatitis
Hepatotoxic drugs

notes

lipase (Pancreatic lipase, Lipoprotein lipase)

Type of test Blood

Normal findings

0–160 units/L or 0–160 units/L (SI units) (Values are method dependent.)

Test explanation and related physiology

The most commonly tested lipase is pancreatic lipase. The most common cause of an elevated serum lipase level is acute pancreatitis. Lipase is an enzyme secreted by the pancreas into the duodenum to break down triglycerides into fatty acids. As with amylase (p. 44), lipase appears in the bloodstream after damage to or disease affecting the pancreatic acinar cells. Lipase is thought to be more specific for the pancreas than amylase.

Other conditions can be associated with elevated lipase levels. Lipase is excreted through the kidneys. Therefore elevated lipase levels are often found in patients with renal failure. Intestinal infarction or obstruction also can be associated with lipase elevation.

In acute pancreatitis, lipase levels increase within several hours of symptom onset, peak at 24 hours, and remain elevated for up to 2 weeks. Another lipase is *Lipoprotein Lipase*. When this enzyme is deficient (as exists in familial lipoprotein lipase deficiency [LPLD]), triglycerides build up in several organs (e.g., skin, bloodstream, muscles, liver, spleen, and brain).

Procedure and patient care

- See inside front cover for Routine Blood Testing.
- Fasting: yes
- Blood tube commonly used: red

Abnormal findings

Acute cholecystitis	Extrahepatic duct obstruction
Acute/chronic relapsing pancreatitis	Pancreatic cancer/pseudocyst
	Peptic ulcer disease
Bowel obstruction or infarction	Renal failure
Cholangitis	Salivary gland inflammation or tumor

notes

lipoprotein-associated phospholipase A$_2$
(Lp-PLA$_2$ PLAC test)

Type of test Blood

Normal findings

Average value for males: 251 ng/mL (range: 131–376)
Average value for females: 174 ng/mL (range: 120–342)

Test explanation and related physiology

Lipoprotein-associated phospholipase A$_2$ (Lp-PLA$_2$) promotes vascular inflammation contributing directly to the atherogenic process. Lp-PLA$_2$ is an independent predictor of cardiovascular disease. When combined with C-reactive protein (CRP) (p. 245), testing for Lp-PLA$_2$ markedly increases the predictive value in determining risks for a cardiac event. An Lp-PLA$_2$ level greater than 200 ng/mL would warrant reclassifying the patient to the next highest risk category, which would require more aggressive use of cholesterol-lowering agents. Lp-PLA$_2$ may play an important role in the progression of atherosclerosis and overall plaque stability.

Lp-PLA$_2$ is also an accurate aid in assessing the risk for ischemic stroke associated with atherosclerosis at all levels of blood pressure.

Procedure and patient care

- See inside front cover for Routine Blood Testing.
- Fasting: no
- Blood tube commonly used: red

Abnormal findings

▲ Increased levels
  Atherosclerosis

notes

lipoproteins (High-density lipoproteins [HDLs, HDL-C], Low density lipoproteins [LDLs, LDL-C], Very-low-density lipoproteins [VLDLs], Lipoprotein (a), Lipoprotein electrophoresis, Lipoprotein phenotyping, Lipid fractionation, Non-HDL cholesterol, Lipid profile) and Apolipoproteins

Type of test Blood
Normal findings
Lipoproteins
HDL
    Male: > 45 mg/dL or > 0.75 mmol/L (SI units)
    Female: > 55 mg/dL or > 0.91 mmol/L (SI units)
LDL
    Adult: < 130 mg/dL
    Children: < 110 mg/dL
VLDL
    7–32 mg/dL

Apolipoproteins
Apo A-I
    Adult/elderly:
        Male: 75–160 mg/dL
        Female: 80–175 mg/dL
    Child:
        5–17 years: 83–151 mg/dL
        6 months-4 years:
            Male: 67–167 mg/dL
            Female: 60–148 mg/dL
        Newborn:
            Male: 41–93 mg/dL
            Female: 38–106 mg/dL
Apo B
    Adult/elderly:
        Male: 50–125 mg/dL
        Female: 45–120 mg/dL
    Child:
        5–17 years:
        Male: 47–139 mg/dL
        Female: 41–132 mg/dL
        6 months-3 years: 23–75 mg/dL
        Newborn: 11–31 mg/dL
Apo A-I/Apo B ratio
    Male: 0.85–2.24
    Female: 0.76–3.23

Lipoprotein (a)
>   White (5th-95th percentiles):
>   Male: 2.2–49.4 mg/dL
>   Female: 2.1–57.3 mg/dL
>   African American (5th-95th percentiles):
>   Male: 4.6–71.8 mg/dL
>   Female: 4.4–75 mg/dL

Test explanation and related physiology

The two important lipid substances in the blood (plasma), lymph, cerebral spinal fluid, and extracellular fluid are cholesterol and triglyceride (see pages 198 and 737). Lipoprotein's (HDL, LDL, and VLDL) primary function is to transport these fatty substances throughout these fluids and into cells of the body. Apolipoproteins are proteins that bind the lipids to form lipoproteins. In addition to stabilizing lipoprotein structure, apolipoproteins interact with lipoprotein cellular membrane receptors and lipid transport proteins, thereby participating in lipoprotein uptake and clearance of cholesterol and triglycerides. Apolipoproteins also act as enzyme cofactors in lipoprotein synthesis. Lipoproteins and apolipoproteins are an accurate predictor of heart and vascular disease.

Tested as a panel called "*lipid profile*," these tests are used to initiate medical interventions and to monitor the response to statin /diet therapy. The lipid profile usually measures total cholesterol, triglycerides, HDL, LDL, and VLDL. HDLs (the majority of which is considered "good cholesterol") are carriers of cholesterol. HDL functions to remove lipids from the endothelium. Most cholesterol carried by LDLs is deposited into the lining of the blood vessels and is associated with an increased risk of arteriosclerotic heart and peripheral vascular disease. Therefore, high levels of LDLs are atherogenic. LDL is difficult to measure and calculated using various formulas. VLDLs, although carrying a small amount of cholesterol, are the predominant carriers of blood triglycerides and are also often calculated.

Apoproteins also act as an atherogenic risk factor. *Apolipoprotein A (apo A),* linked to LDL, forms lipoprotein (a) and is more atherogenic than LDL. *Apolipoprotein B (apo B)* is the major polypeptide component of LDL and chylomicrons and VLDL. The risk of myocardial infarction is determined by apo B lipoproteins alone or *apo B/apo A_1 ratio*, independent from lipid content (cholesterol or triglyceride) or type of lipoprotein (LDL or triglyceride-rich).

Lp(a) (referred to as lipoprotein little a) is a heterogeneous group of lipoproteins consisting of an apo A molecule attached to an apo B molecule. An increased level of Lp(a) may be an independent risk factor for atherosclerosis and is particularly harmful to the endothelium. Serum concentrations of Lp(a) appear to be largely related to genetic factors; diet and statin drugs do not have a major effect on Lp(a) levels. Lp(a) is not routinely included in a lipid profile.

Apolipoprotein E (apo E) is involved in cholesterol transport and is the major lipoprotein in the brain and spinal cord. When diminished in the CSF, cognitive function is decreased. *Apolipoprotein F (apo F)* and *Apolipoprotein M (apo M)* are minor apolipoproteins involved in lipid transfer and metabolism.

Hereditary lipid disorders can result in high levels of LDL-C, triglycerides, Lp(a), and HDL-C. Genetic testing can be important in screening, diagnosis, and potentially in treatment of lipid disorders, particularly for familial hypercholesterolemia (see genetic testing p. 369).

Interfering factors

- Smoking and alcohol ingestion affect some levels.
- Diet can alter values.
- Values are age and sex dependent.
- HDL is elevated in hypothyroid patients and diminished in hyperthyroid patients.
- High triglyceride levels can make LDL calculations inaccurate.

Procedure and patient care

- See inside front cover for Routine Blood Testing.
- Fasting: yes (12–14 hours)
- Blood tube commonly used: red
- **PT** Inform the patient that smoking is prohibited before the test.
- **PT** Inform the patient that dietary indiscretion within the previous few weeks may influence lipoprotein levels.
- **PT** Instruct patients with high lipoprotein levels regarding diet, exercise, and appropriate body weight.

Abnormal findings

▲ **Increased HDL levels**
Excessive exercise
Familial HDL
lipoproteinemia

▼ **Decreased HDL levels**
Familial low HDL
Hepatocellular disease
(e.g., hepatitis,
cirrhosis)
Hypoproteinemia (e.g.,
nephrotic syndrome,
malnutrition)
Metabolic syndrome

▲ **Increased LDL and VLDL levels**
Alcohol consumption
Apoprotein CII deficiency
Chronic liver disease (e.g., hepatitis, cirrhosis)
Familial hypercholesterolemia type IIa
Familial LDL lipoproteinemia
Gammopathies (e.g., multiple myeloma)
Glycogen storage diseases (e.g., von Gierke disease)
Nephrotic syndrome

▲ **Increased apo A-I**
Familial hyperalphalipoproteinemia
Pregnancy
Weight reduction

▲ **Increased apo B**
Coronary artery disease
Diabetes mellitus
Hyperlipoproteinemia (types IIa, IIb, IV, V)

▲ **Increased Lp(a)**
Diabetes mellitus
Familial hypercholesterolemia
Premature vascular disease

▼ **Decreased LDL and VLDL levels**
Familial hypolipoproteinemia
Hyperthyroidism
Hypoproteinemia (e.g., malabsorption, severe burns, malnutrition)

▼ **Decreased apo A-I**
Cholestasis
Chronic renal failure
Coronary artery disease
Diabetes mellitus
Familial hypoalpha-lipoproteinemia

▼ **Decreased apo B**
Chronic anemia
Chronic pulmonary disease
Hyperthyroidism
Malnutrition/weight reduction

▼ **Decreased Lp(a)**
Chronic hepatocellular disease
Malnutrition

notes

liquid biopsy (Fluid biopsy, Fluid phase biopsy, Cell free circulating DNA [cfDNA, ctDNA], Circulating tumor cells)

Type of test Blood, urine, cerebrospinal fluid (CSF)

Normal findings

No abnormal cells or cell nucleic acids

Test explanation and related physiology

The principle supporting liquid biopsy is based on repeated findings that tumors shed molecules and cells into bodily fluids (particularly blood). Since the development of molecular testing laboratory methods, researchers have shown that analyzing these molecules and cells can reveal some of the same and even additional information that tissue biopsies provide. With this additional information, personalized treatment strategies can be developed.

Liquid biopsies are easily obtained through venipuncture or by obtaining a urine specimen. They can track tumors as they develop and change over time. A liquid biopsy may be used to help find cancer at an early stage. Being able to take multiple samples of blood over time may also help doctors understand what kind of molecular changes are taking place in a tumor. Repeated liquid biopsies can be used in surveillance of treated cancer patients to look for treatment response and recurrence.

Different liquid biopsy tests analyze different kinds of tumor material, such as entire circulating free tumor cells (CTCs), circulating tumor DNA (ctDNA), RNA, proteins, and tiny vesicles of nucleic acid molecules called exomes. The tests detect these molecules or cells in various bodily fluids, including blood, urine, CSF, and saliva.

Liquid biopsies are used in lung, colo-rectal, esophageal, gastric, hepatic, pancreatic, head and neck, ovarian, myeloma, lymphoid, and breast cancers. In cardiology, endothelial cells identified in the blood, may indicate myocardial infarction (MI). Cell-free fetal DNA (see cell-free maternal testing, p. 184) is used to identify serious fetal genetic and chromosomal abnormalities.

Another application of liquid biopsy is to identify/follow the course of severe infections e.g., COVID-19. Severe infections can cause significant organ damage highlighted by cell disruption and release of DNA fragments into the bloodstream. cfDNA testing, also, may be more sensitive and more specific in recognizing early rejection of organ transplants.

Procedure and patient care

- See inside front cover for Routine Blood Testing.
- Fasting: no
- Blood tube commonly used: see laboratory for directions

Abnormal findings

Infections diseases, such as endocarditis, opportunistic infections, fungal infections, pneumonia.

Presence of circulating tumor cells

Presence of DNA or RNA fragments of known tumor cells

notes

L

liver biopsy

Type of test Microscopic examination of tissue

Normal findings

Normal liver histology

Test explanation and related physiology

Liver biopsy is a safe, simple, and valuable method of diagnosing pathologic liver conditions. For this study, a specially designed needle is inserted through the abdominal wall and into the liver (Figure L1). A piece of liver tissue is removed for microscopic examination. Percutaneous liver biopsy is used in the diagnosis of various liver disorders (e.g., cirrhosis, hepatitis, drug reaction, granuloma, and tumor). Biopsy is indicated for the following:

- Patients with unexplained hepatomegaly
- Patients with persistently elevated liver enzymes

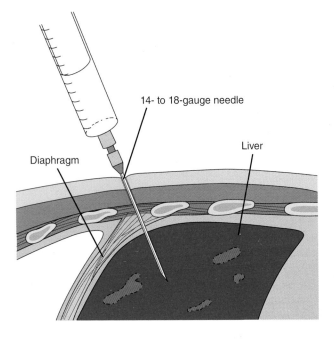

FIG. L1 Liver biopsy. Percutaneous liver biopsy requires the patient's cooperation. The patient must be able to lie quietly and hold his or her breath after exhaling.

The biopsy may be performed by a *blind stick* or directed with the use of computed tomography (CT), magnetic resonance imaging (MRI), or ultrasound.

Contraindications

- Uncooperative patients who cannot remain still and hold their breath during sustained exhalation
- Patients with impaired hemostasis and bleeding disorders
- Patients with obstructive jaundice

Potential complications

- Hemorrhage caused by inadvertent puncture of a blood vessel
- Chemical peritonitis caused by inadvertent puncture of a bile duct, with subsequent leakage of bile
- Pneumothorax caused by improper placement of the biopsy needle into the adjacent chest cavity

Procedure and patient care

Before

PT Explain the procedure to the patient.
- Obtain informed consent.
- Ensure that all coagulation tests are normal.
PT Instruct the patient to keep NPO after midnight on the day of the test.
- Administer sedative medications if ordered.

During

- After injection of a local anesthetic and with mild sedation, and during the patient's sustained exhalation, the physician rapidly introduces the biopsy needle into the liver and obtains liver tissue.
- Occasionally, the biopsy needle is inserted under CT guidance. This is especially useful when tissue from a specific area of the liver is needed.
- Note that this test is performed by a physician in approximately 15 minutes.
PT Inform the patient that he or she may have minor discomfort during injection of the local anesthetic and needle insertion.

After

- After applying a small dressing over the biopsy site, place the patient on his or her right side for approximately 1 to 2 hours. In this position, the liver capsule is compressed against the chest wall, thereby decreasing the risk of hemorrhage or bile leak.

- Assess the patient's vital signs frequently for evidence of hemorrhage and peritonitis.
- Evaluate the rate, rhythm, and depth of respirations. Report chest pain and signs of dyspnea, cyanosis, and restlessness, which may be indicative of pneumothorax.
- PT Tell the patient to avoid coughing or straining, which may cause increased intraabdominal pressure.

Abnormal findings

Abscess
Benign tumor
Cyst
Hepatitis
Infiltrative diseases (e.g., amyloidosis, hemochromatosis, cirrhosis)
Malignant tumor (primary or metastatic)

notes

liver function tests (LFTs, Liver profile, Hepatic function panel)

LFTs can help determine the function of the liver by measuring the level of liver enzymes, proteins, and bilirubin. These tests can help diagnose liver disease, screen for infection, monitor the side effects of medications on the liver, and determine the effectiveness of any treatment. Because certain foods and medications can affect test results, fasting and avoidance of certain medications may be indicated. The panel usually consists of several tests that are run at the same time on a blood sample. These tests are listed here and discussed separately. Sample normal values are shown. Refer to values of the laboratory performing the test.

	Normal values
Liver enzymes	
ALP (alkaline phosphatase, p. 23)	30–120 U/L
ALT (alanine aminotransferase, p. 16)	4–36 U/L
AST (aspartate aminotransferase, p. 105)	0–35 U/L
Proteins	
Albumin (p. 613)	3.5–5 g/dL
Total protein (p. 613)	6.4–8.3 g/dL
Bilirubin (p. 118)	
Total	0.3–1 mg/dL
Direct	0.1–0.3 mg/dL

L

Depending on the laboratory and health-care provider, other tests may be added to the panel. These include the gamma-glutamyl transpeptidase (GGTP or GGT), lactic dehydrogenase (LDH), and prothrombin time (PT) tests.

Test results are often displayed as illustrated (Figure L2).

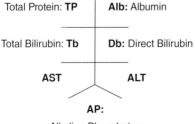

Liver Function Tests

Total Protein: **TP**	**Alb:** Albumin
Total Bilirubin: **Tb**	**Db:** Direct Bilirubin
AST	**ALT**

AP:
Alkaline Phosphatase

FIG. L2 Liver function tests.

liver/spleen scanning (Liver scanning)

Type of test Nuclear scan

Normal findings

Normal size, shape, and position of the liver and spleen

Test explanation and related physiology

This radionuclide procedure is used to outline and detect structural changes of the liver and spleen. Single-photon emission computed tomography (SPECT) has significantly improved the quality and accuracy of liver scanning. With the use of positron emission tomography (PET), anatomic and biochemical changes can be visualized within the liver.

Nuclear liver scan can also identify portal hypertension. Normally, most of the radionuclide administered during a liver scan is taken up by the liver. If the liver-to-spleen ratio is reversed (i.e., the spleen takes up more of the radionuclide), reversal of hepatic blood flow exists as a result of portal hypertension.

Liver/spleen scanning is very rarely indicated because of the increased accuracy of CT and MRI scanning.

Contraindications

- Patients who are pregnant or lactating unless the benefits of testing outweigh the risk of damage to the fetus or infant

Interfering factors

- Barium in the gastrointestinal tract overlying the liver or spleen will produce defects on the scan.

Procedure and patient care

Before

PT Explain the procedure to the patient. See p. xviii for radiation exposure and risks.

PT Tell the patient that no fasting or premedication is required.

PT Assure the patient that he or she will not be exposed to large amounts of radiation.

During

- Note the following procedural steps:
  1. The patient is taken to nuclear medicine, where the radionuclide is administered intravenously.
  2. Thirty minutes after injection, a gamma ray detector is placed over the right upper quadrant of the abdomen.

3. The patient is placed in supine, lateral, and prone positions so that all surfaces of the liver can be visualized.
4. The radionuclide image is recorded digitally.
- Note that this procedure is performed by a technologist in approximately 1 hour. A physician trained in nuclear medicine interprets the results.

PT Tell the patient that the only discomfort associated with this procedure is the (intravenous) injection of the radionuclide.

After

PT Because only tracer doses of radioisotopes are used, inform the patient that no radiation precautions are needed.

Abnormal findings

Abscess of the liver or spleen
Accessory spleen
Cirrhosis
Hemangioma
Hematoma of the liver or spleen
Hepatic or splenic cyst
Infiltrative processes (e.g., sarcoidosis, amyloidosis, tuberculosis, or granuloma of the liver or spleen)
Lacerations of the liver or spleen
Portal hypertension
Primary or metastatic tumor of the liver or spleen
Splenic infarction

notes

lumbar puncture and cerebrospinal fluid examination (LP and CSF examination, Spinal tap, Cerebrospinal fluid analysis)

Type of test Fluid analysis

Normal findings

Pressure: < 20 cm H_2O
Color: clear and colorless
Blood: none
Cells:
    RBC count: 0
    WBC count:
        Total
            Neonate: 0–30 cells/μL
            1–5 years: 0–20 cells/μL
            6–18 years: 0–10 cells/μL
            Adult: 0–5 cells/μL
        Differential
            Neutrophils: 0%-6%
            Lymphocytes: 40%-80%
            Monocytes: 15%-45%
Culture and sensitivity: no organisms present
Protein: 15–45 mg/dL CSF (up to 70 mg/dL in elderly adults and children)
Protein electrophoresis
    Prealbumin: 2%-7%
    Albumin: 56%-76%
    Alpha1 globulin: 2%-7%
    Alpha2 globulin: 4%-12%
    Beta globulin: 8%-18%
    Gamma globulin: 3%-12%
    Oligoclonal bands: none
    Immunoglobulin G (IgG): 0–4.5 mg/dL
Glucose: 50–75 mg/dL CSF or 60%-70% of blood glucose level
Chloride: 700–750 mg/dL
LDH: ≤ 40 units/L (adults), ≤ 70 units/L (neonates)
Lactic acid: 10–25 mg/dL
Cytology: no malignant cells
Serology for syphilis: negative
Glutamine: 6–15 mg/dL

Test explanation and related physiology

By placing a needle in the subarachnoid space of the spinal column, one can measure the pressure of that space and obtain CSF for examination and diagnosis. Lumbar puncture (LP) may also be used therapeutically to inject therapeutic or diagnostic agents and to administer spinal anesthetics. Furthermore, LP may be used to reduce intracranial pressure (ICP) in patients with normal pressure hydrocephalus or in patients with pseudotumor cerebri.

Pressure

By attaching a sterile manometer to the needle used for LP, the pressure within the subarachnoid space can be measured. Because the subarachnoid space surrounding the brain is freely connected to the subarachnoid space of the spinal cord, any increase in ICP will be directly reflected as an increase at the lumbar site. Tumors, infection, hydrocephalus, and intracranial bleeding can cause increased intracranial and spinal pressure.

Color

Normal CSF is clear and colorless. Color differences can occur with hyperbilirubinemia, hypercarotenemia, melanoma, or elevated proteins. A cloudy appearance may indicate an increase in the WBC count or protein. A red tinge to the CSF indicates the presence of blood.

Blood

Normally, CSF contains no blood. Blood may be present because of bleeding into the subarachnoid space or because the needle used in the LP has inadvertently penetrated a blood vessel on the way into the subarachnoid space.

Cells

The number of red blood cells (RBCs) is merely an indication of the amount of blood present within the CSF. Except for a few lymphocytes, the presence of WBCs in the CSF is abnormal. The presence of polymorphonuclear leukocytes (neutrophils) is indicative of bacterial meningitis or cerebral abscess.

Culture and sensitivity

The organisms that cause meningitis or brain abscess can be cultured from the CSF. Organisms found also may include atypical bacteria, fungi, or *Mycobacterium tuberculosis*. A Gram stain (p. 682) of the CSF may give the clinician preliminary information about the causative infectious agent.

Protein

Normally, very little protein is found in CSF because proteins are large molecules that do not cross the blood-brain barrier.

Normally, the proportion of albumin to globulin is higher in CSF than in blood plasma (p. 613) because albumin is smaller than globulin and can pass more easily through the blood–brain barrier.

CSF protein electrophoresis is very important in the diagnosis of CNS diseases. Patients with multiple sclerosis (MS), neurosyphilis, or other immunogenic degenerative central neurologic diseases have elevated immunoglobulins in their CSF. The detection of *oligoclonal gamma globulin bands* is highly suggestive of inflammatory and autoimmune diseases of the CNS, especially MS.

Glucose

The glucose level is decreased when bacteria, inflammatory cells, or tumor cells are present. A blood sample for glucose (p. 386) is usually drawn before the spinal tap is performed.

Chloride

The chloride concentration in CSF may be decreased in patients with meningeal infections, tubercular meningitis, and conditions of low blood chloride levels.

Lactic dehydrogenase

Quantification of LDH (specifically fractions 4 and 5; p. 453) is helpful in diagnosing bacterial meningitis. The sources of LDH are the neutrophils that fight the invading bacteria. When the LDH level is elevated, infection or inflammation is suspected. Diseases directly affecting the brain or spinal cord (e.g., stroke) are also associated with elevated LDH levels.

Lactic acid

Elevated levels indicate anaerobic metabolism associated with decreased oxygenation of the brain. CSF lactic acid is increased in both bacterial and fungal meningitis but not in viral meningitis.

Cytology

Examination of cells found in the CSF can determine whether they are malignant. Tumors in the CNS may shed cells from their surface. These cells can float freely in CSF.

Tumor markers

Increased levels of tumor markers (p. 164) may indicate metastatic tumor.

Serology for syphilis

Latent syphilis is diagnosed by performing one of many presently available serologic tests on CSF. When test results are positive, the diagnosis of neurosyphilis is made, and appropriate antibiotic therapy is initiated.

Glutamine

Elevated glutamine levels are helpful in the detection and evaluation of hepatic encephalopathy and hepatic coma. The glutamine is made by increased levels of ammonia, which are commonly associated with liver failure.

C-reactive protein

Elevated CSF levels of CRP have been useful in the diagnosis of bacterial meningitis. Failure to find elevated CSF levels of CRP appears to be strong evidence against bacterial meningitis.

Contraindications

- Patients with increased ICP. The LP may induce cerebral or cerebellar herniation through the foramen magnum.
- Patients who are anticoagulated due to the risk of epidural hematoma.
- Patients who have severe degenerative vertebral joint disease.
- Patients with infection near the LP site. Meningitis can result.

Potential complications

- Persistent CSF leak, causing severe postural headache
- Puncture of subcutaneous blood vessel during the procedure
- Introduction of bacteria causing meningitis
- Herniation of the brain
- Inadvertent puncture of the spinal cord
- Puncture of the aorta or vena cava
- Transient back pain and pain or paresthesia in the legs

Procedure and patient care

Before

- PT Explain the procedure to the patient.
- Obtain informed consent if required by the institution.
- Perform a baseline neurologic assessment of the legs.
- PT Tell the patient that no fasting or sedation is required.
- PT Instruct the patient to empty the bladder and bowels.
- PT Explain to the patient that he or she must lie very still throughout this procedure. Movement may cause injury.

During

- Note the following procedural steps:
  1. This study can be easily performed at the bedside. The patient is usually placed in the lateral decubitus (fetal) position (Figure L3).

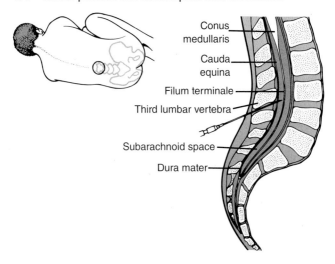

FIG. L3 Patient position for lumbar puncture.

2. The patient is instructed to clasp the hands on the knees to maintain this position. (A sitting position also may be used.)
3. A local anesthetic is injected into the skin and subcutaneous tissues after the site has been aseptically cleaned.
4. A spinal needle containing an inner obturator is placed through the skin and into the spinal canal.
5. The subarachnoid space is entered.
6. The insert (obturator) is removed, and CSF can be seen slowly dripping from the needle.
7. The needle is attached to a sterile manometer, and the pressure (opening pressure) is recorded.
8. Before the pressure reading is taken, the patient is asked to straighten the legs to reduce intraabdominal pressure.
9. Three sterile test tubes are filled with 5 to 10 mL of CSF.
10. The pressure (closing pressure) is measured.

• Note that if blockage in CSF circulation in the spinal subarachnoid space is suspected, a *Queckenstedt-Stookey* test may be performed. For this test, the jugular vein is occluded either manually by digital pressure or by a medium-sized blood pressure cuff inflated to approximately 20 mm Hg. Within 10 seconds after jugular occlusion, CSF pressure should increase from 15 to 40 cm H_2O and then promptly return to normal within 10 seconds after release of the pressure. A sluggish rise or fall of CSF pressure suggests partial blockage of CSF circulation. No rise after 10 seconds suggests a complete obstruction within the spinal canal.

- Note that this procedure is performed by a physician in approximately 20 minutes.
- PT Inform the patient that this procedure is described as uncomfortable or painful by most patients.

After

- Apply digital pressure and a dressing to the puncture site.
- Place the patient in the prone position with a pillow under the abdomen to increase the intraabdominal pressure, which will indirectly increase the pressure in the tissues surrounding the spinal cord. This retards continued CSF flow from the spinal canal.
- PT Encourage the patient to drink increased amounts of fluid with a straw to replace the CSF removed during LP.
- PT Usually keep the patient in a reclining position for 1 hour or up to several hours to avoid the discomfort of potential postpuncture spinal headache. Instruct the patient to turn from side to side as long as the head is not raised.
- Label and number the specimen jars appropriately and deliver them immediately to the laboratory after the test.
- PT Instruct the patient to report numbness, tingling, and movement of the extremities; pain at the injection site; drainage of blood or CSF at the injection site; and the inability to void.

Abnormal findings

Acute demyelinating polyneuropathy
Autoimmune disorder
Brain neoplasm
Cerebral abscess
Cerebral hemorrhage
Coma
Degenerative cord or brain disease
Encephalitis
Hepatic encephalopathy

Meningitis
Metastatic tumor
Multiple sclerosis
Myelitis
Neurosyphilis
Reye syndrome
Spinal cord neoplasm
Subarachnoid bleeding
Tumor
Viral or tubercular meningitis

notes

lung biopsy

Type of test Microscopic examination of tissue

Normal findings

No evidence of pathology

Test explanation and related physiology

This invasive procedure is used to obtain a specimen of pulmonary tissue for a histologic examination by using either an open or a closed technique. The *open method* involves a limited thoracotomy. The *closed technique* includes methods such as transbronchial lung biopsy, transbronchial needle aspiration biopsy, transcatheter bronchial brushing, percutaneous needle biopsy, and video-assisted thoracotomy.

Lung biopsy is indicated to determine the pathology of pulmonary parenchymal disease. Carcinomas, granulomas, infections, and sarcoidosis can be diagnosed. The procedure is also useful in detecting environmental exposures, infections, and familial disease.

Contraindications

- Patients with bullae or cysts of the lung
- Patients with suspected vascular anomalies of the lung
- Patients with bleeding abnormalities
- Patients with pulmonary hypertension
- Patients with respiratory insufficiency

Potential complications

- Pneumothorax
- Pulmonary hemorrhage
- Empyema

Procedure and patient care

Before

PT Explain the procedure to the patient.
- Ensure that informed and signed consent is obtained.
PT Instruct the patient about fasting. The patient may be kept NPO after midnight on the day of the test.
PT Instruct the patient to remain still during the lung biopsy.

During

- Note that the patient's position depends on the method used and that the specimen may be obtained by several methods.

Transbronchial lung biopsy
- This technique is performed via flexible fiberoptic bronchoscopy by using cutting forceps.
- Fluoroscopy is used to ensure proper opening and positioning of the forceps on the lesions.
- Fluoroscopy also permits visualization of the tug of the lung as the specimen is removed.

Transbronchial needle aspiration
- The needle is inserted through the bronchoscope and into the tumor or desired area, where aspiration is performed with the attached syringe (Figure L4).
- The needle is retracted within its sheath, and the entire catheter is withdrawn from the fiberoptic scope.

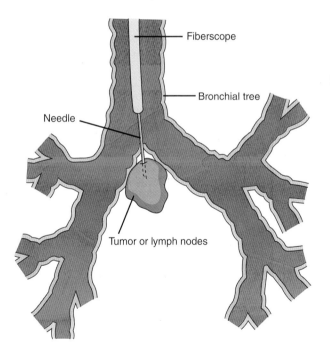

FIG. L4 Transbronchial needle biopsy. The diagram shows a transbronchial needle penetrating the bronchial wall and entering a mass of subcarinal lymph nodes or tumor.

Transbronchial brushing
- A small brush is moved back and forth over the suspicious area in the bronchus or its branches.
- The cells adhere to the brush, which is then removed and used to make microscopic slides.

Percutaneous needle biopsy
- In this method, the biopsy is obtained after using fluoroscopic radiography, ultrasound, or CT scan.
- The procedure is carried out by using a cutting needle or by aspiration with a spinal-type needle.

Open lung biopsy
- The patient is taken to the operating room, and general anesthesia is provided.
- An incision is made into the chest wall.
- After a piece of lung tissue is removed, the lung is sutured.
- Chest tube drainage is used for approximately 24 hours.

Thoracoscopic lung biopsy
- The lung is collapsed with a double-lumen endotracheal tube placed during induction of general anesthesia.
- With the use of a thoracoscope, the lung is grasped, and a piece is cut off with the use of a cutting or stapling device.
- The scope and trocars are removed, and a small chest tube is left in place. The tiny incisions are closed.

- Note that this procedure is performed by a surgeon, radiologist, or pulmonologist in 30 to 60 minutes.
- During the lung biopsy procedure, assess the patient carefully for signs of respiratory distress.

PT Tell patients that most describe this procedure as painful.

After
- Place biopsy specimens in appropriate containers for histologic and microbiologic examination.
- Observe the vital signs frequently for signs of bleeding.
- Obtain a chest x-ray image to check for complications.
- Observe the patient for signs of pneumothorax (e.g., dyspnea, tachypnea, decrease in breath sounds, anxiety, restlessness).

Abnormal findings

Carcinoma
Exposure lung diseases (e.g., black lung, asbestosis)
Granuloma
Infection
Sarcoidosis

notes

lung scan (Ventilation/perfusion scanning [VPS], Pulmonary scintiphotography, V/Q scan)

Type of test Nuclear scan

Normal findings

Diffuse and homogeneous uptake of nuclear material by the lungs

Test explanation and related physiology

This nuclear medicine procedure is used to identify defects in blood *perfusion* of the lung in patients with suspected pulmonary embolism. A homogeneous uptake of particles that fills the entire pulmonary vasculature conclusively rules out pulmonary embolism. If a defect in an otherwise smooth and diffusely homogeneous pattern is seen, a perfusion abnormality exists. This can indicate pulmonary embolism.

The chest x-ray image aids in assessing the perfusion scan because a defect on the perfusion scan seen in the same area as an abnormality on the chest x-ray image does not indicate pulmonary embolism. Rather, the defect may represent pneumonia, atelectasis, effusion, and so on. However, when a perfusion defect occurs in an area of the lung that is normal on a chest x-ray study, pulmonary embolus is likely.

Specificity of a perfusion scan also can be enhanced by performance of a ventilation scan, which detects parenchymal abnormalities in ventilation (e.g., pneumonia, pleural fluid, emphysematous bullae). The *ventilation scan* reflects the patency of the pulmonary airways by using xenon gas or Tc-diethylenetriamine pentaacetic acid (DTPA) as an aerosol. When vascular obstruction (embolism) is present by perfusion scan, ventilation scans demonstrate a normal wash-in and wash-out of radioactivity from the embolized lung area. If parenchymal disease (e.g., pneumonia) is responsible for the perfusion abnormality, however, wash-in or wash-out will be abnormal. Therefore whereas the mismatch of perfusion and ventilation findings is characteristic of embolic disorders, the match is indicative of parenchymal disease. When ventilation and perfusion scans are performed synchronously, this is called a *ventilation/perfusion ($\dot{V}/\dot{Q}$) scan*.

Contraindications

- Patients who are pregnant unless the benefits outweigh the risks

Interfering factors

PT Pulmonary parenchymal problems (e.g., pneumonia, emphysema, pleural effusion, tumors) will give the picture of a perfusion defect and simulate pulmonary embolism.

Procedure and patient care

Before

PT Explain the procedure to the patient. See p. xviii for radiation exposure and risks.

• Obtain informed consent if required by the institution.

PT Assure the patient that he or she will not be exposed to large amounts of radioactivity because only tracer doses are used.

PT Tell the patient that no fasting or sedation is required.

During

• Note the following procedural steps for a V/Q scan:
   1. The patient is taken to the nuclear medicine department.

Ventilation scan
   2. The patient breathes the tracer through a face mask.
   3. Ventilation scans require a cooperative patient.
   4. Technetium-diethylenetriaminepentaacetic acid images are usually done before perfusion images and require patient cooperation with deep breathing.

Perfusion scan
   5. The patient is given a peripheral IV injection of radionuclide-tagged macroaggregated albumin (MAA).
   6. While the patient lies in the appropriate position, a gamma ray detector records radionuclide uptake.
   7. The patient is placed in the supine, prone, and various lateral positions, which allow for anterior, posterior, lateral, and oblique views, respectively.
   8. The results are interpreted by a nuclear medicine physician.

• Note that this test is usually performed by a technologist in approximately 30 minutes.

PT Tell the patient that no discomfort is associated with this test other than the peripheral venipuncture.

After

PT Tell the patient that no radiation precautions are needed.

Abnormal findings

Asthma
Atelectasis
Bronchitis
Chronic obstructive pulmonary
   disease

Emphysema
Pneumonia
Pulmonary embolism
Tuberculosis
Tumor

notes

luteinizing hormone (LH assay, Lutropin) and follicle-stimulating hormone (FSH) assay

Type of test Blood
Normal findings

	LH (IU/L)	FSH (IU/L)
Adult		
Male	1.24–7.8	1.42–15.4
Female		
Follicular phase	1.68–15	1.37–9.9
Ovulatory peak	21.9–56.6	6.17–17.2
Luteal phase	0.61–16.3	1.09–9.2
Postmenopause	14.2–52.3	19.3–100.6
Child		
(age 1–10 years)		
Male	0.04–3.6	0.3–4.6
Female	0.03–3.9	0.68–6.7

(Values may vary, depending on laboratory method.)

Test explanation and related physiology

LH and FSH are glycoproteins that are produced in the anterior pituitary gland. These two hormones then act on the ovary or testes. Spot urine tests for LH have become useful in the evaluation and treatment of infertility. Because LH is rapidly excreted into the urine, the plasma LH surge that precedes ovulation by 24 hours can be recognized quickly and easily. This is used to indicate the period when a woman is the most fertile. The best time to obtain a urine specimen is between 11 AM and 3 PM. Usually, the woman begins to test her urine on the 10th day after the onset of her menses and continues to do so daily. Home kits in which a color change as an endpoint are used to make this process more convenient.

An LH surge in blood levels indicates that ovulation has taken place. Daily samples of serum LH around the woman's midcycle can detect the LH surge, which is believed to occur on the day of maximal fertility.

A more accurate method to evaluate ovarian function is by ovarian reserve testing (see p. 537).

Interfering factors

- Patients with hCG-producing tumors and hypothyroid patients may have falsely high LH levels.

Procedure and patient care

- See inside front cover for Routine Blood Testing.
- Fasting: no
- Blood tube commonly used: red
- Note that the patient may also perform LH assays at home using a home urine test or a 24-hour urine test.

Abnormal findings

▲ **Increased levels**

Anorchia

Castration

Complete testicular
  feminization syndrome

Hypogonadism

Menopause

Ovarian dysgenesis (Turner
  syndrome)

Pituitary adenoma

Polycystic ovaries

Precocious puberty

Testicular dysgenesis
  (Klinefelter syndrome)

▼ **Decreased levels**

Anorexia nervosa

Hypothalamic failure

Malnutrition

Pituitary failure

Stress

notes

lyme disease test

Type of test Blood

Normal findings

Borrelia burgdorferi antibody Enzyme Immunoassay (Lyme index value)

    < 0.9 = negative
    0.91–1.09 = equivocal
    > 1.1 = positive

Western blot

$\geq$ 5 different IgG antibodies reactive = positive
$\geq$ 2 different IgM antibodies reactive = positive
PCR: negative
CSF: negative

Test explanation and related physiology

Lyme disease is a bacterial infection caused by a spirochete called *B. burgdorferi*. This is the most common tickborne disease. The spirochete is spread by a bite from a black-legged tick *(Ixodes pacificus)* or deer tick *(Ixodes scapularis)*. These ticks normally dwell on animals, such as deer, horses, chipmunks, and squirrels, that are found in wooded areas.

Screening serologic studies are performed for the detection of Lyme disease. ELISA is the best diagnostic test for Lyme disease antibodies. This test determines titers of specific IgM and specific IgG antibodies to the *B. burgdorferi* spirochete. Levels of specific IgM antibody peak during the third to sixth week after disease onset and then gradually decline. Titers of specific IgG antibodies are generally low during the first several weeks of illness, reach maximal levels in 4 to 6 months, and often remain elevated for years.

Acute and convalescent sera can be tested to verify the diagnosis with a significant rise in positive antibody titers. Positive or equivocal ELISA screening test results should not be interpreted as truly positive until verified with a confirmatory Western blot assay. The Western blot antibody assay can identify specifically the IgG or the IgM antibody. However, the screening test or Western blot for *B. burgdorferi* antibodies may be falsely negative in early stages of Lyme disease, including the period when cry thema migrans rash is apparent. Also, it is important to note that the compromised immune state of patients with chronic Lyme disease interferes with production of these antibodies.

Interfering factors

- Previous infection with *B. burgdorferi* can cause positive sero-logic testing results.
- Other spirochete diseases (syphilis or leptospirosis) can cause false-positive results.

Procedure and patient care

- See inside front cover for Routine Blood Testing.
- Fasting: no
- Blood tube commonly used: red

Abnormal findings

Lyme disease

notes

magnesium

Type of test Blood

Normal findings

Total Magnesium
Adult: 1.3–2.1 mEq/L or 0.65–1.05 mmol/L (SI units)
Child: 1.4–1.7 mEq/L
Newborn: 1.4–2 mEq/L

Possible critical values (Total Magnesium)

< 0.5 mEq/L or > 3 mEq/L
Ionized Magnesium: 1.5–2.5 mg/dl or 0.4–0.6 mmol/L
Urine: 12–199 mg/24hrs

Test explanation and related physiology

Most organ functions depend on magnesium. It is especially important to monitor magnesium levels in cardiac patients. Low magnesium may increase cardiac irritability and aggravate cardiac arrhythmias. Hypermagnesemia retards neuromuscular conduction and is demonstrated as cardiac conduction slowing.

Magnesium deficiency occurs in patients who are malnourished. Increased magnesium levels most commonly are associated with ingestion of magnesium-containing antacids. Because most of the serum magnesium is reabsorbed by the kidneys, chronic renal diseases cause decreased magnesium levels.

Interfering factors

• Hemolysis should be avoided when collecting this specimen.

Procedure and patient care

• See inside front cover for Routine Blood Testing.
• Fasting: no
• Blood tube commonly used: red

Abnormal findings

▲ **Increased levels**
Addison disease
Hypothyroidism
Ingestion of magnesium-
   containing antacids or salts
Renal insufficiency
Uncontrolled diabetes

▼ **Decreased levels**
Alcoholism
Chronic renal disease
Diabetic acidosis
Hypoparathyroidism
Malabsorption
Malnutrition

M

notes

magnetic resonance imaging (MRI, Nuclear magnetic resonance imaging [NMRI])

Type of test Magnetic field study

Normal findings

No evidence of pathology

Test explanation and related physiology

MRI is a noninvasive diagnostic scanning technique that provides valuable information about the body's anatomy by placing the patient in a magnetic field. MRI does not require exposure to ionizing radiation.

MRI is useful in the evaluation of the following areas:

- Head (brain and surrounding structures)
- Spine (including spinal cord and surrounding structures)
- Mediastinum (including heart and great vessels)
- Abdomen and pelvis (including liver, gallbladder, kidneys, pancreas, prostate)
- Breast
- Musculoskeletal (including joints, soft tissues, ligaments, and bones)

MRI of the brain and meninges is accurate in identifying benign and malignant neoplasms. It is also able to identify vascular pathology such as ischemic and hemorrhagic stroke, AVM, aneurysm, and venous thrombosis. It can identify infections such as abscess, cerebritis, encephalitis, meningitis, AIDS, and herpes. It identifies white matter diseases such as MS and other demyelinating disorders. It shows trauma such as epidural hematoma, contusion, and subdural hematoma. It also shows congenital malformations and hydrocephalus.

Magnetic resonance spectroscopy (MRS) is a diagnostic tool used to show metabolic changes that result from disease and to monitor the effect of therapy. Spectroscopy can identity infection, epilepsy, neurodegenerative disease (Alzheimer, Parkinson, Huntington), multiple sclerosis, hypoxia, acute stroke, and intracranial neoplasms.

MRI musculoskeletal (MSK) is an unsurpassed imaging technique for evaluating joint disorders, fractures, ligaments, tendons, cartilage, osteonecrosis, bone marrow disorders, bone and soft tissue tumors, inflammatory changes, edema, and avascular necrosis. MSK examinations include hip, knee, ankle, foot, shoulder, elbow, wrist, and long bones of the arms and legs.

MRI of the breast is more sensitive than mammography or ultrasonography. MRI of the breast is used for accurate localized staging of breast cancer. Increasingly, abbreviated breast MRI protocols are being used for screening breast examinations, especially in high risk women. MRI of the breast is helpful for preoperative surgical staging and for the identification of postoperative positive margins. This study is particularly helpful in differentiating postoperative scar tissue from breast cancer recurrence. MRI of the breast is the most accurate method of determining abnormalities (such as rupture) of a breast implant. With the addition of a needle-guiding system to the MRI, breast tumors can be nonoperatively and accurately localized and biopsied.

Significant improvement in *MRI of the heart* and great vessels has moved this procedure into the mainstream of clinical cardiology. Cardiac MRI is considered the procedure of choice in the evaluation of pericardial disease and intracardiac and pericardiac masses, for imaging the right and left ventricles and pulmonary vessels, and for assessing many forms of congenital heart disease, especially after corrective surgery. The ventricle size, shape, and blood volumes can be evaluated. Cardiac valvular abnormalities, cardiac septal defects, and suspected intracardiac or pericardiac masses or thrombi can be identified. Pericardial disease (e.g., pericarditis or effusion) is easily identified. Ventricular muscle changes from ischemia or infarction can be determined. Finally, advanced MRI techniques are able to evaluate the coronary vessels directly.

Phase-contrast magnetic resonance imaging (PC-MRI) of the heart quantifies velocity and blood flow in the great arteries. Information obtained includes cardiac outputs of the left and right ventricles, regurgitant volumes and fraction of the aortic and pulmonary valves, and shunt ratio. Stress cardiac MRI can be performed using nitrates, dobutamine, and adenosine.

MRI of the abdomen is used to evaluate the liver, kidneys, spleen, pancreas, gallbladder, adrenal glands, bowel, and aorta. MRI of the pelvis is used for evaluation of bone, soft tissue, bladder, ovaries, uterus, ureters, rectum, fetus in utero, and the prostate gland. *MRI of the liver* has improved significantly with the use of a gadolinium-like contrast agent called gadoxetate. Imaging with this agent provides extremely sharp imaging that can identify liver and biliary tumors smaller than 1 cm.

Magnetic resonance cholangiopancreatography (MRCP) allows noninvasive imaging of the liver, bile ducts, gallbladder, pancreas, and pancreatic duct. It is used to:

M

- Identify tumors, stones, inflammation, or infection.
- Evaluate the cause of pancreatitis.
- Help in the diagnosis of unexplained abdominal pain.
- Provide a less invasive alternative to endoscopic retrograde cholangiopancreatography (ERCP).

Magnetic resonance enterography (MRE) is used to evaluate the small bowel in patients with inflammatory bowel disease. It is also helpful in determining extraluminal bowel pathology.

Magnetic resonance imaging of the prostate gland is helpful in identifying and staging prostate cancer. This imaging is not only anatomical but can also discriminate cancer cells from normal cells through the use of *dynamic contrast-enhanced MRI (DCE-MRI)*. The MRI of the prostate can be used to indicate the need for a prostate biopsy, locate suspicious areas for biopsy, delineate the extent and aggressiveness of cancer, and identify recurrent cancer.

MRI of the spine is the most sensitive imaging test for evaluating the spine. *MRI of the cervical or lumbar spine* is commonly used to determine the cause of neck or back pain, respectively. Enhancement with gadolinium helps distinguish between new infection or inflammation and scarring in patients with prior back surgery.

MRI can detect or assess the following:
- Spine anatomy and alignment
- Birth defects in vertebrae or spinal canal
- Trauma to bones, discs, ligaments, or spinal cord
- Disc or joint disease
- Compression fractures
- Inflammation of vertebrae, disc, spinal cord, or nerve roots
- Tumors or infection in the spinal cord or surrounding soft tissue

Using different MRI protocols, an *MRI myelogram* can be performed. Herniated discs are easily seen and graded as to their compression on the nerves. The *upright MRI* can scan patients in their positions of symptoms (e.g., pain or numbness) including weight-bearing positions such as sitting, standing, or bending. The upright MRI can provide diagnostic images of the cervical spine, the lumbar spine, and the joints over their full range of motion (e.g., cervical flexion/extension). The front-open and top-open design of the upright MRI system nearly eliminates possible claustrophobia and accommodates larger patients.

Magnetic resonance venography (MRV) provides images for the diagnosis of venous abnormalities. It can be used to diagnose deep vein thrombosis and is a good alternative to the more invasive contrast venography (p. 793) and ultrasound venous duplex scan (p. 762). MRV is also used in the diagnosis of cerebral venous thrombosis by demonstrating absence of flow in the cerebral venous sinuses.

Magnetic resonance angiography (MRA) is a noninvasive procedure for viewing possible blockages in arteries. MRA has been useful in evaluation of the cervical carotid artery and large-caliber intracranial arterial and venous structures. Cardiac abnormalities, aortic aneurysm, and anatomic variants can be identified. This procedure also has proved useful in the noninvasive detection of intracranial aneurysms and vascular malformations, especially in renal artery stenosis.

Potential complications

• Gadolinium-based contrast agents have been linked to the development of nephrogenic systemic fibrosis (NSF) or nephrogenic fibrosing dermopathy (NFD). A creatinine, blood urea nitrogen, and/or estimated glomerular filtration rate may be obtained, especially on adults older than the age of 60 years.

Contraindications

• Patients who are extremely obese (usually > 300 lb)
• Patients who are confused or agitated
• Patients who require continuous life-support equipment because most monitoring equipment cannot be used inside the scanner room. Magnet-adaptive equipment is only available at some locations.
• Patients with implantable metal objects (e.g., pacemakers, infusion pumps, aneurysm clips, inner ear implants, and metal fragments in one or both eyes) because the magnet may move the object in the body and injure the patient.

Interfering factors

• Movement during the scan may cause artifacts on MRI images.
• Metals, implants, piercings, braces, permanent retainers may cause artifacts in the images.

Procedure and patient care

Before

PT Explain the procedure to the patient.
PT Inform the patient that there is no exposure to radiation.
• Obtain informed consent if required by the institution.
PT Tell parents of young patients that they may need to change into a patient gown or scrubs for the MRI Exam. They may

read or talk to a child in the scanning room during the procedure. There is no risk of radiation from the procedure.

PT If available, show the patient a picture of the scanning machine and encourage verbalization of anxieties. Some patients may experience claustrophobia. If possible, an open MRI system can be used for these patients.

PT Instruct the patient to remove all metal objects. The magnetic field can damage watches, cellphones, and credit cards.

PT Tell the patient to remove any transdermal medication patches (such as nicotine). Some patches have an aluminum or foil backing that can cause tissue burns.

PT Tell the patient that during the procedure he or she may hear a knocking sound. Earplugs are used.

PT Inform the patient that fluid and food restrictions may be required before MRI.

PT For comfort, instruct the patient to empty the bladder before the test.

During

- Note the following:
  1. The patient usually lies on a platform that slides into a tube containing the cylinder-shaped tubular magnet. However, patients can be scanned in sitting, standing, or bending positions with an upright MRI.
  2. For cardiac MRI, electrocardiography leads are applied.
  3. The patient is instructed to remain very still during the procedure. The patient may be asked to perform short breath-holds during the exam.
  4. During the scan, the patient can talk to and hear the staff via microphone or earphones placed in the scanner.
  5. Gadolinium-based contrast agents for MRI examinations are administered if clinical findings are indicated and ordered by a physician or radiologist.
- Note that a qualified radiologic technologist performs this procedure in approximately 30 minutes.

PT Tell the patient that the only discomfort associated with this procedure may be lying still on a hard surface and a possible tingling sensation in teeth containing metal fillings. An injection may be needed for administration of the contrast medium.

After

PT Inform the patient to drink plenty of water post examination if they received contrast.

Abnormal findings

Brain

Aneurysm
Arteriovenous malformation
Atrophy of the brain
Cerebral tumor
Cerebrovascular accident
Hemorrhage
Multiple sclerosis
Subdural hematoma

Heart

Cardiac or pericardial masses
Congenital heart defects (e.g., septal defects)
Diseases of the great vessels
Intracardiac thrombus
Myocardial ischemia or infarction
Pericarditis or effusion
Valvular disease
Ventricular dilation, dysfunction, or hypertrophy

Other

Abscess
Bone destructive lesion
Degenerative vertebral discs
Edema
Joint disorder
Kidney stones or gallstones
Tumor (primary or metastatic)

M

notes

malaria testing

Type of test Blood

Normal findings

No parasites noted on blood smear; negative rapid antigen test

Possible critical values

Blood smear parasitemia $\geq 5\%$

Test explanation and related physiology

Malaria is a disease caused by parasites endemic throughout most of the tropics. *Plasmodium falciparum* causes most disease, followed by *Plasmodium vivax. Plasmodium malariae* and *Plasmodium ovale* are less common. Malaria is transmitted via the bite of an infected female *Anopheles* mosquito. The initial symptoms of malaria are nonspecific and vary with parasite species, epidemiology, immunity, and age. Forms of diagnosis include light microscopy (blood smear), rapid diagnostic tests (RDTs), and molecular techniques.

Blood smear examination via light microscopy is the standard for diagnosing malaria. If malaria is suspected and the initial smear is negative, additional smears should be prepared and examined over the next 2–3 days.

RDTs for detection of malaria parasite antigens should be used if microscopy is not readily available. They give results rapidly (<1 hour), require no electricity or laboratory technology, and can be performed by health workers with limited training.

Molecular techniques for detection of genetic material are limited to research settings. Nucleic acid tests (by polymerase chain reaction) are used to study antimalarial drugs, vaccines, and other diagnostic agents.

Procedure and patient care

- See inside front cover for Routine Blood Testing
- Fasting: no
- Collect a drop of blood from a fingerstick or collect venipuncture blood in the appropriate test tube. Check with lab.
- For microscopy, apply blood to a glass microscopy slide.
- For RDTs, place blood on a test strip.
- PT Smears should be prepared as soon as possible after blood collection.

Abnormal findings

Malaria

notes

mammography (Mammogram)

Type of test X-ray

Normal findings

Category 1: Negative
Category 2: Benign findings noted
Category 3: Probably benign; short-term follow-up is suggested
Category 4: Suspicious findings; further evaluation is indicated
Category 5: Cancer is highly suspected
Category 6: Known breast cancer
Category 0: Abnormality noted. More imaging is needed

Test explanation and related physiology

Mammography can identify cancers of the breast. In many cases, breast cancers can be detected before they become palpable.

Mammography also can detect other diseases of the breast such as acute suppurative mastitis, abscess, fibrocystic changes, cysts, benign tumors (e.g., fibroadenoma), and intraglandular lymph nodes.

Mammograms can be more thoroughly evaluated with magnified views, deeper views, or tomo-mammography

Mammography can also be used to locate a mammographically identified (i.e., not palpable) lesion for biopsy. Nonsurgical needle biopsy with a *stereotactic biopsy* device is directed by mammography.

Breast tomosynthesis (3D mammography) increases sensitivity of the test. MRI of the breast (p. 491) is more sensitive than mammography, but is less specific.

The frequency and ages of asymptomatic women that benefit most from screening mammography is debated although most professional organizations are recommending testing annually after the age of 40.

Breast tissue density is also evaluated by mammography. Dense breast tissue diminishes the accuracy of mammography while, at the same time, women with dense breasts are at a increased risk for breast cancer.

Contraindications

- Patients who are pregnant unless benefits outweigh risks
- Women younger than age 25 years

Interfering factors

- Talc powder and deodorant can imply calcification.

- Jewelry worn around the neck can preclude total visualization.
- Breast augmentation implants prevent total visualization of the breast. However, implants can be displaced so the native breast tissue can be imaged.
- Previous breast surgery can alter or distort the findings.

Procedure and patient care

Before

PT Explain the procedure to the patient. See p. xviii for radiation exposure and risks.

PT Inform the patient that some discomfort may be experienced during breast compression. Premenopausal women with very sensitive breasts may choose to schedule their mammogram 1 to 2 weeks after their menses.

PT Tell the patient that no fasting is required.

PT Explain that a minimal radiation dose will be used.

PT Instruct the patient to disrobe above the waist and put on an x-ray gown.

- Markers will be placed on any skin bump that may be interpreted as an abnormality on the x-ray image.

During

- Images of the breasts are obtained individually in the craniocaudal and medial-lateral oblique views. Direct lateral, spot compressed, and magnification views may also be performed.
- Note that mammography is performed by a radiologic technologist in approximately 10 minutes. The x-ray images are interpreted by a radiologist.

After

PT No aftercare is needed.

Abnormal findings

Benign tumor (e.g., fibroadenoma)
Breast abscess
Breast cancer
Breast cyst
Fibrocystic changes
Suppurative mastitis

notes

marijuana (THC) test (Cannabinoid or cannabis testing, Tetrahydrocannabinol [THC] testing)

Type of test Blood or saliva

Normal findings

No THC metabolites detected

Test explanation and related physiology

Marijuana contains many chemical compounds, called *cannabinoids*, that interact with the body. The main mind-altering cannabinoid in marijuana is THC (delta-9-tetrahydrocannabinol). The body breaks THC down into several inactive metabolites (e.g., THC-COOH, 11-nor-carboxy-delta-9-tetrahydrocannabinol). Because the metabolites of THC stay in the body for a longer period of time than THC does, *substance abuse testing* (p. 693) detects the presence of THC-COOH or other metabolites in urine.

Anything that contains THC has the potential to be detected as THC or THC-COOH in a marijuana test. Because of the accuracy and validity inherent in blood and saliva testing, this test is considered more accurate than screening the urine for cannabis metabolites. Advantages of saliva testing are that it can be done anytime, saliva is immediately available, and it can be done in front of the person collecting the specimen. This makes saliva tests difficult to falsify.

This test is used if an individual:
- Is being treated in an addiction recovery or chemical dependency program
- Is being treated for chronic pain, to ensure that the person is taking medication as prescribed
- Is involved in an accident that an emergency room physician suspects may be due to drug intoxication
- Is suspected of drug abuse or is known to use illegal drugs
- Is pregnant or has recently given birth, especially if the patient is thought to be at risk for drug abuse or has a newborn baby exhibiting certain characteristic behaviors
- Is an applicant for a life insurance policy, as this is part of an overall health evaluation
- Is being evaluated through employment drug testing

Drug testing for legal, forensic, or employment purposes requires a strictly controlled sample collection with the custody of a sample continuously documented to maintain a legal "chain of custody."

M

Detection times for marijuana vary widely depending on an individual's metabolism, the dose, and frequency of use. Testing can indicate use anywhere from 3 days to more than 30 days prior to testing. Heavy users of marijuana may test positive for even longer than 30 days after last use.

Procedure and patient care

Before

- Be sure that the patient is aware of all of his or her legal rights regarding testing.

During

- See inside front cover for Routine Blood Testing.
- Fasting: No
- Blood tube commonly used: Red, grey, green, or lavender
- For saliva testing, a small swab is placed in the mouth. When soaked, it is placed into a device for analysis.

After

- Ensure the "chain of custody" is maintained throughout the sample handling process.

Abnormal findings

THC use

notes

maternal screen testing (Maternal triple screen, Maternal quadruple screen)

Type of test Blood or urine

Normal findings

Low probability of fetal defects

Test explanation and related physiology

These tests are provided to pregnant women early in pregnancy to identify potential birth defects or serious chromosomal or genetic abnormalities. These screening tests may indicate the potential for the presence of fetal defects (particularly trisomy 21 [Down syndrome] or trisomy 18). They may also indicate increased risk for neural tube defects (e.g., myelomeningocele, spina bifida) or abdominal wall defects (omphalocele or gastroschisis).

Maternal screening is routinely offered to all pregnant women, usually in their second trimester of pregnancy. If the screening test results are positive, more accurate definitive testing such as blood tests, chorionic villus sampling (p. 202), or amniocentesis (p. 39) is recommended.

There are several variations of this test available. See Table M1.

The maternal triple screen test offers a 50% to 80% chance of detecting pregnancies with trisomy 21. The quadruple screen is now routinely recommended and is combined with fetal nuchal translucency (FTN). These tests are most accurately performed during the second trimester of pregnancy, more specifically between the 14th and 24th weeks (ideal 16th and 18th weeks).

M

TABLE M1   Maternal screening tests

Test name	Timing	Tests commonly performed
Double test	15–20 weeks	hCG, AFP
Triple test	15–20 weeks	hCG, AFP, estriol
Quadruple test	15–20 weeks	AFP, estriol, hCG, inhibin A
Combined test	12 weeks	Nuchal translucency, PAPP-A, hCG
Integrated test	12 and 20 weeks	Nuchal translucency, PAPP-A (12 weeks), AFP, estriol, hCG, inhibin A (20 weeks)

First trimester screening for genetic defects is an option for pregnant women. This testing would include fetal nuchal translucency combined with the beta subunit of hCG, and PAPP-A. A low level of PAPP-A may indicate an increased risk for having a stillborn baby.

With trisomy 21, second trimester absolute maternal serum levels of AFP and unconjugated estriol are about 25% lower than normal levels, and maternal serum hCG is approximately two times higher than the normal hCG level. The results of the screening are expressed in *multiples of median (MoM)*. AFP and urinary estriol (E_3) values during pregnancies with trisomy 21 are lower than those associated with normal pregnancies, which means that values lower than the mean are lower than 1 MoM. The hCG value for trisomy 21 is higher than 1 MoM. The MoM, fetal age, and maternal weight are used to calculate the possible risk for chromosomal abnormalities. All of the previously named maternal screening tests are discussed elsewhere in this book. For the sake of thoroughness, inhibin A is discussed here.

Inhibin A levels in maternal serum remain relatively constant through the 15th to 18th week of pregnancy. Inhibin A is important in the control of fetal development. Maternal serum levels of inhibin A are twice as high in pregnancies affected by trisomy 21 as in unaffected pregnancies. Inhibin A concentrations are significantly lower in women with normal pregnancies than in women with pregnancies that result in spontaneous abortions.

Procedure and patient care

Before
PT Explain the procedure to the patient.
• Allow the patient to express her concerns and fears.

During
• Most of these tests can be done with a venous blood sample in a red-top tube. The hCG and estriol can also be tested by collecting a urine sample.

After
PT Provide the results during a personal consultation.
PT Assist the patient in scheduling and obtaining more accurate diagnostic testing if the results are positive.

Abnormal findings
Positive screening tests (trisomy 21, trisomy 18, neural tube defects, abdominal wall defects)

Meckel diverticulum nuclear scan

Type of test Nuclear medicine

Normal findings

No increased uptake of radionuclide in the right lower quadrant of the abdomen

Test explanation and related physiology

Meckel diverticulum usually occurs in the ileum approximately 2 feet proximal to the ileocecal valve. Approximately 20% to 25% of Meckel diverticulum is lined internally by ectopic gastric mucosa. This gastric mucosa can secrete acid and cause ulceration of the intestinal mucosa nearby. Bleeding, inflammation, and intussusception are other potential complications of this congenital abnormality.

Both normal gastric mucosa within the stomach and ectopic gastric mucosa in Meckel diverticulum concentrate ^{99m}Tc pertechnetate. Therefore, one can expect to see a hot spot in the right lower quadrant of the abdomen at about the same time as the normal stomach mucosa. This is a very sensitive and specific test for this congenital abnormality.

Procedure and patient care

Before

- PT Explain the procedure to the patient. See p. xviii for radiation exposure and risks.
- PT Advise the patient to refrain from eating or drinking anything for 6 to 12 hours before the examination.
- A histamine H_2-receptor antagonist is usually given for 1 to 2 days before the scan. This blocks secretion of the radionuclide from the ectopic gastric mucosa and improves visualization of Meckel diverticulum.

During

- The patient lies in a supine position, and a large-view nuclear detector camera is placed over the patient's abdomen to identify nuclear material after intravenous injection.
- Images are taken at 5-minute intervals for 1 hour.
- Patients may be asked to lie on the left side to minimize the excretion of the radionuclide from the normal stomach, flooding the intestine with radionuclide and precluding visualization of Meckel diverticulum.

M

- Occasionally glucagon is provided to prolong intestinal transit time and avoid downstream contamination with the radionuclide.
- Occasionally gastrin is given to increase the uptake of the radionuclide by the ectopic gastric mucosa.
- There is no pain associated with this test.

After

- The patient is asked to void, and a repeat image is obtained. This is to ensure that Meckel diverticulum has not been hidden by a distended bladder.
- **PT** Because only tracer doses of radioisotopes are used, inform the patient that no precautions need to be taken by others against radiation.

Abnormal findings

Meckel diverticula

notes

mediastinoscopy

Type of test Endoscopy

Normal findings

No abnormal mediastinal lymph node tissue

Test explanation and related physiology

Mediastinoscopy is a surgical procedure in which a rigid mediastinoscope (a lighted instrument scope) is inserted through a small incision made at the suprasternal notch. The scope is passed into the superior mediastinum to inspect the mediastinal lymph nodes and to remove biopsy specimens. Because these lymph nodes receive lymphatic drainage from the lungs, their assessment can provide information on intrathoracic diseases (e.g., carcinoma, granulomatous infections, and sarcoidosis). Tumors occurring in the mediastinum (e.g., thymoma or lymphoma) can also be biopsied through the mediastinoscope. With improved CT scan of the chest (p. 231), diagnostic mediastinoscopy is rarely used.

Potential complications

- Puncture of the esophagus, trachea, or blood vessels

Procedure and patient care

Before

PT Explain the procedure to the patient.
- Ensure that the physician has obtained the informed consent.
- Provide preoperative care as with any other surgical procedure.
- Keep the patient NPO (nothing by mouth) after midnight on the day of the test.

During

- After general anesthesia, an incision is made in the suprasternal notch.
- The mediastinoscope is passed through this incision and into the superior mediastinum.
- Abnormalities are biopsied.
- Note that this procedure is performed by a surgeon in approximately 1 hour.

PT Inform the patient that he or she is asleep during the procedure.

M

After

- Provide postoperative care as with any other surgical procedure.
- Assess the patient for mediastinal crepitus on auscultation, which may indicate mediastinal air from pneumothorax or the bronchus or esophagus.
- Assess the patient for cough or shortness of breath, which may indicate a pneumothorax.
- Observe the patient for hypotension and tachycardia, which may indicate bleeding from the biopsy site or the great vessels.
- Evaluate the patient for hoarseness, which may indicate injury to the recurrent laryngeal nerve.

Abnormal findings

Infection
Primary or metastatic tumor
Sarcoidosis
Thymoma
Tuberculosis

notes

metal testing (lead, arsenic, mercury)

Type of test Blood

Normal findings

< 10 mcg/dL for lead

Critical values for lead

Child (≤ 15 years): ≥ 20 mcg/dL
Adult (≥ 16 years): ≥ 70 mcg/dL

Test explanation and related physiology

Lead exposure, indicated by elevated blood lead levels, can result in permanent damage to most parts of the body. Children younger than 6 years of age are the most likely to be exposed and affected by lead. Blood lead levels are the best test for detecting and evaluating recent acute and chronic exposure. Blood lead samples are used to screen for exposure and to monitor the effectiveness of treatment.

Toxicity to heavy metals (e.g., *arsenic, mercury, cadmium, copper, cobalt*) and trace elements (e.g., *aluminum, chromium, antimony, bismuth, selenium, silver, zinc*) can also be tested. Suitable specimens for metal testing include blood, serum, urine, bones, teeth, tissue, or hair.

Procedure and patient care

- See inside front cover for Routine Blood Testing.
- Fasting: no
- Blood tube commonly used: verify with laboratory
- A finger stick can be performed to obtain 1 mL of blood.
- The blood sample is usually sent to a central diagnostic laboratory. The results are available in about 7 to 10 days.

Abnormal findings

▲ Increased levels

Exposure to lead, other heavy metals, and trace elements

notes

metanephrine, plasma free (Fractionated metanephrines)

Type of test Blood

Normal findings

Normetanephrine: < 0.5 nmol/L or 18–111 pg/mL by high-performance liquid chromatography (HPLC)

Metanephrine: < 0.9 nmol/L or 12–60 pg/mL by HPLC

Test explanation and related physiology

Pheochromocytomas are potentially lethal tumors. They produce several catecholamines that can cause episodic or persistent hypertension that is unresponsive to conventional treatment. This blood test measures the amount of metanephrine and normetanephrine, which are metabolites of epinephrine and norepinephrine, respectively.

If the concentrations of the free metanephrines are normal in the blood, then it is very unlikely that a patient has a pheochromocytoma. In about 80% of patients with pheochromocytoma, the magnitude of increase in plasma free metanephrines is so large that the tumor can be confirmed with close to 100% probability. Intermediate concentrations of normetanephrine and metanephrine are considered indeterminate. Urinary testing may clarify indeterminate findings.

Whenever the normetanephrine or metanephrine concentration exceeds the indeterminate range, the presence of pheochromocytoma is highly probable and should be located via imaging techniques. Pheochromocytoma suppression and provocative testing (p. 562) may assist in identifying this tumor.

Interfering factors

- Increased levels may be caused by caffeine or alcohol.
- Vigorous exercise, stress, and starvation may cause increases.

Procedure and patient care

- See inside front cover for Routine Blood Testing
- PT Explain if any dietary or medicinal restrictions.
- Fasting: yes
- Blood tube commonly used: chilled lavender-top or pink-top
- The patient may be asked to lie down and rest quietly for 15 to 30 minutes before sample collection.
- The blood sample may be collected while supine.

Abnormal findings
▲ **Increased levels**
   Pheochromocytoma

notes

M

methemoglobin (Hemoglobin M)

Type of test Blood

Normal findings

0.06–0.24 g/dL or 9.3–37.2 μmol/L (SI units)
0.4%-1.5% of total hemoglobin

Possible critical values

> 40% of total hemoglobin

Test explanation and related physiology

Methemoglobin is formed during the production of normal adult hemoglobin. If oxygenation of the iron component in the protohemoglobin occurs without subsequent reduction of the heme iron back to its Fe^{+2} form as exists in normal hemoglobin, excess methemoglobin accumulates. The oxidized iron form in methemoglobin is unable to combine with oxygen to carry the oxygen to the peripheral tissues. Therefore the oxyhemoglobin dissociation curve is shifted to the left, resulting in cyanosis and hypoxia.

Methemoglobinemia can be congenital or acquired. Acquired methemoglobinemia is a result of ingestion of nitrates (e.g., from well water) or such drugs as phenacetin, sulfonamides, isoniazid, local anesthetics, and some antibiotics.

Interfering factors

- Tobacco use and carbon monoxide poisoning are associated with increased methemoglobin levels.

Procedure and patient care

- See inside front cover for Routine Blood Testing.
- Fasting: no
- Blood tube commonly used: green
- Methemoglobin is very unstable. Place the specimen in an ice slush immediately after collection.
- Be prepared to provide oxygen support and close monitoring in the event the patient becomes increasingly hypoxic.

Abnormal findings

Methemoglobinemia (hereditary or acquired)

notes

microalbumin (MA)

Type of test   Urine

Normal findings

MA: < 2 mg/dL
MA/creatinine ratio:
   Males: < 17 mg/g creatinine
   Females: < 25 mg/g creatinine

Test explanation and related physiology

Microalbuminuria refers to an albumin concentration in the urine that is greater than normal but not detectable with routine protein testing. Normally, only small amounts of albumin are filtered through the renal glomeruli, and that small quantity can be reabsorbed by the renal tubules. However, when the increased glomerular permeability of albumin overcomes tubular reabsorption capability, albumin is spilled in the urine. Preceding this stage of disease is a period of microalbuminuria that would normally go undetected. Therefore MA is an early indication of renal disease.

For a patient with diabetes, the amount of albumin in the urine is related to duration of the disease and the degree of glycemic control. MA is the earliest indicator for the development of diabetic complications (nephropathy, cardiovascular disease [CVD], and hypertension).

All patients with diabetes older than the age of 12 and less than 70 years should be screened annually for MA. This can be done through a spot urine specimen by using a semiquantitative Micral Urine Test Strip. If MA is present, the test should be repeated two more times. If two of three MA urine test results are positive, a quantitative measurement should be performed. The preferred specimen is a 24-hour collection, but a 10-hour overnight collection (9 p.m.-7 a.m.) or a random collection are acceptable.

Correcting albumin for creatinine excretion rates has value with respect to diabetic renal involvement. An *albumin/creatinine* ratio from a random urine specimen is a valid screening tool. Twenty-four-hour excretion over 30 mg/24 hours or an excretion rate over 20 mcg/min is considered abnormal.

The presence of MA in people without diabetes is an early indicator of lower life expectancy from CVD and hypertension. Nondiabetic nephropathies also may be associated with microalbuminuria. Life insurance underwriters are increasingly using MA testing to indicate life expectancy.

M

Interfering factors

- Urinary tract infection, blood, or acid–base abnormalities can cause elevated MA levels.

Procedure and patient care

- See inside front cover for Routine Urine Testing.
- If the urine specimen contains vaginal discharge or bleeding, a clean-catch or midstream specimen will be needed.
- Ensure that the urine sample is at room temperature.
- If using a Micral Urine Test Strip:
  1. Dip the test strip into the urine for 5 seconds.
  2. Allow the strip to dry for 1 minute.
  3. Compare the strip with the color scale on the label.
- If a 24-hour urine collection is requested, the specimen should be refrigerated.
- PT If the results are positive, inform the patient that the test should be repeated in 1 week.

Abnormal findings

▲ **Increased levels**

Cardiovascular disease
Diabetes mellitus
Hemoglobinuria
Hypertension
Myoglobinuria
Nephropathy
Urinary bleeding

notes

microglobulin (Beta$_2$-microglobulin [β$_2$m], Alpha-1-microglobulin, Retinol binding protein)

Type of test Blood, urine, fluid analysis

Normal findings

Beta$_2$-microglobulin:
  Blood: 0.7–1.8 mcg/mL
  Urine: ≤ 300 mcg/L
  Cerebrospinal fluid (CSF): 0–2.4 mg/L
Retinol binding protein:
  Urine: < 163 mcg/24 hours
Alpha-1-microglobulin:
  Urine: < 50 years: < 13 mg/g creatinine
  ≥ 50 years: < 20 mg/g creatinine

Test explanation and related physiology

β$_2$m is increased in patients with malignancies (especially B-cell lymphoma, leukemia, or multiple myeloma), chronic infections, and chronic severe inflammatory diseases.

β$_2$m, alpha-1-microglobulin, and retinol binding proteins pass freely through glomerular membranes and are almost completely reabsorbed by renal proximal tubule cells. Because of extensive tubular reabsorption, under normal conditions very little of these proteins appear in the final excreted urine. Therefore an increase in the urinary excretion of these proteins indicates proximal tubular disease or toxicity or impaired proximal tubular function. Therefore these proteins are helpful in differentiating among various types of renal disease. For example, in patients with aminoglycoside toxicity, heavy metal nephrotoxicity, or tubular disease, protein urine levels are elevated. Excretion is increased 100 to 1000 times normal levels in cadmium-exposed workers. This test is used to monitor these workers.

β$_2$m is particularly helpful in the differential diagnosis of renal disease. If blood and urine levels are obtained simultaneously, one can differentiate glomerular from tubular disease.

Interfering factors

- β$_2$m is unstable in acid urine.

Procedure and patient care

Blood

- See inside front cover for Routine Blood Testing
- Fasting: preferred, not required
- Blood tube commonly used: red-top

Urine
- See inside front cover for Routine Urine Testing. Follow guidelines for 24-hour collection.
- A random urine test can be collected when corrected for creatinine.

Abnormal findings

▲ **Increased urine levels**
    Drug-induced renal toxicity
    Heavy metal-induced renal disease
    Lymphomas, leukemia, myeloma
    Renal tubule disease
▲ **Increased serum levels**
    Chronic inflammatory processes
    Glomerular renal disease
    Lymphomas, leukemia, myeloma
    Renal transplant rejection
    Viral infections, especially HIV and cytomegalovirus

notes

Mycoplasma pneumoniae testing

Type of test Blood

Normal findings

IgG
  ≤ 0.9 (negative)
  0.91–1.09 (equivocal)
  ≥ 1.1 (positive)
IgM
  ≤ 0.9 (negative)
  0.91–1.09 (equivocal)
  ≥ 1.1 (positive)
IgM by IFA
  Negative (reported as positive or negative)
M. pneumoniae PCR; negative

Test explanation

Several diseases have been associated with the *M. pneumoniae* infection, including pharyngitis, tracheobronchitis, pneumonia, and inflammation of the tympanic membrane. *M. pneumoniae* accounts for approximately 20% of all cases of pneumonia. These infections may be associated with cold agglutinin syndrome (p. 215).

Positive IgM results are consistent with acute infection, although there may be some cross-reactivity associated with other *Mycoplasma* infections. A single positive IgG result only indicates previous immunologic exposure. *Mycoplasma* nucleic acid polymerase chain reaction (PCR) from a respiratory tract sample provides more exact evidence of active infection.

Procedure and patient care

- See inside front cover for Routine Blood Testing.
- Fasting: no
- Blood tube commonly used: red
- Avoid undue cooling of the specimen that may lead to agglutination.

Abnormal findings

Mycoplasma infection

notes

M

myelography (Myelogram)

Type of test   X-ray with contrast

Normal findings

Normal spinal canal

Test explanation and related physiology

By placing radiopaque dye into the subarachnoid space of the spinal canal, the contents of the canal can be radiographically outlined. Cord tumors, meningeal tumors, metastatic spinal tumors, herniated intravertebral discs, and arthritic bone spurs can be readily detected by this study. These lesions appear as canal narrowing or as varying degrees of obstruction to the flow of the contrast media within the subarachnoid space. The entire canal (from lumbar to cervical areas) can be examined. This test is indicated in patients with severe back pain or localized neurologic signs that suggest the canal as the location of these injuries. Because this test is usually performed by lumbar puncture (LP; p. 474), all the potential complications of that procedure exist.

MRI or CT of the spine (p. 234) are more common modalities for imaging the spine and its contents.

Contraindications

- Patients with multiple sclerosis because exacerbation may be precipitated by myelography
- Patients with increased intracranial pressure because LP may cause herniation of the brain
- Patients with infection near the LP site because this may precipitate bacterial meningitis
- Patients who are allergic to iodinated contrast material

Potential complications

- Headache
- Meningitis
- Herniation of the brain
- Seizures
- Allergic reaction to iodinated contrast media
- Hypoglycemia or acidosis may occur in patients with poor renal function who are taking metformin and receive iodinated contrast.

Procedure and patient care

Because this study is rarely performed, please review instructions at the facility performing the procedure.

Abnormal findings

Arthritic bone spurs
Arthritic lumbar stenosis
Astrocytoma
Avulsion of nerve roots
Cervical ankylosing spondylosis
Cord tumor
Cysts
Herniated intravertebral discs
Meningeal tumor
Meningioma
Metastatic spinal tumor
Neurofibroma

notes

M

myoglobin

Type of test Blood

Normal findings

< 90 mcg/L or < 90 mcg/L (SI units)

Test explanation and related physiology

Myoglobin is an oxygen-binding protein found in cardiac and skeletal muscle. Increased levels, which indicate cardiac muscle injury or death, occur in about 3 hours. Although this test is more sensitive than creatine phosphokinase (CPK) isoenzymes (p. 247), it is not as specific. The benefit of myoglobin over CPK-MB is that it may become elevated earlier in some patients.

Disease or trauma of the skeletal muscle also causes elevations in myoglobin. Because myoglobin is excreted in the urine and is nephrotoxic, urine levels must be monitored in patients with high levels. Myoglobin may turn the urine red.

Interfering factors

- Increased myoglobin levels can occur after IM injections.

Procedure and patient care

- See inside front cover for Routine Blood Testing.
- Fasting: no
- Blood tube commonly used: red

Abnormal findings

▲ **Increased levels**
  Malignant hyperthermia
  Muscular dystrophy
  Myocardial infarction
  Rhabdomyolysis
  Skeletal muscle inflammation
    (myositis)
  Skeletal muscle ischemia
  Skeletal muscle trauma

▼ **Decreased levels**
  Polymyositis

notes

natriuretic peptides (Atrial natriuretic peptide [ANP], Brain natriuretic peptide [BNP], N-terminal fragment of pro-brain [B-type] natriuretic peptide [NT–pro-BNP], C-type natriuretic peptide [CNP], Ventricular natriuretic peptide, CHF peptides)

Type of test   Blood

Normal findings

ANP: 22–77 pg/mL or 22–77 ng/L (SI units)
BNP: < 100 pg/mL
NT-pro-BNP: < 300 pg/mL
Critical values
   BNP: > 400 pg/mL (Heart failure likely)

Test explanation and related physiology

Natriuretic peptides (NPs) are used to identify and stratify patients with congestive heart failure (CHF). There are three major NPs: ANP, BNP, and CNP. BNP has been implicated in the pathophysiology of hypertension, congestive heart failure (CHF), and atherosclerosis. BNP is released in response to atrial and ventricular stretch, respectively. BNP, in particular, correlates well to left ventricular pressures. As a result, BNP is a good marker for CHF. The higher the levels of BNP are, the more severe the CHF. This test is used in urgent care settings to aid in the differential diagnosis of shortness of breath (SOB). If BNP is elevated, the SOB is because of CHF. If BNP levels are normal, the SOB is pulmonary and not cardiac.

Furthermore, BNP is a helpful prognosticator and is used in CHF risk stratification. CHF patients whose BNP levels do not rapidly return to normal with treatment experience a significantly higher risk for mortality in the ensuing months than do those whose BNP levels rapidly normalize with treatment.

In some laboratories, BNP is measured as an *N-terminal fragment of pro-brain (B-type) natriuretic peptide (NT-pro-BNP)*. Screening diabetics for BNP elevation to determine the risk for cardiac diseases is helpful. BNP is also elevated in patients with prolonged systemic hypertension and in patients with acute myocardial infarction (MI).

Interfering factors

- BNP levels are generally higher in healthy women than healthy men.
- BNP levels are higher in older patients.
- BNP levels are elevated for 1 month after cardiac surgery.

N

Procedure and patient care

- See inside front cover for Routine Blood Testing.
- Fasting: no
- Blood tube commonly used: lavender

Abnormal findings

▲ **Increased levels**

    Congestive heart failure
    Cor pulmonale
    Heart transplant rejection
    Myocardial infarction
    Systemic hypertension

notes

neuron-specific enolase (NSE)

Type of test   Blood

Normal findings

< 8.6 mcg/L

Test explanation and related physiology

NSE is present in neuroendocrine cells and amine precursor uptake and decarboxylation (APUD) cells. Elevated NSE concentrations are observed in patients with neuroblastoma, pancreatic islet cell carcinoma, medullary thyroid carcinoma, pheochromocytoma, and other neuroendocrine tumors.

NSE levels are frequently increased in patients with small cell lung cancer (SCLC) and infrequently in patients with non-SCLC (p. 164, tumor markers). NSE can be used to monitor disease progression and management in SCLC. Levels of NSE can occasionally be elevated in benign disorders such as pneumonia and benign hepatobiliary diseases.

Procedure and patient care

- See inside front cover for Routine Blood Testing.
- Fasting: no
- Blood tube commonly used: red

N

Abnormal findings

▲ **Increased levels**

APUD tumors

Neuroblastoma

Small cell lung cancer

notes

neutrophil antibody screen (Granulocyte antibodies, Polymorphonucleocyte antibodies [PMN ab], Antigranulocyte antibodies, Antineutrophil antibodies, Neutrophil antibodies, Leukoagglutinin)

Type of test Blood

Normal findings

Negative for neutrophil antibodies

Test explanation and related physiology

Neutrophil antibodies are antibodies directed toward white blood cells (WBCs). They develop during blood transfusions or transplacental bleeds and sometimes in patients with autoimmune disorders. Patients who experience a *transfusion reaction* despite complete compatibility testing before blood administration should have a neutrophil antibody screen to see if WBC incompatibility is the source of the reaction. This test is most commonly a part of posttransfusion antibody screening, which is a battery of testing performed if a transfusion reaction is suspected. It is also used in infants in the evaluation of unexplained neutropenia and in patients with suspected or known autoimmune disease.

Most commonly, in blood transfusion reactions, the recipient has antibodies to the donor WBCs and experiences a fever during transfusion. More severe, however, is the reaction when the donor plasma contains antibodies to the recipient's WBCs. This nonhemolytic reaction can lead to severe transfusion reactions, including acute pulmonary failure *(transfusion-related acute lung injury [TRALI])* and multiorgan system failure.

Interfering factors

- Recent administration of dextran
- Recent administration of intravenous (IV) contrast media
- Blood transfusion in the past 3 months

Procedure and patient care

- See inside front cover for Routine Blood Testing.
- Fasting: no
- Blood tube commonly used: red or lavender

Abnormal findings

Alloimmune neonatal neutropenia
Autoimmune neutropenia
TRALI

notes

newborn metabolic screening

Type of test   Blood

Normal findings

Negative

Possible critical values

Positive for any of the tests

Test explanation and related physiology

Newborn screening (NBS) is the practice of testing every newborn for certain harmful or potentially fatal disorders that are not otherwise apparent at birth. The Recommended Uniform Screening Panel (RUSP) is a list of disorders recommended for testing by the government. In most states, this testing is mandatory. NBS tests take place in the first 12 to 48 hours of life. Disorders that may be detected through screening include endocrine and hematologic diseases.

Shortly after a child's birth, a sample of blood is obtained from a heel stick. The sample may be a *blood spot*. It is generally recommended that the sample be taken *after* the first 24 hours of life. Some tests such as the one for phenylketonuria (PKU) may not be as sensitive until the newborn has ingested an ample amount of the amino acid phenylalanine, which is a constituent of both human and cow milk, and after the postnatal thyroid surge has subsided. This is generally after about 2 days.

Tandem mass spectrometry can detect the blood components that are elevated in certain disorders, and it is capable of screening for more than 20 inherited metabolic disorders with a single test. Disorders typically included in screening include phenylketonuria, congenital hypothyroidism, galactosemia, sickle cell anemia, biotinidase deficiency, congenital adrenal hyperplasia, maple syrup urine disease, homocystinuria, tyrosinemia, cystic fibrosis, toxoplasmosis, and X-linked adrenoleukodystrophy.

Certain other rare disorders can also be detected and may include Duchenne muscular dystrophy, HIV, and neuroblastoma. Hematologic disorders such as glucose-6-phosphate dehydrogenase (G6PD) deficiency and thalassemia can also be identified.

Most states require newborns' hearing to be screened before they are discharged from the hospital. The hearing test involves placing a tiny earphone in the baby's ear and measuring his or her response to sound (p. 322, evoked potentials).

N

Interfering factors

- Premature infants may have false-positive results because of delayed development of liver enzymes.
- Infants tested before 24 hours of age may have false-negative.

Procedure and patient care

Before

PT Inform the parents about the purpose and method of the test.

- Assess the infant's feeding patterns before performing the test. An inadequate amount of protein ingested before performing the test can cause false-negative results.

During

- Place a few drops of blood from a heel stick in each circle on the filter paper.

After

PT Inform the parents that if test results are positive they will be notified by their healthcare provider, and further testing or treatment will be recommended.

Abnormal findings

Endocrine diseases
Hematologic diseases
Metabolic diseases

notes

nicotine and metabolites (Nicotine, Cotinine, 3-Hydroxy Cotinine, Nornicotine, Anabasine)

Type of test Urine/blood

Normal findings

	Unexposed nontobacco user (ng/mL)	Passive exposure (non-tobacco user) (ng/mL)	Abstinent user for > 2 weeks (ng/mL)	Active tobacco product user (ng/mL)
Urine				
Nicotine	< 2	< 20	< 30	1000–5000
Cotinine	< 5	< 20	< 50	1000–8000
3-OH-Cotinine	< 50	< 50	< 120	3000–25,000
Nornicotine	< 2	< 2	< 2	30–900
Anabasine	< 3	< 3	< 3	3–500
Serum				
Nicotine	< 2	< 2	< 2	30–50
Cotinine	< 2	< 8	< 2	200–800
3-OH-Cotinine	< 2	< 2	< 2	100–500

N

Test explanation and related physiology

Nicotine is metabolized into cotinine and 3-hydroxy cotinine, which are measurable in urine and serum. In addition to nicotine and metabolites, tobacco products also contain other alkaloids (anabasine and nornicotine). These tests are used to assess compliance with smoking cessation programs and to qualify for surgical procedures. They are also used by insurance companies to determine whether the applicant is a smoker.

Cotinine and 3-hydroxy cotinine are typically detectable for several days to up to 1 week after the use of tobacco. Because the level of these metabolites in the blood is proportionate to the amount of exposure to tobacco smoke, it is a valuable indicator of tobacco smoke exposure. Nicotine and its metabolites can be measured in the serum, urine, and other biofluids (most commonly the saliva). Cotinine is found in urine from 2 to 4 days after tobacco use. Blood cotinine will increase no matter how the tobacco is used (smoked, chew, dip, or snuff products). Nicotine levels have an *in vivo* half-life of approximately 2 hours, which is too short to be useful as a marker of smoking status.

Anabasine (only measured in the urine) is present in tobacco products but not nicotine replacement therapies. Nicotine, cotinine, 3-hydroxy cotinine, and nornicotine are also elevated by the use of any of the nicotine replacement gum, patch, or pill products. The presence of anabasine greater than 10 ng/mL or nornicotine greater than 30 ng/mL in urine indicates current tobacco use, irrespective of whether the subject is on nicotine replacement therapy. The presence of nornicotine without anabasine is consistent with use of nicotine replacement products. Passive exposure to tobacco smoke can cause accumulation of nicotine metabolites in nontobacco users. Urine cotinine has been observed to accumulate up to 20 ng/mL from passive exposure. Neither anabasine nor nornicotine accumulates from passive exposure. Because hydration status and renal function may affect urinary cotinine results, a spot urine cotinine test is accompanied by a spot urine creatinine.

For smokers, another method of determining tobacco use is *expired carbon monoxide testing*. Again, a relatively short half-life (~4 hours) limits the reliability and accuracy. Furthermore, carbon monoxide testing is unable to detect the use of smokeless tobacco.

Interfering factors

- Menthol cigarettes may *increase* cotinine levels because the menthol retains cotinine in the blood for a longer time.
- Diluted or adulterated urine may alter results.

Procedure and patient care

Before

PT Explain the procedure to the patient and indicate the type of specimen needed.

- Obtain an accurate history of recent tobacco use.

During

Blood

- Collect venous blood in a red-top, lavender-top (EDTA), or pink-top (K_2EDTA) tube. See inside front cover for Routine Blood Testing.

Urine
- Immediately transport the specimen to the laboratory.
- Obtain a random spot urine specimen of at least 5 mL. See inside front cover for Routine Urine Testing.

Saliva
- Ask the patient to spit at least 1 mL of saliva into a container.
- Alternatively, dental gauze rolls can be placed in the mouth for 15 minutes and then placed in a storage container.

After
- Keep the specimens in a cool place if they cannot be transported to the laboratory immediately.

Abnormal finding

Tobacco exposure

notes

N

5′-nucleotidase

Type of test Blood

Normal findings

0–1.6 units at 37° C or 0–1.6 units at 37° C (SI units)

Test explanation and related physiology

5′-Nucleotidase is an enzyme specific to the liver. The 5′-nucleotidase level is elevated in patients with liver diseases, especially those associated with cholestasis. It provides information similar to alkaline phosphatase (ALP; p. 23). However, ALP is not specific to the liver. When doubt as to the cause of an elevated ALP exists, 5′-nucleotidase is recommended. If that enzyme is elevated along with the ALP, the source of the pathology is certainly in the liver. If the 5′-nucleotidase is normal in the face of an elevated ALP, the source of pathology is outside the liver. Gamma-glutamyl transpeptidase (GGTP; p. 361). is used similarly because it is also specific to the liver.

Procedure and patient care

- See inside front cover for Routine Blood Testing.
- Fasting: no
- Blood tube commonly used: red

Abnormal findings

▲ **Increased levels**

  Bile duct obstruction
  Cholestasis
  Cirrhosis
  Hepatic necrosis, ischemia, tumor
  Hepatitis
  Hepatotoxic drugs

notes

obstruction series

Type of test X-ray

Normal findings

No evidence of bowel obstruction
No abnormal calcifications
No free air

Test explanation and related physiology

The obstruction series is a group of x-ray images performed on the abdomen of patients with suspected bowel obstruction, paralytic ileus, perforated viscus, kidney stones, or foreign body ingestion. Sometimes, pathology such as abdominal abscess and appendicitis can be indentified. This series of images usually consists of at least two x-ray studies. The *posteroanterior (PA) erect abdominal* image includes visualization of both diaphragms. The image is examined for evidence of free air under either diaphragm, which is pathognomonic for a perforated viscus. This view is also used to detect air–fluid levels within the intestine; the presence of an air fluid level is compatible with bowel obstruction or paralytic ileus. Occasionally patients are too ill to stand erect. In this case an x-ray image can be taken with the patient in the *left lateral decubitus* position.

The *anteroposterior (AP) supine abdominal* x-ray study is similar to a *KUB (kidney, ureter, bladder)* film. A calcification within the course of the ureter could indicate a kidney or ureteral stone. A gas-filled, distended bowel is compatible with bowel obstruction or paralytic ileus.

This x-ray study can also be used as a *scout image* before performing GI or abdominal x-ray studies that use contrast.

The *PA erect chest* radiograph is typically performed as part of the obstruction series because sometimes chest pathology can present as abdominal pain. Also, it is more sensitive for diagnosing pneumoperitoneum.

Contraindications

• Patients who are pregnant unless the benefits outweigh the risk to the fetus

Interfering factors

• Previous GI barium contrast study

Procedure and patient care

Before

PT Explain the procedure to the patient. See p. xviii for radiation exposure and risks.

• Ensure that all radiopaque clothing has been removed.

PT Remind the patient that no GI contrast will be used.

During

• Although the procedure varies from facility to facility, usually a supine abdominal x-ray image, erect abdominal image, and perhaps a lower erect chest image are taken.

• Note that the obstruction series is performed in minutes in the radiology department by a radiologic technologist; however, it can be performed at the bedside with a portable x-ray machine. A radiologist interprets the images.

PT Tell the patient that no discomfort is associated with this study.

After

• No special aftercare is needed.

Abnormal findings

Abdominal abscess
Abdominal aortic aneurysm
Abdominal aortic calcification
Abnormal position of the
  kidneys
Appendicolithiasis
Bladder distention
Bowel obstruction

Kidney stone
Organomegaly
Paralytic ileus
Perforated viscus
Peritoneal effusion or ascites
Presence of a foreign body
Soft tissue masses

notes

octreotide scan (Carcinoid nuclear scan, Neuroendocrine nuclear scan)

Type of test   Nuclear scan

Normal findings

No evidence of increased uptake throughout the body

Test explanation and related physiology

Octreotide scans are used to identify and localize neuroendocrine primary and metastatic tumors. These scans are indicated on patients with known neuroendocrine tumors.

Most neuroendocrine tumors have a somatostatin receptor on the cellular membrane. Octreotide is an analog of somatostatin. When combined with a radiopharmaceutical, the radiolabeled octreotide will attach to the somatostatin receptors of the neuroendocrine tumor cells. This test is used to identify primary and metastatic neuroendocrine tumors. It is also used to monitor the course of the disease.

Many different types of hormone-producing tumors can be detected by this scan, most notably carcinoid, gastrinoma, insulinoma, glucagonoma, pheochromocytoma, and small cell lung cancer. Other abnormalities can pick up octreotide, including granulomatous infections, rheumatoid arthritis, and non-hormonal cancers (breast, lymphoma, and non-small cell lung cancers).

Contraindications

- Patients who are pregnant or lactating because of risk of damage to the fetus or infant

Interfering factors

- Barium in the GI tract overlying the liver or spleen. Barium produces defects that may be mistaken for masses.

Procedure and patient care

Before

PT Explain the procedure to the patient. See p. xviii for radiation exposure and risks.

PT Tell the patient that no fasting is required.

PT Assure the patient that he or she will not be exposed to large amounts of radiation because only tracer doses are used.

- If an iodinated radionuclide is to be used, ensure that the patient does not have an allergy to iodine.

O

- If an iodinated radionuclide is to be used, an iodine preparation may be given prior to testing. This will avoid uptake of the radionuclide by the thyroid gland.
- **PT** If the patient has been receiving octreotide as a form of antineoplastic treatment, this must be discontinued before scanning. Inform the patient.

During

- Note the following procedural steps:
1. The patient is taken to nuclear medicine, where the radionuclide is administered intravenously.
2. One hour after injection, a gamma ray detector or camera is successively placed over the entire body.
3. The patient is placed in supine, lateral, and prone positions.
4. The radionuclide image is recorded. Single-photon emission tomography (SPECT) images may also be performed.
5. After 4 hours, the patient is given a strong laxative to clear the octreotide from the bowel.
6. Repeat scanning is performed at 2, 4, 24, and 48 hours after administration of the octreotide.
- Note that the imaging procedure is performed by a trained technologist in approximately ½ hour. A nuclear medicine physician interprets the results.
- **PT** The only discomfort associated with this procedure is the intravenous injection of the radionuclide.

After

- **PT** Because tracer doses of radioisotopes are used, inform the patient that no radiation precautions are needed.

Abnormal findings

Carcinoid tumors
Granulomatous infections (e.g., sarcoidosis and tuberculosis)
Neuroendocrine tumors

notes

osmolality, blood (Serum osmolality)

Type of test Blood

Normal findings

Adult/elderly: 285–295 mOsm/kg H_2O or 285–295 mmol/kg (SI units)

Child: 275–290 mOsm/kg H_2O

Possible critical values

< 265 mOsm/kg H_2O
> 320 mOsm/kg H_2O

Test explanation and related physiology

Osmolality measures the number of dissolved particles in serum/plasma per unit volume. As the amount of free water in the blood increases or the number of particles decreases per unit volume of serum, osmolality decreases. As the amount of water in the blood decreases or the number of particles per unit volume increases, osmolality increases. Osmolality increases with dehydration and decreases with overhydration.

The simultaneous use of urine osmolality (see next test) helps in the interpretation and evaluation of problems involving osmolality.

The serum osmolality test is useful in evaluating fluid and electrolyte imbalance. The test is very helpful in the evaluation of seizures, ascites, hydration status, acid–base balance, suspected antidiuretic hormone (ADH) abnormalities, and suspected poisoning. Osmolality is also helpful in identifying the presence of organic acids, sugars, and ethanol.

The measured osmolality should not exceed the predicted by more than 10 mOsm/kg. A difference of more than 10 mOsm/kg is considered an *osmolal gap* or *delta gap*. Another measure providing similar data is the ratio of serum sodium to osmolality.

Osmolality may have a role in evaluation of coma patients. Values greater than 385 mOsm/kg H_2O are associated with stupor in patients with hyperglycemia. When values of 400 to 420 mOsm/kg are detected, grand mal seizures can occur. Values greater than 420 mOsm/kg can be lethal.

Interfering factors

• Diseases such as cerebrovascular accident or brain tumors may interfere with test results through inappropriate secretion of ADH.

Procedure and patient care

- See inside front cover for Routine Blood Testing.
- Fasting: no
- Blood tube commonly used: red
- For pediatric patients, draw blood from a heel stick.

Abnormal findings

▲ **Increased levels**

Azotemia
Dehydration
Diabetes insipidus
Hypercalcemia
Hyperglycemia
Hypernatremia
Hyperosmolar nonketotic
  hyperglycemia
Ingestion of ethanol, methanol,
  or ethylene glycol
Ketosis
Mannitol therapy
Renal tubular necrosis
Severe pyelonephritis
Shock
Uremia

▼ **Decreased levels**

Hyponatremia
Overhydration
Paraneoplastic
  syndromes
  associated with
  lung carcinoma
Syndrome of
  inappropriate
  antidiuretic
  hormone
  (SIADH) secretion

notes

osmolality, urine (Urine osmolality)

Type of test Urine

Normal findings

12- to 14-hour fluid restriction: > 850 mOsm/kg H_2O (SI units)

Random specimen: 50–1200 mOsm/kg H_2O, depending on fluid intake, or 50–1200 mmol/kg (SI units)

Test explanation and related physiology

Osmolality is the measurement of the number of dissolved particles in a solution. It is a more exact measurement of urine concentration than specific gravity.

Osmolality is used in the precise evaluation of the concentrating and diluting abilities of the kidney. With normal fluid intake and normal diet, a patient will produce a urine of about 500 to 850 mOsm/kg water. The normal kidney can concentrate a urine to 800 to 1400 mOsm/kg. With excess fluid intake, a minimal osmolality of 40 to 80 mOsm/kg can be obtained. With dehydration, the urine osmolality should be three to four times the plasma osmolality.

Osmolality is used in the evaluation of kidney function and the ability to excrete ammonium salts. Osmolality may be used as part of the urinalysis when the patient has glycosuria or proteinuria or has had tests that use radiopaque substances. In these situations, the *urine osmolar gap* increases because of other organic osmolar particles. The urine osmolar gap is the sum of all the particles predicted or calculated to be in the urine (electrolytes, urea, and glucose) compared with the actual measurement of the osmolality.

Normally, the osmolar gap is 80 to 100 mOsm/kg of H_2O. The urine osmolality is more easily interpreted when the serum osmolality (see previous study) is simultaneously performed. More information concerning the state of renal water handling or abnormalities of urine dilution or concentration can be obtained if urinary osmolality is compared with serum osmolality and if urine electrolyte studies are performed. Normally, the ratio of urine osmolality to serum osmolality is 1 to 3, reflecting a wide range of urine osmolality.

Procedure and patient care

- See inside front cover for Routine Urine Testing.
- PT Tell the patient that no special preparation is necessary for a random urine specimen.
- PT Inform the patient that preparation for a fasting urine specimen may require a high-protein diet for 3 days before the test.

PT Instruct the patient to eat a dry supper the evening before the test and to drink no fluids until the test is completed the next morning.
- Preferably, collect a first-voided urine specimen for a random sample.
- Indicate on the laboratory request the patient's fasting status.

Abnormal findings

▲ **Increased levels**

Acidosis
Addison disease
Congestive heart failure
Hepatic cirrhosis
Hypernatremia
Shock
SIADH secretion

▼ **Decreased levels**

Aldosteronism
Diabetes insipidus
Excess fluid intake
Hypercalcemia
Hypokalemia
Renal tubular necrosis
Severe pyelonephritis

notes

ovarian reserve testing (Inhibin b, Anti-müllerian hormone [AMH], Antral follicular count [AFC], Clomiphene citrate challenge test [CCCT])

Type of test Blood

Normal values

Inhibin b

Females

≤12 years: <183 pg/mL

13–41 years regular cycle (follicular phase): <224 pg/mL

42–51 years regular cycle (follicular phase): <108 pg/mL

13–51 years regular cycle (luteal phase): <80 pg/mL

>51 years (postmenopausal): <12 pg/mL

Anti-müllerian hormone

Females

<3 years: 0.11–4.2 ng/mL

20–24 years: 1.2–12 ng/mL

>55 years: <0.03 ng/mL

Clomiphene citrate challenge test

Day 3 estradiol <80 pg/mL

Day 3 or day 10 FSH above normal (see FSH, p. 485.)

Antral follicular count

14–21 follicles

Test explanation and related physiology

As fertility decreases with age and couples delay having children, increasing numbers of couples seek infertility diagnostic evaluation. Women with diminished ovarian reserve have lower pregnancy rates with or without fertility intervention. Elevated basal FSH concentrations are an indicator of diminished ovarian reserve. Low levels of inhibin B and *anti-müllerian hormone (AMH)* are also an indicator of reduced ovarian reserve.

Provocation tests can also be used to determine ovarian reserve. The *clomiphene citrate challenge test (CCCT)* is commonly used. Other provocation tests include the *GnRH agonist (GnRH-a) stimulation test* and the *exogenous FSH stimulation test*. In CCCT, clomiphene citrate (an ovarian stimulant) is administered. In women with properly responsive ovaries, FSH will increase and then will come back to basal levels because of the release of estradiol and inhibin b produced by developing ovarian follicles. In women whose ovarian reserve is poor, the day 10 FSH remains elevated as there is no estradiol or inhibin b to inhibit its FSH release.

Antral follicular count (AFC) is another method to determine ovarian reserve. This is a count of the number of antral (mature) follicles that can be seen on transvaginal ultrasound during a stimulated cycle. AFC is often performed during CCCT.

AMH, like inhibin b, is a hormone produced by the ovaries in mature females. AMH levels in young girls remain low until puberty, when the ovaries begin to produce it and levels increase. AMH and inhibin b will then steadily decline in women over their reproductive years, becoming very low and eventually undetectable after menopause. Therefore, these hormones are indicators of ovarian reserve. AMH is also used in diagnosing polycystic ovary syndrome as AMH produced by the excess ovarian follicles is very high. Inhibin b and AMH are used as tumor markers for ovarian stomal tumors (particularly granulosa cell carcinoma).

Potential complications

- Hot flushes, minor visual disturbances, headaches, mild mood changes

Procedure and patient care

- See inside front cover for Routine Blood Testing.
- Fasting: no
- Blood tube commonly used: red
- Provocative testing with CCCT
    - Day 3 of menstrual cycle
        - Obtain FSH and estradiol
    - Daily on day 5–9 of menstrual cycle
        - Administer 100 mg of clomiphene citrate
    - Day 10 of menstrual cycle
        - Obtain FSH and estradiol
        - Obtain a transvaginal ultrasound

Abnormal findings

Poor ovarian reserve

notes

oximetry (Pulse oximetry, Oxygen saturation)

Type of test Photodiagnostic

Normal findings

$\geq 95\%$

Possible critical values

$\leq 75\%$

Test explanation and related physiology

Oximetry is a noninvasive method of monitoring arterial blood oxygen saturation (Sao_2). The Sao_2 is the ratio of oxygenated hemoglobin to the total amount of hemoglobin. The Sao_2 is expressed as a percentage; for example, a saturation of 95% indicates that 95% of the total hemoglobin attachments for oxygen have oxygen attached to them. The Sao_2 is an accurate approximation of oxygen saturation obtained from an arterial blood gas study (p. 89). By correlating the Sao_2 and the patient's physiologic status, a close estimate of the partial oxygen pressure (Po_2) can be obtained.

Oximetry is typically used for monitoring the patient's oxygenation status during the perioperative period (or any time of heavy sedation) and for patients receiving mechanical ventilation. This test is used in many clinical situations, such as pulmonary rehabilitation programs, stress testing, and sleep laboratories. Oximetry can be used to assess the body's response to various drugs, such as theophylline (which causes bronchodilation) and methacholine (which evokes bronchospasm in people with asthma). This test is commonly used to titrate levels of oxygen on hospitalized patients.

O_2 levels can also be measured in various body tissues. For example, monitors that continuously measure tissue O_2 partial pressures can be attached to a small catheter placed in the brain, heart, or peripheral muscle. *Brain tissue oxygen testing and monitoring* is the most common use of this technology. It is used to monitor the condition of the brain after severe head trauma by measuring cerebral blood flow and pulmonary oxygenation.

Procedure and patient care

Before

PT Explain the procedure to the patient.

PT Tell the patient that no fasting is required.

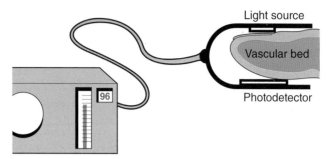

FIG. O1 Oximetry. The pulse oximeter passes a beam of light through the tissue. The amount of light absorbed by the oxygen-saturated hemoglobin is measured by the sensor.

During
- Rub the patient's earlobe, pinna (upper part of the ear), or fingertip to increase blood flow.
- Clip the monitoring probe or sensor to the ear or finger. A beam of light passes through the tissue, and the sensor measures the amount of light the tissue absorbs (Figure O1).
- Note that this study is usually performed at the patient's bedside in a few seconds.
- **PT** Tell the patient that no discomfort is associated with this study.

After
- Note that no special aftercare is needed.

Abnormal findings

▲ **Increased levels**
Hyperventilation
Increased inspired O_2

▼ **Decreased levels**
Hypoxic cardiac diseases
Hypoxic lung diseases
Inadequate O_2 in inspired air
Severe hypoventilation states

notes

pancreatic elastase (PE, EL1, Elastase-1, Fecal Elastase)

Type of test Stool

Normal findings

Stool:
> 200 mcg Elastase/g stool = Normal
100–200 mcg Elastase/g stool = Moderate to slight exocrine pancreatic insufficiency
< 100 mcg Elastase/g stool = Severe exocrine pancreatic insufficiency

Serum:
Less than 3.5 ng/mL

Test explanation and related physiology

PE is a digestive enzyme secreted by the pancreas. In this test, PE is used as a fecal marker to assess exocrine pancreatic function. This test is used to identify maldigestion caused by pancreatic insufficiency. The insufficiency can be caused by chronic pancreatitis, cystic fibrosis, or pancreatic resection. If possible, pancreatic enzyme supplementation should be discontinued before testing. EL1 can also be measured in the serum. Elevated serum levels may indicate pancreatitis. Hypothyroidism is associated with decreased levels.

Interfering factors

• Pancreatic enzyme supplementation can increase results.

Procedure and patient care

Before

PT Explain the procedure to the patient. No preparation is needed.

During

PT Instruct the patient to transfer 5 g of stool to a sterile, plastic, screw-cap container provided by the laboratory. No preservative is needed.

PT Inform the patient that watery, diarrheal stool is not recommended for this test because some dilutions during the assay may give lower EL1 concentrations than are actually present.

After

PT Tell the patient results may take several days if the specimen is sent to an outside reference lab.

Abnormal findings

▼ **Decreased stool levels**
Cholelithiasis
Cystic fibrosis
Diabetes mellitus
Osteoporosis
Pancreatic insufficiency
  (e.g., chronic
  pancreatitis)
Pancreatic resection

▲ **Increased serum levels**
Pancreatitis

▼ **Decreased serum levels**
Hypothyroidism

notes

pancreatic enzymes (Pancreatic secretory test, Amylase, Lipase, Trypsin, Chymotrypsin)

Type of test Fluid analysis

Normal findings

Volume: 2–4 mL/kg body weight
HCO3 (bicarbonate): 90–130 mEq/L
Amylase: 6.6–35.2 units/kg
Trypsin-like immunoreactivity: 10–57 ng/mL
Trypsin: ≥ 1:96
Chymotrypsin: by report

Test explanation and related physiology

Cystic fibrosis (CF) is an inherited disease characterized by abnormal secretion by exocrine glands within the bronchi, small intestines, pancreatic ducts, bile ducts, and skin (see sweat test p. 698 and genetic testing p. 369). Because of this abnormal exocrine secretion, children with CF develop mucus plugs that obstruct their pancreatic ducts and can lead to significant malabsorption, steatorrhea, and diarrhea. The pancreatic enzymes cannot be expelled into the duodenum and therefore are either completely absent or present only in diminished quantities within the duodenal aspirate. Bicarbonate and other neutralizing fluids cannot be secreted from the pancreas.

In this test, secretin and pancreozymin are used to stimulate pancreatic secretion of these enzymes and bicarbonate into the duodenum. The duodenal contents are then aspirated and examined for pH, bicarbonate, and pancreatic enzyme levels. Amylase is the most frequently measured enzyme.

Trypsinogen, another pancreatic exocrine enzyme, is measured in the serum as *trypsin-like immunoreactivity.* This test is used to support the diagnosis of chronic pancreatitis. Levels diminish as exocrine function becomes impaired. It is important to note that serum levels of trypsinogen are used in newborn screening for CF. When levels are elevated, confirmatory tests are done.

When any of these pancreatic enzymes are measured in the serum, they can reflect acute inflammation of the pancreas. Likewise, in patients with burned-out chronic pancreatitis, serum measurements of these pancreatic enzymes are low. Pancreatic enzymes can also be measured in the stool and are more easily accessed for testing. Most commonly *stool for trypsin and chymotrypsin* are tested and are a measure of pancreatic function. Stool for elastase also is a measure of pancreatic function.

Procedure and patient care

Before

PT Explain the procedure to the patient and parents.

PT Instruct the adult patient to fast for 12 hours before testing.

• Determine pediatric fasting times according to the patient's age.

During

• Note the following procedural steps:
  1. With the use of fluoroscopy, a Dreiling tube is passed through the patient's nose and into the stomach.
  2. The distal lumen of the tube is placed within the duodenum and the proximal lumen within the stomach.
  3. Both lumens are aspirated. The gastric lumen is continually aspirated to avoid contamination of the gastric contents in the duodenum aspirate.
  4. A control specimen of the duodenal juices is collected for 20 minutes.
  5. The patient is tested for sensitivity to secretin and pancreozymin by low-dose intradermal injection.
  6. If no sensitivity is present, these hormones are administered intravenously. Secretin can be expected to stimulate pancreatic fluid and bicarbonate secretion. Pancreozymin can be expected to stimulate pancreatic enzyme secretion.
  7. Four duodenal aspirates are collected at 20-minute intervals and placed in the specimen container.
  8. Each specimen is analyzed for pH, volume, bicarbonate, and amylase levels.

• Note that a physician performs this test in the laboratory or at the patient's bedside.

After

• Place the aspirated specimens on ice. Send them to the chemistry laboratory as soon as the test is completed.

• Give appropriate nose and mouth care after removal of the tube.

Abnormal findings

▲ **Increased levels**
Acute pancreatitis

▼ **Decreased levels**
Chronic pancreatitis
Cystic fibrosis
Sprue

notes

pancreatobiliary fish testing

Type of test Microscopic examination

Normal findings

No chromosomal ploidy abnormalities

Test explanation and related physiology

It is sometimes difficult to differentiate benign bile duct strictures from early pancreatobiliary cancer. When a stricture is identified on an endoscopic retrograde cholangiopancreatography (ERCP; p. 301), cancer is a possible cause. If an obvious cancer is not seen at the time of ERCP, a brush is repeatedly swept along the bile duct to obtain duct surface cells for conventional cytology to identify cancer cells. In conventional cytology, the brushing specimens are placed on a slide and stained with a Papanicolaou (PAP) stain. Slides are then interpreted by a cytopathologist to determine whether they show features that are positive for malignancy, suspicious for malignancy, atypical (meaning there are cells that are not normal but cannot be definitely ascribed to a neoplastic process), or negative for malignancy.

With the use of fluorescence *in situ* hybridization (FISH) testing, three chromosome enumeration probes and a gene-specific probe to P16 tumor suppressor gene are able to determine whether more than one pair of chromosomes or P16 genes exists in the cells obtained from the brushings of the bile duct during ERCP. If extra copies of two or more of the chromosomes or P16 genes are evident, the cells are considered to be *polysomic*, which indicates a high chance of malignancy.

Contraindications

• See ERCP.

Potential complications

• See ERCP.

Interfering factors

• Errors in obtaining a good specimen can influence results.

Procedure and patient care

Before

PT Explain the procedure to the patient.

• Obtain informed consent from the patient.

P

- Keep the patient NPO (nothing by mouth) as of midnight the day of the test.
- Follow the procedure for ERCP.

During

- During ERCP, a rounded brush is placed through the accessory lumen of the endoscope and passed repeatedly through the stricture.
- The brush is then swished in a cytology solution for FISH or directly smeared on a slide and preserved for cytology.

After

- Follow the guidelines for ERCP.

Abnormal findings

Biliary sclerosis
Sclerosing cholangitis
Tumor or strictures of the pancreatobiliary duct

notes

Papanicolaou smear (Pap smear, Pap test, Cytologic test for cancer, Liquid-based cervical cytology [LBCC], ThinPrep)

Type of test Microscopic examination

Normal findings

No abnormal or atypical cells

Test explanation and related physiology

A Pap test can detect neoplastic cells in cervical and vaginal secretions. This screening test is based on the fact that normal cells and abnormal cervical and endometrial neoplastic cells are shed into the cervical and vaginal secretions. By examining these secretions microscopically, one can detect early cellular changes associated with premalignant conditions or an existing malignant condition.

The Bethesda System is univerally used to evaluate the cytology of the specimen.

A common method of Pap test specimen collection is *liquid-based cervical cytology (LBCC)*. With this technique, the specimen obtained from the cervix is placed into a preservative solution and is then placed on a slide to be evaluated. The specimen can be split into two parts. The first is evaluated for cytopathology. In the event that cytologic abnormalities of undetermined significance are found that could be better elucidated with further testing, the cells in the second split specimen are used for that testing.

Screening refers to testing for individuals who are at low risk for cervical cancer and who have no prior abnormal test results. There are three main approaches for cervical cancer screening: primary cervical HPV screening (see p. 800), cotesting for HPV and cervical cytology (PAP smear), and PAP alone. While there are no randomized trials comparing the impact of these three methods, multiple professional organizations have created recommendations for cervical cancer screening.

It is important to note that these recommendations change frequently based on newer available data and the effect of HPV vaccinations on the female population.

P

Contraindications

- Patients currently having routine, normal menses because this can alter test interpretation
- Patients with vaginal infections: Cellular changes that may be misinterpreted as dysplastic may transiently occur.

Interfering factors

- A delay in fixing a specimen allows the cells to dry, destroys the effectiveness of the stain, and makes interpretation difficult.
- Using lubricating jelly on the speculum can alter the specimen.
- Douching and tub bathing may wash away cellular deposits.

Procedure and patient care

Before

PT Explain the procedure to the patient.

PT Instruct the patient not to douche or tub bathe during the 24 hours before the Pap test.

PT Instruct the patient to empty her bladder.

PT Tell the patient that no fasting or sedation is required.

During

- Note the following procedural steps:
  1. The patient is placed in the lithotomy position.
  2. A vaginal speculum is inserted to expose the cervix.
  3. Material is collected from the cervical canal.
  4. The specimen can be immediately wiped across a clean glass slide and fixed or placed in the fixative preservative solution.
  5. The specimen is labeled with the patient's name, age, and parity and with the date of her last menstrual period.
- Note that a Pap smear is obtained by a nurse or a physician in approximately 10 minutes.

PT Tell the patient that no discomfort, except for insertion of the speculum, is associated with this procedure.

After

PT Inform the patient that usually she will not be notified unless further evaluation is necessary.

Abnormal findings

Cancer	Infertility
Fungal infection	Parasitic infection
Herpes infection	Reactive inflammatory changes
HPV infection	Sexually transmitted disease

notes

paracentesis (Peritoneal fluid analysis, Ascitic fluid cytology, Peritoneal tap)

Type of test Fluid analysis

Normal findings

Gross appearance: clear, serous, light yellow, < 50 mL
Red blood cells (RBCs): none
White blood cells (WBCs): < 300/μL
Protein: < 4.1 g/dL
Glucose: 70–100 mg/dL
Amylase: 138–404 units/L
Ammonia: < 50 mcg/dL
Alkaline phosphatase
    Adult male: 90–240 units/L
    Female < 45 years: 76–196 units/L
    Female > 45 years: 87–250 units/L
Lactic dehydrogenase (LDH): similar to serum LDH
Cytology: no malignant cells
Bacteria: none
Fungi: none
Carcinoembryonic antigen (CEA): negative

Test explanation and related physiology

Paracentesis is an invasive procedure entailing the insertion of a needle or catheter into the peritoneal cavity (Figure P1) for removal *of* ascitic fluid for diagnostic and therapeutic purposes.

Diagnostically, paracentesis is performed to obtain and analyze fluid to determine the etiology of the peritoneal effusion. Peritoneal fluid is classified as to whether it is a transudate or exudate. This is an important differentiation and is very helpful in determining the etiology of the effusion. *Transudates* are most frequently caused by congestive heart failure, cirrhosis, nephrotic syndrome, myxedema, peritoneal dialysis, and hypoproteinemia. *Exudates* are most often found in infectious or neoplastic conditions.

Therapeutically, this procedure is done to remove large amounts of fluid from the abdominal cavity.

Contraindications

- Patients with coagulation or bleeding abnormalities
- Patients with only a small amount of fluid and extensive previous abdominal surgery

P

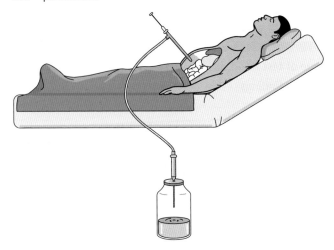

FIG. P1 Paracentesis. A catheter is placed through the skin and abdominal muscle wall and into the peritoneal cavity containing free fluid.

Potential complications
- Hypovolemia if a large volume of peritoneal fluid is removed
- Peritonitis

Procedure and patient care

Before
- PT Explain the procedure to the patient.
- Obtain informed consent for this procedure.
- PT Tell the patient that no fasting or sedation is necessary.
- PT Have the patient empty the bladder before the test.
- Measure abdominal girth.
- Obtain the patient's weight and baseline vital signs.

During
- Note the following procedural steps:
  1. Place the patient in a high Fowler position in bed.
  2. Paracentesis is performed under a strict sterile technique.
  3. Access to the abdominal fluid is obtained by a needle/ catheter attached to a collection device.
- Note that this procedure is performed by a physician. Usually the volume removed is limited to about 4 L at any one time to avoid hypovolemia if the ascites is rapidly reaccumulated.

PT Although local anesthetics eliminate pain at the insertion site, tell the patient that he or she will feel a pressure-like discomfort as the needle is inserted.

After

- Place a small bandage over the needle site.
- Observe the puncture site for bleeding, continued drainage, or signs of inflammation.
- Measure the abdominal girth and weight of the patient; compare with baseline values.
- Monitor vital signs for evidence of hemodynamic changes.
- Occasionally ascitic fluid will continue to leak out of the needle tract after removal of the needle. A suture can stop that. If unsuccessful, a collection bag should be used.

Abnormal findings

Exudate	Transudate
Carcinoma	Abdominal trauma
Lymphoma	Congestive heart failure
Pancreatitis	Hepatic cirrhosis
Peritonitis	Hypoproteinemia
Ruptured viscus	Nephrotic syndrome
Tuberculosis	Peritoneal bleeding
	Portal hypertension

notes

parathyroid hormone (PTH, Parathormone)

Type of test Blood

Normal findings

Intact (whole): 10–65 pg/mL or 10–65 ng/L (SI units)
N terminal: 8–24 pg/mL
C terminal: 50–330 pg/mL

Test explanation and related physiology

This test is useful in establishing a diagnosis of hyperparathyroidism and distinguishing nonparathyroid from parathyroid causes of hypercalcemia. Increased PTH levels are seen in patients with hyperparathyroidism (primary, secondary, or tertiary); in patients with nonparathyroid, ectopic PTH-producing tumors (pseudohyperparathyroidism); or as a normal compensatory response to hypocalcemia in patients with malabsorption or vitamin D deficiency.

It is important to measure serum calcium simultaneous with the measurement of PTH. Most laboratories have a PTH/calcium nomogram, indicating what PTH level is considered normal for each calcium level.

Decreased PTH levels are seen in patients with hypoparathyroidism or as a compensatory response to hypercalcemia in patients with metastatic bone tumors, sarcoidosis, vitamin D intoxication, or milk-alkali syndrome. Surgical ablation of the parathyroids is another cause of hypoparathyroidism.

Procedure and patient care

- See inside front cover for Routine Blood Testing.
- Fasting: yes
- Blood tube commonly used: red
- Obtain a morning blood specimen, because diurnal rhythm affects PTH levels. (Check with the laboratory if the patient works at night.)
- Note that some laboratories require blood in an iced plastic syringe.
- Obtain a serum calcium level determination at the same time if ordered. Serum PTH and serum calcium levels are important in the differential diagnosis.
- Indicate the time the blood was drawn on the laboratory slip because a diurnal rhythm affects test results.

Abnormal findings

▲ **Increased levels**
  Chronic renal failure
  Congenital renal defect
  Hyperparathyroidism
    secondary to adenoma
    or carcinoma of the
    parathyroid gland
  Hypocalcemia
  Kidney carcinoma
  Lung carcinoma
  Malabsorption syndrome
  Non–PTH-producing
    tumors (paraneoplastic
    syndrome)
  Osteomalacia
  Rickets
  Vitamin D deficiency

▼ **Decreased levels**
  Autoimmune destruction of
    the parathyroid glands
  DiGeorge syndrome
  Graves disease
  Hypercalcemia
  Hypomagnesemia
  Hypoparathyroidism
  Metastatic bone tumor
  Milk-alkali syndrome
  Sarcoidosis
  Vitamin D intoxication

notes

P

parathyroid scan (Parathyroid scintigraphy)

Type of test   Nuclear medicine

Normal findings

No increased parathyroid uptake

Test explanation and related physiology

Hypercalcemia can be caused by hyperparathyroidism. Parathyroid hyperplasia, adenoma, or cancer can cause hyperparathyroidism. Parathyroid hyperplasia causes enlargement of all four parathyroid glands. A parathyroid adenoma or cancer, however, causes enlargement of only one parathyroid gland and suppression of the other three glands.

Parathyroids are located most commonly on the lateral borders of the thyroid lobes—two on each side. However, parathyroid anatomic location varies considerably, and they may be located anywhere from the upper neck to the lower mediastinum. Parathyroid scanning is also done immediately before surgery to help the surgeon identify the parathyroid glands and particularly the pathologic glands. In this test, the scan is performed on the parathyroid glands. In the operating room, if the preoperative scan result is abnormal, the surgeon scans the suspect area of the neck with a hand-held gamma ray detector probe. Increased counts are noted in the regions where the parathyroid abnormalities are located.

Contraindications

• Patients who are pregnant

Interfering factors

• Patient movement can alter the quality of the image.
• Recent administration of x-ray contrast material can alter results.
• Iodine-containing foods or drugs can affect results.

Procedure and patient care

Before

PT Explain the procedure to the patient. See p. xviii for radiation exposure and risks.

PT Tell the patient that fasting is usually not required.

During

- Note the following procedural steps for the single tracer double phase (STDP) method.
  1. Technetium-99m sestamibi is injected intravenously.
  2. At 15 minutes and 3 hours, the patient is placed in a supine position. For planar images, the detector is passed over the neck and upper chest area, and the radioactive counts are recorded and displayed.
  3. For SPECT/computed tomography (CT) screening, the patient is placed in the appropriate unit in the supine position.
  4. Initially, the tracer lights up both the thyroid and parathyroid glands. At 3 hours, the tracer remains only in the pathologic parathyroid tissue.
- Note that this study is performed by a technologist and interpreted by a physician in the nuclear medicine department.

PT Tell the patient that no discomfort is associated with testing.

After

PT Assure the patient that the dose of radioactive technetium used in this test is minute and therefore harmless.

Abnormal findings

Aberrantly placed parathyroid tissue in the upper neck, thyroid gland, or mediastinum
Parathyroid adenoma, carcinoma, or hyperplasia

notes

P

Parkinson disease testing

Type of test Microscopic

Normal findings

No peripheral synucleinopathy

Test explanation and related physiology

Synucleinopathy refers to any degenerative disease of the central nervous system in which there is an excessive accumulation of alpha-synuclein (SSA) in the neurons. The synucleinopathies include Parkinson disease (PD), dementia with Lewy bodies, and multiple system atrophy. This test is used to support the diagnosis of PD.

Increased levels of SSA can be detected in the CSF of patients with early Parkinson disease with seed amplification assay.

The DaT scan (Ioflupane I-123) is another method to aid in the diagnosis of PD. This SPECT scan uses a radiopharmaceutical that can visualize striatal dopamine transporters and its function. After intravenous (IV) injection, Ioflupane I-123 reversibly binds to the presynaptic dopamine transporter (DaT) in the striatum and is visualized using single photon emission computed tomography (SPECT). DaT is reduced 50% to 70% in patients with PD. When combined with olfactory testing such as the University of Pennsylvania Smell Identification Test (UPSIT-40) (because most patients with PD lose some sense of smell), the diagnosis of PD can be more strongly confirmed with fewer patients falsely diagnosed as having PD.

Potential complications

- Submandibular gland bleeding, swelling, and inflammation

Procedure and patient care

Before

PT Explain the procedure to the patient.
- Tell the patient no fasting is required

During

- Local anesthesia is used to numb the neck area.
- An otolaryngologist inserts a needle through the skin into the submandibular gland. Three to six needle core biopsies are obtained.

After

- A dressing is applied to the neck area.
- Check the site for bleeding.

Abnormal findings

PD

notes

partial thromboplastin time, activated (APTT, Partial thromboplastin time [PTT])

Type of test Blood

Normal findings

APTT: 30–40 seconds
PTT: 60–70 seconds
Patients receiving anticoagulant therapy: 1.5–2.5 times the control value in seconds

Possible critical values

APTT: > 70 seconds
PTT: > 100 seconds

Test explanation and related physiology

The PTT test is used to assess the intrinsic system and the common pathway of clot formation. PTT evaluates factors I (fibrinogen), II (prothrombin), V, VIII, IX, X, XI, and XII. When any of these factors exist in inadequate quantities, such as in hemophilia A and B or consumptive coagulopathy, PTT is prolonged. Because factors II, IX, and X are vitamin K-dependent factors, biliary obstruction, which precludes GI absorption of fat and fat-soluble vitamins (e.g., vitamin K), can reduce their concentration and thus prolong PTT. Because coagulation factors are made in the liver, hepatocellular diseases will also prolong PTT.

Heparin has been found to inactivate prothrombin (factor II) and prevent the formation of thromboplastin. These actions prolong the intrinsic clotting pathway for approximately 4 to 6 hours after each dose of heparin. Thus heparin is capable of providing therapeutic anticoagulation. The appropriate dose of heparin can be monitored by PTT. Test results are given in seconds, along with a control value.

Activators have been added to PTT test reagents to shorten normal clotting time and provide a narrow normal range. This shortened time is called the *activated* PTT (APTT). Desired ranges for therapeutic anticoagulation are 1.5 to 2.5 times normal (e.g., 70 seconds). The APTT specimen should be drawn 30 to 60 minutes before the patient's next heparin dose is given. If the APTT is less than 50 seconds, the patient may not be receiving therapeutic anticoagulation and need more heparin. An APTT greater than 100 seconds indicates that too much heparin is being given; the risk of serious spontaneous bleeding exists when the APTT is this high. The effects of heparin can be reversed immediately by the administration of protamine sulfate.

APTT is also used to determine *activated protein C (APC) resistance* (p. 325). APC resistance testing is performed in the evaluation of thrombotic patients. A standard APTT test is performed first in the absence of, and then in the presence of, commercially available APC. The APTT is normally prolonged in the presence of APC because of APC's anticoagulant inhibiting coagulation factors VIII and V. An abnormality is detected if the APTT is not prolonged. This results from a resistance to APC, most commonly (80%) caused by an abnormal factor V Leiden.

Procedure and patient care

- See inside front cover for Routine Blood Testing.
- Fasting: no
- Blood tube commonly used: blue
- If the patient is receiving heparin by intermittent injection, plan to draw the blood specimen for the APTT 30 minutes to 1 hour before the next dose of heparin.
- If the patient is receiving continuous heparin, draw the blood at any time.
- Apply pressure to the venipuncture site.
- Assess the patient to detect possible bleeding. Check for blood in the urine and all other excretions and assess the patient for bruises, petechiae, and low back pain.

Abnormal findings

▲ **Increased levels**
Acquired or congenital
clotting factor deficiencies
(e.g., hypofibrinogenemia,
von Willebrand disease,
and hemophilia)
Cirrhosis of the liver
Disseminated intravascular
coagulation (DIC)
Heparin administration
Vitamin K deficiency

▼ **Decreased levels**
Early stages of DIC
Extensive cancer

notes

pepsinogen

Type of test Blood/urine

Normal findings

Pepsinogen I: 28–100 ng/ml
Pepsinogen II: < 22 ng/mL

Test explanation and related physiology

Pepsinogens are secreted in the stomach and are made in the oxyntic gland mucosa of the proximal stomach. When exposed to gastric acid, pepsinogen is converted to pepsin, an active enzyme that is proteolytic and promotes digestion. Patients with gastric atrophy or pernicious anemia (PA) or those who have had a gastrectomy have low levels of pepsinogen I. Pepsinogen I levels are elevated in patients with ulcer disease. Pepsinogen I has been used as a subclinical marker of increased risk for stomach cancer. Pepsinogen I can also be measured in the urine.

Pepsinogen II is made by oxyntic gland mucosa cells that are in the distal stomach and proximal duodenum. Because PA generally affects the proximal stomach, diminished levels of pepsinogen I with normal levels of pepsinogen II are strongly supportive of PA.

Procedure and patient care

- See inside front cover for Routine Blood Testing.
- Fasting: yes
- Blood tube commonly used: red
- PT Tell the patient that antacids or other medications affecting stomach acidity or GI motility should be discontinued, if possible, for at least 48 hours before collection. Verify with the laboratory or health-care provider.

Abnormal findings

▼ **Decreased values**

Chronic gastritis
Gastric atrophy
Peptic ulcer disease
Pernicious anemia

notes

pericardiocentesis (Pericardial tap)

Type of test   Fluid analysis

Normal findings

Less than 50 mL of clear, straw-colored fluid without evidence of any bacteria, blood, or malignant cells

Test explanation and related physiology

Pericardiocentesis, which involves the aspiration of fluid from the pericardial sac with a needle, may be performed for therapeutic and diagnostic purposes. Therapeutically, the test is performed to relieve cardiac tamponade by removing fluid and improving diastolic filling. Diagnostically, pericardiocentesis is performed to remove a sample of pericardial fluid for laboratory examination to determine the cause of the fluid. This is similar to the evaluation described for peritoneal and pleural fluid (p. 549 and p. 705, respectively).

Contraindications

- Patients who are uncooperative because of the risk of lacerations to the epicardium or coronary artery
- Patients with a bleeding disorder. Inadvertent puncture of the myocardium may create bleeding, leading to tamponade.

Potential complications

- Laceration of the coronary artery or myocardium
- Liver laceration caused by inadvertent puncture
- Myocardial infarction
- Needle-induced ventricular arrhythmias
- Pleural infection
- Pneumothorax caused by inadvertent puncture of the lung
- Vasovagal arrest

Procedure and patient care

Before

PT Explain the procedure to the patient.
- Obtain informed consent for this procedure.
- Restrict fluid and food intake for 4 hours (if possible).
- Obtain IV access for infusion of fluids, sedation, and cardiac medications if required.

During

- Note the following procedural steps:
  1. With the patient in the supine position, a needle is inserted into the pericardium after local anesthesia.
  2. An electrocardiographic lead is often attached by a clip to the needle to identify any ST-segment elevations.
  3. Pericardial fluid is aspirated.
  4. Some patients who have recurring cardiac tamponade may require placement of an indwelling pericardial catheter.
  5. With certain types of pericarditis, medications (e.g., antibiotics, antineoplastic drugs, corticosteroids) may be instilled during pericardiocentesis.
- Note that a physician usually performs this procedure in the cardiac catheterization laboratory, operating room, or emergency department in approximately 10 to 20 minutes.
- **PT** Tell the patient that this procedure is associated with very little discomfort.

After

- Closely monitor the patient's vital signs. An increased temperature may indicate infection. Pericardial bleeding would be marked by hypotension or pulsus paradoxus.
- Check the dressing frequently for drainage.
- Label and number the specimen tubes that contain the pericardial fluid and send them to the appropriate laboratories for examination.
- Apply a sterile dressing to the catheter if one has been left for continuing pericardial drainage.
- Establish a closed system if continued pericardial drainage is required.
- Note that to minimize infection, pericardial catheters, if used, are usually removed after 2 days.

Abnormal findings

Blunt or penetrating cardiac trauma	Metastatic cancer
Collagen vascular diseases	Pericarditis
Congestive heart failure	Rupture of ventricular aneurysm
Hypoproteinemia	Uremia

notes

pheochromocytoma suppression and provocative testing (Clonidine suppression test [CST], Glucagon stimulation test)

Type of test Blood

Normal findings

Glucagon stimulation

    Norepinephrine: < 3 times basal levels

Clonidine suppression

    Norepinephrine: > 50% reduction in basal levels or < 500 pg/mL

    Epinephrine: > 50% reduction in basal levels or < 275 pg/mL

    Normetanephrine > 40% reduction in basal levels.

Test explanation and related physiology

In patients with significantly high blood pressure refractory to treatment, the diagnosis of pheochromocytoma or paraganglioma are often considered. When catecholamine levels are excessive (norepinephrine > 2000 pg/mL), the diagnosis is easily made. However, when basal levels are not significantly elevated, it is difficult to differentiate essential hypertension (or other causes of elevated catecholamines) from a functioning pheochromocytoma.

Suppression and provocative tests may be necessary after repeating the testing of blood or urine for other catecholamines. Glucagon can be used as the provocative agent. In patients with pheochromocytoma, the response is accentuated. However, glucagon stimulation offers insufficient diagnostic sensitivity for reliable exclusion or confirmation of pheochromocytoma. Because of this and the risk of hypertensive complications, the test is not routinely used.

More commonly biochemical and radiologic testing is used instead of provocative testing. Clonidine is normally a potent suppressor of catecholamine production, yet it has little to no effect on catecholamines in patients with pheochromocytoma. Testing of metanephrines (p. 508) provides higher diagnostic sensitivity than catecholamine assays in screening for pheochromocytoma. In suppression testing, normetanephrine is the most accurate biochemical to test.

Contraindications

- Hypovolemic/dehydrated patients. Suppression testing may cause a precipitous drop in blood pressure.

Potential complications
- Drowsiness during CST
- Hypotension during CST, especially in patients treated aggressively for hypertension
- Extremely high blood pressure during provocative testing

Procedure and patient care

Before

PT Explain the procedure to the patient.
- Identify the medications being administered before testing.
- The patient must be reclining calmly for 30 minutes before testing.
- The patient must be fasting for at least 10 hours.

During
- Collect a venous blood sample from an antecubital vein in a heparinized tube for determination of basal catecholamine levels.
- Monitor vital signs closely throughout the testing period.

Glucagon provocative test
- Administer a prescribed dose of glucagon intravenously.
- Two minutes later, obtain a blood specimen as described above.

Clonidine suppression test
- Administer a prescribed dose of clonidine orally.
- Three hours later, obtain a blood specimen as described earlier. Place specimen in ice.

After
- Monitor vital signs for at least 1 hour after conclusion of the procedure.

P

Abnormal findings

Pheochromocytoma

notes

phosphate (PO₄, Phosphorus [P])

Type of test Blood

Normal findings

Adult: 3–4.5 mg/dL or 0.97–1.45 mmol/L (SI units)
Elderly: values slightly lower than adult
Child: 4.5–6.5 mg/dL or 1.45–2.1 mmol/L (SI units)
Newborn: 4.3–9.3 mg/dL or 1.4–3 mmol/L (SI units)

Possible critical values

< 1 mg/dL

Test explanation and related physiology

Phosphorus in the body exists in the form of a phosphate. The terms *phosphorus* and *phosphate* are used interchangeably throughout this and other discussions. Most of the phosphate in the body is a part of organic compounds. Only a small part of total body phosphate is inorganic phosphate (i.e., not part of another organic compound). It is the *inorganic* phosphate that is measured when one requests a phosphate, phosphorus, inorganic phosphorus, or inorganic phosphate.

Dietary phosphorus is absorbed in the small bowel. The absorption is very efficient, and only rarely is hypophosphatemia caused by GI malabsorption. Phosphorus levels are determined by calcium metabolism, parathormone (PTH), renal excretion, and, to a lesser degree, intestinal absorption. Because an inverse relationship exists between calcium and phosphorus, a decrease of one mineral results in an increase in the other. The regulation of phosphate by PTH is such that PTH tends to decrease phosphate resorption in the kidney. PTH and vitamin D, however, tend to stimulate phosphate absorption weakly within the gut.

Interfering factors

- Laxatives or enemas containing sodium phosphate can *increase* phosphorus levels.
- Recent carbohydrate ingestion, including IV glucose administration, causes *decreased* phosphorus levels because phosphorus enters the cell with glucose.

Procedure and patient care

- See inside front cover for Routine Blood Testing.
- Fasting: yes
- Blood tube commonly used: red

- If indicated, discontinue IV fluids with glucose for several hours before the test.
- Use a heel stick to draw blood from infants.

Abnormal findings

▲ **Increased levels (hyperphosphatemia)**

Acidosis
Acromegaly
Advanced lymphoma or myeloma
Bone metastasis
Hemolytic anemia
Hypocalcemia
Hypoparathyroidism
Increased dietary or IV intake of phosphorus
Liver disease
Renal failure
Rhabdomyolysis
Sarcoidosis

▼ **Decreased levels (hypophosphatemia)**

Alkalosis
Chronic alcoholism
Chronic antacid ingestion
Diabetic acidosis
Hypercalcemia
Hyperinsulinism
Hyperparathyroidism
Inadequate dietary ingestion of phosphorus
Malnutrition
Osteomalacia (adult)
Rickets (childhood)
Sepsis (gram negative)
Vitamin D deficiency

notes

P

phosphatidylinositol antigen (PI-Linked antigen)

Type of test Blood

Normal findings

RBCs
> Type I (normal expression): 99%-100%
> Type II (partial deficient): 0.00%-0.99%
> Type III (deficient): 0.00%-0.01%

Granulocytes: 0.00%-0.01%

Monocytes: 0.00%-0.05%

Test explanation and related physiology

Paroxysmal nocturnal hemoglobinuria (PNH) is an acquired hematologic disorder characterized by nocturnal hemoglobinuria, chronic hemolytic anemia, thrombosis, pancytopenia, and, in some patients, acute or chronic myeloid malignancies. PNH appears to be a hematopoietic stem cell disorder that affects erythroid, granulocytic, and megakaryocytic cell lines. The abnormal cells in PNH have been shown to lack glycosylphosphatidylinositol (GPI)-linked proteins in RBCs and WBCs. Mutations in the *phosphatidylinositol glycan A (PIGA)* gene have been identified consistently in patients with PNH, thus confirming the biological defect in this disorder.

Flow cytometric immunophenotyping of peripheral blood (WBC and RBC) is performed to evaluate the presence or absence of PI-linked antigens (CD14, FLAER, and/or CD59 antigens), using monoclonal antibodies directed against them. These proteins are absent on the blood cells of patients with PNH. Determination of PI-linked antigens is not only useful in the diagnosis of PNH but also in monitoring of the disease.

Procedure and patient care

- See inside front cover for Routine Blood Testing.
- Fasting: no
- Blood tube commonly used: yellow

Abnormal findings

▼ **Decreased levels**
> PNH

notes

phospholipase A2 receptor antibodies (Anti-pla2r)

Type of test Blood

Normal findings

Negative: < 14 RU/mL
Borderline: 14–19 RU/mL
Positive: ≥ 20 RU/mL

Test explanation and related physiology

   Membranous nephropathy (MN) is a rare disease in which immune complexes deposit at the glomerular basement membrane, causing damage to the filtration barrier, resulting in proteinuria and nephrotic syndrome. Nearly 70% of patients with primary MN (pMN) have autoantibodies directed against the phospholipase A2 receptor (PLA2R). There is also evidence that levels of anti-PLA2R autoantibodies correlate well with disease activity and progression. The presence of anti-PLA2R antibodies can be used to differentiate pMN from other causes of nephrotic syndrome (or secondary membranous nephropathy). Among patients awaiting kidney transplantation, higher levels of anti-PLA2R could predict those more likely for recurrence of pMN after transplantation. Furthermore, successful treatment of pMN will result in reduced PLA2R antibodies. An increase in antibodies would indicate a worsening of the disease.

Procedure and patient care

- See inside front cover for Routine Blood Testing.
- Fasting: no
- Blood tube commonly used: red

P

Abnormal findings

Primary membranous nephropathy (pMN)

notes

phospholipid antibodies (aPL antibodies, aPLA, Anticardiolipin antibodies [aCL Antibodies], ACA, Cardiolipin antibodies, Antiphospholipid antibodies, Beta-2 glycoprotein 1 antibody, Lupus anticoagulant [LA])

Type of test   Blood

Normal findings
Anticardiolipin antibodies
> < 23 GPL (IgG phospholipid units)
> < 11 MPL (IgM phospholipid units)

Beta-2 glycoprotein 1 antibody (IgG and IgM)
> < 15.0 U/mL (negative)
> 15.0–39.9 U/mL (weakly positive)
> 40.0–79.9 U/mL (positive)
> ≥ 80 U/mL (strongly positive)

Test explanation and related physiology
This test is used to diagnose *antiphospholipid syndrome* (APS). APS (*Hughes syndrome*) is characterized by venous or arterial thrombosis and/or adverse pregnancy outcomes (later term miscarriage) in the presence of persistent laboratory evidence of positive antiphospholipid antibodies. APS occurs either as a primary condition or in the setting of an underlying disease, usually systemic lupus erythematosus (SLE).

Antiphospholipid autoantibodies include aCLA, beta-2 glycoprotein 1 antibody, and LA. When the beta-2 GP1 antibody inhibits clot formation in functional coagulation assays, the antibody is called a *lupus anticoagulant* (LA). Antiphospholipid autoantibodies attach to phospholipids of cell membranes and platelets (cardiolipin and glycoproteins). LA will prolong activated partial thromboplastin and prothrombin times. These antibodies can be IgG or IgM immunoglobulins. aPLA can also be seen as a transient finding following infection, drugs (e.g., propranolol, some antibiotics, phenothiazines), or other acute illness. APS may occur with otherwise unexplained mild thrombocytopenia, the prolongation of a blood coagulation test (e.g., activated partial thromboplastin time [aPTT]), or a history of a false-positive serologic test for syphilis [oftentimes uses cardiolipin as an antigen]. In patients with initial positive testing for aPLA, testing should be repeated after at least 12 weeks to confirm persistence of the aCLA, anti-beta2-GPI, or LA test. aPLA may be considered normal in elderly persons.

Interfering factors

- Patients who have or had syphilis infections can have a false-positive result.
- Transient antibodies can occur in patients with infections, AIDS, inflammation, autoimmune diseases, or cancer.

Procedure and patient care

- See inside front cover for Routine Blood Testing.
- Fasting: no
- Blood tube commonly used: Verify with laboratory.

Abnormal findings

▲ **Increased levels**

Acute infection
Elderly persons
Recurrent fetal loss
Syphilis
Systemic lupus erythematosus
Thrombocytopenia
Thrombosis

notes

P

placental growth factor (PGF)

Type of test Blood

Normal findings

Nonpregnant women: < 50 pg/mL
Pregnant women at 22 weeks' gestation: ≥ 200 pg/mL

Test explanation and related physiology

Preeclampsia is one of the most common medical complications of pregnancy and is associated with considerable maternal and neonatal morbidity and mortality. PGF is a protein that is produced during pregnancy by the placental trophoblast. Normally, PGF rises steadily throughout pregnancy to levels exceeding 500 pg/mL. When PGF is tested at 13 to 16 weeks of gestation and it is found to be significantly decreased, the patient is at considerable risk for preeclampsia. Likewise, patients with markedly increased levels of soluble fms-like tyrosine kinase-1 (sFlt-1), which is a known inhibitor of PGF, are also at risk for preeclampsia.

Preeclampsia can be predicted by a combination of factors in the maternal history, including black racial origin, high body mass index, family history of preeclampsia, and personal history of preeclampsia. Screening at risk women with PGF, sFlt-1, PAPP-A (p. 600), and uterine artery Doppler would identify women who would develop early and late preeclampsia. Intensive maternal and fetal monitoring could improve pregnancy outcomes.

Procedure and patient care

- See inside front cover for Routine Blood Testing.
- Fasting: no
- Blood tube commonly used: red

Abnormal findings

▼ **Decreased blood levels**

Hypertension
Preeclampsia

notes

plasminogen (Fibrinolysin)

Type of test Blood

Normal findings

2.4–4.4 Committee on Thrombolytic Agents (CTA) units/mL

Test explanation and related physiology

This test is used to diagnose suspected plasminogen deficiency in patients who have multiple thromboembolic episodes. Plasminogen is a protein involved in the fibrinolytic process of intravascular blood clot dissolution (see Figure C3, p. 212). Plasminogen is converted to plasmin by proteolytic cleavage. Plasmin can destroy fibrin and dissolve clots.

Plasminogen levels are occasionally measured during fibrinolytic therapy (for coronary and peripheral arterial occlusion) and are diminished with full fibrinolysis. Decreased levels of plasminogen are also found in hyperfibrinolytic states. Because plasminogen is made in the liver, patients with cirrhosis or other severe liver diseases can be expected to have decreased levels. Inflammatory conditions may have mild elevations of plasminogens.

Interfering factors

• Pregnancy and eclampsia are associated with elevations.

Procedure and patient care

• See inside front cover for Routine Blood Testing.
• Fasting: no
• Blood tube commonly used: blue

Abnormal findings

▲ **Increased levels**
  Inflammatory conditions
  Pregnancy

▼ **Decreased levels**
  Hyperfibrinolytic state
    (e.g., DIC, fibrinolysis)
  Malnutrition
  Primary liver disease
  Rare congenital
    deficiencies
  Syndrome associated with
    hypercoagulation

notes

plasminogen activator inhibitor 1 antigen/activity (PAI-1)

Type of test   Blood

Normal findings
Antigen assay: 2–46 ng/mL
Activity: < 31.1 IU/mL

Test explanation and related physiology

PAI-1 is a protein that inhibits plasminogen activators (see p. 572). During fibrinolysis, tissue plasminogen activator (tPA) converts plasminogen into plasmin. Plasmin plays a critical role in fibrinolysis by degrading fibrin (see Figure C3, p. 212). PAI-1 is the primary inhibitor of tPA and urokinase plasminogen activator (uPA) in the blood. PAI-1 limits the production of plasmin and keeps fibrinolysis in check.

Elevated levels of PAI-1 are associated with a predisposition to thrombosis, including veno-occlusive disease after bone marrow transplantation or high-dose chemotherapy. Familial thrombosis has been associated with inherited elevation of plasma PAI-1 activity. Increased levels of PAI-1 have also been reported in a number of conditions, including malignancy, liver disease, the postoperative period, septic shock, the second and third trimesters of pregnancy, obesity, coronary heart disease, and restenosis after coronary angioplasty. Increased levels may reduce the effectiveness of antithrombolytic therapy. Patients with insulin resistance syndrome and diabetes mellitus tend to have increased PAI-1 levels.

Low plasma levels of the active form of PAI-1 have been associated with abnormal, clinically significant bleeding. Complete deficiency of PAI-1, either congenital or acquired, is associated with bleeding manifestations that include hemarthroses, hematomas, menorrhagia, easy bruising, and postoperative hemorrhage.

Interfering factors

- Because PAI-1 is an acute-phase reactant, it can become transiently elevated by infection, inflammation, or trauma.
- Levels increase during pregnancy.
- PAI-1 has a circadian rhythm, with the highest concentrations occurring in the morning and the lowest concentrations in the afternoon and evening.

Procedure and patient care

- See inside front cover for Routine Blood Testing.
- Fasting: no
- Blood tube commonly used: light blue
- Discard the first several milliliters of blood if PAI-1 is the only test being drawn. If multiple tests are being drawn, fill the light blue-top tube after any red-top tube.
- Gently invert the blood tube several times after collection.

Abnormal findings

▲ **Increased levels**

Acute coronary syndrome
Coronary artery disease
Diabetes mellitus
Infection
Inflammation
Insulin resistance syndrome
Pregnancy
Restenosis after coronary
  angioplasty
Trauma

▼ **Decreased levels**

Bleeding disorders

notes

P

platelet aggregation test (Ristocetin test)

Type of test   Blood

Normal findings

Dependent on the platelet agonist used

Test explanation and related physiology

Platelet aggregation is an important part of hemostasis. Surrounding an area of acute blood vessel endothelial injury is a clump of platelets. Normal platelets adhere to this area of injury, and through a series of chemical reactions, they attract other platelets to the area. This is platelet aggregation, the first step of hemostasis. After this step, the normal coagulation factor waterfall occurs (see Figure C3, p. 212).

Certain diseases that affect either platelet number or function can inhibit platelet aggregation and prolong bleeding times. If blood is passed through a heart–lung or dialysis pump, platelet injury can occur and reduce aggregation.

Ristocetin is most commonly used to induce platelet agglutination. The agglutination of the patient's blood with the addition of this type of product can help differentiate the disease that may be affecting platelet aggregation.

Interfering factors

- Factors that may cause *increased* platelet aggregation include blood storage temperature, hyperbilirubinemia, hemoglobinemia, hyperlipidemia, and platelet count.

Procedure and patient care

- See inside front cover for Routine Blood Testing.
- Fasting: no
- Blood tube commonly used: blue
- Abnormalities in platelet aggregation can prolong bleeding time, and hematoma at the venipuncture site may occur.

Abnormal findings

Hypoactive platelet aggregation

Various congenital disorders (e.g., Wiskott–Aldrich syndrome, Bernard–Soulier syndrome, glycogen storage, some types of von Willebrand disease)

notes

platelet antibody (Antiplatelet antibody detection)

Type of test Blood

Normal findings

No antiplatelet antibodies identified

Test explanation and related physiology

Immune-mediated destruction of platelets may be caused either by autoantibodies directed against antigens located on the same person's platelets or by alloantibodies that develop after exposure to transfused platelets received from a donor. These antibodies are usually directed to an antigen on the platelet membrane, such as *human lymphocyte antigen (HLA)* (p. 427) or *platelet-specific antigens,* such as *PLA1* and *PLA2.*

Antibodies directed to platelets cause early destruction of the platelets and subsequent thrombocytopenia. Immunologic thrombocytopenia includes the following:

- *Idiopathic thrombocytopenia purpura (ITP).* Platelet-associated IgG antibodies are detected in most of these patients.
- *Posttransfusion purpura.* This is usually associated with an antibody to ABO, HLA, or PLA antigens on the RBC.
- *Maternal–fetal platelet antigen incompatibility (neonatal thrombocytopenia).* This occurs when the fetal platelet contains a PLA1 antigen that is absent in the mother. Neonatal thrombocytopenia can also occur if the mother has ITP autoantibodies that are passed through the placenta and destroy the fetal platelets.
- *Drug-induced thrombocytopenia.* Although a host of drugs are known to induce autoimmune-mediated thrombocytopenia, heparin is the most common and causes heparin-induced thrombocytopenia (HIT). The diagnosis of HIT is confirmed by identifying *heparin-induced thrombocytopenia antibodies (HITAs).*

Other drugs known to cause antiplatelet antibodies include analgesics, antibiotics, cimetidine, diuretics, heavy metals, hypnotics, oral hypoglycemic agents, quinidine-like drugs, and many others.

Interfering factors

- Blood transfusion may cause the development of isoantibodies to HLA antigens on the platelets or RBCs.

Procedure and patient care

- See inside front cover for Routine Blood Testing.
- Fasting: no
- Blood tube commonly used: red

Abnormal findings

▲ **Increased levels**

Drug-induced thrombocytopenia
HIT
Idiopathic thrombocytopenia purpura
Neonatal thrombocytopenia
Paroxysmal hemoglobinuria
Posttransfusion purpura

notes

platelet count (Thrombocyte count)

Type of test Blood

Normal findings

Adult/elderly: 150,000–400,000/mm³ or 150–400 × 10⁹/L (SI units)
Child: 150,000–400,000/mm³
Infant: 200,000–475,000/mm³
Newborn: 150,000–300,000/mm³
Premature infant: 100,000–300,000/mm³

Possible critical values

< 50,000 or > 1 million/mm³

Test explanation and related physiology

The platelet count is a count of the number of platelets (thrombocytes) per cubic milliliter of blood. It is performed on patients who develop petechiae (small hemorrhages in the skin), spontaneous bleeding, or increasingly heavy menses. It is also used to monitor the course of the disease or therapy for thrombocytopenia or bone marrow failure.

Platelet activity is essential to blood clotting. Counts of less than 100,000/mm³ are generally considered to indicate *thrombocytopenia; thrombocytosis (thrombocythemia)* is generally said to exist when counts are greater than 400,000/mm³. Common associative diseases with thrombocytosis are iron-deficiency anemia and malignancy (leukemia, lymphoma, or solid tumors, such as those involving the colon). Thrombocytosis may also occur with polycythemia vera, postsplenectomy syndromes, and a variety of acute/chronic infections or inflammatory processes.

Causes of thrombocytopenia (decreased number of platelets) include the following:

- Reduced production of platelets (secondary to bone marrow failure or infiltration of fibrosis, tumor, and so on)
- Sequestration of platelets (secondary to hypersplenism)
- Accelerated destruction of platelets (secondary to, for example, drugs)
- Consumption of platelets (secondary to DIC)
- Platelet loss from hemorrhage
- Dilution with large volumes of blood transfusions

Interfering factors

- Living at high altitudes may cause increased platelet levels.

- Because platelets can clump together, automated counting is subject to at least a 10% to 15% error.
- Strenuous exercise may cause increased levels.
- Decreased levels may be seen before menstruation.

Procedure and patient care

- See inside front cover for Routine Blood Testing.
- Fasting: no
- Blood tube commonly used: lavender
- If the results indicate that the patient has a serious platelet deficiency, perform the following steps:
  1. Observe the patient for signs and symptoms of bleeding.
  2. Check for blood in the urine and all excretions.
  3. Assess the patient for bruises, petechiae, bleeding from the gums, epistaxis, and low back pain.
  4. Reassess all venipuncture sites for signs of hematoma formation.

Abnormal findings

▲ **Increased levels (thrombocytosis)**
Iron-deficiency anemia
Malignant disorder
Polycythemia vera
Postsplenectomy
  syndrome
Rheumatoid arthritis

▼ **Decreased levels (thrombocytopenia)**
Acute or chronic infection
Cancer chemotherapy
DIC
Hemorrhage
Hypersplenism
Immune
  thrombocytopenia
Inherited
  thrombocytopenia
  disorders
Leukemia and other
  myelofibrosis disorders
Pernicious anemia
Some hemolytic anemias
Systemic lupus
  erythematosus
Thrombotic
  thrombocytopenia

notes

platelet function assay (Platelet closure time, PCT, Aspirin resistance tests, Bleeding time [BT], 11-Dehydro-thromboxane B2)

Type of test Blood, urine

Normal findings

Platelet closure time (blood)
    Collagen/adenosine-5′-diphosphate (CADP): 64–120 seconds
    Collagen/epinephrine (CEPI): 89–193 seconds
11-Dehydro-thromboxane B2 (urine)
    Males: 0–1089 pg/mg of creatinine
    Females: 0–1811 pg/mg of creatinine
Bleeding time (blood)
    1–9 minutes (Ivy method)

Test explanation and related physiology

Platelet dysfunction may be acquired, inherited, or induced by platelet-inhibiting agents. It is clinically important to assess platelet function as a potential cause of a bleeding diathesis (epistaxis, menorrhagia, postoperative bleeding, or easy bruising). Platelet hyperfunction becomes apparent as thrombotic events. Platelet function is important for the monitoring of modern antiplatelet therapies. The most common causes of decreased platelet function are related to uremia, liver disease, von Willebrand disease (vWD), and exposure to such agents as acetyl salicylic acid (ASA, aspirin). Several tests are used to evaluate platelet function. Platelet counts (see p. 577) and volume are often used as a measure of platelet function.

Measurement of *bleeding time* is an older method of determining function. To determine *bleeding time,* a small standard superficial incision is made in the forearm, and the time required for the bleeding to stop is recorded. The *platelet aggregation studies* (p. 574) using any of the many aggregometers is another method to measure function. With the development of automated platelet function analyzer devices, clinical laboratories can easily measure *platelet closure time (PCT)* to quantify platelet function. PCT can differentiate aspirin affects from other causes of platelet dysfunction. This test can also be used to determine resistance of aspirin's therapeutic anticoagulation effects on platelets. This is one of several *aspirin resistance tests* that are performed to determine the effectiveness of aspirin on inhibiting platelet aggregation and thereby protecting the patient from vascular thromboembolic disease (Table P1).

P

TABLE P1 **Platelet closure time**

	Normal	ASA effect	Intrinsic platelet disorders
CEPI membrane	Normal	Abnormal	Abnormal
CADP membrane	Normal	Normal	Abnormal

ASA, Aspirin; *CADP,* collagen/adenosine-5′-diphosphate; *CEPI,* collagen/ epinephrine.

Aspirin resistance can also be determined by measurement of *11-dehydro-thromboxane B2 (11-dTXB2)* in the urine. Thromboxane A2 is produced by activated platelets and still further stimulates platelet activation, platelet aggregation, and vasoconstriction. 11-dTXB2 is the stable, inactive metabolite of thromboxane A2. Urinary 11-dTXB2, therefore is an indication of platelet activation and aggregation. Elevated values are associated with an increased risk of acute ischemic stroke and myocardial infarction. Effective aspirin therapy should reduce the level of this metabolite in the urine. If not, the patient may be aspirin resistant and may be more safely treated with an alternative therapy such as increasing the dosage of aspirin or placing the patient on another antiplatelet medication.

Interfering factors
- Low hematocrit or platelet count can prolong PCT and BT.

Procedure and patient care
- See inside front cover for Routine Blood Testing.
- Fasting: no
- Blood tube commonly used: light blue
- Obtain a drug history to determine whether the patient has recently had aspirin or any other medications that may affect test results.
- For urinary 11-dTXB2, randomly collect 10 mL of urine. No preservative is necessary. See inside front cover for Routine Urine Testing.

Abnormal findings
▲ **Prolonged times or increased values**
   Intrinsic platelet defects
   Bernard–Soulier syndrome
   Glanzmann thromboasthenia
   Hereditary telangiectasia
   Hermansky–Pudlak syndrome

▲ **Prolonged times or increased values**

Some myelodysplastic syndromes
Some myeloid leukemias
Some myeloproliferative neoplasms

Platelet–blood vessel interaction defects
Cushing syndrome
Henoch–Schönlein syndrome
Uremia
von Willebrand disease

▲ **Elevated B2 (11-dTXB2) (on aspirin therapy)**
Increased risk of thromboembolic disease

notes

P

platelet volume, mean (Mean platelet volume [MPV])

Type of test Blood

Normal findings

7.4–10.4 fL

Test explanation and related physiology

The MPV is a measure of the volume of a large number of platelets determined by an automated analyzer. The MPV varies with total platelet production. In cases of thrombocytopenia, despite normal reactive bone marrow (e.g., hypersplenism), the normal bone marrow releases immature platelets to attempt to maintain a normal platelet count. These immature platelets are larger, and the MPV is elevated. When bone marrow production of platelets is inadequate, the platelets that are released are small. This is reflected as a low MPV; in this way, the MPV is useful in the differential diagnosis of thrombocytopenic disorders.

Procedure and patient care

- See inside front cover for Routine Blood Testing.
- Fasting: no
- Blood tube commonly used: lavender
- If the patient is known to have a low platelet count, perform the following steps:
  1. Observe the patient for signs and symptoms of bleeding.
  2. Check for blood in the urine and all excretions.
  3. Assess the patient for bruises, petechiae, bleeding of the gums, epistaxis, and low back pain.

Abnormal findings

▲ Increased levels

B_{12} or folate deficiency
Immune thrombocytopenia
Massive hemorrhage
Myelogenous leukemia
Valvular heart disease

▼ Decreased levels

Aplastic anemia
Chemotherapy-induced myelosuppression
Wiskott–Aldrich syndrome

notes

plethysmography, arterial (Ankle-brachial index [ABI])

Type of test Manometric

Normal findings

< 20 mm Hg difference in systolic blood pressure of the lower extremity compared with the upper extremity

Normal pulse wave amplitude showing a steep upswing; an acute, narrow peak; and a gentler downslope containing a dicrotic notch (normal arterial pulse wave)

Ankle/brachial ratio: 0.9–1.3

Test explanation and related physiology

Plethysmography is usually performed to rule out occlusive disease of the lower extremities; however, it also can identify arteriosclerotic disease in the upper extremities. This test requires one normal extremity against which the other extremities may be compared.

Arterial plethysmography is performed by applying three blood pressure cuffs to the proximal, middle, and distal parts of an extremity. Pressure readings are also taken in the upper arm (brachial) artery. These are then attached to a pulse volume recorder (plethysmograph), and each pulse wave can be displayed. A reduction in amplitude of a pulse wave in any of the three cuffs indicates arterial occlusion immediately proximal to the area where the decreased amplitude is noted. Also, measurements of arterial pressures are performed at each cuff site. A difference in pressure of greater than 20 mm Hg indicates a degree of arterial occlusion in the extremity. A positive result is reliable evidence of arteriosclerotic peripheral vascular occlusion. However, a negative result does not definitely exclude this diagnosis because extensive vascular collateralization can compensate for even a complete arterial occlusion.

An ankle/brachial ratio of less than 0.9 indicates peripheral vascular disease in the lower extremity. Arterial plethysmography can also be performed immediately after exercise to determine whether symptoms of claudication are caused by peripheral vascular occlusive disease.

Although it is not as accurate as arteriography (p. 96), plethysmography is performed without serious complications and can be done for extremely ill patients who cannot be transported to the arteriography laboratory.

P

Interfering factors
- Arterial occlusion proximal to the extremity
- Cigarette smoking can cause transient arterial constriction.

Procedure and patient care

Before
- PT Explain the procedure to the patient.
- PT Tell the patient that no fasting is required.
- PT Inform the patient that this test is painless.
- PT Tell the patient that he or she must lie still.
- Remove all clothing from the patient's extremities.
- PT Instruct the patient to avoid smoking for at least 30 minutes before the test.

During
- Note the following procedural steps:
  1. The patient is placed in the semirecumbent position.
  2. The cuffs are applied to the extremities and then inflated to 65 mm Hg to increase their sensitivity to pulse waves.
  3. The pulse waves are recorded on plethysmographic paper.
  4. The amplitudes and form of the pulse wave of each cuff are measured and compared. A marked reduction in wave amplitude indicates arterial occlusive disease.
- This noninvasive test is usually performed in the vascular laboratory or at the patient's bedside by a vascular technologist in approximately 30 minutes.
- PT Inform the patient that results are usually interpreted by a physician and are available in a few hours.

After
- Encourage the patient to verbalize concerns regarding results.

Abnormal findings
Arterial embolization
Arterial occlusive disease
Arterial trauma
Small vessel diabetic changes
Vascular diseases (e.g., Raynaud phenomenon)

notes

pleural biopsy

Type of test Microscopic examination of tissue

Normal findings

No evidence of pathology

Test explanation and related physiology

This test may be indicated when the pleural fluid obtained by thoracentesis (p. 705) is exudative fluid, which suggests infection, neoplasm, or tuberculosis. The pleural biopsy can distinguish among these disease processes. It is also performed when chest imaging indicates a pleural-based tumor, reaction, or thickening.

Pleural biopsy is the removal of pleural tissue for histologic examination. It is usually performed by a percutaneous needle biopsy. It also can be performed via thoracoscopy. Pleural tissue also may be obtained by an *open pleural biopsy*, which involves a limited thoracotomy and requires general anesthesia.

Contraindications

• Patients with prolonged bleeding or clotting times

Potential complications

• Bleeding or injury to the lung
• Pneumothorax

Procedure and patient care

Before

PT Explain the procedure to the patient.
• Obtain informed consent for this procedure.
PT Tell the patient that no fasting or sedation is required unless an open biopsy is needed.
PT Instruct the patient to remain very still during the procedure. Any movement may cause inadvertent needle damage.

During

• Note the following procedural steps for percutaneous needle biopsy:
  1. The procedure for pleural biopsy is very similar to that described in thoracentesis (see p. 705).
  2. A specialized hook biopsy needle is utilized to obtain one to three biopsy specimens of the pleura.

P

- Note that this procedure is performed by a physician at the patient's bedside, in a special procedure room, or in the physician's office in approximately 30 minutes.
- PT Tell the patient that because of the local anesthetic little discomfort is associated with this procedure.

After
- Apply an adhesive bandage to the biopsy site.
- Note that a chest x-ray is usually taken to detect pneumothorax.
- Observe the patient for signs of respiratory distress (e.g., diminished breath sounds) on the side of the biopsy.
- PT Instruct the patient to report any shortness of breath.
- Observe the patient's vital signs frequently for evidence of bleeding (increased pulse, decreased blood pressure).

Abnormal findings

Neoplasm
Tuberculosis

notes

porphyrins and porphobilinogens

Type of test Urine (fresh and 24 hour)

Normal findings

	Male (mcg/24 hr)	Female (mcg/24 hr)
Total porphyrins	8–149	3–78
Uroporphyrin	4–46	3–22
Coproporphyrin	< 96	< 60

Porphobilinogens: 0–2 mg/24 hr or 0–8.8 μmol/day (SI units)

Test explanation and related physiology

This test is a quantitative measurement of porphyrins and porphobilinogens. Along with measurement of aminolevulinic acid (p. 266), the various forms of porphyria can be identified.

Porphyria is a group of genetic disorders associated with enzyme deficiencies involved with porphyrin synthesis or metabolism. Porphyrins (e.g., uroporphyrin and coproporphyrin) and porphobilinogens are important building blocks in the synthesis of heme. Heme is incorporated into hemoglobin in the erythroid cells. In most forms of porphyria, increased levels of porphyrins and porphobilinogens are found in the urine. Heavy metal (lead) intoxication is also associated with increased porphyrins in the urine.

Urine tests for porphyrins are not as accurate as plasma measurements and pattern identification for the various forms of porphyria. They are accurate, however, in screening for porphyria, especially the intermittent variety. Porphyrin fractionation of erythrocytes and plasma provides specific assays for primary RBC porphyrins. These assays are predominantly used to differentiate the various forms of congenital porphyrias. Plasma measurement of *free erythrocyte protoporphyrin (FEP)* is helpful in the diagnosis of iron-deficiency anemia or lead intoxication.

Procedure and patient care

- See inside front cover for Routine Urine Testing for random and 24-hour collection.
- Protect the specimen from light.
- PT Instruct the patient to avoid alcohol during the collection period.

P

- Keep the 24-hour urine in a light-resistant specimen bottle with a preservative to prevent degradation of the light-sensitive porphyrin.
- PT Encourage the patient to drink fluids during the 24 hours unless contraindicated for medical purposes.

Abnormal findings

▲ **Increased levels**

Lead poisoning

Liver disease

Pellagra

Porphyrias

notes

positron emission tomography (PET scan)

Type of test Nuclear scan, x-ray

Normal findings

No abnormal areas of increased or decreased uptake

Test explanation and related physiology

PET scanning is used in many areas of medicine. The greatest use of PET scan has been for evaluating cancers, heart diseases, and brain disorders.

In PET scanning, radioactive chemicals are administered to the patient. These chemicals are used in the normal metabolic process of the cells of the particular organ being imaged. Positrons emitted from the radioactive chemicals in the organ are sensed by a series of detectors positioned around the patient. The positron emissions are recorded and reconstructed by computer analysis into a high-resolution three-dimensional image indicating a particular metabolic process in a specific anatomic site. A CT scan (p. 231) is performed on the patient at the same time to assist in the development and interpretation of the images created. PET/CT scans provide images representing not only anatomy but also physiology.

Depending on the particular radionuclide used, PET can demonstrate the glucose metabolism, oxygenation, blood flow, and tissue perfusion of any specific area. Pathologic conditions are recognized and diagnosed by metabolic alterations.

Neurology

Pathologic areas of the brain (e.g., cancers) that are more metabolically active more avidly take up fluorodeoxyglucose (FDG) than do normal areas. Because of the high physiologic rate at which glucose is metabolized by normal brain tissue, the detectability of tumors with only modest increases in glucose metabolism, such as low-grade tumors and, in some cases, recurrent tumors, is difficult with FDG.

Epilepsy, PD, and Huntington disease are identified as localized areas of increased metabolic activity indicating rapid nerve firing. Brain trauma resulting in a hematoma or bleeding is evident as decreased metabolic activity in the area of trauma. Stroke can also be identified and its extent determined. Areas of decreased blood flow take up less radioactive H_2O than normal areas and represent areas at risk for stroke.

Alzheimer's disease can be recognized by identifying hypometabolism in multiple areas of the brain (temporal and parietal lobe). PET scanning with amyloid and tau protein specific markers (p. 589) may be helpful in increasing the sensitivity and specificity in diagnosing neurodegenerative diseases such as Alzheimer's disease. A negative PET scan with amyloid imaging eliminates the possibility of Alzheimer's disease in a patient with cognitive impairment. Using Tau protein specific tracers, *Tau PET scans* can identify tau tangles in the brains of people early in the course of Alzheimer's disease and other neurodegenerative disorders.

Cardiology

PET scans of the heart are one of the best tests to indicate decreased blood flow, indicating coronary artery occlusive disease. PET scans are also used when cardiac muscle function is reduced. A PET scan can indicate whether the dysfunction arises from reversible ischemic muscle that would benefit from revascularization or from muscle tissue that is no longer viable.

Oncology

The most commonly used agent in oncology is FDG because increased glucose metabolism is so prevalent in malignant tumors compared with normal or benign pathologic tissue. PET can be used to visualize rapidly growing tumors and indicate their anatomic location. It is used to determine tumor response to therapy, identify recurrence of tumor after surgical removal, and differentiate tumor from other pathologic conditions (e.g., infection). PET is particularly helpful in identifying regional and metastatic spread for a particular tumor. PET has also been particularly useful for identifying metastasis from lung, melanoma, breast, pancreas, colon, lymphoma, and brain cancers.

Rapidly growing tumors are associated with a high metabolic rate and therefore concentrate FDG particularly well. The amount of uptake of FDG is measured by the standardized uptake value (SUV)—the amount of uptake of FDG in tumor compared with the normal tissue in that same area. SUV helps to distinguish between benign and malignant lesions—the higher the SUV, the more likely the tumor is malignant.

PET mammography or positron emission mammography (PEM) is seeing growing use as a tool for diagnostic breast imaging. PEM holds the promise of improving the sensitivity and specificity of routine mammography (p. 497).

Bone

A PET/CT scan with a sodium fluoride F18 injection (^{18}F NaF) scans the entire skeletal system and produces high-resolution images of the bones. These images are used to detect areas of abnormal bone growth associated with tumors. The PET/CT scan of the bone is particularly helpful for patients with prostate or breast cancer. The uptake of ^{18}F NaF in the skeleton reflects sites of increased blood flow and bone remodeling associated with bone injury or metastatic disease. Small parts PET scans are being used for foot inflammatory pathology.

Interfering factors

- Recent use (within 24 hours) of caffeine, alcohol, or tobacco may affect test results.
- Ingestion of a small- to moderate-sized meal can cause a marked uptake of FDG in the gut and muscles, thereby leaving little or no radionuclide to be taken up by tumor.
- Anxiety can cause increased uptake in multiple areas (e.g., neck, upper mediastinum) of the body.
- Mild to moderate exercise can instigate marked uptake of FDG in the muscles, thereby leaving little or no radionuclide to be taken up by tumor. This causes a false-negative result.
- The liver and spleen avidly take up FDG. Therefore these organs are difficult to evaluate on PET imaging.
- FDG is excreted by the urinary system. As a result, the bladder may obscure areas of increased uptake in the pelvis.
- Uptake of FDG can occur in the lymph node basin draining the site of the FDG injection. If PET is being done to stage tumors that could metastasize to those lymph nodes, the FDG should be injected on the contralateral side.

P

Procedure and patient care

Before

PT Explain the procedure to the patient. See p. xviii for radiation exposure and risks.
- Obtain informed consent if required by the institution.
PT Inform the patient that he or she may need to restrict food or fluids for 4 hours on the day of the test.
PT Instruct patients with diabetes to take their pretest dose of insulin at a meal 3 to 4 hours before the test.
PT Tell the patient that no sedatives or tranquilizers should be taken, because he or she may need to perform certain mental activities during the brain PET scan.

PT Tell the patient to empty the bladder before the test for comfort. A Foley catheter may be inserted for PET scanning of the pelvic region.

PT Tell the patient that the only discomfort associated with this study is insertion of the IV line.

• Depending on the organ being evaluated, specific protocols may exist for the examination.

During
• Note the following procedural steps:
  1. The patient is positioned in a comfortable, reclining chair.
  2. The radioactive material can be infused through an IV line.
  3. The gamma rays that penetrate the tissues are recorded outside the body by a circular array of detectors.
  4. Extraneous auditory and visual stimuli are minimized by a blindfold and ear plugs.
  5. If the chest is being scanned, instruct the patient to breathe in a shallow manner until the middle of the chest is reached. Then ask the patient to hold the breath after expiration until the middle of the abdomen is reached.
• Note that a physician performs this procedure with a trained technologist in approximately 40 to 90 minutes.

After
PT Instruct the patient to change position slowly from lying to standing to avoid postural hypotension.

PT Encourage the patient to drink fluids and urinate frequently to aid in removal of the radioisotope from the bladder.

Abnormal findings

Alzheimer disease
Cerebrovascular accident
Coronary artery disease
Dementia
Epilepsy

Huntington disease
Malignant tumor
Myocardial infarction
PD

notes

postcoital test. (Postcoital cervical mucus test, Cervical mucus sperm penetration test)

Type of test Fluid analysis

Normal findings

Cervical mucus adequate for sperm transmission, survival, and penetration

6–20 active sperm per hpf

Test explanation and related physiology

This test consists of a postcoital examination of the cervical mucus to measure the ability of the sperm to penetrate the mucus and maintain motility. This test is used in the evaluation of infertile couples. It evaluates interaction between the sperm and the cervical mucus. It also measures the quality of the cervical mucus. It is performed only after a previously performed semen analysis has been determined to be normal.

This test is performed during the middle of the ovulatory cycle because at this time, the secretions should be optimal for sperm penetration and survival. During ovulation, the quantity of cervical mucus is maximal, but the viscosity is minimal, thus facilitating sperm penetration. The *endocervical mucus sample* is examined for color, viscosity, and tenacity *(spinnbarkeit)*. The fresh specimen is then spread on a clean glass slide and examined for the presence of sperm. Estimates of the total number of sperm and of the number of motile sperm per high-power field are reported.

After the specimen has dried on the glass slide, the mucus can be examined for *ferning*. This pattern is correlated with estrogen activity and is therefore present in all ovulatory women at midcycle. When the cervical mucus is checked again immediately before menstruation, no ferning is found because of progesterone activity.

This test has limited diagnostic potential and poor predictive value. Its use has been associated with increased testing without improvement in pregnancy rates. Furthermore, cervical factor infertility is easily addressed by performing intrauterine inseminations.

Procedure and patient care

Before

PT Explain the procedure to the patient.

PT Inform the patient that basal body temperature recordings should be used to indicate ovulation.

PT Tell the patient that no vaginal lubrication, douching, or bathing is permitted until after the vaginal cervical examination because these factors will alter the cervical mucus.

PT Inform the patient that this study should be performed after 3 days of sexual abstinence.

PT Instruct the patient to remain in bed for 10 to 15 minutes after coitus to ensure cervical exposure to the semen. After resting, the patient should report to her physician for examination of her cervical mucus within 2 hours after coitus.

During

- Note that with the patient in the lithotomy position, the cervix is exposed (similar to a Pap smear) by an unlubricated speculum. The specimen is aspirated from the endocervix and delivered to the laboratory for analysis.
- Note that this procedure is performed by a physician in approximately 5 minutes.

PT Tell the patient that the only discomfort associated with this study is insertion of the speculum.

After

PT Tell the patient how and when she may obtain the test results.

Abnormal findings

Infertility
Suspected rape

notes

potassium, blood (K)

Type of test Blood

Normal findings
Adult/elderly: 3.5–5 mEq/L or 3.5–5 mmol/L (SI units)
Child: 3.4–4.7 mEq/L
Infant: 4.1–5.3 mEq/L
Newborn: 3.9–5.9 mEq/L

Possible critical values
Adult: < 2.5 or > 6.5 mEq/L
Newborn: < 2.5 or > 8 mEq/L

Test explanation and related physiology

Potassium (K) is the major cation within the cell. Because the serum concentration of K is so small, minor changes in concentration have significant consequences. If K is not adequately supplied in the diet (or by IV administration in patients who are unable to eat), serum K levels can drop rapidly.

Serum K concentration depends on many factors, including the following:
- *Aldosterone*. This hormone tends to increase renal losses.
- *Sodium resorption*. As sodium is resorbed, K is lost.
- *Acid–base balance*. Alkalotic states tend to lower serum K levels by causing a shift of K into the cell. Acidotic states tend to raise serum K levels by reversing that shift.

An electrocardiogram may demonstrate peaked T waves, a widened QRS complex, and depressed ST segment in hyperkalemia. Hypokalemia is associated with increased cardiac sensitivity to digoxin, cardiac arrhythmias, flattened T waves, and prominent U waves. The K level should be followed carefully in patients with uremia, Addison disease, vomiting, or diarrhea; in patients on steroid therapy; and in patients taking K-depleting diuretics.

Interfering factors
- Movement of the forearm with a tourniquet in place may increase K levels.
- Hemolysis during venipuncture causes increased levels.

Procedure and patient care
- See inside front cover for Routine Blood Testing.
- Fasting: no
- Blood tube commonly used: red or green

PT Instruct the patient to avoid opening and closing the hand after a tourniquet is applied.
• Evaluate patients for cardiac arrhythmias.

Abnormal findings

▲ **Increased levels (hyperkalemia)**
Acidosis
Acute or chronic renal failure
Aldosterone-inhibiting diuretics
Crush injury to tissues
Dehydration
Excessive dietary intake
Excessive IV intake
Hemolysis
Hypoaldosteronism
Infection
Transfusion of hemolyzed blood

▼ **Decreased levels (hypokalemia)**
Ascites
Burns
Cushing syndrome
Cystic fibrosis
Deficient dietary intake
Deficient IV intake
Diuretics
GI disorders (e.g., diarrhea)
Glucose administration
Hyperaldosteronism
Insulin administration
Licorice ingestion
Renal artery stenosis
Renal tubular acidosis
Surgery
Trauma

notes

potassium, urine (K)

Type of test   Urine (24-hour)

Normal findings

25–100 mEq/L/day or 25–100 mmol/day (SI units)
(Values vary greatly with diet.)

Test explanation and related physiology

K is the major cation within the cell (see previous test). K can be measured in both a spot collection and a 24-hour urine collection. K concentration in the urine depends on many factors. Aldosterone and, to a lesser extent, glucocorticosteroids tend to increase the renal losses of K. Acid–base balance is dependent on K excretion to a small degree. In alkalotic states, hydrogen can be resorbed in exchange for K. The kidneys cannot resorb K. Therefore the intake of K is balanced by kidney excretion.

Interfering factors

• Dietary intake affects K levels.
• Excessive intake of licorice may cause increased levels.

Procedure and patient care

• See inside front cover for Routine Urine Testing.

Abnormal findings

▲ **Increased levels**
  Alkalosis
  Chronic renal failure
  Cushing syndrome
  Diuretic therapy
  Excessive intake of licorice
  Hyperaldosteronism
  Renal tubular acidosis

▼ **Decreased levels**
  Acute renal failure
  Addison disease
  Dehydration
  Diarrhea
  Malabsorption
  Malnutrition
  Vomiting

P

notes

> **prealbumin** (PAB, Thyroxine-binding prealbumin [TBPA], Transthyretin)

Type of test Blood; urine (24-hour); cerebrospinal fluid (CSF) analysis

Normal findings

Serum
> Adult/elderly: 15–36 mg/dL or 150–360 mg/L (SI units)
> Child
> > 14–19 years: 22–45 mg/dL
> > 10–13 years: 22–36 mg/dL
> > 6–9 years: 15–33 mg/dL
> > 1–5 years: 14–30 mg/dL
> > < 5 days: 6–21 mg/dL

Urine (24-hour)
> 0.017–0.047 mg/day

CSF
> Approximately 2% of total CSF protein

Possible critical values

Serum prealbumin levels less than 10.7 mg/dL indicate severe nutritional deficiency.

Test explanation and related physiology

Prealbumin is one of the major plasma proteins. Because prealbumin can bind thyroxine, it is also called *thyroxine-binding prealbumin (TBA)*. However, prealbumin is secondary to thyroxine-binding globulin in the transportation of triiodothyronine (T_3) and thyroxine (T_4). Prealbumin also plays a role in the transport and metabolism of vitamin A.

Because prealbumin levels in serum fluctuate more rapidly in response to alterations in synthetic rate than do those of other serum proteins, clinical interest in the quantification of serum prealbumin has centered on its usefulness as a marker of nutritional status. Its half-life of 1.9 days is much less than the 21-day half-life of albumin (p. 613). Because prealbumin has a short half-life, it is a sensitive indicator of any change affecting protein synthesis and catabolism. For this reason, prealbumin is frequently ordered to monitor the effectiveness of total parenteral nutrition (TPN).

Prealbumin is significantly reduced in hepatobiliary disease because of impaired synthesis. Prealbumin is also a negative acute-phase reactant protein; serum levels decrease in inflammation, malignancy, and protein-wasting diseases of the intestines or kidneys. Because zinc is required for synthesis of prealbumin, low levels occur with a zinc deficiency. Increased levels of prealbumin occur in Hodgkin disease and chronic kidney disease.

Interfering factors

• Coexistent inflammation may make the interpretation of test results impossible.

Procedure and patient care

• See inside front cover for Routine Blood Testing.
• Fasting: no
• Blood tube commonly used: red
• If the patient is going to collect a 24-hour urine specimen, provide a collection bottle. (See guidelines on inside front cover.)

Abnormal findings

▲ **Increased levels**
Chronic kidney disease
Hodgkin disease
Pregnancy
Some cases of nephrotic
syndrome

▼ **Decreased levels**
Burns
Infection
Inflammation
Liver damage
Malnutrition
Salicylate poisoning

notes

P

pregnancy-associated plasma protein-A (PAPP-A)

Type of test Blood

Normal findings

Normal values vary by laboratory and duration of pregnancy

Test explanation and related physiology

Pregnancy-associated plasma protein-A (PAPP-A) is made by the trophoblasts and released into the maternal circulation during pregnancy. Women with low blood levels of PAPP-A at 8 to 14 weeks of gestation have an increased risk of intrauterine growth restriction, trisomy 21, premature delivery, preeclampsia, and stillbirth. This protein rapidly rises in the first trimester of normal pregnancy. However, in Down syndrome-affected pregnancy, serum levels are half that of unaffected pregnancies. Furthermore, low levels of PAPP-A in maternal serum in the first trimester are associated with adverse fetal outcomes, including fetal death in utero and intrauterine growth retardation. This test is commonly used with other pregnancy and screening tests (p. 501).

PAPP-A is present in unstable atherosclerotic plaques, and circulating levels are elevated in acute coronary syndromes, which may reflect the instability of the plaques. PAPP-A is an independent marker of unstable angina and acute myocardial infarction.

Interfering factors

- Levels increase with increased maternal body weight and longer duration of pregnancy.

Procedure and patient care

- See inside front cover for Routine Blood Testing.
- Fasting: no
- Blood tube commonly used: red
- Allow the patient to express her concerns and fears regarding the potential for birth defects.
- **PT** Assist the patient in scheduling and obtaining more accurate diagnostic testing if the results are positive.

Abnormal findings

Coronary atherosclerotic disease

Positive screening tests (trisomy 21, trisomy 18, neural tube defects, abdominal wall defects)

notes

pregnanediol

Type of test   Urine (24-hour)

Normal findings

< 2 years: < 0.1 mg/day
< 9 years: < 0.5 mg/day
10–15 years: 0.1–1.2 mg/day
Adult male: 0–1.9 mg/day
Adult female
    Follicular phase: < 2.6 mg/day
    Luteal: 2.6–10.6 mg/day
    Pregnancy
        First trimester: 10–35 mg/day
        Second trimester: 35–70 mg/day
        Third trimester: 70–100 mg/day

Test explanation and related physiology

Urinary pregnanediol is measured to evaluate progesterone production by the ovaries and placenta. Both serum progesterone levels and the urine concentration of progesterone metabolites (pregnanediol and others) are significantly increased during the latter half of an ovulatory cycle. Pregnanediol is the most easily measured metabolite of progesterone.

Because pregnanediol levels rise rapidly after ovulation, this study is useful in documenting whether ovulation has occurred and, if so, its exact time. During pregnancy, pregnanediol levels normally rise because of the placental production of progesterone. Repeated assays can be used to monitor the status of the placenta in women who are having difficulty becoming pregnant or maintaining a pregnancy. This study is also used to monitor high-risk pregnancies.

Hormone assays for urinary pregnanediol are primarily used today to monitor progesterone supplementation in patients with an inadequate luteal phase. Urinary assays may be supplemented by plasma assays (progesterone assay; p. 606), which are quicker and more accurate.

Procedure and patient care

- See inside front cover for Routine Urine Testing.
- Record the date of the last menstrual period or the week of gestation during pregnancy.

Abnormal findings

▲ **Increased levels**

Adrenocortical hyperplasia
Arrhenoblastoma of ovary
Choriocarcinoma of ovary
Hyperadrenocorticalism
Luteal cysts of ovary
Ovulation
Pregnancy

▼ **Decreased levels**

Amenorrhea
Breast neoplasm
Fetal death
Ovarian hypofunction
Ovarian neoplasm
Placental failure
Preeclampsia
Threatened abortion
Toxemia of pregnancy

notes

primary immunodeficiency genetic testing (PID genetic testing, Genetic testing for PID)

Type of test Microscopic

Normal findings

No immunologic testing abnormalities

Test explanation and related physiology

Primary immunodeficiency disease (PID) testing is used to diagnose, classify, and treat various forms of PID. PIDs encompass over 300 intrinsic defects of immunity, most of which are inheritable. Immunodeficiency diseases can also result from malnutrition, idiosyncratic responses to medications (e.g., cyclosporine, tacrolimus, and phenytoins), or other illnesses. PID can range from severe to mild and can manifest from the neonatal period to adulthood. Common features include frequent infections which may be more severe, recurrent, and harder to manage than expected.

Historically, when a patient presented with a clinical history suspicious for a primary immunodeficiency, the diagnostic process began with a basic immunologic evaluation and subsequent functional studies to identify the specific immunologic defect. Now in PID genetic testing, next-generation sequencing is used to evaluate over 200 genes associated with inherited disorders of the immune system. These targeted genetic testing panels are constantly updated as additional genes become associated with disease. Knowing which gene is affected helps determine the best treatment option. In addition, once the molecular diagnosis is established, the risk of recurrence can be determined. Finally, genetic testing may determine if screening unaffected family members for carrier status is reasonable.

Procedure and patient care

- For diagnostic and proactive testing, obtain 2 mL of saliva. This can be easily provided by patients from home and enables results just as accurate as 4 mL of whole blood.
- PT Warn patients with positive results that they are at risk for infection.

Abnormal findings

Primary immunodeficiency

notes

procalcitonin (PCT, ProCT)

Type of test Blood

Normal findings

Adults and children ≥72 hours old: <0.15 ng/mL
Children <72 hours old: 0.15–20 ng/mL

Possible critical values

>2 ng/mL

Test explanation and related physiology

Procalcitonin (PCT) is a 116-amino-acid peptide that is a prohormone of calcitonin. In the absence of systemic inflammation, PCT is produced by the thyroid neuroendocrine cells and is only released into the blood as calcitonin after getting cleaved by an enzyme. Therefore, PCT is typically undetectable in healthy persons. When faced with proinflammatory stimuli, particularly from bacterial infection, PCT is made and released into the blood by nearly all tissues. Certain fungi, such as *Pneumocystis jirovecii* and *Candida* species, and parasites have also been reported to cause elevations in PCT.

Serum PCT levels rise within 2 to 4 hours of an inflammatory stimulus and typically peak within 24 to 48 hours. Peak levels can correlate with the severity of infection. With resolution of inflammation, PCT levels quickly decline at a predictable rate. Noninfectious causes of systemic inflammation, such as shock, trauma, surgery, burn injury, and chronic kidney disease can also induce PCT production. In these cases, PCT levels rise temporarily to values typically less than 0.5 ng/mL.

Clinically, PCT is most often applied to lower respiratory tract infections; it is elevated in patients with bacterial infections (e.g., community-acquired pneumonia) and is likely normal in patients with viral infections. Therefore, PCT can potentially help guide antibiotic therapy and may help reduce unnecessary antibiotic therapy for viral infections. PCT levels may also serve as a guide for when to discontinue antibiotics in patients with pneumonia. Local bacterial infection or bacterial colonization usually does not elevate PCT. Examples include tonsillitis, minor soft tissue infection, abscess, local appendicitis, and uncomplicated cholecystitis.

The study of PCT is evolving, and the approach to PCT use varies among institutions and experts. It is not meant to be used alone for diagnosing infections. In addition, it may not be available at all institutions.

Interfering factors

- Major stressors that cause systemic inflammation can *elevate* PCT. This includes severe trauma, surgery, cardiac arrest, cardiogenic shock, burns, pancreatitis, intracranial hemorrhage, heat shock, and rhabdomyolysis.
- Certain autoimmune disorders cause *increased* PCT levels.
- Patients with severe renal or liver dysfunction can have *elevated* PCT levels. Levels may decrease after hemodialysis or other treatments.
- Patients with invasive fungal infections or malaria can have *elevated* PCT levels.
- Patients undergoing treatment with medicines that stimulate the release of cytokines will have *elevated* PCT levels.

Procedure and patient care

- See inside front cover for Routine Blood Testing.
- Fasting: no
- Blood tube commonly used: red, green, or lavender

Abnormal findings

▲ **Increased levels**

Autoimmune hepatitis
Bacteremia
Bacterial meningitis
Burns
Community-acquired bacterial pneumonia
Goodpasture syndrome
Islet cell tumors
Kawasaki disease
Major surgery
Medullary thyroid carcinoma
Multiorgan failure
Postpartum
Primary sclerosing cholangitis
Small cell lung carcinoma
Trauma
Viral infections

notes

P

progesterone assay

Type of test Blood

Normal findings

Adult male: 10–50 ng/dL
Adult female
    Follicular phase: < 50 ng/dL
    Luteal: 300–2500 ng/dL
    Postmenopausal: < 40 ng/dL
    Pregnancy
        First trimester: 725–4400 ng/dL
        Second trimester: 1950–8250 ng/dL
        Third trimester: 6500–22,900 ng/dL
Child:
    $\leq$ 15 years: < 20 ng/dL

Test explanation and related physiology

The major effect of progesterone is to induce the development of the secretory phase of the endometrium in anticipation of implantation of a fertilized ovum. Normally, progesterone is secreted by the ovarian corpus luteum after ovulation. Serum progesterone level is significantly increased during the second half of the ovulatory cycle. Normally, blood samples drawn at days 8 and 21 of the menstrual cycle show a large increase in progesterone levels in the latter specimen, indicating that ovulation has occurred. Therefore this study is useful in documenting whether ovulation has occurred and, if so, its exact time. This is very useful information for a woman who has difficulty becoming pregnant.

In pregnancy, progesterone is produced by the corpus luteum for the first few weeks. After that, the placenta begins to make progesterone. Progesterone levels should progressively rise during pregnancy because of placental production. Repeated assays can be used to monitor the status of the placenta in cases of high-risk pregnancy. Progesterone assay is also used today to monitor progesterone supplementation in patients with an inadequate luteal phase to maintain an early pregnancy.

Interfering factors

- Hemolysis caused by rough handling of the sample may affect test results.

Procedure and patient care

- See inside front cover for Routine Blood Testing.
- Fasting: no
- Blood tube commonly used: red
- Indicate the date of the last menstrual period on the laboratory request.

Abnormal findings

▲ **Increased levels**

Adrenocortical hyperplasia
Choriocarcinoma of ovary
Hydatidiform mole of the uterus
Hyperadrenocorticalism
Luteal cysts of ovary
Ovulation
Pregnancy

▼ **Decreased levels**

Amenorrhea
Fetal death
Ovarian hypofunction
Ovarian neoplasm
Placental failure
Preeclampsia
Threatened abortion
Toxemia of pregnancy

notes

P

progesterone receptor assay (PR assay, PRA, PgR)

Type of test   Tumor-specimen analysis

Normal findings

Immunochemistry
   Negative: < 5% of the cells stain for receptors
   Positive: > 5% of the cells stain for receptors
Reverse-transcriptase polymerase chain reaction (RT-PCR)
   Negative: < 5.5 units
   Positive: > 5.5 units

Test explanation and related physiology

The PR assay is used in determination of the prognosis and treatment of breast cancer and, to a lesser degree, other cancers. This assay helps determine whether a tumor is likely to respond to endocrine medical or surgical therapy. The test is done on breast cancer specimens when a primary or recurrent cancer is identified; it is usually done in conjunction with an estrogen receptor (ER) assay (p. 319) to increase the predictability of a tumor response to hormone therapy. Tumor response rates to medical or surgical hormonal manipulation are potentiated if the ER assay is positive. Tumor response rates are as follows:

- ER positive, PR positive: 75%
- ER negative, PR positive: 60%
- ER positive, PR negative: 35%
- ER negative, PR negative: 25%

Procedure and patient care

- Prepare the patient for breast biopsy per routine protocol.
- Record the menstrual status of the patient.
- Record any exogenous hormone the patient may have used during the past 2 months.
- The surgeon obtains tissue.
- This tissue should be placed on ice or in formalin.
- Part of the tissue is used for routine histology. A portion of the paraffin block is sent to a reference laboratory.
- Results are usually available in 1 week.
- Provide routine postoperative care.

Abnormal findings

▲ **Increased levels**
   Hormonally dependent cancer

notes

prolactin levels (PRLs)

Type of test Blood

Normal findings

Adult male: 3–13 ng/mL
Adult female: 3–27 ng/mL
Pregnant female: 20–400 ng/mL

Test explanation and related physiology

Prolactin is a hormone secreted by the anterior pituitary gland (adenohypophysis). In females, prolactin promotes lactation. Its role in males is not clear. During sleep, prolactin levels increase two- to threefold to circulating levels equaling those of pregnant women. With breast stimulation, pregnancy, nursing, stress, or exercise, a surge of this hormone occurs. It is elevated in patients with prolactin-secreting pituitary acidophilic or chromophobic adenomas. To a lesser extent, moderately high prolactin levels have been observed in women with secondary amenorrhea (i.e., postpubertal) and galactorrhea. Paraneoplastic tumors (e.g., lung cancer) may cause ectopic secretion of prolactin as well. In general, very high prolactin levels are more likely to be caused by pituitary adenoma than other causes.

The prolactin level is helpful for monitoring the disease activity of pituitary adenomas. Several *prolactin stimulation tests* (with thyrotropin-releasing hormone or chlorpromazine) and *prolactin suppression tests* (with levodopa) have been designed to help differentiate pituitary adenoma from other causes of prolactin overproduction.

Interfering factors

- Stress from illness, trauma, surgery, seizures, or even the fear of a blood test can elevate levels.

Procedure and patient care

- See inside front cover for Routine Blood Testing.
- Fasting: no
- Blood tube commonly used: red
- PT Inform the patient that blood should be drawn in the morning.
- Transfer the specimen to the laboratory as soon as possible. If a delay occurs, the specimen should be placed on ice.

Abnormal findings

▲ **Increased levels**

Amenorrhea
Anorexia nervosa
Empty sella syndrome
Galactorrhea
Hypothyroidism
Infiltrative diseases of the
  hypothalamus and
  pituitary stalk
Metastatic cancer to the
  pituitary gland
Perineoplastic ectopic
  production of prolactin
Polycystic ovary syndrome
Prolactin-secreting pituitary
  tumor
Renal failure
Stress

▼ **Decreased levels**

Pituitary apoplexy
Pituitary destruction
  from tumor
  (craniopharyngioma)

notes

prostate-specific antigen (PSA, Prostate cancer gene 3 [PCA3], MI-prostate score [MiPS])

Type of test Blood

Normal findings

0–2.5 ng/mL is low
2.6–10 ng/mL is slightly to moderately elevated
10.1–19.9 ng/mL is moderately elevated
≥ 20 ng/mL is significantly elevated

Test explanation and related physiology

PSA is elevated in patients with prostate diseases (e.g., cancer, infection, and benign hypertrophy). PSA can be detected in all men; however, levels can be greatly increased in patients with prostate cancer. The higher the levels, the greater the tumor burden. The PSA assay is also a sensitive test for monitoring response to therapy. Significant elevation in PSA after treatment indicates the recurrence of prostatic cancer.

There is considerable controversy regarding the use of PSA screening for asymptomatic men. A positive screening test result will trigger more aggressive and costly testing. PSA levels may be minimally elevated in patients with benign prostatic hypertrophy (BPH) and prostatitis, and it is sometimes difficult to differentiate benign and malignant prostate disease. To resolve that problem, other measures of PSA have been invented. They include:

- *PSA velocity*: the change in PSA levels per unit time
- *Age-specific PSA*
- *PSA density*: PSA density per unit of the size of the entire prostate or just the transition zone (the part of the prostate that surrounds the urethra)
- *Free PSA*: unbound PSA
- *IsoPSA test*: measures the entire spectrum of PSA isoforms in the blood
- *Pro PSA*: measures several different inactive precursors of PSA
- *Prostate Health Index (PHI)*: using different mathematic formulas to adjust PSA levels
- PSA combined with other prostate cancer-specific biomarkers such as *prostate cancer gene 3 (PCA3)* in urine or the *4 K score test* which measures total PSA with free PSA, intact PSA, and human kallikrein 2 (hK2)
- PSA combined with prostate-specific proteins such as *prostatic-specific membrane antigen (PSMA)* or *early prostate cancer antigen (EPCA)*

P

In 2018, the US Preventive Task Force recommended that for men aged 55 to 69 years, the decision to undergo periodic PSA based screening should be an individual one. For men 70 years and older, screening is not recommended. PSA is also an effective cancer tumor marker, see p. 164.

Interfering factors

- Rectal examinations may elevate PSA levels. The PSA specimen should be drawn before rectal examination of the prostate or several hours afterward.
- Prostatic manipulation by biopsy or transurethral resection of the prostate (TURP) may elevate PSA levels. The test should be done before surgery or 6 weeks afterward.
- Ejaculation within 24 hours of blood testing is associated with elevated PSA levels.
- Recent urinary tract infection or prostatitis can cause elevations of PSA for as long as 6 weeks.

Procedure and patient care

- See inside front cover for Routine Blood Testing.
- Fasting: no
- Blood tube commonly used: red
- MiPS requires collection of the first 20 to 30 mL of voided urine after a digital rectal examination.
- The use of the percent-free PSA demands strict sample handling that is not required with the total PSA. Check for specific guidelines.

Abnormal findings

▲ **Increased levels**

Benign prostatic hypertrophy

Prostate cancer

Prostatitis

notes

protein (Protein electrophoresis, Immunofixation electrophoresis [IFE], Serum protein electrophoresis [SPEP], Albumin, Globulin, Total protein)

Type of test Blood; urine

Normal findings

Adult/elderly

Total protein: 6.4–8.3 g/dL or 64–83 g/L (SI units)

Albumin: 3.5–5 g/dL or 35–50 g/L (SI units)

Globulin: 2.3–3.4 g/dL

Alpha$_1$ globulin: 0.1–0.3 g/dL or 1–3 g/L (SI units)

Alpha$_2$ globulin: 0.6–1 g/dL or 6–10 g/L (SI units)

Beta globulin: 0.7–1.1 g/dL or 7–11 g/L (SI units)

Children

Total protein

Child: 6.2–8 g/dL

Infant: 6–6.7 g/dL

Newborn: 4.6–7.4 g/dL

Premature infant: 4.2–7.6 g/dL

Albumin

Child: 4–5.9 g/dL

Infant: 4.4–5.4 g/dL

Newborn: 3.5–5.4 g/dL

Premature infant: 3–4.2 g/dL

No protein abnormality on electrophoresis

Test explanation and related physiology

Proteins are the most significant component contributing to the osmotic pressure in the vascular space. Albumin and globulin constitute most of the protein in the body and are measured together as the total protein.

Albumin makes up approximately 60% of the total protein. Albumin is synthesized in the liver and is therefore a measure of hepatic function. When disease affects the liver cell, the hepatocyte loses its ability to synthesize albumin. The serum albumin level is greatly decreased. However, because the half-life of albumin is 12 to 18 days, severe impairment of hepatic albumin synthesis may not be recognized until after that period.

Globulins represent all nonalbumin proteins. Alpha$_1$ globulins are mostly alpha$_1$ antitrypsin. Alpha$_2$ globulins include serum haptoglobins, ceruloplasmin, prothrombin, and cholinesterase. Beta$_1$ globulins include lipoproteins, transferrin, plasminogen, and complement proteins; beta$_2$ globulins

P

include fibrinogen. Gamma globulins are the immunoglobulins (antibodies) (p. 438).

Serum albumin and some globulins are measures of nutrition. Malnourished patients, especially after surgery, have a greatly decreased level of serum proteins. Burn patients and patients who have protein-losing enteropathies and uropathies have low levels of protein despite normal synthesis.

In some diseases, albumin is selectively diminished, and globulins are normal or increased to maintain a normal total protein level. These changes, however, can be detected if one measures the *albumin/globulin ratio*. Normally this ratio exceeds 1.

Serum protein electrophoresis (SPEP) can separate the various components of blood protein into bands or zones according to their electrical charge. Several well-established electrophoretic patterns have been identified and can be associated with specific diseases (Table P2).

If a spike is detected, *immunofixation electrophoresis (IFE)* can be done. In general, polyclonal spikes are associated with infectious or inflammatory diseases, whereas monoclonal-specific spikes are often neoplastic.

Protein electrophoresis is also used to evaluate the major protein fractions found in urine. Normally only a small amount of albumin is seen. Urinary protein electrophoresis is useful in classifying the type of renal damage, if present.

Interfering factors

- Prolonged application of a tourniquet can increase both fractions of total proteins.
- Sampling of peripheral venous blood proximal to an IV administration site can result in an inaccurately low protein level. Likewise, massive IV infusion of crystalloid fluid can result in acute hypoproteinemia.

Procedure and patient care

Blood
- See inside front cover for Routine Blood Testing
- Fasting: no
- Blood tube commonly used: gold

Urine
- See inside front cover for Routine Urine Testing.
- Follow guidelines for a 24-hour collection.

TABLE P2 Protein electrophoresis patterns in specific diseases

Pattern	Electrophoresis	Disease
Acute reaction	↓ Albumin ↑ Alpha$_2$ globulin	Acute infections, tissue necrosis, burns, surgery, stress, myocardial infarction
Chronic inflammatory	sl. ↓ Albumin sl. ↑ Gamma globulin N Alpha$_2$ globulin	Chronic infection, granulomatous diseases, cirrhosis, rheumatoid-collagen diseases
Nephrotic syndrome	↓↓ Albumin ↑↑ Alpha$_2$ globulin N ↑ Beta globulin	Nephrotic syndrome
Far-advanced cirrhosis	↓ Albumin ↑ Gamma globulin Incorporation of beta and gamma peaks	Far-advanced cirrhosis
Polyclonal gamma globulin elevation	↑↑ Gamma globulin with a broad peak	Cirrhosis, chronic infection, sarcoidosis, tuberculosis, endocarditis, rheumatoid-collagen diseases
Hypogamma-globulinemia	↓ Gamma globulin with normal other globulin levels	Light-chain multiple myeloma
Monoclonal gammopathy	Thin spikes in the beta (IgA, IgM) and gamma globulins	Myeloma, Waldenström macroglobulinemia, gammopathies

↓, Decreased; ↑, increased; sl. ↓, slightly decreased; sl. ↑, slightly increased; ↓↓, greatly decreased; ↑↑, greatly increased; N, normal.

Abnormal findings

▲ **Increased blood monoclonal immunoglobulins**
Multiple myeloma
Waldenström macroglobulinemia

▲ **Increased blood polyclonal immunoglobulins**
Amyloidosis
Autoimmune diseases
Chronic infection or inflammation
Chronic liver disease

▲ **Increased urine monoclonal immunoglobulins**
Multiple myeloma
Waldenström macroglobulinemia

See also Table P2.

notes

protein C, protein S

Type of test   Blood

Normal findings

Protein S: 60%-130% of normal activity

Protein C: 70%-150% of normal activity

Protein C levels are lower in females and decrease with age in both males and females.

Test explanation and related physiology

The plasma coagulation system is tightly regulated between thrombosis and fibrinolysis. This precise regulation is important. The protein C–protein S system is an important regulator of coagulation. Protein C inhibits the regulation of activated factor VIII and factor V see Figure C3, p. 212). This function of protein C is enhanced by protein S. Congenital deficiencies of these vitamin K-dependent proteins may cause spontaneous intravascular thrombosis. Furthermore, dysfunctional forms of the proteins result in a hypercoagulable state. In addition, nearly 50% of hypercoagulable states are caused by the presence of a factor V (factor V Leiden, p. 325) that is resistant to protein C inhibition. Acquired deficiencies are less commonly symptomatic.

These proteins are vitamin K dependent and are decreased in patients who are taking warfarin, in liver diseases, and in severe malnutrition. These are some of the causes of acquired decreased protein S and C activity. Because complement regulatory proteins are acute phase reactants, autoimmune diseases and other inflammatory diseases are associated with increased binding of protein S causing an acquired protein S deficiency. Affected patients may experience hypercoagulable events. Measurement of *plasma-free protein S antigen* is performed as the initial testing for protein S deficiency.

When decreased activity of these proteins is identified, more testing is required. *Protein C antigen testing (PCAG / Protein C Antigen)* is helpful to distinguish between type I and type II deficiencies. If decreased protein antigen is found, Protein C *(PROC) gene* encodes for protein C and can be evaluated by DNA sequencing.

Interfering factors

- Decreased protein C may occur in the postoperative state.
- Pregnancy or the use of exogenous sex hormones is associated with decreases in proteins C and S.

P

- Active clotting states, such as vein thrombosis, can lower levels of proteins S and C.

Procedure and patient care

- See inside front cover for Routine Blood Testing.
- Fasting: no
- Blood tube commonly used: blue
- **PT** If the patient is found to be deficient in either protein, encourage the patient's family members to be tested, because they may be similarly affected.

Abnormal findings

▼ **Decreased levels**

Arterial or venous thrombosis
Autoimmune diseases
Congenital deficiency of protein C or protein S
DIC
Hypercoagulable states
Inflammation
Malignancy
Pulmonary emboli
Vitamin K deficiency because of drugs or malnutrition
Warfarin

notes

prothrombin time (PT, Protime, International normalized ratio [INR])

Type of test   Blood

Normal findings
(These depend on reagents used for PT.)
11.0–12.5 seconds; 85%-100%
Full anticoagulant therapy: > 1.5–2 times control value; 20%-30%
INR: 0.8–1.1

Possible critical values
20 seconds
INR: > 5.5

Test explanation and related physiology

The PT is used to evaluate the adequacy of the extrinsic system and common pathway in the clotting mechanism. The PT measures the clotting ability of factors I (fibrinogen), II (prothrombin), V, VII, and X. When these clotting factors exist in deficient quantities, PT is prolonged. Many diseases and drugs are associated with decreased levels of these factors. These include the following:

- *Hepatocellular liver disease* Factors I, II, V, VII, IX, and X are produced in the liver. With severe hepatocellular dysfunction, synthesis of these factors will not occur.

- *Obstructive biliary disease* As a result of the biliary obstruction, the bile necessary for fat absorption fails to enter the gut, and fat malabsorption results. Vitamins A, D, E, and K are fat soluble and also are not absorbed. Because the synthesis of factors II, VII, IX, and X depends on vitamin K, these factors will not be adequately produced and serum concentrations will fall.

- *Parenchymal (hepatocellular) liver disease* can be differentiated from obstructive biliary disease by determination of the patient's response to parenteral vitamin K administration. If PT returns to normal after 1 to 3 days of vitamin K administration, one can safely assume that the patient has obstructive biliary disease that is causing vitamin K malabsorption. If, on the other hand, PT does not return to normal with the vitamin K injections, one can assume that severe hepatocellular disease exists and that the liver cells are incapable of synthesizing the clotting factors no matter how much vitamin K is available.

P

- *Oral anticoagulant administration.* Warfarin is used to prevent coagulation in patients with thromboembolic disease. It interferes with the production of vitamin K-dependent clotting factors, which results in a prolongation of PT, as previously described. The adequacy of warfarin therapy can be monitored by following the patient's PT. The ideal INR must be individualized for each patient.

PT test results are usually given in seconds, along with a control value. The control value usually varies somewhat from day to day because the reagents used may vary. The patient's PT should be approximately equal to the control value. Some laboratories report PT values as percentages of normal activity, because the patient's results are compared with a curve representing normal clotting time. Normally, the patient's PT is 85% to 100%.

To have uniform PT results for physicians in different parts of the country and the world, the World Health Organization has recommended that PT results include the use of the *INR* value. The reported INR results are independent of the reagents or methods used. Most hospitals are now reporting PT times in both absolute and INR numbers.

Point-of-care home testing is now available for patients who require long-term anticoagulation with warfarin. Like glucose monitoring, a finger stick is performed. A drop of blood is placed on the testing strip and inserted into the handheld testing device. The PT and INR are provided in a few minutes. The treating physician is notified by phone and any therapeutic changes can be instigated the same day.

Interfering factors

- Alcohol intake can increase PT levels.
- A high-fat diet may decrease PT levels.

Procedure and patient care

- See inside front cover for Routine Blood Testing.
- Fasting: no
- Blood tube commonly used: light blue
- Obtain the blood specimen before the patient is given the daily dose of warfarin.
- PT Teach patients on warfarin to check themselves for bleeding.
- The anticoagulant effect of warfarin can be reversed by the administration of vitamin K.
- PT Instruct patients on warfarin therapy not to take any other medications unless approved by their physician.

Abnormal findings

▲ **Increased levels**
Bile duct obstruction
Cirrhosis
DIC
Hepatitis
Hereditary factor deficiency
Massive blood transfusion
Salicylate intoxication
Vitamin K deficiency
Warfarin ingestion

notes

P

pulmonary angiography (Pulmonary arteriography)

Type of test X-ray with contrast dye

Normal findings

Normal pulmonary vasculature

Test explanation and related physiology

Through an injection of a radiographic contrast material into the pulmonary arteries, pulmonary angiography permits visualization of the pulmonary vasculature. Angiography is used to detect pulmonary embolism when the lung scan yields inconclusive results. This study has mostly been replaced by CT of the chest (p. 231). However, this test is commonly performed if the emboli are voluminous because the emboli can be extracted during testing.

Bronchial angiography can be done to identify bleeding sites in the lungs. For this procedure, catheters are placed transarterially into the orifice of bronchial arteries. Radiopaque material is then injected, and the arteries are visualized. If a bleeding site is identified, the site can be injected with a sclerosing agent to prevent further bleeding.

Contraindications

- Patients with allergies to iodinated dye
- Patients who are pregnant, unless benefits outweigh risks
- Patients with bleeding disorders

Potential complications

- Allergic reaction to iodinated dye
- Hypoglycemia or acidosis may occur in patients who are taking metformin and receive iodine dye.
- Cardiac arrhythmia: Premature ventricular contractions during right-sided heart catheterization may lead to ventricular tachycardia and ventricular fibrillation.

Procedure and patient care

Before

PT Explain the procedure to the patient. See p. xviii for radiation exposure and risks.
- Ensure that written and informed consent for this procedure is obtained.

PT Inform the patient that a warm flush will be felt when the dye is injected.
- Check the patient for allergies to iodinated dyes.
- Determine whether the patient has ventricular arrhythmias.
- Keep the patient NPO after midnight on the day of the test.
- Administer preprocedural medications as ordered.

During
- Note the following procedural steps:
  1. The patient is placed on an x-ray table in the supine position.
  2. A catheter is placed into the femoral vein and passed into the inferior vena cava.
  3. With fluoroscopic visualization, the catheter is advanced into the main pulmonary artery, where the dye is injected.
  4. X-ray images of the chest are immediately taken in timed sequence. This allows all vessels visualized by the injection to be photographed. If filling defects are seen in the contrast-filled vessels, pulmonary emboli are present.
  5. If *bronchial angiography* is performed, the femoral artery is cannulated instead of the vein.
- Note that this test is performed by a physician in approximately 1 hour.
PT During injection of dye, inform the patient that he or she will feel a burning sensation and flush throughout the body.

After
- Observe the catheter insertion site for inflammation, hemorrhage, and hematoma.
- Assess the patient's vital signs for evidence of bleeding.
- Apply cold compresses to the puncture site if needed to reduce swelling or discomfort.

Abnormal findings

Congenital and acquired lesions of the pulmonary vessels (e.g., pulmonary hypertension)
Pulmonary embolism
Tumor

notes

pulmonary function tests (PFTs)

Type of test Airflow assessment

Normal findings

Vary with the patient's age, sex, height, and weight

Test explanation and related physiology

PFTs are performed to detect abnormalities in respiratory function and to determine the extent of any pulmonary abnormality. The main reasons for pulmonary function tests include the following:

- Preoperative evaluation of the lungs and pulmonary reserve
- Evaluation of the response to bronchodilator therapy
- Differentiation between restrictive and obstructive forms of chronic pulmonary disease.
- Determination of the diffusing capacity of the lungs (D_L). Rates are based on the difference in concentration of gases in inspired and expired air.
- Performance of inhalation tests in patients with allergies

PFTs include spirometry, measurement of airflow rates, and calculation of lung volumes and capacities. Exercise pulmonary stress testing can also be performed to provide data concerning the patient's pulmonary reserve.

On the basis of age, height, weight, race, and sex, normal values for the volumes and flow rates can be predicted. If the actual values are greater than 80% of predicted values, the results are considered normal. Spirometry provides information about obstruction or restriction of airflow. If airflow rates are significantly diminished ($< 60\%$ of normal), spirometry can be repeated after bronchodilators are administered by nebulizer.

PFTs include determination of the following:

- *Forced vital capacity (FVC)* is the amount of air that can be forcefully expelled from a maximally inflated lung position. This volume is decreased below the expected value in obstructive and restrictive pulmonary diseases.
- *Forced expiratory volume in 1 second (FEV_1)* is the volume of air expelled during the first second of the FVC. In patients with obstructive disease, airways are narrowed, and resistance to flow is high. Therefore not as much air can be expelled in 1 second, and FEV_1 will be reduced below the predicted value. In restrictive lung disease, FEV_1 is decreased not because of airway resistance but because the amount of air originally inhaled is less. One should therefore measure the *FEV_1/FVC ratio*. A normal value of 80% is found in

patients with restrictive lung disease. In obstructive lung disease, this ratio is considerably less than 80%.

- *Maximal midexpiratory flow (MMEF)* is the maximal rate of airflow through the pulmonary tree during forced expiration. This is also called *forced midexpiratory flow.* MMEF is reduced below expected values in obstructive diseases and normal in restrictive diseases.
- *Maximal volume ventilation (MVV)*, formerly called *maximal breathing capacity*, is the maximal volume of air that the patient can breathe in and out for 1 minute. MVV is decreased below the expected value in both restrictive and obstructive pulmonary disease.

A *comprehensive pulmonary function study* also may include evaluation of the following lung volumes and lung capacities, many of which are illustrated in Figure P2.

- *Tidal volume (TV or V_T)* is the volume of air inspired and expired with each normal respiration.
- *Inspiratory reserve volume (IRV)* is the maximal volume of air that can be inspired from the end of a normal

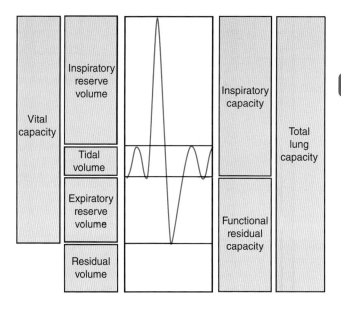

FIG. P2 Relationship of lung volumes and capacities.

inspiration. It represents forced inspiration over and beyond the tidal volume.

- *Expiratory reserve volume (ERV)* is the maximal volume of air that can be exhaled after a normal expiration.
- *Residual volume (RV)* is the volume of air remaining in the lungs after forced expiration.
- *Inspiratory capacity (IC)* is the maximal amount of air that can be inspired after a normal expiration (IC = TV + IRV).
- *Functional residual capacity (FRC)* is the amount of air left in the lungs after a normal expiration (FRC = ERV + RV).
- *Vital capacity (VC)* is the maximal amount of air that can be expired after a maximal inspiration (VC = TV + IRV + ERV).
- *Total lung capacity (TLC)* is the volume to which the lungs can be expanded with the greatest inspiratory effort (TLC = TV + IRV + ERV + RV).
- *Minute volume (MV)*, sometimes called *minute ventilation*, is the volume of air inhaled and exhaled per minute.
- *Dead space.* Dead space is the part of the tidal volume that does not participate in alveolar gas exchange. This would include the air in the trachea.
- *Forced expiratory flow$_{200-1200}$ (FEF$_{200-1200}$)* is the airflow rate of expired air between 200 and 1200 mL during the FVC. This is the portion of the airflow curve that is the most affected by airway obstruction.
- *Forced expiratory flow$_{25-75}$ (FEF$_{25-75}$) is* the airflow rate of expired air between 25% and 75% of the flow during the FVC. This is the part of the airflow curve that is the most affected by airway obstruction.
- *Peak inspiratory flow rate (PIFR)* is the flow rate of inspired air during maximum inspiration. This is used to indicate large (trachea and bronchi) airway disease.
- *Peak expiratory flow rate (PEFR)* is the maximum airflow rate during forced expiration.

Spirometry is the standard method for measuring most relative lung volumes; however, it is incapable of providing information about absolute volumes of air in the lung. Thus a different approach is required to measure RV, FRC, and TLC. Two of the most common methods of obtaining information about these volumes are *body plethysmography* and *gas dilution tests.* Gas dilution or gas exchange studies are used to test *volume of isoflow (VisoV),* which is helpful in identifying early obstructive changes.

Contraindications
- Patients who are in pain because of the inability for deep inspiration and expiration
- Patients who are unable to cooperate

Procedure and patient care

Before

PT Explain the test to the patient.

PT Inform the patient that cooperation is necessary.

PT Instruct the patient not to use bronchodilators (if requested by health-care provider) or smoke for 6 hours before this test.

PT Tell the patient that the use of small-dose meter inhalers and aerosol therapy may be withheld before this study. Verify with health-care provider.

- Measure and record the patient's height and weight before this study to determine the predicted values.

During

- Note the following procedural steps:

Spirometry and airflow rates

1. The patient is taken to the pulmonary function laboratory.
2. The patient breathes through a sterile mouthpiece and into a spirometer to measure and record the values.
3. The patient is asked to inhale as deeply as possible and then forcibly exhale as much air as possible. This is repeated several times (usually two to three times). The two best are used for calculations.
4. From this, the machine computes FVC, FEV_1, FEV_1/FVC, PIFR, PEFR, and MMEF.
5. The patient is asked to breathe in and out as deeply and frequently as possible for 15 seconds. The total volume breathed is recorded and multiplied by 4 to obtain the MVV.
6. The patient is asked to breathe in and out normally into the spirometer and then exhale forcibly from the end tidal volume expiration point. This provides the ERV.
7. The patient is asked to breathe in and out normally into the spirometer and then inhale forcibly from the end-tidal volume expiration point. This provides the IC.
8. The patient is asked to breathe in and out maximally. This is a measure of VC and the calculated TLC.

Gas exchange/diffusing capacity of the lung

- The D_L of CO is usually measured by having the patient inhale a CO mixture.

P

- D_LCO is calculated with an analysis of the amount of CO exhaled compared with the amount inhaled.

Inhalation tests (bronchial provocation studies)

- These tests also may be performed during pulmonary function studies to establish a cause-and-effect relationship in some patients with inhalant allergies.
- The *Provocholine challenge* test is typically used to detect the presence of hyperactive airway diseases. This test would not be indicated for a patient with asthma.
- Care is taken during this challenge test to reverse any severe bronchospasm with prompt administration of an inhalant bronchodilator.

After

- Note that patients with severe respiratory problems are occasionally exhausted after the testing and will need rest.

Abnormal findings

Airway infection	Inhalation pneumonitis
Asthma	Interstitial lung diseases
Bronchiectasis	Neuromuscular disease
Chest wall trauma	Pneumonia
Chronic bronchitis	Postpneumonectomy
Emphysema	Pulmonary fibrosis
Hypersensitivity bronchospasm	Tumor

notes

pyelography (Intravenous pyelography [IVP], Excretory urography [EUG], Intravenous urography [IUG, IVU], Retrograde pyelography, Antegrade pyelography)

Type of test X-ray with contrast

Normal findings

Normal size, shape, and position of the kidneys, renal pelvis, ureters, and bladder

Normal kidney excretory function as evidenced by the length of time for passage of contrast material through the kidneys

Test explanation and related physiology

Pyelography or urography is an x-ray study that uses radiopaque contrast material to visualize the kidneys, renal pelvis, ureters, and bladder. The contrast can be injected intravenously, through a catheter placed into the ureter (retrograde), or through a catheter percutaneously placed into the proximal renal collecting system (antegrade).

IVP is indicated for patients with

- Pain compatible with urinary stones
- Blood in the urine
- Proposed pelvic surgery to locate the ureters
- Trauma to the urinary system
- Urinary outlet obstruction
- A suspected kidney tumor

Today, ultrasonography, computed tomography (CT), and magnetic resonance imaging (MRI) are commonly used for the evaluation of urinary tract diseases as they are more accurate. Contraindications and Potential Complications are derived from the injection of iodinated contrast (see p. 235).

Procedure and patient care

- Information regarding technique is not provided as performance of this test is rare. Follow institution guidelines.

Abnormal findings

Bladder tumor
Congenital abnormality of the urologic tract
Cyst or polycystic disease of the kidney
Extrinsic compression of the collecting system (e.g., caused by tumor, aneurysm)
Hydronephrosis
Kidney tumor

Prostate enlargement
Pyelonephritis
Renal hematoma
Renal laceration
Renal or ureteral calculi
Trauma to the kidneys, ureters, or bladder
Tumor of the collecting system

notes

red blood cell count (RBC count, Erythrocyte count)

Type of test Blood

Normal findings

(RBC × 10^6/µL or RBC × 10^{12}/L [SI units])
Adult/elderly
    Male: 4.7–6.1
    Female: 4.2–5.4
Children
    1–18 years: 4–5.5
    6 months-1 year: 3.5–5.2
    2–6 months: 3.5–5.5
    2–8 weeks: 4–6
    0–13 days: 3.9–6

Test explanation and related physiology

This test is a count of the number of circulating RBCs in 1 mm^3 of peripheral venous blood. The RBC count is routinely performed as part of a complete blood count (CBC).

Normal RBC values vary according to gender and age. Women tend to have lower values than men, and RBC counts tend to decrease with age. When the value is decreased lower than the range of the expected normal value, the patient is said to be anemic. Low RBC values are caused by decreased bone marrow production (e.g., myelofibrosis, leukemia, renal disease, or dietary deficiencies), increased blood loss (e.g., bleeding), or increased RBC destruction (hemolysis).

RBC counts greater than normal can be physiologically induced as a result of the body's requirements for greater oxygen-carrying capacity (e.g., at high altitudes). Diseases that produce chronic hypoxia (e.g., congenital heart disease) also provoke this physiologic increase in RBCs. Polycythemia vera is a neoplastic condition causing uncontrolled production of RBCs.

R

Interfering factors

- Normal decreases are seen during pregnancy because of normal body fluid increases and dilution of the RBCs.
- Persons living at high altitudes have increased RBCs.
- Hydration status: Dehydration factitiously increases the RBC count, and overhydration decreases the RBC count.

Procedure and patient care

- See inside front cover for Routine Blood Testing.
- Fasting: no
- Blood tube commonly used: lavender
- Thoroughly mix the blood with the anticoagulant by tilting the tube.
- Avoid hemolysis.

Abnormal findings

▲ **Increased levels**

Congenital heart disease
Cor pulmonale
Dehydration or
  hemoconcentration
High altitude
Polycythemia vera
Pulmonary fibrosis
Severe chronic obstructive
  pulmonary disease
Thalassemia trait

▼ **Decreased levels**

Advanced cancer
Anemia
Antineoplastic chemotherapy
Bone marrow failure
Chronic illness
Dietary deficiency
Hemoglobinopathy
Hemolysis
Hemorrhage
Leukemia
Lymphoma
Multiple myeloma
Overhydration
Pernicious anemia
Pregnancy
Prosthetic valves
Renal disease
Rheumatoid disease
Subacute endocarditis

notes

red blood cell indices (RBC indices, Blood indices)

Type of test Blood

Normal findings

Mean corpuscular volume (MCV)
    Adult/elderly/child: 80–95 fL
    Newborn: 96–108 fL
Mean corpuscular hemoglobin (MCH)
    Adult/elderly/child: 27–31 pg
    Newborn: 32–34 pg
Mean corpuscular hemoglobin concentration (MCHC)
    Adult/elderly/child: 32–36 g/dL (or 32%-36%)
    Newborn: 32–33 g/dL (or 32%-33%)
Red blood cell distribution width (RDW)
    Adult: 11%-14.5%

Test explanation and related physiology

The RBC indices provide information about the size (MCV and RDW), hemoglobin content (MCH), and hemoglobin concentration (MCHC) of RBCs. This test is routinely performed as part of a CBC. The results of the RBC, hematocrit, and hemoglobin tests are necessary to calculate the RBC indices. When investigating anemia, it is helpful to categorize the anemia according to the RBC indices, as shown in Table R1. Additional information about RBC size, shape, color, and intracellular structure is described in the blood smear study (p. 128).

Mean corpuscular volume

The MCV is a measure of the average volume, or size, of a single RBC and is therefore used in classifying anemias. When the MCV value is increased, the RBC is said to be abnormally large, or *macrocytic*. This is most frequently seen in megaloblastic anemias (e.g., vitamin B_{12} or folic acid deficiency). When the MCV value is decreased, the RBC is said to be abnormally small, or *microcytic*. This is associated with iron-deficiency anemia or thalassemia.

Mean corpuscular hemoglobin

The MCH is a measure of the average amount of hemoglobin in an RBC. Because macrocytic cells generally have more hemoglobin and microcytic cells have less hemoglobin, the causes for these values closely resemble those for the MCV value.

R

TABLE R1   Categorization of anemia according to red blood cell indices

Normocytic,[a] normochromic[b] anemia

Iron deficiency (detected early)

Chronic illness (e.g., sepsis, tumor)

Acute blood loss

Aplastic anemia (e.g., total body therapeutic irradiation)

Acquired hemolytic anemias (e.g., from a prosthetic cardiac valve)

Renal disease (because of the loss of erythropoietin)

Microcytic,[c] hypochromic[d] anemia

Iron deficiency (detected late)

Thalassemia

Lead poisoning

Microcytic, normochromic anemia

Chronic illnesses

Macrocytic,[e] normochromic anemia

Vitamin B_{12} or folic acid deficiency

Phenytoin ingestion

Chemotherapy

Some myelodysplastic syndromes

Myeloid leukemia

Ethanol toxicity

Thyroid dysfunction

---

[a] Normocytic—normal red blood cell (RBC) size.

[b] Normochromic—normal color (normal hemoglobin content).

[c] Microcytic—smaller than normal RBC size.

[d] Hypochromic—less than normal color (decreased hemoglobin content).

[e] Macrocytic—larger than normal RBC size.

Mean corpuscular hemoglobin concentration

The MCHC is a measure of the average concentration or percentage of hemoglobin in a single RBC. When values are decreased, the cell has a deficiency of hemoglobin and is said to be *hypochromic* (frequently seen in iron-deficiency anemia and thalassemia). When values are normal, the anemia is said to be *normochromic* (e.g., hemolytic anemia). RBCs cannot be considered *hyperchromic*. Alterations in RBC shape (spherocytosis), RBC agglutination, and a hemolyzed specimen may cause automated counting machines to indicate MCHC levels higher than normal.

Red blood cell distribution width

The RDW is an indication of the variation in RBC size. It is calculated with a machine by using the MCV and RBC values. Variations in the width of RBCs may be helpful when classifying certain types of anemia. The RDW is essentially an indicator of the degree of *anisocytosis*, a blood condition characterized by RBCs of variable and abnormal size.

Interfering factors

- Abnormal RBC size may affect indices.
- Extremely elevated white blood cell counts may affect RBC indices.
- Large RBC precursors (e.g., reticulocytes; p. 646) cause an abnormally high MCV.
- Marked elevation in lipid levels (> 2000 mg/dL) causes automated cell counters to indicate high hemoglobin levels. MCHC and MCH will be calculated falsely high.

Procedure and patient care

- See inside front cover for Routine Blood Testing.
- Fasting: no
- Blood tube commonly used: lavender

Abnormal findings

▲ **Increased MCV**
Alcoholism
Antimetabolite therapy
Folic acid deficiency
Liver disease
Pernicious anemia

▼ **Decreased MCV**
Anemia caused by chronic illness
Iron deficiency anemia
Thalassemia

▲ **Increased MCH**
Macrocytic anemia

▼ **Decreased MCH**
Hypochromic anemia
Microcytic anemia

▲ **Increased MCHC**
Cold agglutinins
Intravascular hemolysis
Spherocytosis

▼ **Decreased MCHC**
Iron deficiency anemia
Thalassemia

▲ **Increased RDW**
B_{12} or folate deficiency anemia
Hemoglobinopathies (e.g., sickle cell disease)
Hemolytic anemias
Iron deficiency anemia
Posthemorrhagic anemias

R

notes

renal biopsy (Kidney biopsy)

Type of test   Microscopic examination of tissue

Normal findings

No pathologic conditions

Test explanation and related physiology

Biopsy of the kidney affords microscopic examination of renal tissue. Renal biopsy is performed for the following purposes:

- To diagnose the cause of renal disease (e.g., poststreptococcal glomerulonephritis, Goodpasture syndrome)
- To detect primary and metastatic malignancy of the kidney
- To evaluate the degree of rejection after kidney transplantation

Renal biopsy is most often obtained percutaneously (Figure R1). During this procedure, a needle is inserted through the skin and into the kidney to obtain a sample of kidney tissue. The biopsy needle is more accurately placed when guided by computed tomography (CT) scanning, ultrasonography, or fluoroscopy.

Contraindications

- Patients with coagulation disorders because of the risk of excessive bleeding
- Patients with operable kidney tumors because tumor cells may be disseminated during the procedure
- Patients with hydronephrosis because the enlarged renal pelvis can be easily entered and cause a persistent urine leak requiring surgical repair
- Patients with urinary tract infections because the needle insertion may disseminate the active infection

Potential complications

- Hemorrhage from the highly vascular renal tissue
- Inadvertent puncture of the liver, lung, bowel, aorta, and inferior vena cava
- Infection when an open biopsy is performed

Procedure and patient care

Before

PT Explain the procedure to the patient.

- Ensure that written and informed consent is obtained.
- Keep the patient NPO (nothing by mouth) after midnight on the day of the test in the event that bleeding or inadvertent puncture of an abdominal organ may necessitate surgery.

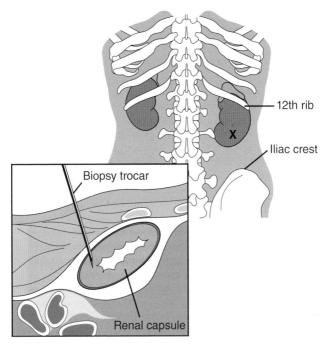

FIG. R1 Renal biopsy. A biopsy needle is placed through the posterior lower chest wall and into the renal parenchyma, from which tissue is extracted.

- Assess the patient's coagulation studies.
- Check the patient's hemoglobin and hematocrit values.
PT Tell the patient that no sedative is required.
- Note that the needle stick may be done at the bedside.
- If CT scanning or ultrasound guidance is used, the needle stick is done in the radiology or ultrasonography department.

During

- Note the following procedural steps:
  1. The patient is placed in a prone position with a sandbag or pillow under the abdomen to straighten the spine.
  2. Under sterile conditions, the skin overlying the kidneys is infiltrated with a local anesthetic (lidocaine).
  3. While the patient holds his or her breath to stop kidney motion, the physician inserts the biopsy needle into the kidney and takes a specimen.

- Note that this procedure is performed by a physician in approximately 10 minutes.
- PT Tell the patient that this procedure is uncomfortable but only minimally if enough lidocaine is used.

After

- After the test, apply a pressure dressing.
- Turn the patient onto his or her back and keep him or her on bed rest for approximately 24 hours.
- Check the patient's vital signs, puncture site, and hematocrit values frequently during the 24-hour period.
- PT Instruct the patient to avoid any activity that increases abdominal venous pressure (e.g., coughing).
- Assess the patient for signs and symptoms of hemorrhage (e.g., decrease in blood pressure, increase in pulse, pallor).
- Evaluate the patient's abdomen for signs of bowel or liver penetration (e.g., abdominal pain and tenderness, abdominal muscle guarding and rigidity, decreased bowel sounds).
- PT Instruct the patient to avoid strenuous exercise or jolting of the kidney for at least 2 weeks.
- PT Instruct the patient to report burning during urination or development of a fever. Either could indicate an infection.
- Inspect all urine specimens for gross hematuria. Usually the patient's urine will contain blood initially, but this generally will not continue after the first 24 hours.
- PT Encourage the patient to drink large amounts of fluid to prevent clot formation and urine retention.

Abnormal findings

Primary and metastatic malignancy of the kidney
Rejection of kidney transplant
Renal disease (e.g., poststreptococcal conditions, glomerulonephritis, lupus nephritis)

notes

renal scanning (Kidney scan, Radiorenography, Radionuclide renal imaging, Nuclear imaging of the kidney, DSMA renal scan, DTPA renal scan, Captopril renal scan)

Type of test   Nuclear scan

Normal findings

Normal size, shape, and function of the kidney

Test explanation and related physiology

Renal scans are used to indicate the perfusion, function, and structure of the kidneys. They are also used to indicate the presence of ureteral obstruction or renovascular hypertension. Because this study uses no iodinated dyes, it is safe to perform on patients who have iodine allergies or compromised renal function. Renal scans are used to monitor renal function in patients with known renal disease. This scan also plays a large part in the diagnosis of renal transplant rejection.

This nuclear procedure provides visualization of the urinary tract after intravenous (IV) administration of a radioisotope.

Renal blood flow (perfusion) scan

This type of renal scan is used to evaluate the blood flow to each kidney. Decreased gamma activity is noted in a kidney with arterial stenosis or renovascular hypertension. Decreased activity relative to the aorta is noted in a transplanted kidney that is experiencing rejection. Localized increased gamma activity is noted in a kidney that contains a hypervascular tumor (cancer).

Renal structural scan

This type of renal scan is performed to outline the structure of the kidney to identify pathology that may alter normal anatomic structure (e.g., tumor, cyst, abscess). Information concerning postrenal transplants can be obtained with this scan.

Renal function scan (Renogram)

Renal function can be determined by documenting the capability of the kidney to take up and excrete a particular radioisotope. A well-functioning kidney can be expected to rapidly assimilate the isotope and then excrete it. A poorly functioning kidney will not be able to take up the isotope rapidly or excrete it in a timely manner. Renal function can be monitored by serially repeating this test and comparing results. Each radioactive tracer is handled by the kidney in a different manner. Different renal functions can be tested according to which isotope is used.

R

Renal hypertension scan

This scan is used to identify the presence and location of renovascular hypertension. It usually uses angiotensin-converting enzyme (ACE) inhibitors such as captopril. The *captopril scan* (captopril renography/scintigraphy) determines the functional significance of a renal artery or arteriole stenosis. These scans may predict the response of the blood pressure to medical treatment, angioplasty, or surgery.

Renal obstruction scan

This scan is performed to identify obstruction of the outflow tract of the kidney caused by obstruction of the renal pelvis, ureter, or bladder outlet. Ultrasound, CT scanning, or magnetic resonance imaging are preferable and more accurate for anatomic abnormalities, tumors, and cysts.

Often several of these scans are combined to obtain the maximum possible information about the renal system. A *triple renal study* may use all of these techniques to evaluate renal blood perfusion, structure, and excretion. Radionuclear scans are also helpful in the evaluation of arterial trauma.

Contraindications

- Patients who are pregnant, unless the benefits outweigh the risks of fetal damage

Procedure and patient care

Before

PT Explain the procedure to the patient. See p. xviii for radiation exposure and risks.
- Remind the patient to void before the scan.
PT Tell the patient that no sedation or fasting is required.
PT Instruct the patient to drink two to three glasses of water before the scan.

During

- Note the following procedural steps:
  1. The unsedated, nonfasting patient is taken to the nuclear medicine department.
  2. After intravenous injection of radionuclide, a gamma ray scintigraphy camera is passed over the kidney area and records the radioactive uptake.
  3. Scans may be repeated at different intervals after the initial isotope injection.
- Note that the duration of this test varies from 1 to 4 hours, depending on the specific information required. Perfusion

scans are done in approximately 20 minutes and functional scans in less than 1 hour. Static structure scans require 20 minutes to 4 hours for completion.

- Note that this study is performed by a nuclear medicine technologist or physician.
- PT Tell the patient that no pain or discomfort is associated with this procedure.
- PT Inform the patient of the need to lie still during this study.

After

- PT Because only tracer doses of radioisotopes are used, inform the patient that no precautions need to be taken against radioactive exposure.
- PT Tell the patient that the radioactive substance is usually excreted from the body within 6 to 24 hours. Encourage the patient to drink fluids.

Abnormal findings

Absence of kidney function
Acute tubular necrosis
Congenital abnormalities
Glomerulonephritis
Pyelonephritis
Renal abscess/cyst/infarction/trauma/tumor
Renal arterial atherosclerosis
Renovascular hypertension
Transplant rejection
Urinary obstruction

notes

R

renin assay, plasma (Plasma renin activity [PRA], Plasma renin concentration [PRC])

Type of test Blood
Normal findings
Plasma renin assay
Adult/elderly
   Upright position, *sodium depleted* (sodium-restricted diet)
      Ages 20–39 years: 2.9–24 ng/mL/hr
      > 40 years: 2.9–10.8 ng/mL/hr
   Upright position, *sodium repleted* (normal sodium diet)
      Ages 20–39 years: 0.6–4.3 ng/mL/hr
      > 40 years: 0.6–3 ng/mL/hr
Child
      15–18 years: < 4.3 ng/mL/hr
      12–15 years: < 4.2 ng/mL/hr
      9–12 years: < 5.9 ng/mL/hr
      6–9 years: < 4.4 ng/mL/hr
      3–6 years: < 6.7 ng/mL/hr
      0–3 years: < 16.6 ng/mL/hr

Renal vein
Renin ratio of involved kidney to uninvolved kidney < 1.4

Test explanation and related physiology

Renin is an enzyme released by the juxtaglomerular apparatus of the kidney into the renal veins in response to hyperkalemia, sodium depletion, decreased renal blood perfusion, or hypovolemia. Renin activates the renin-angiotensin system (Figure R2).

Renin is not actually measured in this test. Plasma renin activity (PRA) measures enzyme ability to convert angiotensinogen to angiotensin I and is limited by the availability of angiotensinogen. The PRA test actually measures, by radioimmunoassay, the rate of angiotensin I generation per unit time.

The PRA test is a screening procedure for the detection of renal-based or renovascular hypertension. The PRA may be supplemented by other tests such as the *renal vein renin assay*. A determination of the PRA and a simultaneous measurement of the plasma aldosterone (p. 19) level are used in the differential diagnosis of primary versus secondary hyperaldosteronism.

Renal vein assays for renin are used to diagnose and lateralize renovascular hypertension—that is, hypertension that is related to

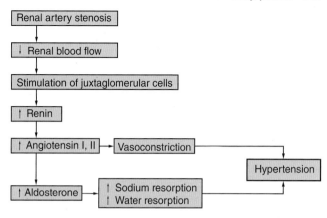

FIG. R2 Physiology of renovascular hypertension.

inappropriately high renin levels from a diseased kidney or a hypo-perfused kidney. The renal veins can be identified using injection of a radiopaque dye into the inferior vena cava. A catheter is placed into each renal vein, and blood is withdrawn from each vein. PRA is determined in each sample. If hypertension is caused by renal artery stenosis or renal pathology, the renal vein renin level of the affected kidney should be 1.5 or more times greater than that of the unaffected kidney or peripheral venous sample. If the levels are the same, the hypertension is not caused by a renovascular source.

The *renin stimulation test* can be performed to more clearly diagnose and distinguish primary and secondary hyperaldosteronism. In this test, PRA is obtained while the patient is in the recumbent position and on a low-salt diet. The PRA is then repeated with the patient on the same diet while the patient is standing erect.

The PRA is assessed as part of the *captopril test* (a screening test for renovascular hypertension). Patients with renovascular hypertension have greater falls in blood pressure and increases in PRA after administration of ACE inhibitors than do those with essential hypertension. For the captopril test, the patient receives an oral dose of captopril (ACE inhibitor) after a baseline PRA test, and blood pressure measurements are then taken. Subsequent blood pressure measurements and a repeat PRA test at 60 minutes are used for test interpretation. This is an excellent screening procedure to determine the need for a more invasive

R

radiographic evaluation (e.g., digital subtraction renal arteriography or bilateral renal arteriography).

Contraindications
• Patients who are allergic to iodinated dye

Potential complications
• Allergic reaction to iodinated dye

Interfering factors
• Renin levels are affected by pregnancy, salt intake, and licorice ingestion.
• Values are higher in patients on low salt diets.
• Posture: Renin is increased in the erect position and decreased in the recumbent position.
• Values are higher early in the day due to diurnal variation.

Procedure and patient care
Before
PT Explain the procedure to the patient.
PT Instruct the patient regarding dietary sodium prior to testing.
PT Instruct the patient to discontinue medications that may interfere with results for 2 to 4 weeks before the test as ordered by the physician.
• Usually draw a fasting blood sample because renin values are higher in the morning.
PT For stimulation tests, instruct the patient regarding sodium intake.
• Ensure that the patient is in the required position before the blood is drawn.

During
• The test is usually performed with the patient in an upright position.
• For the stimulation tests, the blood is drawn in the recumbent and upright positions.
• Collect a venous blood sample in a chilled lavender-top tube.
• Record the patient's position and dietary status and time of day.

After
• Apply pressure to the venipuncture site.
PT Tell the patient that usually a normal diet may be resumed.

Abnormal findings

▲ **Increased levels**
Addison disease
Bartter syndrome
Chronic renal failure
Cirrhosis
Essential hypertension
Hemorrhage
Hyperkalemia
Hypovolemia
Malignant hypertension
Renin-producing renal tumor
Renovascular hypertension
Salt-losing gastrointestinal disease (e.g., diarrhea)

▼ **Decreased levels**
Chronic renal impairment
Congenital adrenal hyperplasia
Ectopic adrenocorticotrophic hormone syndrome
Hypervolemia
Primary hyperaldosteronism
Steroid therapy

notes

reticulocyte count (Retic count) ·

Type of test Blood

Normal findings

Reticulocyte count:
 Adult/elderly/child: 0.5%-2%
 Infant: 0.5%-3.1%
 Newborn: 2.5%-6.5%
Reticulocyte index: 1

Test explanation and related physiology

A reticulocyte is an immature RBC that can be readily identified under a microscope. Normally there are a small number of reticulocytes in the bloodstream. The reticulocyte count is a test for determining bone marrow function and evaluating erythropoietic activity. This test is also useful in classifying anemias.

Increased reticulocyte counts indicate that the marrow is putting an increased number of RBCs into the bloodstream, usually in response to anemia. A normal or low reticulocyte count in a patient with anemia indicates that the marrow response to the anemia by way of production of RBCs is inadequate and perhaps contributing to or the cause of the anemia (as in aplastic anemia, iron deficiency, vitamin B_{12} deficiency, or depletion of iron stores). An elevated reticulocyte count found in patients with a normal hemogram indicates increased RBC production compensating for an ongoing loss of RBCs (hemolysis or hemorrhage).

To determine whether a reticulocyte count indicates an appropriate erythropoietic (RBC marrow) response in patients with anemia and a decreased hematocrit, one should calculate the *reticulocyte index:*

$$\text{Reticulocyte index} = \text{Reticulocyte count (in \%)} \times \frac{\text{Patient's hematocrit}}{\text{Normal hematocrit}}$$

The reticulocyte index in a patient with a good marrow response to the anemia should be 1. If it is lower than 1, even though the reticulocyte count is elevated, the bone marrow response is inadequate in its ability to compensate.

Determination of the *reticulocyte-specific hemoglobin content* (or *reticulocyte hemoglobin equivalent*) is a measure of the mean hemoglobin in reticulocytes. This test indicates the amount of iron available for incorporation into hemoglobin over the previous 3 to 5 days. It is a very reliable test to identify iron deficiency, especially in children or in the face of complex other chronic diseases.

Interfering factors

- Pregnancy may cause an increased reticulocyte count.
- RBCs containing Howell-Jolly bodies look like reticulocytes and can be miscounted by some automated counter machines to be reticulocytes and give a falsely high number of reticulocytes.

Procedure and patient care

- See inside front cover for Routine Blood Testing.
- Fasting: no
- Blood tube commonly used: lavender

Abnormal findings

▲ **Increased levels**

Hemolytic anemia

Hemolytic disease of the newborn

Hemorrhage (3–4 days later)

Leukemias

Postsplenectomy

Pregnancy

Recovery from nutritional anemias

Sickle cell anemia

▼ **Decreased levels**

Adrenocortical hypofunction

Anterior pituitary hypofunction

Aplastic anemia

Chronic infection

Cirrhosis

Folic acid deficiency

Iron-deficiency anemia

Malignancy

Marrow failure

Pernicious anemia

Radiation therapy

notes

R

rheumatoid factor (RF)

Type of test Blood

Normal findings

Negative (< 60 units/mL by nephelometric testing)

Test explanation and related physiology

In rheumatoid arthritis (RA), abnormal immunoglobulin G (IgG) antibodies produced by lymphocytes in the synovial membranes act as antigens. Other IgG and IgM antibodies in the patient's serum react with the fc component of the abnormal synovial antigenic IgG to produce immune complexes. These immune complexes activate the complement system and other inflammatory systems to cause joint damage. The reactive IgM is called *RF.*

Tests for RF are directed toward identification of the IgM antibodies. Approximately 80% of patients with RA have positive RF titers. To be considered positive, RF must be found in a dilution of greater than 1:80; when RF is found in titers less than 1:80, such diseases as systemic lupus erythematosus, scleroderma, and other autoimmune conditions should be considered. Although the normal value is "no rheumatoid factor identifiable at low titers," a small number of normal patients will have RF present at a very low titer. Furthermore, a negative RF does not exclude the diagnosis of RA. RF is not a useful disease marker because its presence does not disappear in patients who are experiencing a remission from the disease symptoms.

Interfering factors

- Elderly patients often have false-positive results.
- Hemolysis or lipemia may cause false-positive results.

Procedure and patient care

- See inside front cover for Routine Blood Testing.
- Fasting: no
- Blood tube commonly used: red

Abnormal findings

▲ **Increased levels**

Chronic hepatitis
Chronic viral infection
Cirrhosis
Dermatomyositis
Infectious mononucleosis
Leukemia
Other autoimmune diseases (e.g., systemic lupus
  erythematosus)
RA
Renal disease
Scleroderma
Subacute bacterial endocarditis
Syphilis
Tuberculosis

notes

R

ribosome P antibodies (Ribosomal P Ab, Anti–ribosome P antibodies)

Type of test Blood

Normal findings

Negative

Test explanation and related physiology

Ribosome P antibodies are used as an adjunct in the evaluation of patients with lupus erythematosus (LE). Antibodies to ribosome P proteins are considered highly specific for LE and have been reported in patients with central nervous system (CNS) involvement (i.e., lupus psychosis). This antibody is therefore an aid in the differential diagnosis of neuropsychiatric symptoms in patients with LE. Because patients with LE may manifest signs and symptoms of CNS diseases, including neuropsychiatric symptoms, the presence of antibodies to ribosome P protein may be useful in the differential diagnosis of such patients. Most patients with LE do not have detectable levels of antibodies to ribosome P protein. But when they do, CNS involvement should be considered possible.

Procedure and patient care

- See inside front cover for Routine Blood Testing.
- Fasting: no
- Blood tube commonly used: red
- Check the venipuncture site for infection. Patients with autoimmune disease have compromised immune systems.

Abnormal findings

▲ Increased levels

Lupus erythematosus

notes

salivary gland nuclear imaging (Parotid gland nuclear imaging)

Type of test Nuclear medicine

Normal findings

Normal function of the salivary gland; no tumor or duct obstruction

Test explanation and related physiology

The ability of the epithelial cells of the salivary glands to transport large pertechnetate ions from the blood and to secrete them into the saliva provides the principle for imaging the salivary glands. The functional capabilities, structural integrity, and location of the glands can be assessed. Usually, the parotid gland alone is visualized. Occasionally, the submandibular glands can be seen.

Indications for salivary gland nuclear imaging include patients with xerostomia (dry mouth), pain, tumors, and possible parotid duct obstruction.

By following the radionuclide immediately after injection, blood flow can be evaluated. In about 10 minutes after injection, gland function becomes obvious by uptake of the radionuclide into the gland. Five to 10 minutes later, one should see secretion of nuclear material into the mouth. Washout demonstrates complete salivary gland excretion. Usually the patient is asked to suck on a lemon to encourage rapid washout. With the development of improved imaging using CT scan or MRI, this test is uncommonly performed.

Contraindications

• Patients who are pregnant unless the benefits outweigh the risks

Interfering factors

• Rinsing the mouth before study may reduce excretion.

Procedure and patient care

Because this test is rarely performed, please review instructions at the facility performing the study.

Abnormal findings

Benign mixed tumors or pleomorphic adenomas
Malignant lesions
Salivary duct obstruction
Sjögren syndrome

notes

semen analysis (Sperm count, Sperm examination)

Type of test Fluid analysis

Normal findings

Volume: 2–5 mL
Liquefaction time: 20–30 minutes after collection
Appearance: Normal
Motile/mL: $\geq 10 \times 10^6$
Sperm/mL: $\geq 20 \times 10^6$
Viscosity: ≥ 3
Agglutination: ≥ 3
Supravital: $\geq 75\%$ live
Fructose: Positive
pH: 7.12–8
Sperm count (density): ≥ 20 million/mL
Sperm motility: $\geq 50\%$ at 1 hour
Sperm morphology: > 30% (Kruger criteria > 14%) normally shaped

Test explanation and related physiology

Semen production depends on the function of the testicles; semen analysis is a measure of testicular function. Gonadotropin-releasing hormone (Gn-RH) stimulates the pituitary to produce follicle-stimulating hormone (FSH) and luteinizing hormone (LH, also called interstitial cell-stimulating hormone). The FSH stimulates the Sertoli cell growth to encourage sperm production. LH stimulates the Leydig cells to produce testosterone, which in turn stimulates the seminiferous tubules to produce sperm. Inadequate sperm production can be the result of primary gonadal failure (because of age, genetic cause [Klinefelter syndrome], infection, radiation, or surgical orchiectomy) or secondary gonadal failure (because of pituitary diseases). These forms of gonadal failure can be differentiated by measuring LH and FSH levels. In primary gonadal failure, LH and FSH levels are increased. In secondary gonadal failure, they are decreased. Stimulation tests using Gn-RH agonists such as leuprolide acetate clomiphene, or human chorionic gonadotropin are also used in the differentiation. Men with *aspermia* (no sperm) or *oligospermia* (< 20 million/mL) should be evaluated endocrinologically for pituitary, thyroid, or testicular aberrations.

Semen analysis is one of the most important aspects of the fertility workup because the cause of a couple's inability to conceive often lies with the man. After 2 to 3 days of sexual abstinence, semen is collected and examined for volume, sperm count, motility, and morphology.

The freshly collected semen is first measured for *volume, pH, and viscosity*. After liquefaction of the white, gelatinous ejaculate, a sperm count is done. Men with very low or very high counts likely are infertile. The motility of the sperm is then evaluated; at least 50% should show rapid (> 25 μm/s at 37° C) or sluggish progressive motility. Morphology is studied by staining a semen preparation and calculating the number of sperm with normal versus abnormal morphology. More exhaustive semen analysis or second-tier testing for male infertility may include sperm functional testing, identification of sperm antibodies (p. 79), and biochemical testing.

Sperm functional tests include:

1. *Sperm–cervical mucus interaction:* This is a postcoital test that evaluates the sperm–cervical mucus interaction. Normal is more than 10 to 20 motile sperm per high-power field (hpf).
2. *Computer-assisted semen analysis:* In this test, several different sperm kinetics are evaluated, including velocities, linearity, and amplitude of sperm head displacement.
3. *Sperm penetration assay (SPA):* This test that offers a biologic assessment of human sperm fertilizing ability.
4. *Hemizona and zona pellucida binding tests:* These include the hemizona assay (HZA) and a competitive intact zona binding assay. These tests evaluate the interaction between the spermatozoa and the zona pellucida of the female egg.

Interruption in sperm DNA integrity is a potential cause of male infertility. DNA fragmentation in sperm increases with age. Therefore, impaired DNA integrity may be an increasing infertility factor among older couples. Testing for DNA integrity include *sperm chromatin structure assay test* and the *sperm DNA fragmentation assay (SDFA) test*. The sperm specimen is considered abnormal if more than 70% of the sperm have abnormal forms.

Sperm biochemical testing includes measurements of zinc, citric acid, glucosidase and the *Hyaluronan binding assay (HBA)*. The HBA is based on the ability of mature, but not immature, sperm to bind to hyaluronan, the main mucopolysaccharide of the egg matrix and a component of human follicular fluid. Hyaluronan-binding capacity is acquired late in the sperm maturation process; immature sperm lack this ability. Therefore a low level of sperm binding to hyaluronan suggests that there is a low proportion of mature sperm in the sample. Similar to the sperm penetration assay, it has been suggested that the HBA assay may be used to determine the need for an intracytoplasmic sperm injection procedure as part of an assisted reproductive technique.

A single sperm analysis, especially if it indicates infertility, is inconclusive because sperm count varies from day to day. A

S

semen analysis should be done at least twice and possibly a third time, 3 weeks apart. A normal semen analysis alone does not accurately assess the male factor unless the effect of the partner's cervical secretion on sperm survival is also determined. Sperm antibody testing (p. 79) is also performed on the specimen.

In addition to its value in infertility workups, semen analysis is also helpful in documenting adequate sterilization after a vasectomy. It is usually performed 6 weeks after the surgery. If any sperm are seen, the adequacy of the vasectomy must be suspect.

Procedure and patient care

Before

- PT Explain the procedure to the patient.
- PT Instruct the patient to abstain from sexual activity for 2 to 3 days before collecting the specimen. Prolonged abstinence before the collection should be discouraged because the quality of the sperm cells, especially their motility, may diminish.
- • Give the patient the proper container for the sperm collection.
- PT Instruct the patient to avoid alcoholic beverages for several days before the collection.
- • For evaluation of the adequacy of vasectomy, the patient should ejaculate once or twice before the day of examination.

During

- • Note that semen is best collected by ejaculation into a clean container. For the best results, the specimen should be collected in the physician's office or laboratory by masturbation.
- PT Note that less satisfactory specimens can be obtained in the patient's home by coitus interruptus or masturbation. Instruct the patient to deliver these home specimens to the laboratory within 1 hour after collection. Tell the patient to avoid excessive heat and cold during transportation of the specimen.

After

- • Record the date of the previous semen emission along with the collection time and date of the fresh specimen.
- PT Tell the patient when and how to obtain the test results.

Abnormal findings

Hyperpyrexia
Infertility
Orchitis
Testicular atrophy
Testicular failure
Vasectomy

notes

serotonin (5-hydroxytryptamine [5-HT], Chromogranin A)

Type of test Blood

Normal findings

Chromogranin A: ≤ 225 ng/mL
Serotonin: ≤ 230 ng/mL

Test explanation and related physiology

The main diseases that may be associated with measurable increases in serotonin are neuroectodermal tumors, in particular tumors arising from EC cells. These tumors are collectively referred to as *carcinoids*. Most symptoms of carcinoid tumors are caused by elevated serotonins (carcinoid syndrome). The carcinoid syndrome consists of flushing, diarrhea, right-sided valvular heart lesions, and bronchoconstriction.

Diagnosis of carcinoid tumors with symptoms suggestive of carcinoid syndrome rests on measurements of serum serotonin, urinary 5-HIAA (5-hydroxyindoleacetic acid, a metabolite of serotonin, see p. 431), and *serum chromogranin A* (a peptide that is cosecreted alongside serotonin by the neuroectodermal cells). Disease progression can be monitored in patients with serotonin-producing carcinoid tumors by measurement of serotonin or chromogranin A in blood.

Chromogranin A also acts as a useful cancer tumor marker (p. 164) for other neuroendocrine neoplasms, including carcinoids, pheochromocytomas, neuroblastomas, medullary thyroid carcinomas, some pituitary tumors, functioning and nonfunctioning islet-cell tumors, and other amine precursor uptake and decarboxylation (APUD) tumors. It can also serve as a sensitive means for detecting residual or recurrent disease in treated patients. Carcinoid tumors, in particular colon and rectal carcinoids, almost always secrete chromogranin A.

Procedure and patient care

- See inside front cover for Routine Blood Testing.
- Fasting: no
- Blood tube commonly used: red

Abnormal findings

▲ **Increased levels**

Carcinoid tumors
Neuroendocrine tumors
Pheochromocytoma
Small cell lung cancer

notes

sexual assault testing (Rape testing)

Type of test   Blood; fluid analysis

Normal findings

No physical evidence of sexual assault

Test explanation and related physiology

The sexual assault victim needs to have psychoemotional support, treatment of any physical injuries, and accurate evidentiary testing. Nearly all acute care centers have protocols in place that provide that care to victims of sexual assault.

The patient is first interviewed in a nonjudgmental manner. A thorough gynecologic history is obtained. A brief summary of the assault (if there was vaginal, oral, or anal penetration) and timing of the assault is important. After 72 hours, very little evidence persists. It is important to ascertain if the victim changed clothing, showered, or used a douche before coming to the hospital. The general demeanor of the patient, status of the clothing, and physical maturation assessment is documented.

The victim's clothes are removed and separately placed in a paper bag for possible DNA sources of the victim's or assailant's body parts. Plastic bags are not used because bacteria may grow in them and can destroy DNA. Photographs of all injuries should be obtained. The victim is then examined for signs of external and internal injuries. A pelvic examination is then performed. A "sexual assault evidence collection kit" (also known as a rape kit, sexual assault kit [SAK], a sexual assault forensic evidence [SAFE] kit, a sexual assault evidence collection kit [SAECK], a sexual offense evidence collection [SOEC] kit, or a physical evidence recovery kit [PERK]) is used to obtain all the needed specimens.

Secretions from any area of penetration are swabbed for sperm (p. 652) or other cells from the assailant. Prostate specific antigen (PSA) (p. 611) is also obtained using this specimen. Cervical secretions are swabbed for sexually transmitted disease (STD) testing. Wet preps may show motile sperm. These anatomic areas along with the anorectal area are swabbed per directions in the kit. In a male victim, penile and anorectal areas are swabbed. Pubic hair is obtained by combing or plucking. STD testing includes syphilis (p. 700), trichomoniasis (p. 659), gonorrhea (p. 659), and chlamydia (p. 194). Later, blood can be tested for human immunodeficiency virus (HIV) (p. 800), hepatitis (p. 795), and pregnancy (p. 425).

Next, blood specimens are obtained for DNA testing. More blood or urine may also be collected for drug testing. After this testing, a more detailed examination of the vagina, cervix, and rectum is performed using a Wood lamp to more easily identify saliva or sperm from the assailant. These areas are examined for subtle injuries from forced penetration. Two methods used to identify these injuries are the toluidine blue dye test and use of a colposcope (p. 223). The *toluidine blue dye test* can also be used to identify recent or healed genital or anorectal injuries. Finally, the fingernails are scraped underneath because they may potentially contain tissue from the assailant. On completion of the examination, the victim is usually interviewed by the police.

Unless medically contraindicated, all victims should be offered antimicrobial therapy to prevent STDs. The use of antiretroviral drugs in the prevention of HIV transmission may be recommended. It may also be advisable to offer victims a hepatitis B vaccination or immunoglobulin.

A pregnancy test should be done before any treatment or drugs are prescribed. If there is a risk of pregnancy, the victims may be offered postcoital contraception if the rape occurred less than 72 hours before examination by the health worker. If it occurred more than 72 hours but less than 7 days before the examination, an intrauterine contraceptive device may be used to prevent pregnancy. Pregnancy testing may be repeated in the succeeding week after the rape.

Clinicians may perform forensic evaluation of an assault perpetrator. Principles for evidentiary examinations are similar to those for victims and require evidence collection kits and strict attention to maintain the chain of evidence. Swabs, hair combing, and fingernail sampling are obtained. Penile swabs should be collected from the shaft, glans, and area under the foreskin; finger swabs should be done in cases of digital penetration of a victim. Bruises, scratches, and bite marks are identified, with swabbing of bites and scratches to identify victim DNA.

Contraindications

• The patient is emotionally unable to undergo testing.

Interfering factors

• Delays in examination after the alleged attack diminish the possibility of identifying meaningful evidence.

Procedure and patient care

Before

PT Explain the procedure and provide emotional support.
- Obtain consent to treat the patient.
- Assess the patient's emotional condition and determine whether the victim is able to undergo sexual assault testing.

During

- Use the SAECK or similar test kit exactly as described to maintain the chain of evidence.
- Refrigerate all blood and urine samples containing biological evidentiary material such as DNA to prevent putrefaction.
- It is important to examine carefully all areas of the body to help corroborate the victim's version of the alleged events.

After

- Notify police of the alleged assault.
- Assess the patient's need for urgent counseling support.

Abnormal findings

Rape
Sexual assault

notes

sexually transmitted disease testing (STD testing)

Type of test   Microscopic examination

Normal findings

No evidence of STD

Test explanation and related physiology

In the United States, common STDs include *Chlamydia*, genital herpes (herpes simplex virus), human papilloma virus (HPV), syphilis, human immunodeficiency virus (HIV), trichomonas, and gonorrhea. In this test discussion, we will concentrate on *Trichomonas vaginalis* and *Neisseria gonorrhoeae*, as all others are discussed elsewhere in this reference book. Early identification of STDs enables sexual partners to obtain treatment as soon as possible and thereby reduce the risk of disease spread. Furthermore, prompt treatment reduces the risk of infertility in women. If the STD result is positive, sexual partners should be evaluated and treated. Performing STD testing is also part of the prenatal workup.

T. vaginalis can cause urethritis, vaginitis, endometritis, pelvic inflammatory disease, pharyngitis, proctitis, epididymitis, prostatitis, and salpingitis. Children born of infected mothers may develop conjunctivitis, pneumonia, neonatal blindness, or neonatal neurologic injury and may even die.

Gonorrhea is caused by the bacterium *N. gonorrhoeae*. Many infections in women are asymptomatic. This organism causes genitourinary infections in women. Because infection in men is commonly associated with symptoms, screening of asymptomatic patients is not indicated. However, in light of the risk for asymptomatic infection in women, screening is recommended for women at high risk for infection. High-risk women include women with previous gonorrhea or other STD, inconsistent condom use, and new or multiple sex partners and women in certain demographic groups such as those in communities with high STD prevalence.

To obtain an appropriate specimen for women, swabs (that are sometimes specific to the particular laboratory) are obtained from the endocervix, vagina, urethra, urine, or a Pap ThinPrep. For men, a swab of the urethra or a urine specimen is used for testing. Generally, urine specimens are less accurate. Rectal and throat swabs are performed in persons who have engaged in anal and oral intercourse. Because rectal gonorrhea accompanies genital gonorrhea in a high percentage of women, rectal cultures are

S

recommended in all women with suspected gonorrhea. Rectal and orogastric specimens should be performed on the neonates of infected mothers.

Serologic testing is available to detect antibodies and other proteins of STD pathogens. However, in some instances, this testing is less accurate. PCR array using biochip technology is able to test for the presence of multiple sexually transmitted infections (STIs) from the same specimen. This test provides excellent accuracy for STI diagnosis within 6 hours. Confirmatory tests may not be necessary. Simultaneous screening for multiple STIs will identify specific viral, protozoan, and bacterial pathogens. It can also identify secondary infections, which may otherwise remain undiagnosed. Through the use of simultaneous multiplex testing, smaller sample volumes are required, enabling faster throughput and rapid patient diagnosis.

Urine/swab samples from home collection can also be used for PCR testing and results provided directly to the patient. (*Home STI testing*).

STD cultures and smears are obtained by a physician or nurse in several minutes during a pelvic examination. Very little discomfort is associated with these procedures.

Interfering factors

- *N. gonorrhoeae* is very sensitive to lubricants and disinfectants.
- Menses may alter test results.
- In women, douching within 24 hours before a cervical culture makes fewer organisms available for culture.
- In men, voiding within 1 hour before a urethral culture washes secretions out of the urethra.
- Fecal material may contaminate an anal culture.

Procedure and patient care

Before

PT Explain the purpose and procedure.
PT Tell the patient that no fasting or sedation is required.

During

Cervical culture

- The female patient is told to refrain from douching and tub bathing before the cervical culture.
- The patient is placed in the lithotomy position, and a vaginal speculum is inserted to expose the cervix (see Figure P1, p. 550).
- Excess cervical mucus is removed with a cotton ball.

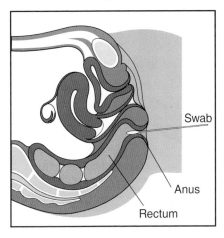

FIG. S1 Rectal culture of the female. Method for obtaining an anorectal culture for sexually transmitted diseases in a female patient.

- A sterile cotton-tipped swab is inserted into the endocervical canal and moved from side to side to obtain the specimen.
- The swab is placed in sterile saline or a transporting fluid obtained from the laboratory.

Anal canal culture
- An anal culture of the female or male patient is taken by inserting a sterile, cotton-tipped swab approximately 1 inch into the anal canal (Figure S1).
- If stool contaminates the swab, a repeat swab is taken.

Oropharyngeal culture
- A throat culture is best obtained by depressing the patient's tongue with a wooden tongue blade and touching the posterior wall of the throat with a sterile cotton-tipped swab.

Urethral culture
- The urethral specimen should be obtained from the male patient before he voids. Voiding within 1 hour before collection washes secretions out of the urethra, making fewer organisms available for culture. The best time to obtain the specimen is before the first morning micturition.
- A culture is taken by inserting a sterile swab gently into the anterior urethra (Figure S2).

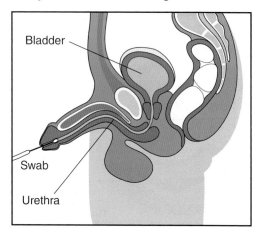

FIG. S2 Urethral culture of the male. Method for obtaining a urethral culture for sexually transmitted diseases in a male patient.

- It is advisable to place the male patient in the supine position to prevent falling if vasovagal syncope occurs during introduction of the cotton swab or wire loop into the urethra.
- The patient is observed for hypotension, bradycardia, pallor, sweating, nausea, and weakness.
- In a male patient, prostatic massage may increase the chances of obtaining positive cultures.

Urine culture

- Obtain the first catch voided specimen in the female patient. (Urine cultures for STD are not helpful in male patients.)

Pap smear ThinPrep

See p. 547.

After

- Place the swabs for gonorrhea in a Thayer-Martin medium and roll them from side to side.
- Label and send the culture bottle to the microbiology laboratory as soon as possible.
- Handle all specimens as though they were capable of transmitting disease.
- Do not refrigerate the specimen.
- Record the collection time, date, source of specimen, patient's age, current antibiotic therapy, and clinical diagnosis.

PT Advise the patient to avoid intercourse and all sexual contact until test results are available.

PT If the culture results are positive, tell the patient to receive treatment and to have sexual partners evaluated.

• Note that repeat cultures should be taken after completion of treatment to evaluate therapy.

Abnormal findings

STDs

notes

S

sialography

Type of test X-ray

Normal findings

No evidence of pathology in the salivary ducts and related structures

Test explanation and related physiology

Sialography is an x-ray procedure used to examine the salivary ducts (parotid, submaxillary, submandibular, and sublingual) and related glandular structures after injection of a contrast medium into the desired duct. This procedure is used to detect calculi, strictures, tumors, or inflammatory disease in patients who complain of pain, tenderness, or swelling in these areas. Also see salivary gland nuclear imaging (p. 651). CT and MRI are more frequently used in the evaluation of salivary glands unless a definitive diagnosis is required.

Contraindications

• Patients with mouth infections

Potential complications

• Allergic reaction to the iodinated contrast media. This rarely occurs because the dye is not administered intravenously.

Procedure and patient care

Because this test is rarely performed, please review instructions at the facility performing the study.

Abnormal findings

Calculi
Inflammatory disease
Strictures
Tumor

notes

sickle cell screen (Sickledex, Hemoglobin [Hgb] S test)

Type of test   Blood

Normal findings

No sickle cells present or no Hgb S identified

Test explanation and related physiology

Both sickle cell disease (homozygous for Hgb S) and sickle cell trait (heterozygous for Hgb S) can be detected by this screening study. Sickle cell anemia results from a genetic homozygous defect and is caused by the presence of Hgb S instead of Hgb A. When Hgb S becomes deoxygenated, it tends to bend in a way that causes the red blood cell (RBC) to assume a sickle shape. Hgb S is found in varying quantities in 8% to 10% of the black population.

The *Sickledex test* is only a screening test. The definitive diagnosis of sickle cell disease or trait is made by Hgb electrophoresis (p. 411) in which Hgb S can be identified and quantified.

Interfering factors

- Any blood transfusions within 3 to 4 months before the sickle cell test may cause false-negative results because the donor's normal hemoglobin may dilute the recipient's Hgb S.
- Polycythemia or paraproteinemias may cause false-positive solubility results.
- Infants younger than 3 months may have false-negative results.

Procedure and patient care

- See inside front cover for Routine Blood Testing.
- Fasting: no
- Blood tube commonly used: lavender
- If the test is positive, further testing is done.
- PT Inform patients with sickle cell anemia that they should avoid situations in which hypoxia may occur.

Abnormal findings

Sickle cell anemia
Sickle cell trait

notes

S

> **skin biopsy** (Cutaneous immunofluorescence biopsy, Skin biopsy antibodies, Skin immunohistopathology, Direct immunofluorescence antibody test)

Type of test Microscopic examination

Normal findings

Normal skin histology

No evidence of immunoglobulin (Ig) G, IgA, or IgM antibody or of complement C3 or fibrinogen

Test explanation and related physiology

Autoimmune skin diseases are associated with autoantibodies in the skin and serum. Direct (testing for antibodies in the skin) immunofluorescence antibody (IFA) is most specific and diagnostic. For this study, a tissue specimen in or around the skin or mucosal lesion is obtained and evaluated by routine histology and by IFA methods for deposition of human immunoglobulins (IgG, IgA, or IgM), complement C3, or fibrinogen components.

Procedure and patient care

Before

PT Explain the procedure to the patient.
• Obtain an informed consent.

During

• The skin area used for biopsy is surgically biopsied.
• A 4-mm punch biopsy or elliptical tissue excision is obtained.

After

• Apply a dry, sterile dressing over the biopsy site.
PT Tell the patient that results may not be available for days.
• Send the specimen to the laboratory immediately after the biopsy is taken.

Abnormal findings

Bullous pemphigoid
Dermatitis herpetiformis
Discoid lupus erythematosus
Pemphigus
Systemic lupus erythematosus

notes

skull x-ray

Type of test   X-ray

Normal findings

Normal skull and surrounding structures

Test explanation and related physiology

An x-ray image of the skull allows for visualization of the bones making up the skull, the nasal sinuses, and any cerebral calcification. Skull x-rays are rarely indicated today because of the availability of CT scanning of the brain (p. 231). However, skull x-rays are still used for determining skull bone suture lines in the evaluation of children with abnormal head shape or size. It is also part of a skeletal survey and may be used to evaluate bony lesions of the scalp.

Procedure and patient care

Before

- PT Explain the procedure to the patient. See p. xviii for radiation exposure and risks.
- PT Instruct the patient to remove all objects above the neck because metal objects and dentures prevent x-ray visualization.
- • Avoid hyperextension and manipulation of the head if surgical injuries are suspected.
- PT Tell the patient that no sedation or fasting is required.

During

- • Note that the patient is taken to the radiology department and placed on an x-ray table. Axial, half-axial, posteroanterior, and lateral views of the skull are usually taken.
- • Note that a technologist takes skull x-rays in a few minutes.
- • Tell the patient that this test is painless.

After

- • If a prosthetic eye is present, note this on the x-ray examination request.

Abnormal findings

Congenital anomaly	Paget disease of bone
Hematoma	Sinusitis
Hemorrhage	Skull fracture
Metastatic tumor	Tumor

notes

sleep studies (Polysomnography [PSG])

Type of test Electrodiagnostic; various

Normal findings

Respiratory disturbance index (RDI): < 5 episodes of apnea per
hour
Normal progress through sleep stages
No interruption in nasal or oral airflow
End-tidal CO_2: 30–45 mm Hg
Oximetry: ≥ 90%; no oxygen desaturation of > 5%
Minimal snoring sounds
Electrocardiogram (ECG): no disturbances in rate or rhythm
No evidence of restlessness
No apnea
Multiple sleep latency test (MSLT): onset of sleep > 9 minutes

Test explanation and related physiology

There are many types of sleep disorders. Sleep studies can
identify the cause of the sleep disorders and indicate appropriate treatment. Sleep studies include polysomnography (PSG) and
testing for wakefulness and sleepiness. A full PSG would include:

- *Electroencephalography* identifies sleep stages (p. 288).
- *Electrooculography* documents eye movements (see electro-
  nystagmography, p. 294).
- *Electromyography (EMG)* demonstrates muscle movement,
  usually of the chin and legs (p. 290).
- *Electrocardiography* determines heart rate and rhythm (p. 284).
- *Chest impedance* monitors respiratory effort.
- *Airflow monitors* measure the airflow pressure in and out of
  the mouth and nose.
- *CO_2 monitors* measure expiratory CO_2 levels.
- *Pulse oximetry* monitors tissue oxygen levels (p. 539).
- *Sound sensors* document snoring sounds.
- *Audiovisual recordings* document restless motion, fitfulness
  and snoring.
- *Esophageal pH probe* is used only if gastroesophageal reflux is
  considered to be a cause of paroxysmal nocturnal dyspnea and
  coughing (p. 310).

On occasions when sleep apnea alone is suspected, a four-
channel PSG is performed. This more simplified test includes
the ECG, chest impedance, airflow monitor, and O_2 oximetry.
Audiovisual recordings are also performed.

A sleep screening study is often performed to see whether full sleep studies are indicated. This is done during sleep using pulse oximetry. If no hypoxia occurs, significant sleep apnea would be rare, and full studies are not indicated.

Sleep apnea can be obstructive or central. Obstructive apnea is by far the most common and is caused by muscle relaxation of the posterior pharyngeal muscles. Breathing stops for 10 to 40 seconds. Central sleep apnea is highlighted by simple cessation of breathing not caused by an obstructed airway. Primary cardiac events that lead to significant and transient reduction in cardiac output can also cause apnea. Apnea from either cause is associated with an increase in heart rate, decreased oxygen levels, change in brain waves, and increased expiratory CO_2. Obstructive apnea is also associated with progressively diminished airflow.

These tests can also be used to determine the success of therapy for sleep disorders. Upon recognition of sleep apnea, often continuous positive airway pressure (CPAP) is begun and pressures titrated to the lowest level that eliminates apneic episodes to less than 10 per hour. In a *split sleep study*, a sleep disorder is diagnosed and then sleep is evaluated using CPAP or a dental fixture for therapy. During that time, appropriate CPAP settings are calibrated to reduce apneic episodes and minimize uncomfortable side effects.

Because of the expense and the psychoemotional difficulties associated with testing in a sleep laboratory, there has been significant growth in unattended *home sleep studies*. The sensors are self-applied by the patient at home following instruction from a technologist or via an instructional video. The monitoring device records airflow, respiratory effort, and oxygen saturation, but not measures of sleep or leg movements.

Interfering factors

- Psychologically induced insomnia associated with being in a sleep center.
- Environmental noises, temperature changes, or other sensations may affect the sleep pattern.
- Times for sleep testing that are different from usual times may affect sleep patterns and should be avoided.

Procedure and patient care

Before

PT Explain the procedure to the patient.

PT Instruct the patient to avoid caffeine for several days before testing if indicated.

S

PT Reassure the patient that monitoring equipment will not interrupt the patient's sleep pattern.

- Allow the patient to express concerns about videotaping and other forms of monitoring.
- Several sleep rating questionnaires are completed by both the patient and his or her sleeping partner.
- Age, weight, and medical history are recorded.

During

- Electrodes for ECG, EEG, and EMG are applied to the patient. Excess hair may need to be shaved on male patients.
- Airflow, oximetry, and impedance monitors are also applied.
- When the patient is comfortable, he or she is allowed to sleep.
- The lights are turned off, and monitoring begins.
- For PSG, the patient is asked to sleep per normal routine.

After

- On completion of the sleep cycle, the monitors and electrodes are removed.
- Test results take several days to collate and interpret.

Abnormal findings

Cardiac sleep apnea
Central sleep apnea
Insomnia
Narcolepsy
Obstructive sleep apnea
Parasomnia
REM disorder
Restless legs syndrome

notes

small bowel follow-through (SBFT, Small bowel enema)

Type of test X-ray with contrast

Normal findings

Normal positioning, motility, and patency of the small intestine
No evidence of intrinsic obstruction or extrinsic compression

Test explanation and related physiology

The SBFT study is performed to identify abnormalities in the small bowel. Usually the patient is asked to drink barium; in patients who cannot drink, barium can be injected through a nasogastric tube. X-ray images are then taken at timed intervals (usually 30 minutes) to follow the progression of barium through the small intestine. Significant delays in transit time of the barium may occur with both benign and malignant forms of obstruction or diminished intestinal motility (ileus). On the other hand, the flow of barium is faster in patients who have hypermotility states of the small bowel (malabsorption syndromes). Failure of the progression through the small bowel can be seen in patients with partial mechanical small bowel obstruction or diminished intestinal motility, as seen in patients with diabetes. Furthermore, SBFT series are helpful in identifying and defining the anatomy of small bowel fistulas.

A more accurate radiographic evaluation of the small intestine is provided by the *small bowel enema*. Unlike the SBFT, in which the barium is swallowed by the patient, during the small bowel enema, the barium is injected into a tube previously passed to the small bowel. This small bowel enema provides better visualization of the entire small bowel because the barium is not diluted by gastric and duodenal fluid. Tumors, ulcers, and small bowel fistulas are more easily identified and defined with the enema.

Contraindications

- Patients with a complete small bowel obstruction
- Patients suspected of having a perforated viscus. Barium should not be used in these patients because it may cause prolonged and recurrent abscesses if it leaks out of the bowel. Gastrografin, a water-soluble contrast medium, can be used if perforation is suspected.

Potential complications

- Barium-induced small bowel obstruction

S

Interfering factors
- Barium in the intestinal tract from a previous barium x-ray image may obstruct adequate visualization of the small bowel.
- Food or fluid in the GI tract

Procedure and patient care

Before
PT Explain the procedure to the patient. See p. xviii for radiation exposure and risks.

PT Instruct the patient not to eat anything for at least 8 hours before the test.

PT Inform the patient that the SBFT series may take several hours. Suggest that the patient bring reading material or some paperwork to occupy his or her time.

During
- Note the following procedural steps for SBFT:
  1. A specially prepared drink containing barium sulfate is mixed as a milkshake, which the patient drinks through a straw.
  2. Usually, an upper GI series is performed concomitantly (p. 765).
  3. The barium flow is followed through the upper GI tract fluoroscopically.
  4. At frequent intervals (15–60 minutes), repeat x-ray images are taken to follow the flow of barium through the small intestine. These images are repeated until barium is seen flowing into the right colon. This usually takes 60 to 120 minutes, but in patients with delayed progression of the barium, the test may take as long as 24 hours to complete.
- Note the following steps for a small bowel enema:
  1. This is usually performed by placing a long weighted tube transorally; however, a tube also can be placed into the upper small bowel endoscopically.
  2. After the tube is in place, a thickened barium mixture is injected through the tube, and x-ray images are serially performed as described for the SBFT.
- Note that this procedure is performed by a radiologist in the radiology department in approximately 30 to 60 minutes.

PT Tell the patient that this test is not uncomfortable.

After
PT Inform the patient of the need to evacuate adequately all the barium. Cathartics (e.g., magnesium citrate) are recommended. Initially, stools will be white and should return to normal color with complete evacuation.

Abnormal findings

Congenital abnormalities (e.g., small bowel atresia, duplication, Meckel diverticulum)

Congenital anatomic anomaly (e.g., malrotation)

Inflammatory small bowel disease (e.g., Crohn disease)

Malabsorption syndromes (e.g., Whipple disease, sprue)

Small bowel intussusception

Small bowel obstruction from adhesions, extrinsic tumors, or hernia

Small bowel obstruction from intrinsic tumors

Small bowel perforation

Small bowel tumor

notes

S

small intestinal bacterial overgrowth test (SIBO test, Lactulose breath test)

Type of test miscellaneous

Normal findings

Change in hydrogen < 20 ppm

Methane peak > 10 ppm

Test explanation and related physiology

Small intestinal bacterial overgrowth (SIBO) is characterized by excessive bacteria or the presence of atypical microbiota in the small intestine. This breath test relies on measurement of gases produced by bacteria in the intestine—hydrogen (H_2) and methane (CH_4)—after ingestion of lactulose in a fasting state. Lactulose is not absorbed by the intestines. Hydrogen gas is exclusively produced by colonic bacteria as a result of fermentation of the lactulose. In SIBO, the abnormal presence of abundant bacteria in the small intestine ferment the malabsorbed lactulose resulting in elevated concentration of exhaled hydrogen. An abnormal rise of hydrogen in the first 90 minutes of testing is positive for SIBO. Elevated exhaled methane is abnormal and is common in patients with irritable bowel disease, chronic constipation, or overeating. CO_2 is routinely measured to determine sample integrity.

Conditions commonly associated with SIBO include irritable bowel syndrome, inflammatory bowel disease, celiac disease, diabetes, and obesity. These patients commonly complain of bloating, gas, pain, diarrhea, constipation, muscle pain (fibromyalgia), and bad breath. Bacterial overgrowth can also be identified by analyzing small intestinal fluid samples during enteroscopy.

In preparation for this test, the patient must wait at least 2 to 4 weeks after colonoscopy or barium enema. No antibiotics, bismuth containing agents, probiotics, stool softeners, laxatives, or antacids should be administered in that same time frame.

Interfering factors

- Patients with lactose intolerance or diseases of maldigestion may have increased levels.

Before

PT Explain the procedure to the patient. Inform the patient that multiple breath samples will be needed.

PT Instruct the patient to fast for 12 hours before testing.

PT Tell the patient to avoid smoking, including second-hand smoke, for at least 1 hour before or during the breath test.

During
- Provide a specified dose of lactulose usually diluted in 8oz of water.
- Collect breath samples at 20 minute intervals up to 60 to 120 minutes.

After
- Indicate actual time of the breath sample and the amount of time after ingestion of the sample.
- Immediately send test specimens to the laboratory.

Abnormal findings

Small bowel bacterial overgrowth

sodium (Na), blood

Type of test Blood

Normal findings

Adult/elderly: 136–145 mEq/L or 136–145 mmol/L (SI units)
Child: 136–145 mEq/L
Infant: 134–150 mEq/L
Newborn: 134–144 mEq/L

Possible critical values

< 120 or > 160 mEq/L

Test explanation and related physiology

Sodium is the major cation in the extracellular space, in which serum levels of approximately 140 mEq/L exist. Therefore sodium salts are the major determinants of extracellular osmolality. The sodium content of the blood is a result of a balance between dietary sodium intake and renal excretion.

Many factors regulate homeostatic sodium balance. Aldosterone causes conservation of sodium by decreasing renal losses. Natriuretic hormone, or third factor, increases renal losses of sodium. Antidiuretic hormone (ADH), which controls the resorption of water at the distal tubules of the kidney, also affects serum sodium levels.

Physiologically, water and sodium are very closely interrelated. As free body water is increased, serum sodium is diluted, and the concentration may decrease. The kidney compensates by conserving sodium and excreting water. If free body water were to decrease, the serum sodium concentration would rise; the kidney would then respond by conserving free water.

Interfering factors

• Recent trauma, surgery, or shock may cause increased levels.

Procedure and patient care

• See inside front cover for Routine Blood Testing.
• Fasting: no
• Blood tube commonly used: red or green

Abnormal findings

▲ **Increased levels (hypernatremia)**

Increased sodium intake
Excessive dietary intake
Excessive sodium in IV
  fluids

Decreased sodium loss
Cushing syndrome
Hyperaldosteronism

Excessive free body water loss
Diabetes insipidus
Excessive sweating
Extensive thermal burns
GI loss
Osmotic diuresis

▼ **Decreased levels (hyponatremia)**

Decreased sodium intake
Deficient dietary intake
Deficient sodium in IV
  fluids

Increased sodium loss
Addison disease
Chronic renal insufficiency
Diarrhea
Diuretic administration
Vomiting or nasogastric
  aspiration

Increased free body water
Congestive heart failure
Excessive IV water intake
Excessive oral water intake
Osmotic dilution
Syndrome of inappropriate
  ADH (SIADH) secretion

Third-space losses of sodium
Ascites
Intraluminal bowel loss
  (ileus or mechanical
  obstruction)
Peripheral edema
Pleural effusion

notes

S

sodium (Na), urine

Type of test Urine (24-hour)

Normal findings

40–220 mEq/day or 40–220 mmol/day (SI units)
Spot urine: > 20 mEq/L
Fractional excretion of sodium (FE_{Na}): 1%-2%

Test explanation and related physiology

This test evaluates sodium balance in the body by determining the amount of sodium excreted in urine over 24 hours. Sodium is the major cation in the extracellular space. Measuring the amount of sodium in the urine is useful for evaluating patients with volume depletion, acute renal failure, adrenal disturbances, and acid–base imbalances. In the setting of acute renal failure, whereas an increased value will indicate acute tubular necrosis, a low value would be typical of prerenal azotemia.

This test is also useful when the serum sodium concentration is low. For example, in patients with hyponatremia caused by inadequate sodium intake, urine sodium will be low. In patients with hyponatremia caused by chronic renal failure, however, urine sodium concentration will be high.

Urine sodium excretions are helpful when the urine output is low (< 500 mL/24 hr). However, a more accurate test to determine the cause of reduced urine output is the FE_{Na}, which is the fraction of sodium actually excreted relative to the amount filtered by the kidney. FE_{Na} is a calculation based on the concentrations of sodium (Na) and creatinine (Cr) in the blood and the urine. FE_{Na} is usually greater than 3% with acute tubular necrosis and severe obstruction of the urinary drainage of both kidneys. It is generally less than 1% in patients with acute glomerulonephritis, hepatorenal syndrome, and states of prerenal azotemia (e.g., congestive heart failure and dehydration). FE_{Na} may also be less than 1% with acute partial urinary tract obstruction.

Interfering factors
- Dietary salt intake may increase sodium levels.
- Altered kidney function may affect levels.

Procedure and patient care
- See inside front cover for Routine Urine Testing.
- If FE_{Na} is ordered, collect a venous blood sample in a gold-top tube for serum creatinine and sodium measurements.

Abnormal findings

▲ **Increased levels**
Adrenocortical insufficiency
Dehydration
Diabetic ketoacidosis
Diuretic therapy
Hypothyroidism
SIADH secretion
Starvation
Toxemia of pregnancy

▼ **Decreased levels**
Aldosteronism
Congestive heart failure
Cushing syndrome
Diaphoresis
Diarrhea
Inadequate sodium intake
Malabsorption
Pulmonary emphysema
Renal failure

notes

S

spinal x-ray (Cervical, Thoracic, Lumbar, Sacral, and Coccygeal x-ray studies)

Type of test X-ray

Normal findings

Normal spinal vertebrae

Test explanation and related physiology

Spinal x-ray studies may be performed to evaluate any area of the spine. They usually include anteroposterior, lateral, and oblique views of these structures. These x-ray images are often done to assess back or neck pain, degenerative arthritic changes, traumatic fractures, tumor metastasis, spondylosis (stress fracture of the vertebrae), and spondylolisthesis (slipping of one vertebral disc on the other). Cervical spinal x-ray studies may be performed in cases of multiple trauma to ensure that there is no fracture before the patient is moved or the neck is manipulated. However, CT scan is more commonly used to ensure that there is no cervical fracture. Spinal x-rays are very helpful in evaluating children and adults for spinal alignment abnormalities (e.g., kyphosis, scoliosis). Magnetic resonance imaging is another very accurate method of evaluating the spine.

Contraindications

• Patients who are pregnant unless benefits outweigh risks

Procedure and patient care

Before

PT Explain the procedure to the patient. See p. xviii for radiation exposure and risks.

PT Instruct the patient to remove any metal objects covering the area to be visualized.

• Immobilize the patient if a spinal fracture is suspected. Apply a neck brace if a cervical spine fracture is suspected.

PT Tell the patient that no fasting or sedation is required; however, if a fracture is suspected, the patient may be kept NPO.

During

• Note that the patient is placed on an x-ray table. Anterior, posterior, lateral, and oblique x-ray images are taken of the desired area on the spinal cord. These same views can also be obtained with the patient in the standing position.

- Note that a radiologic technologist takes spinal x-ray images in a few minutes.
PT Tell the patient that no discomfort is associated with testing.

After

- Note that positioning and patient activity depend on test results.

Abnormal findings

Degenerative arthritis changes
Metastatic tumor invasion
Scoliosis
Spondylolisthesis
Spondylosis
Suspected spinal osteomyelitis
Traumatic or pathologic fracture

notes

S

sputum culture and sensitivity (C&S, Culture and Gram stain)

Type of test Sputum

Normal findings

Normal upper respiratory tract

Test explanation and related physiology

Sputum cultures are obtained to determine the presence of pathogenic bacteria in patients with respiratory infections (e.g., pneumonia). A *Gram stain* is the first step in the microbiologic analysis of sputum. Staining of sputum provides an opportunity to classify bacteria as gram positive or gram negative. This may be used to guide drug therapy until the culture and sensitivity (C&S) report is complete. The sputum sample is then applied to a series of bacterial culture plates. The bacteria that grow on those plates 1 to 3 days later are then identified. Determinations of bacterial sensitivity to various antibiotics are done to identify the most appropriate antimicrobial drug therapy. This is done by observing a ring of growth inhibition around an antibiotic plug in the culture medium.

Sputum for C&S should be collected before antimicrobial therapy is initiated unless the test is being performed to evaluate the effectiveness of medications already being given. Preliminary reports are usually available in 24 hours. Cultures require at least 48 hours for completion. Sputum cultures for fungus and *Mycobacterium tuberculosis* may take 6 to 8 weeks.

Procedure and patient care

Before

- PT Explain the procedure for sputum collection to the patient.
- PT Remind the patient that sputum must be coughed up from the lungs and that saliva is not sputum.
- • Hold antibiotics until after the sputum has been collected.
- • If an elective specimen is to be obtained, give the patient a sterile sputum container on the night before the sputum is to be collected so that the morning specimen may be obtained on arising.
- PT Instruct the patient to rinse out his or her mouth with water before the sputum collection to decrease contamination of the sputum by particles in the oropharynx.

During

- Note that sputum specimens are best when the patient first awakens in the morning and before eating or drinking.
- Collect at least 1 teaspoon of sputum in a sterile sputum container.
- Usually obtain sputum by having the patient cough after taking several deep breaths.
- If the patient is unable to produce a sputum specimen, stimulate coughing by lowering the head of the patient's bed or giving the patient an aerosol administration of a warm hypertonic solution, if ordered.
- Note that other methods to collect sputum include endotracheal aspiration, fiberoptic bronchoscopy, and transtracheal aspiration.

After

PT Inform the patient to notify the nurse as soon as the sputum is collected.
- Label the sputum and send it to the lab as soon as possible.
- Note any current antibiotic therapy on the request.

Abnormal findings

Atypical bacterial infection (e.g., tuberculosis)
Bacterial infection (e.g., pneumonia)
Viral infection

notes

S

sputum cytology

Type of test Sputum

Normal findings

Normal epithelial cells

Test explanation and related physiology

Tumors in the pulmonary system frequently slough cells into the sputum. When the sputum is gathered, the cells are examined. If the cytologic test result is positive, malignant cells are seen, indicating a lung tumor. If only normal epithelial cells are seen, either no malignancy exists or any existing tumor is not shedding cells. Therefore a positive test result indicates malignancy; a negative test result means nothing.

Bronchoscopy and percutaneous lung biopsy have supplanted the need for sputum cytology to a large degree. Now its greatest use is in patients who have an abnormal chest x-ray result, productive cough, and nothing visible on bronchoscopy.

Procedure and patient care

Before

- PT Explain the procedure for sputum collection to the patient.
- PT Remind the patient that sputum must be coughed up from the lungs and that saliva is not sputum.
- Give the patient a sterile sputum container on the night before so that the morning specimen may be obtained on arising.

During

- Sputum specimens are collected as described in the previous study.
- Usually collect sputum on three separate occasions.

After

- PT Instruct the patient to notify the nurse as soon as the sputum is collected.
- Label the specimen, and send it to the laboratory as soon as possible.

Abnormal findings

Malignancies

notes

stool cancer screening (Stool for occult blood, Stool for OB, Fecal occult blood test [FOBT], Fecal immunotest [FIT], DNA stool sample, Colon cancer screening)

Type of test Stool

Normal findings

No occult blood within stool

Test explanation and related physiology

Stool-based testing for colorectal cancer is used for colorectal cancer screening of asymptomatic individuals. These tests can find occult blood or tumor DNA within a stool sample. Tumors of the intestine grow into the lumen and are subjected to repeated trauma by the fecal stream. Eventually the friable neovascular tumor ulcerates and bleeding occurs. Most often, bleeding is so slight that gross blood is not seen in the stool. Guaiac is the most commonly performed chemical assay.

Occult blood (OB) can be detected by immunochemical methods detecting the globin portion of hemoglobin. These tests are called *fecal immunochemical test (FIT)* or *immunochemical fecal occult blood test (iFOBT)*. Immunochemical methods may fail to recognize OB from the upper GI tract because the globin is digested by the time it gets in the stool. Benign and malignant GI tumors, ulcers, inflammatory bowel disease, arteriovenous malformations, diverticulosis, and hematobilia (hemobilia) can all cause OB in the stool. Other more common abnormalities (e.g., hemorrhoids, swallowed blood from oral or nasopharyngeal bleeding) may also cause OB in the stool.

The *DNA stool sample test* may be more sensitive than guaiac testing in the detection of significant colorectal precancerous, benign and malignant tumors. Because most precancerous polyps do not bleed, they can be missed by FOBT. In contrast, precancerous polyps shed cells that contain abnormal DNA. This test is an easy-to-use home kit to collect a stool sample and mail it to a laboratory for analysis. Screening of gastrointestinal cancer often requires dietary restrictions and/or stool handling. A sensitive and specific blood test is available. Cytosine residues in an altered gene called *SEPT9 (Septin 9)* may become methylated in colorectal cancer tissue. This methylated SEPT9 can be detected in the patient's blood and indicates colorectal cancer. Also, *liquid biopsy* (p. 466) may offer another form of blood test for colorectal screening by detecting circulating tumor cells in the blood. It is important to note that screening colonoscopy (p. 223) is the most effective method to detect asymptomatic colorectal cancer and can also prevent the development of those cancers by removal of benign polyps prior to their turning into cancer.

Regular screening, beginning at age 50 years, can reduce the number of people who die of colorectal cancer by as much as 60%.

Interfering factors

- Vigorous exercise
- Bleeding gums after a dental procedure
- Ingestion of red meat within 3 days before testing
- Ingestion of peroxidase-rich fruits and vegetables (turnips, artichokes, mushrooms, radishes, horseradishes, broccoli, bean sprouts, cauliflower, oranges, bananas, cantaloupes, and grapes) may affect results.
- Diarrhea or blood in the urine or stool (e.g., bleeding hemorrhoids, rectal bleeding, or menstruation)

Procedure and patient care

Before

- PT Explain the procedure to the patient.
- PT Instruct the patient to refrain from eating any red meat for at least 3 days before the test.
- PT Instruct the patient to refrain from drugs known to interfere with OB testing.
- PT Instruct the patient as to the method of obtaining appropriate stool specimens. Tests may be done at home and mailed.
- PT Instruct the patient not to mix urine with the stool specimen.
- PT Inform the patient as to the need for multiple specimens obtained on separate days to increase the test's accuracy.
- Note that in some centers a high-residue diet is recommended to increase the abrasive effect of the stool.
- Be gentle in obtaining stool by digital rectal examination (DRE). A traumatic digital examination can cause a false-positive stool, especially in patients with prior anorectal disease, such as hemorrhoids.

During

Hemoccult slide test

- Place a stool sample on one side of guaiac paper.
- Place two drops of developer on the other side.
- Note that bluish discoloration indicates OB in the stool.

Tablet test

- Place a stool sample on the developer paper.
- Place a tablet on top of the stool specimen.

- Put two or three drops of tap water on the tablet and allow it to flow onto the paper.
- Note that bluish discoloration indicates OB in the stool.

DNA Home Test
- Place the bracket on the toilet and add the container.
- After moving the bowels, place a small stool sample in the smaller tube.
- Place preservative on the stool in the larger container of stool.
- Replace the top on the container and mail both the container and the smaller tube to the address on the enclosed label.

After

PT Inform the patient of the results.
- If the tests are positive, ask if the patient violated any of the preparation recommendations.

Abnormal findings

Diverticulosis	Inflammatory bowel disease
Esophagitis	Ischemic bowel disease
Gastritis	Polyps
GI trauma	Recent GI surgery
GI tumor	Ulcer
Hemorrhoids	Varices

notes

S

stool culture (Stool for culture and sensitivity [C&S], Stool for ova and parasites [O&P])

Type of test Stool

Normal findings

Normal intestinal flora

Test explanation and related physiology

Normally, stool contains many bacteria and fungi. The more common organisms include *Enterococcus, Escherichia coli, Proteus, Pseudomonas, Staphylococcus aureus, Candida albicans, Bacteroides,* and *Clostridium.* Bacteria are indigenous to the bowel. Sometimes normal stool flora can become pathogenic if overgrowth of the bacteria occurs as a result of antibiotics (e.g., *Clostridium difficile*), immunosuppression, or overaggressive catharsis. *Salmonella, Shigella, Campylobacter, Yersinia,* pathogenic *E. coli, Clostridium,* and *Staphylococcus* are acquired bacteria that can infect the bowel. Parasites also may affect the stool. Common parasites are *Ascaris* (hookworm), *Strongyloides* (tapeworm), and *Giardia* (protozoans). Identification of any of these pathogens in the stool incriminates that parasite as the etiology of the infectious enteritis.

Infections of the bowel from bacteria, virus, or parasites usually present as diarrhea, excessive flatus, and abdominal discomfort. Patients who have been drinking well water, have been on prolonged antibiotics, or have traveled outside of the United States are especially susceptible. Rapid multiplex panel PCR detection of the most common agents of bacterial, viral, and parasitic enteric infections directly from stool specimens is sensitive, specific, and provides same-day results, obviating the need for culture, antigen testing, microscopy.

Interfering factors

- Urine may inhibit the growth of bacteria. Therefore urine should not be mixed with the feces during collection.
- Recent barium studies may obscure the detection of parasites.

Procedure and patient care

Before

PT Explain the method of stool collection to the patient.

PT Instruct the patient not to mix urine or toilet paper with the stool specimen.

During

PT Instruct the patient to defecate into a clean bedpan.
• Place a small amount of stool in a sterile collection container.
• Send mucus and blood streaks with the specimen.
• If a rectal swab is to be used, wear gloves and insert the cotton-tipped swab at least 1 inch into the anal canal. Then rotate the swab for 30 seconds and place it into the clean container.

Tape test
• Use this test when pinworms *(Enterobius)* are suspected.
• Place clear tape in the patient's perianal region. (This is especially helpful in children.)
• Because the female worm lays her eggs at night around the perianal area, apply the tape before bedtime and remove it in the morning before the patient gets out of bed.
• Press the sticky surface of the tape directly to a glass slide and examine microscopically for pinworm ova.

After

• Handle the stool specimen carefully as though it were capable of causing infection.
• Note any antibiotics that the patient may be taking.
• Promptly send the stool specimen to the laboratory. Delays in transfer of the specimen may affect viability of the organism.
• Note that some enteric pathogens occasionally take as long as 6 weeks to isolate.
• When pathogens are detected, maintain isolation of the patient's stool until therapy is completed.

Abnormal findings

Bacterial enterocolitis
Parasitic enterocolitis
Protozoan enterocolitis

S

notes

stool for leukocytes (White blood cell stool test, Fecal leukocyte stain, Stool for white cells)

Type of test Stool

Normal findings

≤ 2/hpf

Test explanation and related physiology

Leukocytes are not normally seen in stools in the absence of infection or inflammatory bowel diseases. Fecal leukocytosis is a response to infection with microorganisms that invade tissue or produce toxins. This leads to tissue damage of the bowel wall, generating a vigorous leukocyte infiltration. This test is used to identify intestinal infections, diarrheal diseases, or inflammatory bowel diseases.

Fecal leukocytes are commonly found in patients with bacterial infections such as *Shigella*, *Campylobacter*, *Salmonella*, *Yersinia*, or *Clostridium* spp. Amebiasis is also associated with fecal leukocytes. The greater the number of leukocytes, the greater the likelihood of infection. Diarrhea caused by most parasites (e.g., *Giardia*) or by viral infections (e.g., Norwalk, rotaviruses, or adenoviruses) do not cause leukocytes in the stool. Therefore a negative fecal leukocyte test result does not rule out other potential problems.

Procedure and patient care

Before

PT Explain the procedure to the patient.

PT Tell the patient that no fasting is needed.

During

- Collect a random stool specimen at least the size of a walnut. Liquid stool may be used.
- Carefully follow instructions on container. Fresh, ECOFIX-preserved, or polyvinyl alcohol-preserved stool must be sent to the laboratory.

After

PT Tell the patient that results will be available within 1 to 2 days.

Abnormal findings

Infectious colitis such as cholera, *C. difficile*, *Salmonella*, etc.
Inflammatory bowel diseases such as ulcerative colitis, or Crohn disease

notes

Streptococcus serologic testing (Antistreptolysin O titer [ASO], Antideoxyribonuclease-B titer, [Anti-DNase-B, ADNase-B, ADB], *Streptococcus* group B antigen detection, Streptozyme)

Type of test   Blood, cerebrospinal fluid (CSF)

Normal findings

Antistreptolysin O titer
    Adult/elderly: ≤ 160 Todd units/mL
    Child:
        5–12 years: 170–330 Todd units/mL
        2–4 years: ≤ 160 Todd units/mL
        6 months-2 years: ≤ 50 Todd units/mL
        Newborn: similar to mother's value
Antideoxyribonuclease-B titer
    Adult: ≤ 85 Todd units/mL or titer ≤ 1:85
    Child:
        School age: ≤ 170 Todd units/mL or titer ≤ 1:170
        Preschool age: ≤ 60 Todd units/mL or titer ≤ 1:60
Streptozyme
    Titer < 1:100
Streptococcus group B antigen
    None detected

Test explanation and related physiology

Infection by group A *Streptococcus* is unique because it can be followed by a serious nonpurulent complication (e.g., rheumatic fever, scarlet fever, glomerulonephritis). Serologic tests are used primarily to determine whether a previous group A *Streptococcus* infection (pharyngitis, pyodermia, pneumonia) has caused a poststreptococcal disease. These poststreptococcal diseases occur after the infection and after a period of latency during which the patient is asymptomatic.

These antibodies are directed against streptococcal extracellular products that are primarily enzymatic proteins. Serial rising titers of these antibodies over several weeks followed by a slow fall in titers are more supportive of the diagnosis of a previous streptococcal infection than is a single titer.

One such extracellular enzyme produced by streptococcus is called *streptolysin O,* which has the ability to destroy (lyse) RBC corpuscles. The streptolysin O is antigenic, stimulating the immunologic production of a neutralizing *ASO antibody.* ASO appears in the serum 1 week to 1 month after the onset of a streptococcal infection. A high ASO titer is not specific for

S

a certain type of poststreptococcal disease (i.e., rheumatic fever versus glomerulonephritis) but merely indicates that a streptococcal infection is or has been present.

Like the ASO titer, *ADB* is used to detect previous streptococcal infections. Although this test may be more sensitive than the ASO titer, it is not used alone in the evaluation of streptococcal infections because its results are too variable.

The *Streptozyme* assay detects antibodies to multiple extracellular antigens of group A *Streptococcus,* including antistreptolysin O, antistreptokinase, and antihyaluronidase. Approximately 80% of specimens positive by streptozyme have antistreptolysin O, and 10% have antistreptokinase and/or antihyaluronidase. The remaining 10% of positive samples are apparently caused by ADB antibodies or other streptococcal extracellular antigens.

Streptococcus group B antigens accumulate in CSF, serum, or urine and provide a direct qualitative detection of bacterial antigens. These antigens indicate acute infection and are not related to poststreptococcal sequelae as described previously. Confirmatory diagnosis of streptococcal infection is done by cultures (p. 710).

Interfering factors

- Increased beta-lipoprotein levels inhibit streptolysin O and give a falsely high ASO titer.

Procedure and patient care

- See inside front cover for Routine Blood Testing.
- Fasting: no
- Blood tube commonly used: red

Abnormal findings

▲ Increased levels

Acute glomerulonephritis
Acute rheumatic fever
Bacterial endocarditis
Scarlet fever
Streptococcal infection
Streptococcal pyoderma

notes

Type of test Urine, blood, various

Normal findings

Negative

Test explanation and related physiology

Substance abuse testing is used mostly by employers and law enforcement agencies. Industrial testing is used at the time of preemployment, prepromotion, annual physical examination, after an accident when there is reasonable suspicion, or for random testing or follow-up treatment surveillance.

Most commonly, a drug screen is performed to detect small amounts of any number of metabolites of commonly used drugs. If the screen result is positive, a more accurate and quantitative test is performed on the same specimen. Drug screens are available for a variety of drug categories. The most common are listed in Table S1. Alcohol testing is most commonly used by law enforcement (see ethanol, p. 320). Not only is drug testing helpful in identifying users, it also acts as a deterrent. Athletes can be tested for anabolic hormones, stimulants, diuretics, beta-blockers, street drugs, antiestrogens, erythropoietin, and beta-2 agonists that may unfairly improve their performance. Health and life insurance companies routinely test for illicit drugs.

Until recently, substance abuse testing has used urine exclusively as the sample of choice. Urine drug testing is generally inexpensive. Urine is easily obtained, and it contains a large amount of drug metabolites. More important, whereas urine can identify drug usage for several days after the last usage, blood testing reflects drug usage only during the past few hours.

Saliva, breath, hair, and sweat are becoming increasingly important and accurate specimens for specific drug testing. These testing methods are very expensive, however. Hair samples detect the presence of drugs used during the past 3 months. In addition, hair and nail samples may be used to detect or document exposure to arsenic and mercury.

Ideally, all urine specimens should be observed. Unannounced testing is another way to improve validity. Therefore the urine sample is tested for odor, color, temperature, creatinine, pH, and specific gravity to ensure that it is a proper specimen. Results can be affected by genetic disorders in drug metabolism (e.g.,

TABLE S1   **Typical multipanel drug screen**

Drugs or drug classes	Screen	Confirmation[a]
Amphetamines	300 ng/mL	200 ng/mL
Barbiturates	200 ng/mL	50 ng/mL
Benzodiazepines	200 ng/mL	20 ng/mL
Cocaine	150 ng/mL	50 ng/mL
Marijuana	20 ng/mL	5 ng/mL
MDMA (Ecstasy)	500 ng/mL	200 ng/mL
Methadone	150 ng/mL	10 ng/mL
Opiates	300 ng/mL	5 ng/mL
Oxycodone	100 ng/mL	5 ng/mL
Phencyclidine	25 ng/mL	10 ng/mL
Propoxyphene	300 ng/mL	10 ng/mL

[a] Confirmatory tests are more sensitive and can detect metabolites at lower levels.

CYP2D6 or catechol-O-methyltransferase) and drug receptor variations (e,g., opiod receptor exon 1). This must be considered in result interpretation.

Toxicology screening tests for drug overdose and poisoning (e.g., lead and carbon monoxide) are best performed on blood. Results indicate current drug levels, which are used to determine or alter therapy.

Interfering factors
- Poppy seeds can cause positive opiate results.
- Secondhand marijuana smoke can cause positive THC results.
- Detergents, bicarbonates, salt tablets, and blood can all foil accurate drug testing in a urine specimen.

Procedure and patient care
Before
PT Explain the procedure to the patient or significant others.
- If the specimen is obtained for medicolegal testing, ensure that the patient or family member has signed a consent form.
- Obtain a list of prescription medicines that the patient is taking that may alter or confuse screening results.
- Carefully assess the patient for respiratory distress.

During
- Collect blood and urine samples as designated by the lab.

- Urine specimens for substance abuse testing are usually collected in the presence of a healthcare provider.
- Be sure that the patient does not alter the urine specimen.
- For hair testing, cut 50 strands of hair from the scalp.
- A second confirmatory specimen may be obtained (and is used if results are positive).
- Collect gastric contents as indicated by the specific institution. A nasogastric tube is required.

After

- Apply pressure to the venipuncture site.
- If indicated, refer the patient for appropriate counseling.
- Follow the chain of custody for the specimen as provided by standard guidelines of the institution.
- Place the specimen in the required container for delivery.
- Check the temperature of urine specimens within 3 minutes after voiding. The temperature should be between 97° and 99° F.
- The specimen may be sent to a nationally certified laboratory for federal workers or workplace testing. Local hospital laboratories are often able to test for many drugs.

Abnormal findings

Positive drug level

notes

S

swallowing examination (Videofluoroscopy swallowing examination)

Type of test X-ray with contrast

Normal findings

Normal swallowing function and complete clearing of radio-graphic material through the upper digestive tract

Test explanation and related physiology

This test is performed to identify problems that exist in a patient who is unable to swallow. Problems in swallowing may result from local structural diseases such as tumors, upper esophageal diverticula, inflammation, extrinsic compression of the upper GI tract, or surgery on the oropharyngeal tract. Motility disorders of the upper GI tract (e.g., Zenker diverticulum) and neurologic disorders (e.g., stroke syndrome), Parkinson disease, and neuropathies also may cause difficulty in swallowing. Videofluoroscopy of the swallowing function allows a speech pathologist to delineate more clearly the exact pathology in the swallowing mechanism. This procedure then can be used to determine the most appropriate treatment and teach the patient the proper swallowing technique.

This test is performed by asking the patient to swallow barium or a barium-containing meal. With the use of videofluoroscopy, the swallowing function is visualized and documented. Morphologic abnormalities and functional impairment can be identified easily using the slow-frame progression and reversal that is available with videofluoroscopy. Although this test is similar to the barium swallow (p. 109), finer details of swallowing can be evaluated with the use of videofluoroscopy.

Contraindications

- Patients who aspirate their saliva are not candidates for this swallowing examination because they will require nonswallowing methods of alimentation.

Procedure and patient care

Before

PT Explain the procedure to the patient. See p. xviii for radiation exposure and risks.

PT Explain to the patient that no preparation is required.

During

- In the radiology department, the patient is asked to swallow a barium-containing meal. The consistency of the meal will be determined by the speech therapist and radiologist. The food may be liquid, semisoft (e.g., applesauce), or solid (e.g., a tea biscuit). While the patient is swallowing, videofluoroscopy is recorded in both the lateral and the anterior positions.
- The video is then examined by the radiologist and speech pathologist.

After

- No catharsis is required.

Abnormal findings

Achalasia
Cancer
Diffuse esophageal spasms
Extrinsic compression
Neuromuscular disorder
Oral pharyngeal inflammation
Upper GI motility disorder (e.g., stroke syndrome, Parkinson disease, peripheral neuropathy)
Zenker diverticulum

notes

S

sweat test (Sweat electrolyte test, Sweat chloride test, Sweat conductivity test, Iontophoretic sweat test)

Type of test Fluid analysis

Normal findings

Sodium values in children
> Normal: < 70 mEq/L
> Abnormal: > 90 mEq/L
> Equivocal: 70–90 mEq/L

Chloride values in children
> Normal: < 50 mEq/L
> Abnormal: > 60 mEq/L
> Equivocal: 50–60 mEq/L

Test explanation and related physiology

Patients with cystic fibrosis (CF) have increased sodium and chloride contents in their sweat. CF is an inherited disease characterized by abnormal secretion by exocrine glands in the bronchi, small intestines, pancreatic ducts, bile ducts, and skin (sweat glands). Increased sodium, chloride, and water stay in the cells and cause thick secretions in the ducts of multiple organs. Increased concentrations of these electrolytes exist in the sweat of patients with CF. Sweat induced by electrical current *(pilocarpine iontophoresis)* is collected, and its sodium and chloride contents are measured. In most circumstances just the chloride needs to be tested. Sodium usually mirrors chloride.

This test can also be used to screen children or siblings of CF patients for the disease. Almost all patients with CF have sweat sodium and chloride contents two to five times greater than normal values. In patients with suspicious clinical manifestations, these levels are diagnostic of CF.

Sweat direct measurement testing is the preferred confirmatory test for CF. Measuring the *sweat conductivity* by using a commercial analyzer is easier and is most used as a screening test for CF.

Molecular genotyping for the CFTR gene (see genetic testing, p. 369) is used for carrier identification, prenatal diagnosis in at-risk pregnancies and newborn screening programs for CF.

Procedure and patient care

Before

PT Explain the procedure to the patient and parents.

PT Tell the patient and parents that no fasting is required.

During

- Note the following procedural steps:
    1. For iontophoresis, a low-level electrical current is applied to the test area (the thigh in infants and the forearm in older children).
    2. Pilocarpine hydrochloride is applied to the positive electrode to induce sweating. The negative electrode is saturated with a bicarbonate solution.
    3. Paper disks are used to collect the sweat.
    4. The paper disks are weighed and sent for sodium and chloride analysis.
- Note that a technologist performs the sweat test in approximately 90 minutes in the laboratory or at the bedside.
- **PT** Inform the patient that the electrical current is small and no discomfort or pain is generally associated with this test.

After

PT Initiate extensive education and counseling for the patient and parents if the results indicate CF.

Abnormal findings

CF

notes

S

---

syphilis detection test (Serologic test for syphilis [STS], Venereal Disease Research Laboratory [VDRL], Rapid plasma reagin [RPR], Fluorescent treponemal antibody test [FTA])

Type of test Blood

Normal findings

Negative or nonreactive

Test explanation and related physiology

Serologic tests are used to diagnose and to document successful therapy for syphilis. Syphilis is caused by the spirochete *Treponema pallidum* that cannot be isolated in culture. Two groups of antibodies form the basis for these tests. The first and older of these tests detects a nontreponemal antibody called *reagin,* which reacts to phospholipids similar to lipids in the membrane of *T. pallidum.* The nontreponemal antibody tests are relatively nonspecific and lack sensitivity. These antibodies would be detected by the *Wassermann test, VDRL test,* or *RPR test.* These test results become positive after 2 weeks from the patient's inoculation with *T. pallidum* and return to normal after adequate treatment is administered. The test result is positive in nearly all primary and secondary stages of syphilis and in two-thirds of patients with tertiary syphilis. Screening for syphilis is usually done during the first prenatal checkup for pregnant women using the VDRL or RPR. VDRL is the only test that can be used on cerebral spinal fluid (CSF) when evaluating neurosyphilis. They are also used to document the success of treatment.

If these nontreponemal serologic test results are positive, the diagnosis must be confirmed by the second type of syphilis test, called *Treponema test,* such as the *FTA absorption test (FTA-ABS)* or the *microhemagglutination assay (MHA-TP).* These tests for a more specific antibody are more accurate than the VDRL and RPR tests. The FTA-ABS and MHA-TP are technically simple to perform, but they are labor intensive and require subjective interpretation by testing personnel. In contrast, the syphilis IgG *enzyme immunoassay (EIA)* is a treponemal test for the detection of IgG class antibodies.

During early primary syphilis, the first antibodies to appear are IgM, with IgG antibodies reaching significant titers later in the primary phase. As the disease progresses into the secondary phase, IgG *T. pallidum* antibodies reach peak titers. *T. pallidum* IgG antibodies persist indefinitely, regardless of the course of the disease. If syphilis IgG and/or IgM is positive, results can be confirmed with FTA or MHA testing. The IgG- and IgM-specific antibodies assist in determining the etiology of neonatal syphilis. IgM does not pass through the placenta and, if positive, indicates active neonatal infection.

Interfering factors

- Excessive hemolysis and gross lipemia may affect test results.
- Excess chyle in the blood may interfere with the test results.
- Many conditions cause false-positive results when VDRL and RPR tests are used. Some of these conditions include *Mycoplasma* pneumonia, malaria, acute bacterial and viral infections, autoimmune diseases, and pregnancy.
- Recent ingestion of alcohol may alter the test results.

Procedure and patient care

- See inside front cover for Routine Blood Testing.
- Fasting: verify with laboratory
- Blood tube commonly used: red
- Check with the laboratory regarding fasting requirements. Some prefer collecting the specimen before meals. Some laboratories request that the patient refrain from alcohol for 24 hours before the blood test.
- PT If the test result is positive, instruct the patient to inform recent sexual contacts so that they can be evaluated.
- PT If the test result is positive, be sure the patient receives the appropriate antibiotic therapy.

Abnormal findings

Syphilis

notes

S

testosterone (Dihydrotestosterone [DHT])

Type of test Blood

Normal findings

Free testosterone, pg/mL

Male	Female
	Postmenopausal: 0.6–3.8
Tanner stage I: ≤ 3.7	Tanner stage I: < 2.2
Tanner stage II: 0.3–21	Tanner stage II: 0.4–4.5
Tanner stage III: 1–98	Tanner stage III: 1.3–7.5
Tanner stage IV: 35–169	Tanner stage IV: 1.1–15.5
Tanner stage V: 41–239	Tanner stage V: 0.8–9.2

% Free testosterone
Adult male: 1.6%-2.9%
Adult female: 0.1%-0.3%

Total testosterone, ng/dL

Age	Male	Female
7 months-9 years (Tanner stage I)	< 30	< 30
10–13 years (Tanner stage II)	< 300	< 40
14–15 years (Tanner stage III)	170–540	< 60
16–19 years (Tanner stage IV, V)	250–910	< 70
20 years and above	280–1080	< 70

Dihydrotestosterone
Adult male: 240–650 pg/mL
Adult female: ≤ 300 pg/mL

Test explanation and related physiology

Testosterone levels are used to evaluate ambiguous sex characteristics, precocious puberty, virilizing syndromes in the female, and infertility in the male. This test can also be used as a tumor marker for rare tumors of the ovary and testicle.

Androgens include dehydroepiandrosterone (DHEA), androstenedione, and testosterone. DHEA is produced in the adrenal glands during cortisol and aldosterone formation, and it is also produced *de novo* by the testes or the ovaries. DHEA is the precursor of androstenedione, which is the precursor of testosterone (and estrogen).

Testosterone levels vary by sex and stage of maturity (indicated by Tanner stage). Physiologically, testosterone stimulates spermatogenesis and influences the development of male secondary sex characteristics. Overproduction of this hormone in a young male may cause precocious puberty. This can be caused by testicular, adrenal, or pituitary tumors. Overproduction of this hormone in females causes masculinization, which is manifested as amenorrhea and excessive growth of body hair (hirsutism). Ovarian and adrenal tumors/hyperplasia and medications (e.g., danazol) are all potential causes of masculinization in the female. Reduced levels of testosterone in the male suggest hypogonadism or Klinefelter syndrome.

Dihydrotestosterone (DHT) is the principal androgen made in body tissues, particularly the prostate. Levels of DHT remain normal with aging, despite a decrease in the plasma testosterone. Measurement of this hormone is useful in monitoring patients receiving 5 alpha-reductase inhibitor therapy, such as finasteride or chemotherapy, which may affect prostate function. It is also useful in evaluating patients with possible 5 alpha-reductase deficiency.

There are several *testosterone stimulation tests* that can be performed to more accurately evaluate hypogonadism. Human chorionic gonadotropin, clomiphene, and GnRH can be used to stimulate testosterone secretion.

17-Ketosteroids (17-KS) are metabolites of the testosterone and nontestosterone androgenic sex hormones that are excreted in the urine.

11-oxoandrogens (11-ketotestosterone, 11-hydroxytestosterone, and 11-hydroxyandrostenedione) are only made in the adrenal gland of men and women and are used in the identification and surveillance of particular disease states. They are elevated in patients with congenital adrenal hyperplasia and can be used to monitor therapy of this disease. Testicular adrenal-rest tumors (TARTs) in men can be identified and treatment monitored with 11 oxo-androgen testing. 11-ketotestosterone has been shown to be in excess in polycystic ovary syndrome. Measuring 11-ketotestosterone as a marker of adrenal-specific androgens will provide additional information for monitoring GnRH agonist treatment prostate cancer.

Procedure and patient care

- See inside front cover for Routine Blood Testing.
- Fasting: no
- Blood tube commonly used: red

- Because testosterone levels are the highest in the early morning hours, blood should be drawn in the morning.

Abnormal findings

▲ **Increased levels (male)**

Adrenocortical tumor
Congenital adrenal
  hyperplasia
Encephalitis
Hyperthyroidism
Idiopathic sexual precocity
Pinealoma
Testicular or extragonadal
  tumor
Testosterone resistance
  syndromes

▼ **Decreased levels (male)**

Cryptorchidism
Hepatic cirrhosis
Klinefelter syndrome
Orchidectomy
Primary and secondary
  hypogonadism
Trisomy 21 (Down
  syndrome)

▲ **Increased levels (female)**

Adrenal tumor
Congenital adrenocortical hyperplasia
Idiopathic hirsutism
Ovarian tumor
Polycystic ovaries
Trophoblastic tumor

notes

thoracentesis and pleural fluid analysis (Pleural tap)

Type of test Fluid analysis

Normal findings

Gross appearance: Clear, serous, light yellow, 50 mL
Red blood cells (RBCs): None
White blood cells (WBCs): < 300/mL
Protein: < 4.1 g/dL
Glucose: 70–100 mg/dL
Amylase: 138–404 units/L
Alkaline phosphatase
    Adult male: 90–240 units/L
    Female: < 45 years: 76–196 units/L
    Female: > 45 years: 87–250 units/L
Lactic dehydrogenase (LDH): Similar to serum LDH
Cytology: No malignant cells
Bacteria: None
Fungi: None
Carcinoembryonic antigen (CEA): < 5 ng/mL

Test explanation and related physiology

Thoracentesis is an invasive procedure that entails insertion of a needle into the pleural space for removal of fluid (Figure T1). Pleural fluid is removed for diagnostic and therapeutic purposes. *Therapeutically,* it is done to relieve pain, dyspnea, and other symptoms of pleural pressure. Removal of this fluid also permits better radiographic visualization of the lung. *Diagnostically,* thoracentesis is performed to obtain and analyze fluid to determine the etiology of the pleural effusion.

Pleural fluid is classified according to transudate or exudate. *Transudates* are most frequently caused by congestive heart failure, cirrhosis, nephrotic syndrome, and hypoproteinemia. *Exudates* are most often found in inflammatory, infectious, or neoplastic conditions. However, collagen vascular disease, pulmonary infarction, trauma, and drug hypersensitivity also may cause an exudative effusion.

Pleural fluid is usually evaluated for the following features.

Gross appearance

The color, optical density, and viscosity are noted as the pleural fluid appears in the aspirating syringe. Empyema is characterized by the presence of a foul odor and thick, puslike fluid. An opalescent, pearly fluid is characteristic of chylothorax.

T

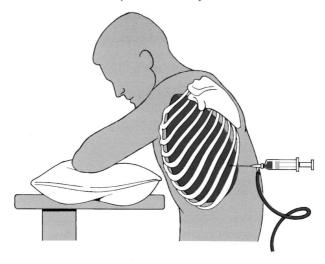

FIG. T1 Thoracentesis. A needle is placed through the chest wall and into the fluid contained in the pleural cavity. A special one-way valve system is placed between the needle and the syringe to allow aspiration of fluid when the plunger of the syringe is pulled back and diversion of the fluid to a container when the plunger is pushed in.

Cell counts

The WBC and differential counts are determined. A WBC count exceeding 1000/mL is suggestive of an exudate. The predominance of polymorphonuclear leukocytes usually is an indication of an acute inflammatory condition (e.g., pneumonia). When more than 50% of the WBCs are small lymphocytes, the effusion is usually caused by TB, or tumor. The presence of RBCs may indicate neoplasms, TB, or intrathoracic bleeding.

Protein content

Whereas total protein levels greater than 3 g/dL are characteristic of exudates, transudates usually have a protein content of less than 3 g/dL. The *albumin gradient* between serum and pleural fluid can differentiate better between the transudate and exudate natures of pleural fluid than can the total protein content. The total protein ratio (fluid/serum) has been considered to be another accurate criterion differentiating transudate from exudate.

Lactic dehydrogenase

A pleural fluid/serum LDH ratio greater than 0.6 is typical of an exudate. An exudate is identified with a high degree of accuracy if the pleural fluid/serum protein ratio is greater than 0.5 and the pleural fluid/serum LDH ratio is greater than 0.6.

Glucose

Usually pleural glucose levels approximate serum levels. Low values appear to be a combination of glycolysis by the extra cells and impairment of glucose diffusion because of damage to the pleural membrane. Values less than 60 mg/dL are occasionally seen in TB, or malignancy and typically occur in rheumatoid arthritis and empyema.

Amylase

In a malignant effusion, the amylase concentration is slightly elevated. Amylase levels above the normal range are seen when the effusion is caused by pancreatitis or rupture of the esophagus associated with leakage of salivary amylase.

Triglyceride

Measurement of triglyceride levels is an important part of identifying chylous effusions. These effusions are usually produced by obstruction or transection of the lymphatic system caused by lymphoma, neoplasm, trauma, or recent surgery.

Gram stain and bacteriologic culture

These tests are routinely performed when bacterial pneumonia or empyema is a possible cause of the effusion.

Cultures for *Mycobacterium tuberculosis* and fungus

Tuberculosis is less often a cause for pleural effusion in the United States today than it was. Fungus may be a cause of pulmonary effusion in patients with compromised immunologic defenses.

Cytology

A cytologic study is performed to detect tumor cells in patients with malignant effusions. Breast and lung are the two most common tumors; lymphoma is the third.

Carcinoembryonic antigen

Pleural fluid CEA levels are elevated in various malignant (gastrointestinal, breast) conditions (p. 164).

Special tests

The pH of pleural fluid is usually 7.4 or greater. The pH is typically less than 7.2 when empyema is present. The pH may be 7.2 to 7.4 in TB, or malignancy.

In some instances, the rheumatoid factor (p. 648) and the complement levels (p. 226) are also measured in pleural fluid.

Pleural fluid antinuclear antibody (ANA) levels and pleural fluid/serum ANA ratios are often used to evaluate pleural effusion secondary to systemic lupus erythematosus.

When tuberculosis (TB) is suspected, the effusion can be tested for *Adenosine Deaminase (ADA)*. ADA is an enzyme in lymphocytes and myeloid cells. ADA levels are elevated in inflammatory effusions caused by bacterial infections, granulomatous inflammation (e.g., tuberculosis, sarcoidosis), malignancy, and autoimmune diseases (e.g., lupus, vasculitis). ADA cannot distinguish between latent and active TB.

Contraindications

• Patients with significant thrombocytopenia

Potential complications

• Pneumothorax because of puncture of the visceral pleura or entry of air into the pleural space
• Interpleural bleeding because of puncture of tissue or a blood vessel
• Hemoptysis caused by needle puncture of a pulmonary vessel or by inflammation
• Reflex bradycardia and hypotension
• Pulmonary edema
• Seeding of the needle track with tumor

Procedure and patient care

Before

PT Explain the procedure to the patient.
• Obtain informed consent for this procedure.
PT Tell the patient that no fasting or sedation is usually necessary.
PT Inform the patient that movement or coughing should be minimized to avoid inadvertent needle damage.
• Administer a cough suppressant before the procedure if the patient has a troublesome cough.

During

• Note the following procedural steps:
  1. The patient is usually placed in an upright position, with the arms and shoulders raised and supported.
  2. The thoracentesis is performed under strict sterile technique.
  3. The needle insertion site, which is determined by percussion, auscultation, and examination of a chest x-ray image, ultrasound scan, or fluoroscopy, is aseptically cleansed and anesthetized locally.

4. The needle is positioned in the pleural space, and the fluid is withdrawn with a syringe and a three-way stopcock.

5. A short catheter may be inserted into the pleural space for fluid aspiration.

- Monitor the patient's pulse for reflex bradycardia and evaluate the patient for diaphoresis and a feeling of faintness.
- Note that this procedure is performed by a physician at the patient's bedside, in a procedure room, or in the physician's office in less than 30 minutes.
- PT Tell the patient that he or she may feel a pressure-like pain when the pleura is entered and the fluid is removed.

After

- Place a small bandage over the needle site. Usually turn the patient on the unaffected side for 1 hour to allow the pleural puncture site to heal.
- Send the labeled specimen promptly to the laboratory.
- Obtain a chest x-ray to check for pneumothorax.
- Monitor the patient's vital signs.
- Observe the patient for coughing or expectoration of blood (hemoptysis), which may indicate trauma to the lung.
- Evaluate the patient for signs and symptoms of pneumothorax, tension pneumothorax, subcutaneous emphysema, and pyogenic infection (e.g., tachypnea, dyspnea, diminished breath sounds, anxiety, restlessness, fever).

Abnormal findings

Exudate
Collagen vascular disease
Drug hypersensitivity
Empyema
Lymphoma
Pancreatitis
Pneumonia
Pulmonary infarction
Ruptured esophagus
TB, effusion
Tumors

Transudate
Cirrhosis
Congestive heart failure
Hypoproteinemia
Nephrotic syndrome
Trauma

T

notes

throat and nose cultures and sensitivity

Type of test Microscopic examination

Normal findings

Negative

Test explanation and related physiology

Because the throat and nose are normally colonized by many organisms, cultures of these areas serve only to isolate and identify a few particular pathogens (e.g., streptococci, meningococci, gonococci, *Bordetella pertussis, Corynebacterium diphtheriae*).

Streptococci are most often sought on a throat culture because beta-hemolytic streptococcal pharyngitis may be followed by rheumatic heart disease or glomerulonephritis. This type of streptococcal infection most frequently affects children between the ages of 3 and 15 years.

Rapid immunologic tests *(strep screens)* with antiserum against group A streptococcus antigen are very accurate. With these kits, the streptococcus organism can be identified directly from the swab specimen without culture in about 15 minutes.

Nasal and nasopharyngeal cultures are often done to screen for infections and carrier states caused by various other organisms, such as *Staphylococcus aureus, Haemophilus influenzae, Neisseria meningitidis,* respiratory syncytial virus (RSV), and viruses causing rhinitis. Health-care workers in the operating room and newborn nursery may have these cultures to screen potential sources of spread when an outbreak occurs in a hospital setting.

About 5% of hospitalized patients carry *methicillin resistant staphylococcus aureus (MRSA)* in their nose or on their skin. However, people who are simply colonized won't necessarily develop a serious infection. These patients can, however, act as carriers of the bacterium to others who may experience invasive MRSA infections. MRSA is most commonly identified by nasal swab cultures. Unfortunately, it takes 48 hours to identify MRSA in cultures. *Bacteriophage technology* is able to detect MRSA more quickly – as early as 6 hours. This new technology offers health care providers an advantage when trying to prevent and contain the spread of antibiotic resistant bacteria.

All cultures should be performed before antibiotic therapy is initiated. Otherwise, the antibiotic may interrupt the growth of the organism in the laboratory. Most organisms take approximately 24 hours to grow in the laboratory, and a preliminary report can be given at that time. Occasionally, 48 to 72 hours is required for growth and identification of the organism.

Procedure and patient care

Before

PT Explain the procedure to the patient.

During

- Obtain a *throat culture* by depressing the tongue with a wooden tongue blade and touching the posterior wall of the throat and areas of inflammation, exudation, or ulceration with a sterile cotton swab. Two swabs are preferred. Growth of streptococcus from both swabs is more accurate, and the second swab can also be used in the strep screen. Avoid touching any part of the mouth. Place the swabs in a sterile container.
- Obtain a *nasal culture* by gently raising the tip of the nose and inserting a flexible swab into the nares. Rotate the swab against the side of the nares. Remove the swab and place it in an appropriate culture tube.
- Obtain a *nasopharyngeal culture* by gently raising the tip of the nose and inserting a flexible swab along the bottom of the nares. Guide this swab until it reaches the posterior pharynx. Rotate the swab to obtain secretions and then remove it. Place the swab in an appropriate culture tube.

After

- Label all specimens and send them immediately to the microbiology laboratory.

Abnormal findings

Bacterial pathogens (e.g., streptococci)
H. influenzae bacteria
Respiratory syncytial virus

notes

T

thromboelastography (Thromboelastometry)

Type of test Blood

Normal findings

5.3–12.4 dynes/cm²

Possible critical value

> 12.4 dynes/cm²

Test explanation and related physiology

Trauma, infection, and inflammation all activate the blood's clotting system, which depends on the interaction of two separate systems: enzymatic proteins (clotting factors, intrinsic and extrinsic systems) and platelets. The two systems work in concert to plug defects in the broken vessels. If a particular clotting factor is dysfunctional or absent, as in hemophilia, an insufficient amount of fibrin forms. Similarly, massive consumption of clotting factors in a trauma situation decreases the amount of fibrin formed. Inadequate numbers of platelets resulting from trauma, surgery, or chemotherapy also decrease platelet aggregation, as do genetic disorders, uremia, or medication therapy. Ultimately, reduced fibrin formation or platelet aggregation results in clots of inadequate tensile strength and reduced elastography. This *hypo*coagulable state is associated with excessive bleeding. Conversely, endothelial injury, stasis, cancer, genetic diseases, or other *hyper*coagulable states lead to thrombosis formation, causing thromboembolic events.

This test is used to determine platelet function (p. 579) and to identify patients who are hypercoagulable and may experience a thromboembolic phenomenon when immobile (e.g., after surgery or trauma). It is also used to determine hyperfibrinolysis as a cause of hypocoagulability. This test can determine the percent of platelet inhibition instigated by drugs such as heparin, aspirin, and antiplatelet drugs.

Procedure and patient care

- See inside front cover for Routine Blood Testing.
- Fasting: no
- Blood tube commonly used: red
- Remember that abnormalities in platelet aggregation can prolong bleeding time.

Abnormal findings

Hypocoagulability
    Anticoagulation
    Factor deficiency
    Increased fibrinolysis
    Platelet function abnormalities
    Thrombocytopenia

Hypercoagulability
    Factor V Leiden abnormality
    Genetic hypercoagulability
    Idiopathic hypercoagulability
    Protein S/C abnormality

notes

T

thrombosis indicators
fibrin monomers (Fibrin degradation products [FDPs], Fibrin split products [FSPs])
fibrinopeptide A (FPA)
prothrombin fragment (F1 + 2)

Type of test Blood

Normal findings

FDP: < 10 mcg/mL or < 10 mg/L (SI units)
FPA
    Male: 0.4–2.6 mg/mL
    Female: 0.7–3.1 mg/mL
F1+2: 7.4–103 mcg/L or 0.2–2.8 nmol/L

Possible critical values

FDP: > 40 mcg/mL

Test explanation and related physiology

Identification of FDPs, FPA, and F1 + 2 is mostly used to document that fibrin clot formation and therefore thrombosis is occurring in patients. These tests support the diagnosis of disseminated intravascular coagulation (DIC). The D-dimer test (p. 264) is more commonly used to identify DIC or other forms of thrombosis. These tests also provide an indication of the effectiveness of anticoagulation therapy. Finally, they are used to support the diagnosis and follow treatment for hypercoagulable states.

F1 + 2 is liberated when prothrombin is converted to thrombin in reaction 4 of secondary hemostasis (see Figure C3, p. 212). FPA is released into the bloodstream from alpha and beta chains of fibrinogen during its conversion to fibrin.

Measurement of FDPs is an indicator of the activity of the fibrinolytic system. Whenever a fibrin clot or primarily fibrinogen degenerates, fragment monomers called FDPs (X, D, E, and Y) result. These, therefore, are indirect evidence of thrombosis and/or DIC. FDPs also are increased with other secondary fibrinolytic disorders. Thrombolytic therapy used to treat vascular thrombosis is associated with increased FDPs. Streptokinase or urokinase stimulates the conversion of plasminogen to plasmin.

These products of hemostasis and fibrinolysis also may be elevated in patients with extensive malignancy, tissue necrosis, trauma surgery, or gram-negative sepsis.

Interfering factors

- Traumatic venipunctures may increase FPA levels.
- Surgery or massive trauma is associated with increased levels.
- Menstruation may be associated with increased FDP levels.

Procedure and patient care

- See inside front cover for Routine Blood Testing.
- Fasting: no
- Blood tube commonly used: verify with laboratory
- Avoid prolonged use of a tourniquet.
- Draw the sample before initiating heparin therapy.
- Avoid excessive agitation of the blood sample.

Abnormal findings

▲ Increased levels

Advanced malignancy
Antithrombin III deficiency
Deficiency in proteins S
  and C
DIC
Heart or vascular surgery
Massive trauma
Postoperative states
Severe inflammation
Thromboembolism
Thrombosis

▼ Decreased levels

Anticoagulation therapy

notes

T

thyroglobulin (Tg, Thyrogen-stimulated thyroglobulin)

Type of test Blood
Normal findings

Age	Male, ng/mL	Female, ng/mL
12 years and older	0.5–53	0.5–43
1–11 years	0.6–50.1	0.5–52.1
0–11 months	0.6–5.5	0.5–5.5

Test explanation and related physiology

Thyroglobulin is the protein precursor of thyroid hormone and is made by both normal, well-differentiated, benign thyroid cells and thyroid cancer cells. Because thyroglobulin is normally only made by thyroid cells, it serves as a useful readout for the presence or absence of thyroid cells, especially after thyroid cancer surgery. This test is primarily used as a tumor marker for well-differentiated thyroid cancers (p. 164, Tumor markers).

If postoperative Tg levels are low, very little thyroid tissue remains. Tg can also be used as a tumor marker for thyroid cancer. Rising levels of Tg may indicate recurrence.

After thyroidectomy, thyroid hormone replacement is required for normal metabolic function. Endogenous stimulation of any residual thyroid cells is minimal in these patients. As a result, Tg and endogenous thyroid hormones are low.

Thyrogen-stimulated testing has eliminated the need for withdrawal of thyroid hormone medications and provides a safe and effective method to elevate TSH levels so that even minimal levels of Tg can be detected. This allows patients to undergo periodic thyroid cancer follow-up evaluations while avoiding the often debilitating side effects of hypothyroidism.

Thyrogen is a highly purified recombinant source of human TSH. Thyrogen raises serum TSH levels and thereby stimulates Tg production. Normal thyroid-remnant and well-differentiated thyroid tumors display a greater (> 10-fold) serum Tg response to TSH stimulation. If, after thyroid surgery, thyrogen-stimulated Tg levels are elevated, either a significant amount of normal thyroid gland was left in the neck or metastatic disease exists.

Thyrogen stimulation is also used for patients undergoing I^{131} whole-body scanning for metastatic thyroid cancer. Now, with the use of Thyrogen, the ill effects of hormone withdrawal are not experienced.

In patients with thyroid cancer an aspirate from a cervical lymph node can be tested for the presence of thyroglobulin if there is suspicion that thyroid cancer has spread to the lymphatic system.

Interfering factors
- Levels are decreased in less well-differentiated thyroid cancers.
- Thyrogen stimulation of Tg levels is less in patients whose tumors do not have TSH receptors or whose tumors cannot make Tg.

Procedure and patient care
- See inside front cover for Routine Blood Testing.
- Fasting: no
- Blood tube commonly used: serum separator
- Determine whether the patient is to have a whole-body nuclear scan along with the Tg blood test.
- If thyrogen stimulation is to be used:
  1. Administer thyrogen intramuscularly to the buttock every 24 hours for two or three doses as ordered.
  2. Collect a venous blood sample in a gold-top (serum separator) tube after 3 days.
- For radioiodine imaging:
  1. The nuclear medicine technologist will administer the radioiodine 24 hours after the final thyrogen injection.
  2. Scanning is usually performed 48 hours after radioiodine administration.
  3. Scanning times for single (spot) images of body regions may be obtained.

Abnormal findings
▲ **Increased levels**
   Metastatic thyroid cancer
   Residual thyroid tissue in the neck

T

notes

thyroid fine needle aspiration biopsy (FNAB, Skinny-needle thyroid biopsy, Fine-needle aspiration [FNA])

Type of test Microscopic examination of tissue

Normal findings

Benign

Test explanation and related physiology

FNAB is used to obtain tissue to rule out cancer in a "cold" (does not light up on a thyroid scan) thyroid nodule or cyst of a patient whose thyroid function is normal. In FNAB, samples of thyroid tissue are obtained by placing a very thin needle into the thyroid nodule and obtaining small pieces of thyroid tissue that are then examined microscopically. The Bethesda System for Reporting Thyroid Cytopathology is used to provide the results of the biopsy. The implied risk of malignancy for each diagnostic category is shown in the following table.

Diagnosis	Chance of malignancy with surgical biopsy, %
Nondiagnostic	1–4
Benign	0–3
Atypia	5–15
Follicular neoplasm	15–30
Suspicious	60–75
Malignant	> 97

FNAB samples can be challenging to interpret and produce indeterminate results in 15% to 30% of cases. Approximately 70% to 80% of the time, the nodules prove to be benign for cancer by surgical pathology.

Contraindications

- Patients with coagulation disorders because of the risk of excessive bleeding
- Patients with hyperthyroidism, because the needle insertion may instigate thyroid storm and toxic nodular goiters are not malignant.

Potential complications

- Hemorrhage from the highly vascular thyroid tissue
- Cyst formation in the thyroid gland
- Infection when an open biopsy is performed

Procedure and patient care

Before

PT Explain the procedure to the patient.
• Ensure that the physician obtains informed consent.
PT Inform the patient that no fasting is required.
PT Tell the patient that no sedative is required.
• Note that the needle stick may be done at the bedside.
• If ultrasound guidance is to be used, note that the needle stick is performed in the radiology or ultrasonography department.

During

• Note the following procedural steps:
  1. The patient is placed in a supine position with a sandbag or pillow under the shoulder to hyperextend the neck.
  2. Under sterile conditions, the skin overlying the thyroid is infiltrated with a local anesthetic (lidocaine).
  3. If the nodule can be felt, a biopsy can be performed in the doctor's office. When the nodule is not palpable, ultrasound is used to help guide the biopsy.
  4. The patient holds her or his breath while the needle is rocked gently to obtain as much tissue as possible.
  5. The needle is then withdrawn and tissue is placed on a glass slide.

After

• Apply pressure over the thyroid area to minimize bleeding.
• Note that a physician performs this procedure in approximately 10 minutes.

Abnormal findings

Malignancy

notes

T

thyroid scanning (Thyroid scintiscan)

Type of test Nuclear scan

Normal findings

Normal size, shape, position, and function of the thyroid gland
No areas of decreased or increased uptake

Test explanation and related physiology

Thyroid scanning allows the size, shape, position, and physiologic function of the thyroid gland to be determined with the use of radionuclear scanning.

Thyroid nodules are easily detected by this technique. Nodules are classified as functioning (warm/hot) or nonfunctioning (cold), depending on the amount of radionuclide taken up by the nodule. A functioning nodule could represent a benign adenoma or a localized toxic goiter. A nonfunctioning nodule may represent a cyst, carcinoma, nonfunctioning adenoma or goiter, lymphoma, or localized area of thyroiditis.

Scanning is useful in patients with
- A neck or substernal mass.
- A thyroid nodule.
- Hyperthyroidism.
- Metastatic tumors without a known primary site.
- A well-differentiated form of thyroid cancer. Areas of metastasis may show up on whole-body nuclear scans.

Thyroid scanning is usually preceded by a thyroid uptake scan. An iodine-123 capsule is given to the patient 6 to 24 hours before measuring iodine uptake. After uptake counts are obtained, Tc 99m^{04} is administered intravenously. Scan images are then obtained as described earlier.

Another form of thyroid scan is called the *whole-body thyroid scan*. This scan is performed on patients who have previously had a thyroid cancer treated. An iodine-131 capsule or solution, Tc 99m^{04}, or iodine-123 is given orally, and the entire body is scanned to look for metastatic thyroid tissue. A hot spot indicates recurrent tumor. This test is routinely performed (every 1–2 years) on patients who have had a thyroid cancer larger than 1 cm.

Contraindications
- Patients who are allergic to iodine
- Patients who are pregnant unless benefits outweigh risks

Potential complications

- Radiation-induced oncogenesis. This complication is minimized if technetium or low-radioactive iodine isomers are used instead of iodine-131.

Interfering factors

- Iodine-containing foods, such as dairy products, shellfish, sushi, kelp, seaweed, and iodized salt.
- Recent administration of x-ray contrast agents

Procedure and patient care

Before

PT Explain the procedure to the patient. See p. xviii for radiation exposure and risks.
- Check the patient for allergies to iodine.
PT Instruct the patient about medications that need to be restricted for weeks before the test (e.g., thyroid drugs, medications containing iodine).
PT If indicated, instruct the patient about iodine-containing foods to avoid for about one week prior to testing.
- Obtain a history concerning previous contrast x-ray studies, nuclear scanning, or intake of any thyroid-suppressive or antithyroid drugs.
PT Tell the patient that fasting is usually not required.

During

- Note the following procedural steps:
  1. A standard dose of iodine-123 is usually given to the patient by mouth 6 to 24 hours before scanning. The capsule or solution is tasteless.
  2. Iodine uptake is measured. IV technetium is administered, and thyroid imaging is performed 2 hours later.
  3. At the designated time, the patient is placed in a supine position, and anterolateral images of the thyroid area are obtained. The whole-body imaging protocol is somewhat different.
  4. The radioactive counts are recorded and displayed.
- Note that this study is performed by a radiologic technologist in less than 30 minutes and is then interpreted by a nuclear medicine physician.
PT Tell the patient that no discomfort is experienced.

After

PT Usually the dose of radioactivity used in this test is minimal and considered harmless. No isolation and no special urine

precautions are needed. However, if higher doses of radionuclide are used, isolation for 24 hours may be recommended.

Abnormal findings

Adenoma
Carcinoma
Cyst
Graves disease
Hashimoto thyroiditis
Hyperthyroidism
Hypothyroidism
Lymphoma
Metastasis
Plummer disease
Thyroiditis
Toxic and nontoxic goiter

notes

thyroid-stimulating hormone (TSH, Thyrotropin, TRH stimulation test)

Type of test   Blood

Normal findings

Adult: 0.4–4.2 μU/mL or 0.4–4.2 mU/L (SI units)
Newborn: 3–18 μU/mL or 3–18 mU/L
Cord: 3–12 μU/mL or 3–12 mU/L
(Values vary among laboratories.)

Test explanation and related physiology

The TSH concentration aids in differentiating primary from secondary hypothyroidism. Pituitary TSH secretion is stimulated by hypothalamic thyroid-releasing hormone (TRH). Low levels of triiodothyronine and thyroxine (T_3 and T_4) are the underlying stimuli for TRH and TSH. Therefore a compensatory elevation of TRH and TSH occurs in patients with primary hypothyroid states such as surgical or radioactive thyroid ablation; patients with burned-out thyroiditis, thyroid agenesis, idiopathic hypothyroidism, or congenital hypothyroidism; and patients taking antithyroid medications.

In secondary hypothyroidism, the function of the hypothalamus or pituitary gland is faulty because of tumor, trauma, or infarction. Thus TRH and TSH cannot be secreted, and plasma levels of these hormones are near 0 despite low T_3 and T_4 levels.

The *TRH stimulation test* is sometimes used to stimulate low levels of TSH to identify primary from secondary hypothyroidism in cases in which TSH is low. However, this test is not commonly used because extremely low levels of TSH can be identified now with the use of immunoassays.

The TSH test is used as well to monitor exogenous thyroid replacement. The goal of thyroid replacement therapy is to provide an adequate amount of thyroid medication so that TSH secretion is in the low normal range, indicating a euthyroid state. This test is also done to detect primary hypothyroidism in newborns with low screening T_4 levels. TSH and T_4 levels are frequently measured to differentiate pituitary from thyroid dysfunction. A decreased T_4 with a normal or elevated TSH level can indicate a thyroid disorder. A decreased T_4 with a decreased TSH level can indicate a pituitary disorder.

T

Interfering factors
- Severe illness may cause decreased TSH levels.

Procedure and patient care
- See inside front cover for Routine Blood Testing.
- Fasting: no
- Blood tube commonly used: red
- Use a heel stick to obtain blood from newborns.

Abnormal findings

▲ **Increased levels**
Congenital hypothyroidism
Large doses of iodine
Pituitary TSH-secreting
  tumor
Primary hypothyroidism
  (thyroid dysfunction)
Severe and chronic illnesses
Thyroid agenesis
Thyroiditis

▼ **Decreased levels**
Hyperthyroidism
Pituitary hypofunction
Secondary
  hypothyroidism
  (pituitary dysfunction)

notes

thyroid-stimulating hormone stimulation test
(TSH stimulation test)

Type of test Blood

Normal findings

Increased thyroid function with administration of exogenous TSH

Test explanation and related physiology

The TSH stimulation test is used to differentiate *primary* (or thyroidal) hypothyroidism from *secondary* (or hypothalamic-pituitary) hypothyroidism. Normal people and patients with hypothalamic-pituitary hypothyroidism can increase thyroid function when exogenous TSH is given. However, patients with primary thyroidal hypothyroidism do not; their thyroid glands are inadequate and cannot function no matter how much stimulation they receive. Patients with less than a 10% increase in radioactive iodine uptake (RAIU) or less than a 1.5 mcg/dL rise in T_4 are considered to have a primary cause for their hypothyroid state. If the initially low uptake is caused by inadequate pituitary stimulation of an intrinsically normal thyroid gland, the RAIU should increase at least 10% and the T_4 level should rise 1.5 mcg/dL or more. This is characteristic of secondary hypothyroidism.

Procedure and patient care

- See inside front cover for Routine Blood Testing.
- Fasting: no
- Blood tube commonly used: Verify with laboratory.
- Obtain baseline levels of RAIU or T_4 (p. 729) as indicated.
- Administer the prescribed dose of TSH intramuscularly for 3 days, as ordered.
- Repeat the levels of RAIU or T_4 as indicated.

Abnormal findings

Primary (thyroidal) hypothyroidism
Secondary (hypothalamic-pituitary) hypothyroidism

T

notes

thyroid-stimulating immunoglobulins (TSIs, Long-acting thyroid stimulator [LATS], Thyroid-binding inhibitory immunoglobulin [TBII], Thyrotropin receptor antibody, Thyroid-stimulating hormone receptor [TSHR] antibodies)

Type of test Blood

Normal findings

TSI: < 130% of basal activity
TBII: < 10% inhibition

Test explanation and related physiology

TSIs represent a group of immunoglobulin G (IgG) antibodies directed against the thyroid cell receptor for TSH and are associated with autoimmune thyroid disease states, such as chronic thyroiditis and Graves disease. These autoantibodies bind and transactivate the TSHRs. This instigates stimulation of the thyroid gland independent of the normal feedback-regulated TSH stimulation. This, in turn, will stimulate the release of thyroid hormones from the thyroid cells. Some patients with Graves disease also have TSHR-blocking antibodies, which do not transactivate the TSHR.

The use of these antibodies is helpful in the evaluation of patients for whom the diagnosis of Graves disease is confused by conflicting data (e.g., subclinical Graves hyperthyroidism).

Because TSIs can cross the placenta, they may be found in neonates whose mothers have Graves disease.

Procedure and patient care

- See inside front cover for Routine Blood Testing.
- Fasting: no
- Blood tube commonly used: red or gold
- Hemolysis may interfere with interpretation of test results.

Abnormal findings

▲ Increased levels

Graves disease
Hashimoto thyroiditis
Hyperthyroidism

Malignant exophthalmos
Neonatal thyrotoxicosis

notes

thyrotropin-releasing hormone stimulation test (TRH stimulation test, Thyrotropin-releasing factor stimulation test [TRF stimulation test])

Type of test Blood

Normal findings

Baseline TSH: < 10 µU/mL
Stimulated TSH: more than double the baseline

Test explanation and related physiology

The TRH stimulation test assesses the anterior pituitary gland via its secretion of TSH in response to an IV injection of TRH. After the TRH injection, the normally functioning pituitary gland should secrete TSH. In hyperthyroidism, either a slight or no increase in the TSH level is seen because pituitary TSH production is suppressed by the direct effect of excess circulating T_4 and T_3 on the pituitary gland. A normal result is considered reliable evidence for excluding the diagnosis of thyrotoxicosis. Since the development of very sensitive radioimmunoassay for TSH, the TRH stimulation test is no longer required to diagnose hyperthyroidism. However, it still has a role in the evaluation of pituitary deficiency.

In addition to assessing the responsiveness of the anterior pituitary gland, this test aids in the detection of primary, secondary, and tertiary hypothyroidism. The TRH test also may be useful in differentiating primary depression from manic-depressive psychiatric illness and from secondary types of depression. In primary depression, whereas the TSH response is blunted in most patients, patients with other types of depression have a normal TRH-induced TSH response.

Interfering factors

• Pregnancy may increase the TSH response to TRH.

Procedure and patient care

• See inside front cover for Routine Blood Testing.
• Fasting: no
• Blood tube commonly used: verify with laboratory
PT Instruct the patient to discontinue thyroid preparations for 3 to 4 weeks before the TRH test, if indicated.
• Administer a prescribed IV bolus of TRH.
• Obtain venous blood samples at intervals and measure for TSH levels.

Abnormal findings

Acute starvation
Hyperthyroidism
Hypothyroidism
Old age (especially in men)
Pregnancy
Psychiatric primary depression

notes

thyroxine, total and free (T₄, Thyroxine screen, FT₄)

Type of test Blood

Normal findings

Free T_4:
    Adult: 0.8–2.8 ng/dL or 10–36 pmol/L (SI units)
    2 weeks-20 years: 0.8–2 ng/dL or 10–26 pmol/L (SI units)
    0–4 days: 2–6 ng/dL or 26–77 pmol/L (SI units)

Total T_4:
    Adult male: 4–12 mcg/dL or 59–135 nmol/L (SI units)
    Adult female: 5–12 mcg/dL or 71–142 nmol/L (SI units)
    Adult > 60 years: 5–11 mcg/dL or 64–142 nmol/L (SI units)
    Pregnancy: 9–14 mcg/dL or 117–181 nmol/L (SI units)
    10–15 years: 5–12 mcg/dL or 72–151 nmol/L (SI units)
    5–10 years: 6–13 mcg/dL or 83–172 nmol/L (SI units)
    1–5 years: 7–15 mcg/dL or 94–194 nmol/L (SI units)
    1–12 months: 8–16 mcg/dL or 101–213 nmol/L (SI units)
    1–2 weeks: 10–16 mcg/dL or 126–214 nmol/L (SI units)
    1–3 days: 11–22 mcg/dL or 152–292 nmol/L (SI units)

Test explanation and related physiology

The two main hormones secreted by the thyroid gland are thyroxine, which contains four atoms of T_4 and T_3 (p. 739). More than 90% of thyroid hormone is made up of T_4. Thyroid hormones circulate primarily bound to carrier proteins (e.g., TBG, albumin, or transthyretin); a small fraction circulates unbound (free). Ninety-nine percent of T_4 is bound to proteins. Total T_4 measurements consist of both the bound and unbound fractions. Free T_4 is a measure of unbound metabolically active T_4. Thyroxine tests are used to determine thyroid function. Greater than normal levels indicate hyperthyroid states, and subnormal values are seen in hypothyroid states. T_4 and TSH are used to monitor thyroid replacement and suppressive therapy.

Pregnancy and hormone replacement therapy increase TBG and may cause total T_4 to be falsely elevated, suggesting that hyperthyroidism exists when in fact the patient is euthyroid. If the free T_4 is measured in these patients, it would be normal, indicating that free T_4 is a more accurate indicator of thyroid function than total T_4. In cases in which TBG is reduced (e.g., hypoproteinemia), the total T_4 is likewise reduced, suggesting hypothyroidism. Measurement of free T_4 would indicate normal

T

levels and thereby discount the abnormal total T_4 as merely a result of the reduced TBG and not as a result of hypothyroidism.

Procedure and patient care

- See inside front cover for Routine Blood Testing.
- Fasting: no
- Blood tube commonly used: red
- PT If indicated, instruct the patient to stop exogenous T_4 medication 1 month before testing.

Abnormal findings

▲ **Increased levels**

Acute thyroiditis
Congenital
  hyperproteinemia
Factitious hyperthyroidism
Familial dysalbuminemic
  hyperthyroxinemia
Graves disease
Hepatitis
Pregnancy
Struma ovarii
Thyroid cancer
Toxic multinodular goiter
Toxic thyroid adenoma

▼ **Decreased levels**

Cirrhosis
Congenital hypothyroidism
Cushing syndrome
Hashimoto thyroiditis
Hypothalamic failure
Iodine insufficiency
Myxedema
Pituitary insufficiency
Renal failure
Surgical ablation of the
  thyroid
Thyroid agenesis
TSH receptor defects

notes

thyroxine-binding globulin (TBG, Thyroid binding globulin)

Type of test Blood

Normal findings

Age	Male (mg/dL)	Female (mg/dL)
1–5 days	2.2–5.9	2.2–5.9
1–11 months	3.1–5.6	3–5.6
1–9 years	2.5–5	2.5–5
10–19 years	2.1–4.6	2.1–4.6
> 20 years	1.2–2.5	1.4–3

Oral contraceptive use: 1.5–5.5 mg/dL
Pregnancy (third trimester): 4.7–5.9 mg/dL

Test explanation and related physiology

TBG is the major thyroid hormone protein carrier. When it is elevated, total T_3 and total T_4 are also elevated. This may give the false indication that the patient has hyperthyroidism when in fact the patient just has elevated TBGs. When total T_4 is elevated, one must ascertain whether that elevation is caused by an elevation in TBG or a real elevation in T_4 alone, which is associated with hyperthyroidism.

The most common causes of elevated TBGs are pregnancy, hormone replacement therapy, and the use of oral contraceptives. Decreased TBGs are commonly associated with other causes of hypoproteinemia (e.g., nephrotic syndrome).

Procedure and patient care

- See inside front cover for Routine Blood Testing.
- Fasting: no
- Blood tube commonly used: red
- List on the laboratory slip any drugs that may affect test results.

Abnormal findings

▲ Increased levels

Acute intermittent porphyria
Estrogen-producing tumors
Estrogen replacement
  therapy
Genetic increased TBG
Infectious hepatitis
Pregnancy

▼ Decreased levels

Major stress
Malnutrition
Ovarian failure
Protein-losing enteropathy
Protein-losing nephropathy
Testosterone-producing
  tumors

T

notes

TORCH test

The term *TORCH* (toxoplasmosis, other, rubella, cytomegalovirus, herpes) has been applied to maternal infections with recognized detrimental effects on the fetus. TORCH testing refers to the testing for IgG (indicating past infection) and IgM (indicating recent infection) antibodies to the particular infectious agents described. Included in the category of *other* are such infections as syphilis. All of these tests are discussed separately:

- Toxoplasmosis, p. 735
- Rubella, p. 795
- Cytomegalovirus, p. 795
- Herpes virus, p. 799

The direct effects of these infections may be immediate or delayed. A majority of infants infected by toxoplasmosis in utero are asymptomatic at birth with neurologic sequelae appearing later in life. Prenatal rubella infections, on the other hand, may severely damage the fetus, causing congenital heart disease and mental retardation. Congenital cytomegalovirus infections can result in infant death, hearing loss, cerebral palsy, mental retardation, or chorioretinitis. Neonatal herpes infection (can occur in utero or during birth) presents as localized infection to the skin, eye, and mouth (SEM) or as disseminated infection (involving multiple organs, such as the liver, lung, adrenal glands, or brain). The earlier these infections are recognized, the earlier they can be treated or steps can be made to preclude the long-term effects of the disease. Other effects of TORCH infections on the fetus may be indirect and precipitate abortion or premature labor.

notes

total blood volume (TBV, Red blood cell [RBC] volume)

Type of test Nuclear scan

Normal findings

Approximately 70 mL per kg of body weight

Test explanation and related physiology

Measurement of TBV is performed using radionuclides. This measurement is an accurate indicator of true plasma (liquid components of blood) measurement. Based on the patient's height, weight, gender, and body composition, TBV can determine whether the measured volumes are high or low compared with what would be ideal for the particular patient. The report indicates actual volumes for TBV and RBCs that deviate from normal.

This information may be useful in the following clinical circumstances:

- *Congestive heart failure.* The amount of fluid overload can be calculated, and diuresis can be more appropriately determined.
- *Presurgery.* The patient's fluid status can be accurately determined as can RBC status.
- *Acutely ill patients.* There are often large fluid shifts in these patients, and TBV may help in guiding IV fluid replacement.
- *Azotemia.* Measurement of TBV will indicate if azotemia is prerenal (hypovolemia) or primary renal.
- *Hypertension.* TBV may indicate plasma volume overload versus vascular constriction.
- *Anemia.* TBV and RBC volumes can indicate the extent of anemia that otherwise could be affected by fluid status, etc.

Procedure and patient care

Before

PT Explain the procedure and tell the patient that no fasting is required.

T

During

- Obtain venous access.
- Fifteen minutes after radionuclide injection, the first venous blood sample is collected in a red-top tube.
- Similar venous blood samples are obtained every 5 minutes for a total of five samples.

After

- Apply pressure to the IV site upon removal after extracting the last sample.

Abnormal findings

▲ **Increased levels**
    Congestive heart failure
    Hypertension
    Hypervolemia
    Polycythemia vera
    Primary renal disease

▼ **Decreased levels**
    Acute bleeding
    Anemia
    Dehydration
    Hypovolemia

notes

toxoplasmosis antibody titer

Type of test   Blood

Normal findings

Ig G titers < 1:16 indicate no previous infection.

Ig G titers 1:16–1:256 are usually prevalent in the general population.

Ig G titers > 1:256 suggest recent infection.

Ig M titers > 1:256 indicate acute infection.

Test explanation and related physiology

Toxoplasmosis is a protozoan disease caused by *Toxoplasma gondii*, which is found in poorly cooked or raw meat and in cat feces. The Centers for Disease Control and Prevention recommends that patients who are pregnant be serologically tested for this disease.

The presence of antibodies before pregnancy indicates prior exposure and chronic asymptomatic infection. The presence of these antibodies probably ensures protection against congenital toxoplasmosis in the child. Fetal infection occurs if the mother acquires toxoplasmosis after conception and passes it to the fetus through the placenta. Repeat testing of pregnant patients with low or negative titers may be done before the 20th week and before delivery to identify antibody converters and determine appropriate therapy (e.g., therapeutic abortion at 20 weeks, treatment during the remainder of the pregnancy, or treatment of the newborn). Hydrocephaly, microcephaly, chronic retinitis, and seizures are complications of congenital toxoplasmosis.

Procedure and patient care

- See inside front cover for Routine Blood Testing.
- Fasting: no
- Blood tube commonly used: red

Abnormal findings

Toxoplasmosis infection

notes

transferrin receptor (TfR) assay

Type of test Blood

Normal findings

Men: 2–5 mg/L
Women: 1.9–4.4 mg/L

Test explanation and related physiology

Both iron metabolism and transport are altered in chronic illness. Differentiation of the anemia of chronic disease from iron deficiency anemia is by measurement of the serum TfR.

TfR assists with absorption of iron into cells. TfR is increased when erythropoiesis is enhanced. The concentration of cell surface TfR is carefully regulated by TfR mRNA, according to the internal iron content of the cell and its individual iron requirements. Whereas iron-deficient cells contain increased numbers of receptors, receptor numbers are downregulated in iron-replete cells.

An increased mean TfR concentration is noted in patients with iron-deficiency anemia compared with patients with anemia secondary to chronic disease. TfR is also useful in distinguishing iron-deficiency anemia from situations that are commonly encountered in childhood, adolescence, and during pregnancy when iron stores are uniformly low to absent. When iron-deficiency anemia coexists with anemia of chronic disease, TfR concentrations increase secondary to the underlying iron deficiency, thus avoiding the need for a bone marrow examination.

Interfering factors

- Individuals who live at high altitudes have a reference range higher than normal.
- Results are related to ethnicity. Individuals of African descent can be expected to have higher levels.

Procedure and patient care

- See inside front cover for Routine Blood Testing.
- Fasting: no
- Blood tube commonly used: red or green

Abnormal findings

▲ **Increased plasma TfR**
Erythropoietin therapy
Iron-deficiency anemia
Reticulocytosis

▼ **Decreased plasma TfR**
Hemochromatosis

notes

triglycerides (TGs)

Type of test Blood
Normal findings
Adult/elderly
  Male: 40–160 mg/dL or 0.45–1.81 mmol/L (SI units)
  Female: 35–135 mg/dL or 0.40–1.52 mmol/L (SI units)
Child/adolescent

Age, years	Male, mg/dL	Female, mg/dL
0–5	30–86	32–99
6–11	31–108	35–114
12–15	36–138	41–138
16–19	40–163	40–128

Possible critical values
> 400 mg/dL

Test explanation and related physiology
  TGs are a form of fat that exists in the bloodstream. They are transported by very-low-density lipoproteins (VLDLs) and low-density lipoproteins (LDLs). TGs are produced in the liver by using glycerol and other fatty acids as building blocks. TGs act as a storage source for energy. When TG levels in the blood are in excess, TGs are deposited into the fatty tissues. TGs are a part of a lipid profile that also evaluates cholesterol (p. 198) and lipoproteins (p. 462). A lipid profile is performed to assess the risk of coronary and vascular disease.

Interfering factors
- Ingestion of fatty meals may cause increased TG levels.
- Ingestion of alcohol may cause increased levels.
- Pregnancy may cause increased levels.

Procedure and patient care
- See inside front cover for Routine Blood Testing.
- Fasting: yes (12–14 hours)
- Blood tube commonly used: red
- **PT** Tell the patient to avoid alcohol for 24 hours before the test.
- **PT** Inform the patient that dietary indiscretion for as long as 2 weeks before this test will influence results.
- **PT** Instruct the patient with increased TG levels regarding diet, exercise, and appropriate weight.

Abnormal findings

▲ **Increased levels**

Alcoholic cirrhosis
Glycogen storage disease
High-carbohydrate diet
Hyperlipidemias
Hypertension
Hypothyroidism
Myocardial infarction
Nephrotic syndrome
Poorly controlled diabetes
Pregnancy
Risk of arteriosclerotic
  occlusive coronary disease
  and peripheral vascular
  disease

▼ **Decreased levels**

Hyperthyroidism
Malabsorption syndrome
Malnutrition

notes

triiodothyronine (T_3 radioimmunoassay)

Type of test Blood

Normal findings

>50 years: 40–180 ng/dL or 0.6–2.8 nmol/L (SI units)
20–50 years: 70–205 ng/dL or 1.2–3.4 nmol/L (SI units)
16–20 years: 80–210 ng/dL
11–15 years: 80–215 ng/dL
6–10 years: 95–240 ng/dL
1–5 years: 105–270 ng/dL
1–11 months: 105–245 ng/dL
1–3 days: 100–740 ng/dL

Reversed T_3: 10–24 ng/dL

Test explanation and related physiology

As with the thyroxine (T_4) test, the serum T_3 test is an accurate measure of thyroid function. T_3 is less stable than T_4 and occurs in minute quantities in the active form. Only about 7% to 10% of thyroid hormone is composed of T_3. Seventy percent of that T_3 is bound to proteins (TBG and albumin). Abnormal levels (high or low) of thyroid hormone-binding proteins (primarily albumin and TBG) may cause abnormal T_3 concentrations in euthyroid patients. This test is a measurement of total T_3 (i.e., the free and the bound T_3). Generally, when the T_3 level is below normal, the patient is in a hypothyroid state.

In severe nonthyroidal diseases, T_3 levels are decreased because conversion of T_4 to T_3 in the liver is diminished. This makes T_3 levels less useful in indicating hypothyroid states. Instead, there is peripheral conversion of T_4 to T_3. This form of T_3 is called *reverse T_3 (rT_3)*. Elevated rT_3 levels associated with reduced T_3 have been observed in starvation, anorexia nervosa, severe trauma and hemorrhagic shock, hepatic dysfunction, postoperative states, severe infection, and burn patients (i.e., "sick euthyroid" syndrome).

Furthermore, there is considerable overlap between hypothyroid states and normal thyroid function. Because of this, T_3 levels are mostly used just to assist in the diagnosis of hyperthyroid states. T_3 levels are frequently low in sick or hospitalized euthyroid patients. An elevated T_3 level indicates hyperthyroidism, especially when the T_4 is also elevated.

T

Interfering factors

- T$_3$ values are increased in pregnancy.

Procedure and patient care

- See inside front cover for Routine Blood Testing.
- Fasting: no
- Blood tube commonly used: red
- Determine whether the patient is taking any exogenous T$_3$ medication because this will affect test results.
- Withhold drugs that may affect results, if ordered.

Abnormal findings

▲ **Increased levels**

Acute thyroiditis
Congenital
  hyperproteinemia
Factitious hyperthyroidism
Graves disease
Hepatitis
Plummer disease
Pregnancy
Struma ovarii
Toxic thyroid adenoma

▼ **Decreased levels**

Cirrhosis
Congenital hypothyroidism
Cushing syndrome
Hypothalamic failure
Hypothyroidism
Iodine insufficiency
Liver diseases
Myxedema
Pituitary insufficiency
Protein malnutrition and
  other protein-depleted
  states (e.g., nephrotic
  syndrome)
Renal failure
Thyroid surgical ablation

notes

troponins (Cardiac-specific troponin T [cTnT], Cardiac-specific troponin I [cTnI], High-sensitivity troponin [hsTnT, hs-cTn])

Type of test Blood

Normal findings

Cardiac troponin T: < 0.1 ng/mL
Cardiac troponin I: < 0.03 ng/mL
hsTnT :
  < 22 ng/L for men
  < 14 ng/L for women

Test explanation and related physiology

This test is used to assist in the evaluation of patients with suspected acute coronary ischemic syndromes. Cardiac troponin T (cTnT) and cardiac troponin I (cTnI) are structural proteins in the heart that are released into circulation following myocardial injury. In addition to improving the diagnosis of acute ischemic disorders, troponins are also valuable for risk stratification in patients with unstable angina and pulmonary embolism.

Cardiac troponins become elevated as early as 2 to 3 hours after myocardial injury. Levels of cTnI may remain elevated for 7 to 10 days after myocardial infarction, and cTnT levels may remain elevated for up to 14 days. *High sensitivity troponins (hs-cTn)* detect concentrations of troponins at much lower concentrations, thereby detecting infarction earlier in the process (as early as 90 minutes). High senstivity troponins speed the triage of patients with suspected myocardial infarction. They also detect small changes sooner than senstive troponins. The pattern of change in the troponin helps to differentiate acute coronary syndrome from other causes of elevated troponin. Therefore, the troponin is repeated one to three hours after the first test for high sensitivity assay (or three to six hours for sensitive assay).

Cardiac troponins are used in the following cardiac clinical situations:

- Diagnosis of myocardial infarct and estimation of infarct size. Peak troponin levels correlate with infarct size. Late cardiac troponin levels are inversely related to left ventricular ejection fraction.
- Evaluation of patient with unstable angina.
- Detection of reperfusion associated with coronary recanalization.
- Detection of perioperative myocardial infarction.
- Evaluation of the severity of pulmonary emboli. Elevated levels may indicate more severe disease and the need for thrombolytic therapy.

- Congestive heart failure. Persistently elevated troponins indicate continued ventricular strain.

Elevations of troponin T do not necessarily indicate the presence of an ischemic mechanism. Many other disease states are associated with elevations of troponin T via mechanisms different from those that cause injury in patients with acute coronary syndromes. These include cardiac trauma (e.g., contusion, cardioversion, defibrillation), congestive heart failure, hypertension, hypotension, pulmonary embolism, renal failure, and myocarditis.

Interfering factors

- Troponin levels are also elevated in tachyarrhythmias, heart failure, hypertensive emergencies, critical illness, myocarditis, Takotsubo cardiomyopathy, structural heart disease, aortic dissection, pulmonary embolism/pulmonary hypertension, and renal dysfunction.

Procedure and patient care

- See inside front cover for Routine Blood Testing.
- Fasting: no
- Blood tube commonly used: yellow or green
- PT Discuss with the patient the need and reason for frequent venipuncture in diagnosing myocardial infarction.
- If a qualitative immunoassay is to be done at the bedside, whole blood is obtained in a micropipette and placed in the sample well of the testing device. A red or purple color in the read zone indicates that 0.2 ng/mL or more of cardiac troponin is present in the patient's blood.

Abnormal findings

▲ **Increased levels**

Congestive heart failure
Myocardial infarction
Myocardial injury
Pulmonary embolism
Renal disease
Trauma

notes

tuberculosis testing (Acid-fast bacillus [AFB] smear, Interferon gamma release assay [IGRA], Lipoarabinomannan [LAM] assay, Mycobacteria growth indicator tube [MGIT], Nucleic acid amplification [NAA] testing, Quantiferon-TB gold in-tube plus [QFT-GIT Plus] assay, Purified protein derivative [PPD] test, Tuberculosis [TB] culture, Tuberculin skin test [TST], T-SPOT, TB assay, Xpert MTB/RIF test)

Type of test Microbiology culture, blood, sputum, fluid, skin, urine

Normal findings:

Negative for TB
TST: Negative; reaction < 5 mm

Test explanation and related physiology

Mycobacterium tuberculosis infects a significant portion of the world population. Therefore, diagnosing tuberculosis quickly and effectively is valuable for minimizing transmission and for initiating treatments. The diagnosis of pulmonary TB is definitively established by isolation of *M. tuberculosis* from a bodily secretion culture or tissue culture such as sputum, bronchoalveolar lavage, pleural effusion, pleural biopsy or lung biopsy. Patients who are suspected of having tuberculosis should have sputum samples sent for culture, AFB smear, and NAA testing. In addition, a TST or IGRA may be performed.

All clinical specimens suspected of containing mycobacteria should be cultured by *conventional culture* techniques. This is the most sensitive tool for detection of TB. Culture is also used for drug susceptibility testing and for species identification. Rapid culture techniques such as *mycobacteria growth indicator tube (MGIT)* uses liquid culture to assess whether mycobacteria grow in the absence or presence of various antituberculosis drugs. These results are available more rapidly than conventional solid culture. The microscopic *sputum AFB smear* detects acid-fast bacilli on stained sputum smears. It is the most rapid and inexpensive TB diagnostic tool.

Molecular methods are available for detection of *M. tuberculosis* DNA and common mutations associated with drug resistance. All molecular tests for TB and drug resistance must be confirmed by culture. *Nucleic acid amplification (NAA) tests* are a type of molecular tests that can be used for rapid TB diagnosis (within 24–48 hours). These tests amplify a specific nucleic acid sequence that can be detected by a nucleic acid probe. One example of this type of test is the *Xpert MTB/RIF test*.

T

The urine *LAM (lipoarabinomannan) assay* is a commercially available point-of-care test that detects LAM, a component of the bacterial cell walls, present in some people with active TB. It is particularly helpful in settings with high incidence of TB and HIV. The test is simple and shows results in 25 minutes.

The *tuberculin skin test (TST)* and *interferon-gamma release assays (IGRAs)* are tests that can be used to diagnose latent TB. The TST is also referred to as the *PPD (purified protein derivative) test* because a PPD of the tubercle bacillus is injected intradermally during this test. If the patient has latent TB, lymphocytes will recognize the PPD antigen and cause a local skin reaction. The skin must be re-evaluated in 48–72 hours to assess for reaction. If the patient is not infected, no reaction will occur. This test is contraindicated in patients with known active TB or in those who have received Bacille Calmette-Guérin (BCG) immunization.

IGRAs are in vitro blood tests of cell-mediated immune response to *M. tuberculosis.* They measure T-cell release of interferon-gamma following stimulation by antigens specific to *M. tuberculosis.* Like the TST, they cannot distinguish between latent infection and active TB and should not be used for diagnosis of active TB. They can, however, be used for patients with prior BCG vaccination and do not require follow up as compared with the TST. Two specific IGRAs are the *Quantiferon-TB Gold In-Tube Plus (QFT-GIT Plus)* assay that uses whole blood for testing and the *T-SPOT.TB* assay which uses separated peripheral blood.

Interfering factors

- A false-negative result can be due to the stage of infection, comorbid conditions that affect immune function, or other individual immunologic factors.

Procedure and patient care

Before

PT Explain the procedure to the patient.

PT Tell the patient that no fasting is required.

- Assess the patient for a previous history of TB and BCG immunization. Report a positive history to the physician.

During

- For sputum or AFB smear collection, it is best to induce sputum production in the morning until about 5 mL is collected. Often, several samples are collected over the course of several days. Send the specimen to the lab for evaluation.

Conventional cultures and drug susceptibility can take days to weeks to result. Rapid sputum tests can provide results within 24 hours.

- For TST, prepare the patient's forearm with alcohol and allow it to dry. Then intradermally inject the PPD. A skin wheal will occur. Record the time at which the PPD was injected.
- For blood, use the specialized collection tubes as directed by the lab. This typically involves collecting 1 mL of whole blood via venipuncture into each specified tube. IGRA results can be available in 24 to 48 hours.

After

PT Instruct the patient as to appropriate isolation of sputum and other body fluids to avoid potential spread of suspected TB.

PT If the patient's results are positive, educate the patient on the necessary follow-up studies, such as chest radiography and sputum cultures. Ensure that the physician is notified.

- For TST: Read the results in 48 to 72 hours. Measure the area of induration (not redness) in millimeters.

Abnormal findings

Atypical mycobacterial nontuberculosis disease
Latent tuberculosis
Tuberculosis infection

notes

T

> **tumor analysis** (DNA ploidy status, S-phase fraction, Cathepsin D, HER-2 [c erbB2, neu] protein, p53 protein, Ki67 protein)

Type of test Microscopic examination

Normal findings

DNA ploidy

Aneuploid is unfavorable.
Diploid is favorable.

S-phase fraction

> 5.5% is unfavorable.
< 5.5% is favorable.

HER-2 protein

IHC method: 0 to 1 +
FISH method: < 2 copies/cell
Oncotype DX method: < 10.7 units

Cathepsin D

> 10% is unfavorable.
< 10% is favorable.

p53 protein

> 10% is unfavorable.
< 10% is favorable.

Ki67 protein

> 20% is unfavorable.
10% to 20% is borderline.
< 20% is favorable.

Test explanation and related physiology

The most important predictor of recurrent cancer is stage of disease. However, some patients whose tumors have been completely removed and who have no evidence of lymph node metastasis will also develop recurrence. It is important to accurately predict the patients who are destined for recurrence so that they can be selected for systemic therapy. These tests are routinely used for breast cancer analysis. Many of these prognostic tumor indicators can also be found in other tumors and provide similar information.

DNA ploidy status and S-phase fraction

These are measurements of the rapidity with which the cells in a breast cancer grow.

Cathepsin D

This protein catabolic enzyme was found to be absent in resting breast tissue but significantly elevated in malignant tissue.

HER-2 (c erbB2, neu) protein

HER-2/neu, which stands for *human epidermal growth factor receptor 2*, is a protein associated with worse clinical outcomes.

The *HER-2* gene can act as a target for an antineoplastic monoclonal antibody drug such as trastuzumab.

p53 protein

The *p53* gene is a tumor suppressor gene that is overexpressed in more aggressive breast cancer cells.

Ki67 protein

The *Ki67* gene encodes the synthesis for the Ki67 protein that is associated with worse clinical outcomes.

Interfering factors

- Delay in tissue fixation may cause deterioration of marker proteins and may produce lower values.
- Preoperative use of some chemotherapy agents may cause *decreased* levels of some marker proteins.

Procedure and patient care

- The physician obtains tumor tissue through biopsy or surgical extirpation and the tissue is immediately delivered to the pathology department without any additional preservative.
- Result are usually available in 3–7 days.

Abnormal findings

Unfavorable test results indicating a risk of cancer reoccurrence

notes

T

ultrasound of the abdomen (Abdominal ultrasound, Abdominal sonogram)

Type of test Ultrasound

Normal findings

Normal abdominal aorta, liver, gallbladder, bile ducts, pancreas, kidneys, ureters, and bladder

Test explanation and related physiology

Ultrasonography provides accurate visualization of the abdominal aorta, liver, gallbladder, pancreas, bile ducts, kidneys, ureters, and bladder. Real-time ultrasound provides an accurate picture of the organ being studied (Figure U1).

The *kidney* is ultrasonographically evaluated to diagnose and locate renal cysts, to assess renal arterial and venous patency, to detect suspected congenital abnormalities, to differentiate renal cysts from solid renal tumors, to demonstrate renal and pelvic calculi, to document hydronephrosis, and to guide invasive procedures. Ultrasound of the urologic tract is also used to detect malformed or ectopic kidneys and perinephric abscesses. Renal transplantation surveillance is possible with ultrasound.

Endourethral urologic ultrasound can also be performed through a stent that has a transducer at its end. The stent probe can be advanced into the bladder where the depth of a tumor into the bladder wall can be measured. In the ureter, stones, tumors, or extraurethral compression can be identified and localized. Finally, in the proximal ureter, renal tumors or cysts can be delineated.

One of the most common uses of ultrasound is the measurement of post void urinary bladder residual. This is a measurement of the amount of urine after micturition. This test can be easily performed at the bedside or in doctor's office with a portable ultrasound unit.

Pelvic, obstetric, prostate, and testes ultrasound are discussed on pp. 754, 757, and 759.

The *abdominal aorta* can be assessed for aneurysmal dilation. In an aortic dissection, a dissection flap can be detected by abdominal US. However, if a flap is not detected, a dissection cannot be ruled out, and another form of imaging is required (see TEE, p. 281, and CTA, p. 232).

Ultrasound is used to detect cystic structures of the *liver* (e.g., benign cysts, hepatic abscesses, and dilated hepatic ducts) and solid intrahepatic tumors (primary and metastatic). Hepatic ultrasound also can be performed intraoperatively to provide the

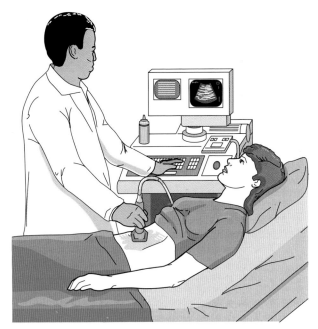

FIG. U1 Ultrasound of the abdomen.

locations of small, nonpalpable hepatic tumors or abscesses. The *gallbladder* and *bile ducts* can be visualized and examined for evidence of gallstones, polyps, or bile duct dilation. The *pancreas* is examined for evidence of tumors, pseudocysts, acute inflammation, chronic inflammation, or pancreatic abscesses. Because this study requires no contrast material and has no associated radiation, it is especially useful in patients who are allergic to contrast, have diminished renal function, or are pregnant. Fasting may be preferred, but it is not mandatory.

Interfering factors

- Barium limits transmission of ultrasonic waves. For this reason, ultrasonography of the abdomen should be performed before any barium contrast studies.
- Large amounts of gas in the bowel distort visualization of abdominal organs because bowel gas reflects sound.
- Obesity may affect the results of the study because sound waves are altered by fatty tissue.

U

- The quality of the ultrasound image and the sufficiency of the study depend to a very large part on the abilities of the ultrasound technologist performing the study.

Procedure and patient care

Before

PT Explain the procedure to the patient.

PT Tell the patient that fasting may or may not be required, depending on the organ to be examined.

During

- Note the following procedural steps:
  1. The patient is placed on the ultrasonography table in the prone or supine position, depending on the organ to be studied.
  2. Gel is applied to the patient's skin to enhance sound wave transmission and reception.
  3. A transducer is placed over the skin.
  4. Pictures are taken of the reflections from the organs.
- The test is completed in about 1 hour, usually by an ultrasound technologist, and is interpreted by a radiologist.

PT Tell the patient that this procedure causes no discomfort.

After

- Remove the gel from the patient's skin.
- Note that if a biopsy is done, refer to biopsy of the specific organ (e.g., liver or kidney biopsy).

Abnormal findings

Abdominal aorta

Aneurysm

Abdominal cavity

Abscess

Ascites

Bile ducts

Dilation

Gallstone

Stricture

Tumor

Gallbladder

Gallstone

Polyps

Tumor

Kidney
Glomerulonephritis
Hydronephrosis
Perirenal abscess
Perirenal hematoma
Pyelonephritis
Renal calculi
Renal cysts
Renal tumor
Ureteral obstruction

Liver
Abscess
Intrahepatic dilated bile ducts
Tumor

Pancreas
Abscess
Cysts
Inflammation
Pseudocysts
Tumor

notes

U

ultrasound of the breast (Breast ultrasonography, Ultrasound mammography, Breast sonogram)

Type of test Ultrasound

Normal findings

BIRADS I, II

Test explanation and related physiology

Ultrasound examination of the breast is diagnostically performed to determine whether a mammographic abnormality or a palpable lump is a cyst (fluid-filled) or a solid tumor (benign or malignant). It is also used in screening for breast cancer in women whose breasts are dense on mammography.

Ultrasonography of the breast is used to:

- Differentiate cystic from solid breast lesions.
- Identify masses in women with breast tissue too dense for accurate mammography.
- Monitor a cyst to determine whether it enlarges or disappears.
- Measure the size of a tumor.
- Evaluate the axilla in women who are newly diagnosed with breast cancer.

Ultrasonography is also useful for examination of symptomatic breasts in women in whom the radiation of mammography is potentially harmful. These include:

- Pregnant women. Radiation may be harmful to the fetus.
- Women younger than age 25 years, who may be at greater oncologic risk from the radiation of mammography.

With high-quality diagnostic ultrasonography, the characteristics of an abnormality can be evaluated and a reasonable prediction can be made whether it is malignant. Diagnostic accuracy is improved when breast ultrasonography is combined with mammography (p. 497).

Ultrasound can be used to locate and accurately direct percutaneous biopsy probes to a nonpalpable breast abnormality for biopsy or aspiration. Ultrasound is painless, harmless, and without any radiation effects on the breast tissue.

Procedure and patient care

Before

PT Explain the procedure to the patient.

PT Assure the patient that no discomfort is associated with this study.

PT Inform the patient that no fasting or sedation is required before the tests.

During

- The patient is placed in a partially rolled position to one side, and the transducer is directly applied to the breast using contact gel to improve sound transmission.
- Note that this test is performed by an ultrasound technician in approximately 15 minutes.

After

- After the test is completed, the gel is removed.

Abnormal findings

Abscess
Cancer
Cyst
Fibroadenoma
Fibrocystic disease
Hematoma

notes

U

ultrasound of the pelvis (Pelvic ultrasonography, Obstetric ultrasonography, Vaginal ultrasound)

Type of test Ultrasound

Normal findings

Normal fetal and placental size and position. Normal blood flow to ovaries

Test explanation and related physiology

Ultrasound examination of the pelvis evaluates the female genital tract and fetus. Pelvic ultrasonography can be performed with the transducer placed on the anterior abdomen (see Figure U1, p. 749) or in the vagina with a vaginal probe. Vaginal ultrasound adds accuracy in identifying paracervical, endometrial, and ovarian pathology that otherwise may not be detected with the anterior abdominal probe. Using color Doppler evaluation during pelvic ultrasound is also part of the standard evaluation.

Pelvic ultrasonography may be useful in the *obstetric patient* in the following circumstances:

- Making an early diagnosis of pregnancy
- Identifying multiple pregnancies
- Differentiating a tumor from a normal pregnancy
- Determining fetal head circumference to assist in calculating the age of the fetus
- Measuring the rate of fetal growth
- Identifying placental abnormalities
- Diagnosing ectopic pregnancy
- Providing a realistic image of the fetus using three- or four-dimensional imaging
- Evaluating the kidneys and upper collecting system
- Localizing the placenta before amniocentesis
- Making a differential diagnosis of various uterine and ovarian enlargements (e.g., polyhydramnios)

Ultrasonography is a very accurate and easily performed screening test to recognize risks of fetal abnormalities (see amniotic fluid index, p. 333). *Fetal nuchal translucency (FNT)* is an ultrasound measurement of subcutaneous edema in the neck region of the fetus. It is performed at 10 to 14 weeks of gestation. Major heart defects, trisomy 21, and other genetic defects are associated with increased edema in this location at this age of gestation. With FNT, these abnormalities can be identified earlier in the pregnancy.

Pelvic ultrasonography is used in the *nonpregnant woman* to monitor the endometrium in patients who take tamoxifen and to aid in the diagnosis of the following:

- Ovarian cyst or tumor
- Ovarian torsion
- Tubo-ovarian abscess
- Uterine fibroids or cancer
- Pelvic inflammatory disease (PID)
- Thickened uterine endometrium (stripe) (caused by cancer, hyperplasia, and so on)

Pelvic ultrasonography is widely used in the evaluation of endometrial abnormalities, abnormal uterine bleeding, and infertility of the female. *Saline infusion sonography (SIS)* is a simple and inexpensive method to determine patency of the uterus and tubes. In SIS, saline is injected under ultrasound guidance. This provides better visualization of any intrauterine abnormalities. Air bubbles are then injected and imaged through the tubes to demonstrate patency.

When a woman is unable to visualize or palpate the string of an intrauterine device (IUD), ultrasound is used in *localization of a contraceptive device.*

Contraindications

- Patients with latex allergy require a latex free probe cover.

Interfering factors

- Patients who have had recent GI contrast studies because barium creates severe distortion of reflective sound waves
- Patients with air-filled bowels because gas does not transmit the sound waves well

Procedure and patient care

Before

PT Explain the procedure to the patient.

PT Tell the patient that no fasting or sedation is required.

PT Assure the patient that this study has no known deleterious effects on maternal or fetal tissues.

PT If the radiologist requests a full bladder for the procedure, give the patient 16 ounces of water or another liquid 1 hour before abdominal ultrasonography, and instruct the patient *not* to void until after the procedure is completed.

U

During

- Note the following procedural steps:
  1. In the ultrasound room, the patient is placed in the supine position on the examining table.

2. The ultrasonographer applies a gel to the abdomen to enhance sound transmission.
3. A transducer is passed over the skin.
4. If a vaginal probe is used, it is inserted via the vagina and angled to identify the various parts of the pelvis.
5. Pictures are taken of the reflections.

- Note that this procedure is performed in approximately 20 minutes.

After

- Remove the gel from the patient's skin.

Abnormal findings

Abdominal pregnancy
Abnormal fetal position
Abruptio placentae
Abscesses
Cysts
Fetal anomalies
Fetal death
Hydatidiform mole of the uterus
Hydrocephalus of the fetus
Intrauterine growth retardation
Multiple pregnancy
Neoplasm of the ovaries, uterus, or fallopian tubes
Ovarian torsion
Placenta previa
Polyhydramnios
Tubal pregnancy

notes

ultrasound of the prostate/rectum (Prostate/rectal sonogram)

Type of test Ultrasound

Normal findings

Normal size, contour, and consistency of the prostate gland

Test explanation and related physiology

Rectal ultrasonography of the prostate is a very valuable tool in the early diagnosis of prostate cancer. When combined with rectal digital examination and prostate-specific antigen (p. 611), very small prostate cancers can be identified. Prostate/rectal sonography is also helpful in evaluating the seminal vessels and other perirectal tissue.

Ultrasound is very helpful in guiding the direction of a prostate biopsy (Figure U2) and in quantitating the volume of prostate cancer. The ultrasound images direct the placement of needles to the areas of suspicion; however, ultrasound is not specific enough to accurately indicate cancerous from normal prostate tissue. MRI of the prostate is far more sensitive and specific for the location of prostate cancers but because the confines of space in an MRI machine,

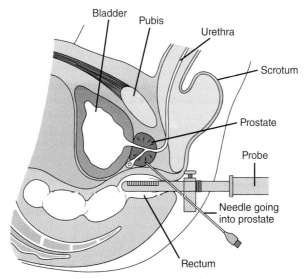

FIG. U2 Rectal ultrasonography. Diagram demonstrating transrectal biopsy of the prostate.

U

prostate biopsy cannot be performed. Computerized software can "fuse" detailed MRI scans with live, real-time ultrasound images of the prostate. A patient first undergoes an MRI scan. Then prostate ultrasound is performed. As the probe scans the prostate, the fusion software provides an overlaid MRI image of the same area of the prostate, giving a detailed 3-D ultrasound/MRI view of the prostate gland and where the suspicious tissue is located for biopsy. This method is called a *fusion biopsy of the prostate.*

When radiation therapy implantation is required for treatment, ultrasonography is used to map the exact location of the prostate cancer. Rectal ultrasonography is very helpful in staging rectal cancers as well. The depth of transmural involvement and presence of extrarectal extension can be accurately assessed.

Contraindications

• Patients with latex allergy require a latex free probe cover.

Interfering factors

• Stool within the rectum

Procedure and patient care

Before

PT Explain the procedure to the patient.

PT Instruct the patient that a small-volume rectal enema may be required approximately 1 hour before the examination.

During

• The patient is placed in the left lateral decubitus position.
• A digital rectal examination may be performed to assess the prostate gland or rectal tumor.
• A draped and lubricated ultrasound probe is placed in the rectum.
• Scans are performed in various spatial planes.

After

• Provide the patient with tissue material to cleanse the perianal area.

Abnormal findings

Benign prostatic hypertrophy
Intrarectal or perirectal tumor
Perirectal abscess
Prostate abscess
Prostate cancer
Prostatitis
Seminal vesicle tumor

ultrasound of the scrotum (US Testicles, Scrotal ultrasound, Ultrasound of testes)

Type of test   Ultrasound

Normal findings

Normal size, shape, and configuration of the testicles. Normal blood flow to testicles.

Test explanation and related physiology

Present uses for scrotal ultrasound include:

- Evaluation of scrotal masses
- Measurement of testicular size
- Evaluation of scrotal trauma
- Evaluation of scrotal pain and identification of torsion of the testicle
- Evaluation of occult testicular neoplasm
- Surveillance of primary or metastatic testicular neoplasms
- Follow-up for testicular infections
- Location of undescended testicles

The testicle and extratesticular intrascrotal tissues are examined. Both benign and malignant tumors can be identified with ultrasound. Benign abnormalities such as testicular abscess, orchitis, testicular infarction, and testicular torsion also can be identified. Extratesticular lesions such as hydrocele (fluid in the scrotum), hematocele (blood in the scrotum), and pyocele (pus in the scrotum) can be identified.

Ultrasonography of the scrotum is the preferred method to identify torsion of the testicle. Ultrasonography is a very accurate method of identifying microlithiasis in the testicles. When identified, microcalcifications in the testicle indicate a marked increased risk for testicular cancer. Calcifications can also occur after orchitis or trauma. In most cases, both testicles are routinely imaged during the ultrasound examination.

The use of color Doppler is helpful in determining blood flow to the testicle. If there is torsion of the testicle, color Doppler will indicate markedly reduced blood flow; immediate surgical exploration would be required. Conversely, ultrasound can also show increased blood flow to the epididymis as a result of reperfusion if a testis has detorsed.

There is little discomfort associated with testicular ultrasound. It is usually performed by an ultrasound technologist and interpreted by an ultrasound physician.

U

Procedure and patient care

Before

PT Explain the procedure to the patient.
PT Tell the patient that no fasting is required.

During

- Note the following procedural steps:
  1. Careful examination of the scrotum is performed by the physician. Usually a short history is obtained.
  2. The scrotum is supported by a towel or cradled by the examiner's gloved hand.
  3. Gel is applied to the scrotum. This enhances sound wave transmission and reception.
  4. Thorough scanning in the sagittal, transverse, and oblique projections is performed.
- The test takes approximately 20 to 30 minutes.

After

- Remove the gel from the patient's scrotum.

Abnormal findings

Benign testicular tumor
Cryptorchidism
Epididymitis
Hematocele
Hematoma
Hydrocele
Malignant testicular tumor
Occult testicular tumor
Pyocele
Scrotal hernia
Spermatocele
Testicular infection (orchitis)
Testicular torsion
Varicocele

notes

ultrasound of the thyroid (US Thyroid, Thyroid echogram, Thyroid sonogram)

Type of test   Ultrasound

Normal findings

Normal size, shape, and position of the thyroid gland

Test explanation and related physiology

Ultrasound examination of the thyroid gland distinguishes cystic from solid thyroid nodules. If the nodule is found to be purely cystic (fluid filled), the fluid can simply be aspirated and surgery avoided. If the nodule has a mixed or solid appearance, however, a tumor may be present, and FNA (p. 718) surgery may be required. This study may be repeated at intervals to determine the response of a thyroid mass to medical therapy.

Procedure and patient care

Before

PT Explain the procedure to the patient.

PT Tell the patient that breathing or swallowing will not be affected by the placement of a transducer on the neck.

PT Inform the patient that a lubricant will be applied to the neck to ensure effective transmission of sound waves.

PT Tell the patient that no fasting or sedation is required.

During

- Note the following procedural steps:
  1. The patient is taken to the ultrasonography department and placed in the supine position with the neck hyperextended.
  2. Gel is applied to the patient's neck.
  3. A sound transducer is passed over the nodule.
  4. Photographs are taken of the image displayed.
- A technologist usually performs this study in about 15 to 60 minutes and a radiologist evaluates the results.

PT Tell the patient that no discomfort is associated with this study.

After

- Assist the patient in removing the lubricant from the neck.

Abnormal findings

Cyst

Goiter

Thyroid adenoma

Thyroid carcinoma

Tumor

U

notes

ultrasound vascular studies (Venous doppler ultrasound, Venous duplex scan, Intravascular ultrasound [IVUS], Ultrasound extremities)

Type of test Ultrasound

Normal findings

Venous

A normal Doppler venous signal with spontaneous respiration
Normal venous system without evidence of occlusion

Arterial

Normal arterial Doppler signal with systolic and diastolic components
No reduction in blood pressure in excess of 20 mm Hg compared with the normal extremity
A normal ankle-to-brachial arterial blood pressure index of 0.85 or greater
No evidence of arterial occlusion

Test explanation and related physiology

Vascular ultrasound studies are used to identify occlusion or thrombosis of the veins or arteries of an extremity. Patency is demonstrated with Doppler ultrasound by detecting moving red blood cells (RBCs) in the vessel.

Vascular duplex scanning combines the benefits of Doppler with B-mode scanning. With this technique, one is able to directly visualize areas of vascular narrowing or occlusion. The degree of occlusion is measured as percentage of the entire lumen.

Color Doppler ultrasound (CDU) can be added to arterial duplex scanning. This allows visualization of stenotic areas based on velocity or direction of blood flow in a particular area of the artery.

Duplex scanning is routinely used to identify venous thrombosis *(venous duplex scan)* in patients suspected of having deep vein thrombosis (DVT) in an extremity. It is more rapidly performed and interpreted than venography (p. 793) or MRV (p. 492). B-mode imaging assesses the compressibility of the vein. Normal veins collapse with the application of pressure using the ultrasound probe; thrombosed veins do not collapse.

With a single-mode transducer, blood flow can be heard audibly as a swishing noise. With single-mode arterial Doppler studies, peripheral arteriosclerotic occlusive disease of the extremities can be easily located. By slowly deflating blood pressure cuffs placed on the thigh, calf, and ankle, systolic pressure in the arteries of the extremities can be accurately measured by detecting the first evidence of blood flow with the Doppler transducer. Normally systolic blood pressure is slightly higher in the arteries of the arms than in the legs. If the difference in blood pressure exceeds 20 mm Hg, occlusive disease is believed to exist immediately proximal to the area tested. Lower extremity arterial bypass graft patency can also be assessed with Doppler ultrasound.

Percutaneous *intravascular ultrasound (IVUS)* can be used to study the progression, stabilization, and potential regression of coronary atherosclerosis using a specially made intravascular transducer. IVUS permits imaging of the lumen size, vessel wall structure, and any atheroma that may be present. It allows characterization of atheroma size, plaque distribution, and lesion composition. This procedure is predominantly used in the coronary artery; however, it can also be used to determine the extent of obstruction in other vessels (e.g., iliac/inferior vena cava).

Interfering factors

- Venous or arterial occlusive disease proximal to the testing site
- Cigarette smoking because nicotine can cause constriction of the peripheral arteries and alter the results

Procedure and patient care

Before

PT Explain the procedure to the patient.

PT Inform the patient that this is a painless procedure.

- Remove all clothing from the extremity to be examined.

PT Instruct the patient to abstain from cigarette smoking for at least 30 minutes before the test.

During

- Note the following procedural steps:

Venous studies

1. Gel is applied to the skin overlying the venous system of the extremity in multiple areas.
2. Usually, for the lower extremity, the deep venous system is identified in the ankle, calf, thigh, and groin.
3. The characteristic "swishing" sound of the blood flow indicates a patent venous system.
4. Both the superficial and deep venous systems can be evaluated.

Arterial studies

1. These are performed with the use of blood pressure cuffs, which are placed around the thigh, calf, and ankle.

2. A conductive gel is applied to the skin overlying the artery distal to the cuffs.
3. The proximal cuff is inflated to a level higher than systolic blood pressure in the normal extremity.
4. The Doppler ultrasound transducer is placed immediately distal to the inflated cuff.
5. The pressure in the cuff is slowly released.
6. The highest pressure at which blood flow is detected by the characteristic "swishing" Doppler signal is recorded as the blood pressure of that artery.
7. The test is repeated at each successive level.
8. When the ankle pressure is divided by the arm (brachial artery) pressure, this is known as the ankle brachial index (ABI). If the ABI is less than 0.85, significant arterial occlusive disease exists within the extremity.

• Note that these studies are usually performed in the vascular laboratory or radiology department and take approximately 30 to 60 minutes.

After

• Encourage the patient to verbalize his or her concerns.
• Remove the transducer gel from the extremity.
PT Inform the patient that the physician must interpret the studies and that results will be available in a few hours.

Abnormal findings

Arterial aneurysm
Embolic arterial occlusion
Small or large vessel arterial occlusive disease
Small vessel arterial occlusive disease (as in diabetes)
Spastic arterial disease (e.g., Raynaud phenomenon)
Venous occlusion secondary to thrombosis or thrombophlebitis
Venous varicosities

notes

upper gastrointestinal x-ray study (Upper GI series, UGI)

Type of test X-ray with contrast

Normal findings

Normal size, contour, patency, filling, positioning, and transit of barium through the lower esophagus, stomach, and upper duodenum

Test explanation and related physiology

The upper GI study consists of a series of x-ray images of the lower esophagus, stomach, and duodenum, usually with barium sulfate as the contrast medium. When there is concern about leakage of x-ray contrast through a perforation of the GI tract, however, Gastrografin (a water-soluble contrast) is used. This test can be performed in conjunction with a barium swallow or a small bowel series (pp. 109 and 671), which can precede or succeed the upper GI study, respectively.

The purpose of this examination is to detect ulcerations, tumors, inflammations, and anatomic malpositions (e.g., hiatal hernia) in these organs. Obstruction of the upper GI tract is also easily detected. With the development of improved imaging using CT scan or MRI, this test is uncommonly performed.

Contraindications

- Patients with complete bowel obstructions
- Patients suspected of upper GI perforation. Water-soluble Gastrografin should be used instead of barium.
- Patients who are uncooperative because of the necessity of frequent position changes

Potential complications

- Aspiration of barium
- Constipation or partial bowel obstruction caused by inspissated barium in the small bowel or colon

Interfering factors

- Previously administered barium may block visualization.
- Incapacitated patients cannot assume the multiple positions required for the study.
- Food and fluid in the stomach give the false impression of filling defects within the stomach, precluding adequate evaluation of the gastric mucosa.

U

Procedure and patient care

Because this test is rarely performed, we recommend identifying local healthcare instructions for testing.

Abnormal findings

Benign gastric tumor (e.g., leiomyoma)

Congenital abnormalities (e.g., duodenal web, pancreatic rest, malrotation syndrome)

Duodenal cancer

Duodenal diverticulum

Duodenal ulcer

Esophageal cancer

Esophageal diverticula

Esophageal varices

Extrinsic compression by pancreatic pseudocysts, cysts, pancreatic tumors, or hepatomegaly

Gastric cancer

Gastric inflammatory disease (e.g., Ménétrier disease)

Gastric ulcer (benign and malignant)

Gastritis

Hiatal hernia

Perforation of the esophagus, stomach, or duodenum

notes

urea breath test (UBT, *Helicobacter pylori* breath test)

Type of test Other

Normal findings

< 50 dpm (if ^{14}C is used)

< 3% (if ^{13}C is used)

Test explanation and related physiology

This test is used to detect *Helicobacter pylori* infections. It is indicated in patients who have recurrent or chronic gastric or duodenal ulceration or inflammation. When the *H. pylori* infection is successfully treated, the ulcer or inflammation will usually heal.

There are several serologic and microscopic methods of detecting *H. pylori* (see *Helicobacter pylori* antibodies test, p. 403). The UBT is the noninvasive test of choice for diagnosis of *H. pylori* infection. It is based on the capability of *H. pylori* to metabolize urea to CO_2 because of the organism's capability to produce a large amount of urease. In the breath test, carbon (^{13}C)-labeled urea is administered orally. The urea is then absorbed through the gastric mucosa. If *H. pylori* is present, the urea will be converted to $^{13}CO_2$. The $^{13}CO_2$ is then taken up by the capillaries in the stomach wall and delivered to the lungs, where it is exhaled. The labeled carbon can be measured by gas chromatography or a mass spectrometer.

This test has been simplified to the point that two breath samples collected before and 30 minutes after the ingestion of urea in a liquid form suffice to provide reliable diagnostic information. Labeling urea with ^{13}C is becoming increasingly popular because it is a nonradioactive isotope of ^{14}C and is innocuous. It can be safely used in children and women of childbearing age. See also Lactose tolerance test, p. 456.

Interfering factors

- Dietary constituents with a natural abundance of ^{13}C, such as maize, cane, and corn flour, can cause increased levels.

U

Procedure and patient care

Before

PT Explain the procedure to the patient.

PT Instruct the patient to abstain from oral intake for 6 hours before testing.

PT When providing the isotopic urea to the patient, instruct the patient as to proper administration (per laboratory routine).

During

- Several minutes after the patient has swallowed the carbon dose, provide the patient with 2 oz of water.
- Breath samples are collected in any one of a number of gas collection devices depending on how and when the sample will be analyzed.

After

PT Instruct the patient to resume medications and normal diet.

PT If radioactive carbon was used, instruct the patient to drink plenty of fluids to facilitate excretion of the radioisotope.

Abnormal findings

H. pylori infection

notes

uric acid, blood, and urine

Type of test Blood, urine

Normal findings

Blood

Adult

    Male: 4–8.5 mg/dL or 0.24–0.51 mmol/L

    Female: 2.7–7.3 mg/dL or 0.16–0.43 mmol/L

Child: 2.5–5.5 mg/dL or 0.12–0.32 mmol/L

Newborn: 2–6.2 mg/dL

Physiologic saturation threshold: > 6 mg/dL or > 0.357 mmol/L

Therapeutic target for gout: < 6 mg/dL or < 0.357 mmol/L

Urine

250–750 mg/24 hr or 1.48–4.43 mmol/day (SI units)

Possible critical values

Blood: > 12 mg/dL

Test explanation and related physiology

Uric acid is a nitrogenous compound that is a product of purine (a DNA building block) catabolism. Uric acid is excreted to a large degree by the kidney and to a smaller degree by the intestinal tract. When uric acid levels are elevated (hyperuricemia), the patient may have gout.

Causes of hyperuricemia can be overproduction or decreased excretion of uric acid (e.g., kidney failure). Overproduction of uric acid may occur in patients with a catabolic enzyme deficiency that stimulates purine metabolism or in patients with cancer in whom purine and DNA turnover is great. Other causes of hyperuricemia may include alcoholism, leukemia, metastatic cancer, multiple myeloma, hyperlipoproteinemia, diabetes mellitus, renal failure, stress, lead poisoning, and dehydration caused by diuretic therapy. Ketoacids (as occur in diabetic or alcoholic ketoacidosis) may compete with uric acid for tubular excretion and may cause decreased uric acid excretion. Many causes of hyperuricemia are undefined and therefore labeled as *idiopathic*.

Uric acid can become supersaturated in the urine and crystallize to form kidney stones that can block the renal system.

U

Urinary excretion of uric acid depends on uric acid levels in the blood, along with glomerular filtration and tubular secretion of uric acid into the urine. Uric acid is less well saturated in alkaline urine. As the urine pH rises, more uric acid can exist without crystallization and stone formation. Therefore when a person is known to have high uric acid in the urine, the urine can be alkalinized by ingestion of a strong base to prevent stone formation.

Interfering factors

- Stress may cause increased uric acid levels.
- Recent use of x-ray contrast agents may cause decreased serum levels.
- Recent use of x-ray contrast may increase uric acid levels in the urine.

Procedure and patient care

Before

PT Explain the procedure to the patient.
- Follow the institution's requirements regarding fasting.

During

Blood
- Collect a venous blood sample in a red-top tube.

Urine
PT Instruct the patient to begin the 24-hour urine collection after voiding. Discard the initial specimen and start the 24-hour timing at that point.
- See inside front cover for Routine Urine Testing.

After

Blood
- Apply pressure to the venipuncture site.

Urine
- Transport the urine specimen promptly to the laboratory.

Abnormal findings

▲ **Increased blood levels (hyperuricemia)**

Acidosis (ketotic or lactic)
Alcoholism
Cancer chemotherapy
Chronic renal disease
Genetic inborn error in purine metabolism
Gout
Hemolysis
Hyperlipoproteinemia
Hypothyroidism
Idiopathic
Increased ingestion of purines
Leukemia
Metastatic cancer
Multiple myeloma
Rhabdomyolysis (e.g., heavy exercise, burns, crush injury, epileptic seizure, or myocardial infarction)
Shock or chronic blood volume depletion states
Toxemia of pregnancy

▼ **Decreased blood levels**

Fanconi syndrome
Lead poisoning
Wilson disease
Yellow atrophy of the liver

▲ **Increased urine levels**

Cancer chemotherapy
Gout
High purine diet
Lead toxicity
Leukemia
Metastatic cancer
Multiple myeloma

▼ **Decreased urine levels**

Acidosis (ketotic or lactic)
Chronic alcohol ingestion
Eclampsia
Kidney disease

notes

U

urinalysis (UA)

Type of test Urine

Normal findings

Appearance: clear
Color: amber yellow
Odor: aromatic
pH: 4.6 to 8 (average 6)
Protein
    0–8 mg/dL
    50–80 mg/24 hr (at rest)
    < 250 mg/24 hr (exercise)
Specific gravity
    Adult: 1.005–1.03 (usually 1.01–1.025)
    Newborn: 1.001–1.02
Leukocyte esterase: negative
Nitrites: negative
Ketones: negative
Crystals: negative
Casts: none
Glucose
    Fresh specimen: negative
    24-hour specimen: 50–300 mg/day or 0.3–1.7 mmol/day (SI
        units)
White blood cells (WBCs): 0–4 per high-power field
WBC casts: none
Red blood cells (RBCs): ≤ 2
RBC casts: none

Test explanation and related physiology

A total urinalysis involves multiple routine tests on a urine specimen. This specimen is not necessarily a clean-catch specimen. However, if urinary tract infection (UTI) is suspected, often a midstream clean-catch specimen is obtained. Some of this urine is also cultured (p. 783) if the urinalysis indicates infection. Abnormalities detected by urinalysis may reflect either urinary tract diseases (e.g., infection, glomerulonephritis, loss of concentrating capacity) or extrarenal disease processes (e.g., glucosuria in diabetes, proteinuria in monoclonal gammopathies, bilirubinuria in liver disease).

Urinalysis routinely includes remarks about the color, appearance, and odor of the urine. The pH is determined. The urine is tested for the presence of proteins, glucose, ketones, blood, and leukocyte esterase. The urine is examined microscopically for RBCs, WBCs, casts, crystals, and bacteria.

Appearance and color

Urine appearance and color are noted as part of routine urinalysis. The appearance of a normal urine specimen should be clear. Cloudy urine may be caused by the presence of pus, RBCs, or bacteria; however, normal urine also may be cloudy because of ingestion of certain foods. The color indicates the concentration of the urine and varies with specific gravity. Dilute urine is straw colored, and concentrated urine is deep amber. Dark yellow urine may indicate the presence of urobilinogen or bilirubin. *Pseudomonas* organisms may produce green urine. Beets may cause red urine, and rhubarb can color the urine brown. Many frequently used drugs also may affect urine color.

Odor

Determination of urine odor is a part of routine urinalysis. The aromatic odor of fresh, normal urine is caused by the presence of volatile acids. Urine of patients with diabetic ketoacidosis has the strong, sweet smell of acetone. In patients with UTIs, the urine may have a very foul odor. Patients with a fecal odor to their urine may have an enterovesical fistula.

pH

Urine pH is affected by diet, medications, systemic acid–base disturbances, and renal tubular function. An alkaline pH is obtained in a patient with alkalemia. Also, bacteria, UTI, or a diet high in citrus fruits or vegetables may cause an increased urine pH. Slightly acidic urine is normal. Normal average pH is 7.0, slightly acidic compared with average blood pH of 7.4. However, acidic urine is observed in patients with acidemia, which can result from metabolic or respiratory acidosis, starvation, dehydration, or a diet high in meat products or cranberries. The urine pH is useful in identifying crystals in the urine and determining the predisposition to form a given type of stone.

Protein

Protein is a sensitive indicator of glomerular and tubular renal function. Normally, less than 30 mg of protein per day is in urine. This is not detectable in the routine protein analysis. Microalbumin can be detected, however (p. 511). If the glomerular filtration membrane is injured, protein seeps out into the filtrate and then into the urine. If tubular disease exists, protein is not reabsorbed and is present in the urine. If proteinuria persists at a significant rate, the patient can develop interstitial edema. The combination of proteinuria and edema is known as the nephrotic syndrome.

U

Proteinuria (usually albumin) is probably the most important indicator of renal disease. The urine of all pregnant women is routinely checked for proteinuria, which can be an indicator of preeclampsia. In addition to screening for nephrotic syndrome, urinary protein also screens for complications of diabetes mellitus, glomerulonephritis, amyloidosis, and multiple myeloma (see test for Bence Jones protein, p. 112).

If significant protein is noted at urinalysis, a 24-hour urine specimen should be collected to measure the quantity of protein. This estimate is usually performed with a urine creatinine. The normal *protein/creatinine ratio* is less than 0.15.

Glucose

This can be an effective screening test for the presence of glucose in the urine that may identify diabetes mellitus or other causes of glucose intolerance (see glucose, p. 392).

Glucose is filtered from the blood by the glomeruli of the kidney. Normally, all of the glucose is resorbed in the proximal renal tubules. When the blood glucose level exceeds the capability of the renal threshold to resorb the glucose (normally ~180 mg/dL), it begins to spill over into the urine (glycosuria). As the blood glucose level increases further, greater amounts of glucose are spilled into the urine.

Osmolality

This is measured during routine urinalysis (p. 772).

Specific gravity

Specific gravity is a measure of the concentration of particles, including wastes and electrolytes, in the urine. A high specific gravity indicates concentrated urine; a low specific gravity indicates dilute urine. Specific gravity refers to the weight of the urine compared with that of distilled water (which has a specific gravity of 1.000). Particles in the urine give it weight or specific gravity.

Specific gravity is used to evaluate the concentrating and excretory power of the kidney. It is also a measurement of the hydration status of the patient. An overhydrated patient will have a more dilute urine with a lower specific gravity. The specific gravity of the urine in a dehydrated patient can be expected to be abnormally high. Specific gravity correlates roughly with osmolality.

Leukocyte (WBC) esterase

Leukocyte (WBC) esterase is a screening test used to detect leukocytes in the urine. When positive, this test indicates a UTI.

This examination uses chemical testing with a leukocyte esterase dipstick; a shade of purple is considered a positive result. Some laboratories have established screening protocols in which a microscopic examination is performed only if a leukocyte esterase test is positive.

Nitrites

Like the leukocyte esterase test, the nitrite test is a screening test for the identification of UTIs. This test is based on the principle that many, but not all, bacteria produce an enzyme called *reductase,* which can reduce urinary nitrates to nitrites. Chemical testing is done with a dipstick containing a reagent that reacts with nitrites to produce a pink color, thus indirectly suggesting the presence of bacteria. A positive test result indicates the need for a urine culture. Nitrite screening enhances the sensitivity of the leukocyte esterase test to detect UTIs.

Ketones

Normally no ketones are present in the urine; however, a patient with poorly controlled diabetes who is hyperglycemic may have massive fatty acid catabolism. Ketones (beta-hydroxybutyric acid, acetoacetic acid, and acetone) are the end products of this fatty acid breakdown. As with glucose, ketones (predominantly acetoacetic acid) spill over into the urine when the blood levels of patients with diabetes are elevated. This test for ketonuria is also important in evaluating ketoacidosis associated with alcoholism, fasting, starvation, high-protein diets, and isopropanol ingestion. Ketonuria may occur with acute febrile illnesses, especially in infants and children.

Bilirubin and urobilinogen

Bilirubin is a major constituent of bile. If bilirubin excretion is inhibited, conjugated (direct) hyperbilirubinemia will result (p. 118). Conjugated bilirubin is water soluble and can be excreted into the urine. Therefore bilirubin in urine suggests disease affecting bilirubin metabolism after conjugation or with defects in excretion (e.g., gallstones). Unconjugated bilirubin caused by prehepatic jaundice will not be excreted in the urine because it is not water soluble.

Bilirubin is excreted by way of the bile ducts into the bowel. There, some of the bilirubin is transformed into *urobilinogen* by the action of bacteria in the bowel. Most of the urobilinogen is excreted from the liver back into the bowel, but some is excreted by the kidneys.

U

Crystals

Crystals found in urinary sediment on microscopic examination indicate that renal stone formulation is imminent, if not already present. Urea crystals occur in patients with high serum uric acid levels (gout). Phosphate and calcium oxalate crystals occur in the urine of patients with parathyroid abnormalities or malabsorption states. The type of crystal found varies with the disease and the pH of the urine.

Casts

Casts are rectangular clumps of materials or cells that are formed in the renal distal and collecting tubules, where the material is maximally concentrated. These clumps of material and cells take on the shape of the tubule, thus the term *cast*. Casts are usually associated with some degree of proteinuria and stasis in the renal tubules. There are several kinds of casts.

Hyaline casts are conglomerations of protein and indicate proteinuria. A few hyaline casts are normally found, especially after strenuous exercise or dehydration.

Granular casts result from the disintegration of cellular material into granular particles within a WBC or epithelial cell cast. Granular casts are found after exercise and in patients with various renal diseases.

Fatty casts are made up of lipids and are associated with glomerular disease or the nephrotic syndrome or nephrosis.

Waxy casts may be cell casts, hyaline casts, or renal failure casts. Waxy casts represent further degeneration of granular casts. They are associated with chronic renal failure.

Epithelial cells can enter the urine anywhere along the process of urinary excretion. The presence of occasional epithelial cells is not remarkable. Large numbers, however, are abnormal and can conglomerate into *tubular (epithelial) casts.*

Normally, few WBCs are found in urine sediment on microscopic examination. The presence of five or more WBCs in the urine indicates a UTI involving the bladder, kidney, or both. *WBC casts* are most commonly found in infections of the kidney, such as acute pyelonephritis.

Any disruption in the blood–urine barrier will cause RBCs to enter the urine. The bleeding can be microscopic or gross hematuria. Patients with more than three RBCs per high-power field should be considered to have microhematuria and hence be evaluated for possible pathologic causes. *RBC casts* suggest glomerulonephritis. RBC casts are also seen in patients with acute tubular necrosis, pyelonephritis, renal trauma, or renal tumor.

Interfering factors

Appearance and color
- Sperm in the urethra can cause the urine to appear cloudy.
- Urine that has been refrigerated for longer than 1 hour can become cloudy.
- Certain foods affect urine color.
- Urine darkens with prolonged standing because of oxidation of bilirubin metabolites.
- Many drugs, given the right environment, can alter the color of urine.

Odor
- Some foods (e.g., asparagus) produce a characteristic odor.
- When urine stands for a long time and begins to decompose, it has an ammonia-like smell.

pH
- Urine pH becomes alkaline on standing, because of the action of urea-splitting bacteria, which produce ammonia.
- The urine pH of an uncovered specimen will become alkaline because carbon dioxide vaporizes from the urine.
- Dietary factors affect urine pH.

Protein
- Transient proteinuria may be associated with severe emotional stress, excessive exercise, and cold baths.
- Radiopaque contrast media administered within 3 days may cause false-positive results for proteinuria.
- Urine contaminated with prostate or vaginal secretions commonly causes proteinuria.
- Diets high in protein can cause proteinuria.
- Highly concentrated urine may have a higher concentration of protein than more dilute urine.
- Hemoglobin may cause a positive result with the dipstick method.
- Bence Jones protein may not appear with the dipstick method.

Specific gravity
- Recent use of radiographic dyes increases specific gravity.
- Cold temperatures cause falsely high specific gravity.

Leukocyte esterase
- False-positive results may occur in specimens contaminated by vaginal secretions that contain WBCs.
- False-negative results may occur in specimens containing high levels of protein or ascorbic acid.

U

Ketones
- Special diets (carbohydrate-free, high-protein, high-fat) may cause ketonuria.

Bilirubin and urobilinogen
- Bilirubin is not stable in urine, especially when exposed to light.
- pH can affect urobilinogen levels. Alkaline urine indicates higher levels; acidic urine may show lower levels.

Crystals
- Radiographic contrast media may cause urinary crystals.

WBCs
- Vaginal discharge may contaminate the urine specimen and factitiously cause WBCs in the urine.

RBCs
- Strenuous physical exercise may cause RBC casts.
- Traumatic urethral catheterization may cause RBCs.
- Overaggressive anticoagulant therapy or bleeding disorders tend to cause RBCs in the urine without concomitant disease.

Procedure and patient care

Before

PT Explain the procedure to the patient.

During
- Collect a fresh urine specimen in a urine container.
- If the urine specimen contains vaginal discharge or bleeding, a clean-catch or midstream specimen will be needed. This requires cleaning of the urinary meatus with an antiseptic preparation to reduce contamination of the specimen by external organisms. For the *midstream collection*, use the following procedural steps indicated on p. 784.
- For ketones, this test can be performed immediately after collection with a dipstick.
- With a Ketostix, dip the reagent into the urine specimen and remove it. Read the strip in 15 seconds by comparing it with the color chart.
- For urine specific gravity, a first-voided specimen is the best.
- For protein, the first-voided specimen is the best; however, occasionally a 24-hour urine collection is preferred.
- See inside front cover for Routine Urine Testing.

After
- Transport the urine specimen to the laboratory promptly.

- If the specimen cannot be processed immediately, refrigerate it. If the urine cannot be tested within 2 hours of collection, a preservative should be used.
- If a 24-hour urine collection is requested, the specimen should be refrigerated, or a preservative should be used.
- Casts will break up as urine is allowed to sit. Urine examinations for casts should be performed on fresh specimens.

Abnormal findings

Appearance and color
Bacteria
Certain foods (e.g., beets, carrots)
Dehydration
Diabetes insipidus
Drug therapy
Excessive sweating
Fever

Jaundice
Overhydration
Pathologic conditions (e.g., bleeding from the kidney)
Pus
Red blood cells

Crystals
Drug therapy
Renal stone formation
UTI

Epithelial casts
Acute renal allograft rejection
Eclampsia
Ethylene glycol intoxication

Glomerulonephritis
Heavy-metal poisoning

Fatty casts
Chronic renal disease
Diabetic nephropathy

Glomerulonephritis
Nephrotic syndrome

Glucose
▲ **Increased levels**
Diabetes mellitus
Hereditary defects in metabolism of other reducing substances (e.g., galactose, fructose, pentose)
Nephrotoxic chemicals (e.g., carbon monoxide, mercury, lead)
Pregnancy
Renal glycosuria

Granular casts

Acute tubular necrosis
Chronic lead poisoning
Glomerulonephritis
Nephrosclerosis
Pyelonephritis

Reaction after exercise
Renal transplant rejection
Stress
UTI

Hyaline casts

Chronic renal failure
Congestive heart failure
Fever
Glomerulonephritis

Proteinuria
Pyelonephritis
Strenuous exercise
Stress

Ketones

After anesthesia
Anorexia nervosa
Dehydration
Excessive aspirin ingestion
Fasting
Febrile illnesses in infants
  and children
High-protein diets

Isopropanol ingestion
Ketoacidosis of alcoholism
Prolonged vomiting
Starvation
Uncontrolled diabetes
  mellitus
Weight reduction diets

Leukocyte esterase

Possible UTI

Nitrites

Possible UTI

Odor

Hepatic failure
Infection
Ketonuria
Maple syrup urine disease
Phenylketonuria

Rectal fistula
UTI

pH

▲ **Increased levels**

Diuretic therapy
Gastric suction
Metabolic alkalosis
Renal failure with inability
  to form ammonia
Renal tubular acidosis
Respiratory alkalosis
Urea-splitting bacteria
UTI
Vegetarian diet
Vomiting

▼ **Decreased levels**

Diabetes mellitus
Diarrhea
Metabolic acidosis
Pyrexia
Respiratory acidosis
Sleep
Starvation

Protein

▲ **Increased levels**

Amyloidosis
Bacterial pyelonephritis
Bladder tumor
Congestive heart failure
Diabetes mellitus
Diabetic glomerulosclerosis
Galactosemia
Glomerulonephritis
Goodpasture syndrome
Heavy-metal poisoning

Malignant hypertension
Multiple myeloma
Nephrotic syndrome
Nephrotoxic drug therapy
Polycystic kidney disease
Preeclampsia
Renal vein thrombosis
Systemic lupus
  erythematosus

Red blood cells and casts

▲ **Increased RBC levels**

Acute tubular necrosis
Cystitis
Glomerulonephritis
Interstitial nephritis
Prostatitis
Pyelonephritis
Renal stones
Renal trauma
Renal tumor
Traumatic bladder
  catheterization

▲ **Increased RBC cast levels**

Glomerulonephritis
Goodpasture syndrome
Malignant hypertension
Renal infarct
Sickle cell anemia
Subacute bacterial
  endocarditis
Systemic lupus
  erythematosus
Vasculitis

U

Specific gravity
▲ **Increased levels**
Decrease in renal blood
flow (as in heart failure,
renal artery stenosis, or
hypotension)
Dehydration
Diarrhea
Excessive sweating
Fever
Glycosuria and proteinuria
Pituitary tumor or trauma
that causes syndrome of
inappropriate antidiuretic
hormone (SIADH)
Vomiting
Water restriction
X-ray contrast dye

▼ **Decreased levels**
Diabetes insipidus
Diuresis
Glomerulonephritis
Hypothermia
Overhydration
Pyelonephritis
Renal failure

Waxy casts
Chronic renal disease
Chronic renal failure
Diabetic nephropathy
Glomerulonephritis

Malignant hypertension
Nephrotic syndrome
Renal transplant rejection

White blood cells and casts
▲ **Increased WBC levels**
Bacterial infection in the
urinary tract

▲ **Increased WBC cast levels**
Acute pyelonephritis
Glomerulonephritis
Lupus nephritis

notes

urine culture and sensitivity (C&S)

Type of test Urine; microscopic

Normal findings

Negative: < 10,000 bacteria per milliliter of urine
Positive: > 100,000 bacteria per milliliter of urine

Test explanation and related physiology

Urine cultures and sensitivities are obtained to determine the presence of pathogenic bacteria in patients with suspected UTIs. An important part of any routine culture is to assess the *sensitivity* of any bacteria that are growing in the urine to various antibiotics. The physician can then more appropriately recommend the correct antibiotic therapy.

Most often, UTIs are limited to the bladder. However, the kidneys, ureters, bladder, or urethra can be the source of infection. All cultures should be performed before antibiotic therapy is initiated; otherwise the antibiotic may interrupt the growth of the organism in the laboratory. Most organisms require at least 24 hours to grow in the laboratory, and a preliminary report can be given at that time. Usually 48 to 72 hours is required for growth and identification of the organism. With DNA sequencing through PCR or nanopore technology, the infecting bacteria can be identified and antibiotic sensitivity can be available within 4 hours of testing, allowing effective antibiotic therapy to be instigated very soon after testing.

To save money, urine cultures are usually done only if the urinalysis suggests a possible infection (e.g., increased number of WBCs, bacteria, high pH, positive leukocyte esterase).

Interfering factors

- Contamination of the urine with stool, vaginal secretions, hands, or clothing will cause false-positive results.

Procedure and patient care

Before

PT Explain to the patient the procedure for obtaining a clean-catch (midstream) urine collection.
- Hold antibiotics until after specimen collection.
- Provide the patient with the necessary supplies.

During

- Note that a *clean-catch* or *midstream urine* collection is required for C&S testing. This requires cleansing of the urinary meatus

U

with an antiseptic preparation to reduce contamination of the specimen by external organisms. Then the cleansing agent must be completely removed, or it will contaminate the urine specimen. The midstream collection is obtained by

1. Having the patient begin to urinate in a bedpan, urinal, or toilet and then stop urinating (this washes the urine out of the distal urethra)
2. Correctly positioning a sterile urine container, into which the patient voids 3 to 4 oz of urine
3. Capping the container
4. Allowing the patient to finish voiding

- Note that *urinary catheterization* may be needed for patients unable to void.
- For patients with an *indwelling urinary catheter*, obtain a specimen by aseptically inserting a syringe into the sampling port on the catheter. (Usually the catheter tubing distal to the puncture site needs to be clamped for 15–30 minutes before the aspiration of urine to allow urine to fill the tubing. After the specimen is withdrawn, the clamp is removed.)
- Note that *suprapubic aspiration* of urine is a safe method of obtaining urine in neonates and infants. The abdomen is prepared with an antiseptic, and a 25-gauge needle is inserted into the suprapubic area 1 inch above the symphysis pubis. Urine is aspirated into the syringe and then transferred to a sterile urine container.
- Note that for patients with a *urinary diversion* (e.g., an ileal conduit), catheterization should be done through the stoma.
- Urine should *not* be collected from an ostomy pouch.

After

- Transport the specimen to the laboratory immediately (at least within 30 minutes).
- Notify the physician of any positive results so that appropriate antibiotic therapy can be initiated.

Abnormal findings

UTI

notes

urodynamic studies (Uroflowmetry, Urine flow studies, Cystometry, Cystometrogram [CMG], Urethral pressure profile [UPP], Urethral pressure measurements)

Type of test Manometric

Normal findings

Normal sensations of fullness and temperature
Normal pressures and volumes
Maximal cystometric capacity
    Male: 350–750 mL
    Female: 250–550 mL
Intravesical pressure when bladder is empty: usually < 40 cm H_2O
Detrusor pressure: < 10 cm H_2O
Residual urine: < 30 mL

Maximal urethral pressures in normal patients

Age (years)	Male (cm H_2O)	Female (cm H_2O)
> 64	35–105	35–75
45–64	40–123	40–100
25–44	35–113	31–115
< 25	37–126	55–103

Test explanation and related physiology

    These tests are used to measure pressures and urine volume of the bladder and urethra in order to identify patients who have bladder function problems. Urodynamic tests usually include urine flow studies, postvoid residual (PVR) urine measurement, and CMG. They are used in patients with bladder outlet obstruction, urinary incontinence, and questionable neurogenic bladder. They are also used to document progress with treatment.

    Both the motor and sensory function of the bladder are evaluated. During CMG, water is used to assess the first sensation of filling, fullness, and urinary urge. Bladder compliance and the presence of uninhibited detrusor contractions (i.e., phasic contractions) can also be noted during this filling CMG. Abdominal leak point pressure (ALPP) is useful in determining the etiology of urinary stress incontinence. The neuromuscular function of the bladder is assessed by measuring the efficiency of the detrusor muscle, intravesical pressure and capacity, and the bladder's response to thermal stimulation. Because urodynamic

U

studies have a wide range of normal, urodynamic findings of significance must be associated with reproduction of the patient's symptoms.

Cystometry can determine whether a bladder function abnormality is caused by neurologic, infectious, or obstructive diseases. Cystometry is indicated to elucidate the causes of bladder outlet obstruction or frequency and urgency. It is also part of the evaluation for incontinence, persistent residual urine, vesicoureteral reflux, severe nocturnal enuresis, motor and sensory disorders affecting the bladder, and the effect of certain drugs on bladder function.

Uroflowmetry is the simplest of the urodynamic techniques, being noninvasive and requiring uncomplicated and relatively inexpensive equipment. It measures the volume of urine expelled from the bladder per second. If the rate is reduced, outflow obstruction can be documented and measured. Nomograms of maximal flow versus voided volume may be used for accurate test result interpretation, taking into account the patient's gender and age. Urine flowmeters provide a permanent graphic recording.

UPP is often performed with urine flow studies. UPP is the fluid pressure that would hypothetically be required to force open the collapsed urethra and allow urine to flow. The urethral pressure varies from point to point within the urethra. Thus, a graph of urethral pressure against distance along the urethra is determined. It is used to document reduced urethral pressures in incontinent patients. It is also used to indicate the degree of compression applied to the urethra from an abnormally enlarged prostate (which will increase UPP value).

Urodynamic studies are performed by a urologist in approximately 45 minutes and are often performed at the same time as cystoscopy. The only discomfort is that associated with the urethral catheterization.

Contraindications

- UTIs because of the possibility of false results and the potential for the spread of infection.

Procedure and patient care

Before

PT Explain the purpose and the procedure to the patient. Instruct the patient to arrive with a full bladder.
- Obtain informed consent.
PT Tell the patient that no fluid or food restrictions are needed.

- Assure the patient that he or she will be draped to prevent unnecessary exposure.
- Assess the patient for signs and symptoms of UTI.
- PT Instruct the patient not to strain while voiding because the results can be skewed.

During

- Note the following procedural steps:
  1. Cystometry, usually performed in a urologist's office or a special procedure room, begins with the patient being asked to void.
  2. The amount of time required to initiate voiding and the size, force, and continuity of the urinary stream are recorded. The amount of urine, the time of voiding, and the presence of any straining, hesitancy, or terminal urine dribbling are also recorded.
  3. Next the bladder is tested for post void residual (see ultrasound of the pelvis, p. 754).
  4. A standing cough stress test is performed.
  5. The patient is placed in a lithotomy or supine position.
  6. A dual lumen catheter is inserted through the urethra and into the bladder.
  7. Residual urine volume is measured and recorded.
  8. Thermal sensation is evaluated by the instillation of approximately 30 mL of room-temperature saline solution into the bladder followed by an equal amount of warm water. The patient reports any sensations.
  9. This fluid is withdrawn from the bladder.
  10. The urethral catheter is connected to a cystometer to monitor bladder pressure. Sterile water, normal saline solution, or carbon dioxide gas is slowly introduced into the bladder at a controlled rate, usually with the patient in a sitting position. While the bladder is slowly filled, pressures are simultaneously recorded. This is called a cystometrogram.
  11. Patients are asked to indicate the first urge to void and then when they have the feeling that they must void. The bladder is full at this point.
  12. The pressures and volumes are plotted on a graph.
  13. ALPP to investigate for stress urinary incontinence are obtained by asking the patient to perform the Valsalva maneuver in gradients (i.e., mild, moderate, strong) followed by cough (i.e., mild, moderate, strong).

U

14. The patient is asked to void around the catheter, and the maximal intravesical voiding pressure is recorded.

15. The bladder is drained for any residual fluid or gas. If no additional studies are to be done, the urethral catheter is removed.

16. For urethral pressures, fluid or gas is instilled through the catheter, which is withdrawn while pressures along the urethral wall are obtained

- Note that pelvic floor sphincter electromyography (p. 290) can be performed to evaluate the urethral sphincter in cases of incontinence.

PT Throughout the study, ask the patient to report any sensations, such as pain, flushing, sweating, nausea, bladder filling, and an urgency to void.

- Note that certain drugs may be administered during the cystometric examination to distinguish between underactivity of the bladder because of muscle failure and underactivity associated with denervation. Cholinergic drugs (e.g., bethanechol) may be given to enhance the tone of a flaccid bladder. Anticholinergic drugs (e.g., atropine) may be given to promote relaxation of a hyperactive bladder. If these drugs are to be given, the catheter is left in place. After these drugs are given, the examination is repeated 20 to 30 minutes later using the first test as a control value. The information obtained with the drugs assists in deciding whether drugs will be effective treatment.

After

- Observe the patient for any manifestations of infection (e.g., elevated temperature, chills, or dysuria).
- Examine the urine for hematuria. Notify the physician if the hematuria persists after several voidings.
- Provide a warm sitz bath or tub bath for the patient's comfort if desired.

Abnormal findings

Bladder obstruction, infection, or hypertonicity
Diminished bladder capacity
Neurogenic bladder
Prostatic obstruction secondary to benign prostatic hypertrophy
    or cancer
Urinary incontinence

notes

uroporphyrinogen-1-synthase

Type of test Blood

Normal findings

1.27–2 mU/g of hemoglobin or 81.9–129.6 units/mol Hgb (SI units)

Test explanation and related physiology

Porphyria is a group of genetic disorders characterized by an accumulation of porphyrin products, usually in the liver. This group of disorders results from enzymatic deficiencies in synthesis of heme (a part of hemoglobin). Acute intermittent porphyria is the most common form of the liver porphyrias; it is caused by a deficiency in uroporphyrinogen-1-synthase (also called porphobilinogen deaminase). This enzyme is necessary for erythroid cells to make heme.

This enzyme is significantly reduced during the acute and latent phases of this disorder. It is important to identify this deficiency to prevent acute bouts of porphyria. See porphyrins and porphobilinogens on p. 587.

Procedure and patient care

- See inside front cover for Routine Blood Testing.
- Fasting: no
- Blood tube commonly used: purple
- Because this test is based on the hemoglobin measurement, concurrently obtain a hemoglobin level on the patient.
- Indicate on the laboratory slip if the patient is having symptoms of acute porphyria.

Abnormal findings

▼ Decreased levels
  Acute intermittent porphyria

notes

U

vanillylmandelic acid (VMA), homovanillic acid (HVA), and catecholamines (Epinephrine, Norepinephrine, Metanephrine, Normetanephrine, Dopamine)

Type of test Urine (24-hour)

Normal findings

VMA

Adult/elderly: < 6.8 mg/24 hr or < 35 µmol/24 hr (SI units)
Adolescent: 1–5 mg/24 hr
Child: 1–3 mg/24 hr
Infant: < 2 mg/24 hr
Newborn: < 1 mg/24 hr

HVA

≥15 years (adults): not applicable
10–14 years: < 12 mg/g creatinine
5–9 years: < 9 mg/g creatinine
2–4 years: < 13.5 mg/g creatinine
1 year: < 23 mg/g creatinine
< 1 year: 35 mg/g creatinine

Catecholamines

Free catecholamines
    < 100 mcg/24 hr or < 590 nmol/day (SI units)
Epinephrine
    Adult/elderly: < 20 mcg/24 hr or < 109 nmol/day (SI units)
    Child
        0–1 year: 0–2.5 mcg/24 hr
        1–2 years: 0–3.5 mcg/24 hr
        2–4 years: 0–6 mcg/24 hr
        4–7 years: 0.2–10 mcg/24 hr
        7–10 years: 0.5–14 mcg/24 hr
Norepinephrine
    Adult/elderly: <100 mcg/24 hr or <590 nmol/day (SI units)
    Child
        0–1 year: 0–10 mcg/24 hr
        1–2 years: 0–17 mcg/24 hr
        2–4 years: 4–29 mcg/24 hr
        4–7 years: 8–45 mcg/24 hr
        7–10 years: 13–65 mcg/24 hr
Dopamine
    Adult/elderly: 65–400 mcg/24 hr

Child
    0–1 year: 0–85 mcg/24 hr
    1–2 years: 10–140 mcg/24 hr
    2–4 years: 40–260 mcg/24 hr
    > 4 years: 65–400 mcg/24 hr
Metanephrine
    < 1.3 mg/24 hr or < 7 μmol/day (SI units)
Normetanephrine
    15–80 mcg/24 hr or 89–473 nmol/day (SI units)

Test explanation and related physiology

This 24-hour urine test is a screening test for the diagnosis of catecholamine-producing tumors such as neuroblastoma, pheochromocytoma, and other rare adrenal and neural crest tumors. Likewise, neural crest tumors such as neuroblastoma can also hypersecrete catecholamines. Dopamine is the precursor of epinephrine and norepinephrine. HVA is a metabolite of dopamine. Metanephrine and normetanephrine are catabolic products of epinephrine and norepinephrine, respectively. VMA (3-methoxy-4-hydroxymandelic acid) is the product of catabolism of both metanephrine and normetanephrine. In pheochromocytoma, one or all of these substances will be present in excessive quantities in a 24-hour urine collection. These hormones may be measured singularly in the urine, but the collective metabolic end products, HVA and VMA, are more easily detected because their concentrations are much higher than any one catecholamine component.

VMA and HVA are primarily used as a screening test for neural crest tumors. These urinary tests can also be used to monitor tumor activity. CT scanning or MRI is the preferred technique for localizing pheochromocytomas.

Interfering factors

- *Increased* levels of VMA may be caused by certain foods (e.g., tea, coffee, cocoa, vanilla, chocolate).
- Vigorous exercise, stress, and starvation may cause *increases.*
- Falsely *decreased* levels of VMA may be caused by uremia, alkaline urine, and radiographic iodine contrast agents.

Procedure and patient care

Before

PT Explain the procedure to the patient.
PT For 2 or 3 days before the 24-hour collection for VMA and throughout the collection, place the patient on a VMA-restricted diet. Generally, instruct the patient to avoid coffee,

V

tea, bananas, chocolate, cocoa, licorice, citrus fruit, all foods and fluids containing vanilla, and aspirin.

PT Inform the patient of the need to avoid taking antihypertensive medications, and sometimes all medications, during this period and possibly even longer.

During

PT See inside front cover for Routine Urine Testing.

• Collect the 24-hour urine specimen using a preservative.

After

• Send the specimen to the laboratory promptly.

• Allow the patient to have foods and drugs that were restricted in preparation for the test.

Abnormal findings

▲ **Increased levels**

Ganglioblastomas

Ganglioneuromas

Neuroblastomas

Pheochromocytomas

Severe stress/acute anxiety

Strenuous exercise

notes

venography of lower extremities (Phlebography, Venography)

Type of test X-ray with contrast

Normal findings

No evidence of venous thrombosis or obstruction

Test explanation and related physiology

Venography is an x-ray study designed to identify and locate thrombi within the veins of extremities and to assess the status of a vein prior to surgery or a bypass procedure. During this study, dye is injected into the venous system of the affected extremity. X-ray images are then taken at timed intervals to visualize the venous system. Obstruction to the flow of dye or a filling defect within the dye-filled vein indicates that thrombosis exists. A positive study accurately confirms the diagnosis of venous thrombosis; however, a normal study, although not as accurate, does make the diagnosis of venous thrombosis very unlikely. Venography is also used to identify venous stenosis caused by external obstruction or indwelling catheter-induced thrombosis.

Often both extremities are studied, even though only one leg is suspected of containing deep vein thrombosis. The normal extremity is used for comparison with the involved extremity. A venous ultrasound (p. 762) is more commonly done for evaluation of DVT.

Contraindications

- Patients with severe edema of the legs
- Patients who are uncooperative
- Patients who are allergic to iodinated contrast material
- Patients with renal failure

Potential complications

- Allergic reaction to intravenous contrast
- Renal failure, especially in elderly people who are chronically dehydrated or may have a mild degree of renal failure
- Subcutaneous dye infiltration, causing cellulitis and pain
- Venous thrombophlebitis caused by the contrast material
- Bacteremia caused by a break in a sterile technique
- Venous embolism caused by dislodgment of a deep vein clot induced by the contrast injection
- Lactic acidosis may occur in patients who are taking metformin and receiving contrast. The metformin should be held the day of the test to prevent this complication.

V

Procedure and patient care

Before

PT Explain the procedure to the patient. See p. xviii for radiation exposure and risks.

PT Obtain informed consent for this procedure.

• Assess the patient for allergies to iodinated contrast media.

• If needed, provide appropriate pain medication.

PT Ensure that the patient is appropriately hydrated before testing.

During

• Note the following procedural steps:
  1. The patient is taken to the radiology department and placed in a supine position on the x-ray table.
  2. Catheterization of a superficial vein on the foot is performed. This may require a surgical cutdown.
  3. An iodinated contrast material is injected into the vein.
  4. X-ray images are taken to follow the course of the contrast material up the leg.
  5. A tourniquet is frequently placed on the leg to prevent filling of the superficial saphenous vein. As a result, all of the dye goes toward filling the deep venous system, which contains the most clinically significant thrombosis that can embolize.

• Note that a radiologist performs this study in approximately 30 to 90 minutes.

PT The dye may cause the patient to feel a warm flush. Occasionally, mild degrees of nausea, vomiting, or skin itching also may occur.

After

• Continue appropriate hydration of the patient.

• Observe the puncture site for infection, cellulitis, or bleeding.

• Assess the patient's vital signs for signs of bacteremia.

Abnormal findings

Acute deep vein thrombosis
Obstructed venous systems

notes

virus testing (COVID-19, Cytomegalovirus, Epstein-Barr, Mononucleosis, Hepatitis, Herpes, HIV, Human papilloma, Human T-cell lymphotropic, Parvovirus, Rabies, Rubella, Rubeola, Varicella, Zika)

Type of test Microscopic, blood

Normal findings

Negative for viral antibody or antigen
No virus isolated in culture

Test explanation and related physiology

This test is used to diagnose active, chronic, and past viral diseases. It is also used to document successful treatment of and immunity to viral diseases. Testing for a virus is indicated when a person develops viral symptoms especially after suspected exposure to a particular virus.

Testing is also performed for epidemiologic reasons to identify a viral outbreak and its extent/origins. Finally, testing can indicate immunity after exposure to the virus or a vaccination.

Most viral infections have common symptoms that are flulike and include fever, lethargy, headache, and body aches. Respiratory viruses will additionally commonly cause a cough, runny nose, or shortness of breath. Gastrointestinal viruses may cause nausea, vomiting, or diarrhea. If a person shows signs of viral disease and has had a possible exposure, he or she should be isolated and supportive treatment should be initiated. After a definitive diagnosis is made, recent contacts should be identified, tested, and quarantined.

Definitive diagnoses of viral diseases can be made by:
- Nucleic acid amplification tests (NAAT-PCR) to identify nucleic acid particles
- Serologic tests identifying antibodies to a specific virus or other protein viral antigenic parts.
- Culture of the virus

Viral genetic material may stay in the body for up to 90 days and this testing is most accurate. It is considered the gold standard for many viruses. Test accuracy depends on viral load (generally measured by the quantity of viral nucleic acid in the specimen). Testing is performed in the laboratory and results may take several days. Rapid PCR testing to specific protein parts of the virus is available for many viral diseases and can be performed at home by the patient. Results are usually available in 15 minutes. These at-home tests are not as reliable as NAAT testing.

V

Viral testing is often performed as panel testing, for example, respiratory virus panel. This panel, typically performed on a nasopharyngeal swab, can detect multiple viruses/viral subtypes (e.g., COVID-19, influenza B, influenza A). Testing results can be obtained in 30 minutes.

When the virus is no longer present in great enough numbers in a patient's blood, nucleic acid testing methods will no longer be effective. The detection of antibodies can confirm exposure and infection. Serologic testing can identify IgM, IgG, or IgA antibodies to a virus several days to months after viral infection.

Growth and identification of the virus from a viral culture provides a definitive diagnosis when positive. Because viral load is always greatest in the early stages of the disease, cultures obtained in the first few days after symptoms begin offer the best chance of identifying the infective virus. Blood, sputum, tissue, and other body fluids are acceptable specimens to be tested. Viral cultures take 1 to 2 days to be reported.

COVID, Flu, RSV

COVID-19 (SARS-COV-2, Novel coronavirus 2), Influenza A and B, Respiratory Syncytial Virus (RSV), SARS coronavirus (SARS-CoV), and *MERS coronavirus (MERS-CoV)* are all contagious respiratory illnesses associated with malaise, fever, chills, cough, runny nose, aches and pains, and shortness of breath. Illness can progress to pneumonia and respiratory failure. Older people and those with underlying medical conditions or immunosuppression are more likely to develop serious illness. Infections are acquired by contact with body secretions. The *COVID-Flu panel nasal assay* is a real-time RT-PCR assay intended for the simultaneous qualitative detection and differentiation of nucleic acid from COVID-19, influenza A virus, and/or influenza B virus and is commonly used as first-line testing. Lower respiratory tract specimens also have high sensitivity. Although viral vaccinations can cause positive serologic antibody tests, they do not influence the results of PCR antigen or nucleic acid tests.

Cytomegalovirus (CMV)

CMV infections usually occur in the fetus, during early childhood, and in the young adult. Immunocompromised patients are at increased risk. Transplant patients, and AIDS patients are particularly susceptible. Infections are acquired by contact with body secretions or urine. Blood transfusions are a common form of spread for CMV. CMV is the most common congenital infection.

Pregnant mothers can get the disease during pregnancy, or a previous CMV infection can become reactivated. Approximately 10% of infected newborns exhibit permanent damage, usually mental retardation or auditory damage. Fetal infection can cause microcephaly, hydrocephaly, cerebral palsy, intellectual disability, or death. The term TORCH (p. 732) (toxoplasmosis, other, rubella, cytomegalovirus, herpes) (see p. 732) has been applied to infections with recognized detrimental effects on fetuses.

Nucleic acid detection is the standard for diagnosing CMV infection. Serology provides indirect evidence of recent or prior CMV infection. Testing is used to diagnose active disease and to monitor response to therapy. Conventional and rapid method (Shell) cultures from a variety of body fluids and tissue are most useful in the diagnosis of congenital CMV.

Epstein-Barr Virus (EBV)

EBV is a herpesvirus (human herpes virus 4) that affects 90% to 95% of adults worldwide. It is the primary cause of infectious mononucleosis and has a latency phase that persists for life in most adults. In some people, it is associated with the development of B-cell lymphomas, T-cell lymphomas, Burkitt lymphoma, Hodgkin lymphoma, and nasopharyngeal carcinomas. In symptomatic patients, EBV should be confirmed with a heterophile *antibody test* or through EBV-specific antibodies. EBV DNA can be detected in blood and throat swabs. The majority of EBV infections can be diagnosed by solely testing the patient's serum for heterophile antibodies (*rapid latex slide agglutination test* or *mononucleosis rapid test [monospot test]*). Detectable levels of the heterophile antibody can usually be expected to occur between the sixth and tenth day after the onset of symptoms.

EBV-specific antibodies can be used in a patient when the heterophile test is negative or when a complication of EBV is suspected. The following tests can more precisely define the acuity of the infection:

- Epstein-Barr viral capsid antigen (VCA)IgM - early in disease
- Epstein-Barr viral capsid antigen (VCA)IgG- mid phase, persists for life
- IgG antibodies to EBV nuclear antigen (EBNA) – mid phase, persists for life
- IgG antibodies to EBV early antigen (EA) – at onset of illness

Ebola Virus

Ebola virus disease (EVD) is a deadly disease that most commonly affects people from Africa. It is caused by an infection with a group of viruses called Ebolavirus. Ebola virus then spreads to other people through direct contact with body fluids of a person who is sick with or has died from EVD. Symptoms include fever, aches and pains, fatigue, diarrhea, and vomiting.

Diagnosis is made by testing body fluids for viral nucleic acids. An *Ebola Rapid Antigen Test* is also available. The ability to use this test to promptly make a diagnosis provides more rapid isolation and treatment that can be lifesaving.

Additionally, this test could be used on cadavers to support safe and dignified burials while helping to reduce the risk of transmission.

Hepatitis Virus

The most common types of hepatitis are hepatitis A, hepatitis B, and hepatitis C. Hepatitis D and hepatitis E viruses are much less common. Many people with hepatitis are asymptomatic. If symptoms occur with an acute infection, fever, malaise, loss of appetite, and abdominal pain are seen. Symptoms of chronic viral hepatitis can take decades to develop.

Hepatitis A virus (HAV) infection is usually a self-limited virus that does not become chronic. It is highly contagious. During active infection, HAV is excreted in the stool and transmitted via fecal–oral route by person-to-person contacts or by contamination of food and drink. The HAV virus can also be detected directly by measuring HAV RNA in the serum of patients suspected of acute infection. It can be detected earlier than HAV-Ab/IgM and is more sensitive in the early phase of HAV infection.

Hepatitis B virus (HBV) infection has a long incubation period of 1 to 6 months. Testing for HBV should be performed in people who have signs and symptoms of acute or chronic hepatitis.

It is also used in asymptomatic patients who are at high risk of HBV exposure or high risk of adverse outcomes from infection. This includes pregnant women and babies born to HBV-infected mothers, immunosuppressed patients, persons born in areas of high HBV prevalence, persons with HIV or hepatitis C virus, IV drug users, men who have sex with men, patients with end-stage renal disease, inmates of correctional facilities, and donors of blood, plasma, organ, tissue, or semen. HBV, also called the Dane particle, is made up of an inner core surrounded by an outer capsule. The outer capsule contains the hepatitis B surface antigen (HBsAg). The inner core contains HBV core antigen (HBcAg). The hepatitis B e-antigen (HBeAg) is also found in the core. Antibodies to these antigens are called HBsAb, HBcAb, and HBeAb. In addition to testing for serum antigens and antibodies of hepatitis B, tests for hepatitis B DNA have been developed to test for HBV replication/viral load. The major clinical role of serum HBV DNA assays in patients with chronic HBV infection is to determine candidacy for antiviral therapy.

Hepatitis C (HCV) infection causes a variety of nonspecific symptoms in most individuals. Untreated, up to 30% of patients with chronic HCV progress to cirrhosis and end-stage liver disease over the course of several decades. It is now recommended that individuals born between 1945 and 1965 (Baby Boomers) be tested for hepatitis C. Treatments are available that can cure hepatitis C.

Diagnostic tests for HCV include tests to detect antibodies for hepatitis C (HCV-Ab or anti-HCV) and tests to detect or quantify HCV RNA. Several rapid immunoassay tests are also available to test for HCV-Ab. These tests can be run on finger stick blood, serum, plasma, and oral fluid. Results are generally available in less than 30 minutes.

Hepatitis D virus (HDV or delta virus) is caused by a defective virus and requires the presence of HBV for infection.

Hepatitis E virus (HEV) is one of the most common causes, yet least diagnosed etiologies, of acute viral hepatitis. Transmission can occur through contaminated food and water, blood transfusions, and through mother-to-child transmission (perinatal).

Herpes Virus

Herpes virus *(Herpes simplex, HSV, Herpes genitalis)* can be classified as either type 1 or type 2. Type 1 is primarily responsible for oral lesions (blisters on the lips, or "cold sores") or even corneal lesions. HSV 2 is a sexually transmitted viral infection of the urogenital tract. It is important to know that this virus is not the causative agent of herpes zoster (see varicella virus, below). Because most infants become infected as they pass through a birth canal containing HSV, determining its presence at or before delivery is necessary. Congenital infections may result in problems such as microcephaly, chorioretinitis, and intellectual disability in the newborn. Disseminated neonatal herpes virus infections carry a high incidence of infant mortality.

If active genital lesions are present, culture of the fluid in the skin lesion is still the standard method to make the diagnosis. Serologic tests are more conveniently available for detection of HSV 1 and HSV 2 antibodies. HSV DNA PCR assays have emerged as a more sensitive method to confirm HSV infection

V

in clinical specimens obtained from genital ulcers, cerebrospinal fluid, and mucocutaneous sites. PCR differentiates HSV-1 and HSV-2.

Human Immunodeficiency Virus (HIV)

There are two active types of *human immunodeficiency viruses (HIV)*, types 1 and 2. Viral infection with HIV is the cause of *acquired immunodeficiency syndrome (AIDS)*. Immunoassay testing identifies antibodies developed as a result of HIV infections.

Nucleic acid tests identify RNA (or DNA) specific to HIV. Serologic screening tests for HIV include tests to detect HIV antigens or antibodies to HIV. Rapid HIV fingerstick screening produces results in less than 1 hour. HIV RNA qualitative testing is used to screen donor blood products. Insurance companies also commonly use it to exclude AIDS risks. Blood, oral fluids, urine, and other body fluids are adequate specimens for testing.

Persons known to be at increased risk of HIV infection include homosexual males, infants of HIV-positive mothers, IV drug abusers, persons involved in transactional sex, recipients of infected blood products, and women with an at-risk male partner or with multiple male partners.

See HIV drug resistance testing, (p. 416) and HIV RNA quantification (viral load), (p. 417).

Human Papilloma Virus (HPV)

A *HPV* test is performed to identify genital infection in a woman with an abnormal PAP smear (p. 547). Some strains of HPV cause condylomata genital warts and low-grade cervical changes, such as mild dysplasia. Some HPV infections produce no signs or symptoms. As a result, infected persons are frequently unaware that they are carriers, and transmission occurs unknowingly. High-risk strains are associated with intraepithelial neoplasia and are more likely to progress to severe lesions and cervical cancer. HPV is found in almost all cases of oral/pharyngeal malignancies worldwide.

HPV testing is typically included as a part of regular screening with a Pap test. HPV DNA screen with cytology triage (Pap/ThinPrep [p. 547]), if positive, is more accurate than conventional cervical cancer screening using Pap/ThinPrep alone. HPV is also the leading cause of oropharyngeal cancers.

HPV can be detected by testing for HPV viral DNA or by testing for specific viral proteins such as E6 and E7 oncogenes. HPV can be quantitated by HPV RNA testing and thereby more accurately indicate active disease. Appropriate testing specimens include cervical or oral fluids. HPV-induced tumors can also reveal the presence of HPV.

Human T-cell Lymphotropic Virus (HTLV)

Several forms of HTLV, a human retrovirus, affect humans. HTLV-I is associated with adult T-cell leukemia, lymphoma, myelopathy and uveitis. HTLV-II is associated with adult hairy-cell leukemia, lung, skin, and neurologic disorders.

HTLV transmission is similar to HIV transmission (e.g., body fluid contamination, intravenous drug use, sexual contact, breastfeeding).

Blood and organ donors are routinely tested for the presence of anti-HTLV-I/II protein antibodies. HTLV-I/II viral DNA is also available but less commonly used.

Monkey Pox Virus

Monkeypox (Mpox) is a viral illness caused by the monkeypox virus, a species of Orthopoxvirus. Common symptoms of mpox are a skin rash, mucosal lesions, fever, headache, muscle aches, back pain, low energy, and swollen lymph nodes. Mpox is transmitted to humans through physical contact with someone who is infected.

Detection of viral DNA is the preferred laboratory test for mpox. The best diagnostic specimens are taken directly from the rash. In the absence of skin lesions, testing can be done on oropharyngeal, anal, or rectal swabs. Testing blood for antibodies is not useful because this does not distinguish between different orthopoxviruses.

Parvovirus B19 Virus

Many of the severe manifestations of *Parvovirus B19* relate to the ability of the virus to infect and lyse RBC precursors in the bone marrow. *Erythema infectiosum* is the most common manifestation of parvovirus B19 infection and occurs predominantly in children.

This pathogen is also referred to as fifth disease or academy rash. Serologic testing for parvovirus B19-specific antibodies is done. Fetal infection may be recognized by hydrops fetalis and the presence of B19 DNA in amniotic fluid or fetal blood.

Rabies Virus

Identification and documentation of the presence of *rabies virus-neutralizing antibody* are important for veterinary healthcare workers and others who may be or may have been exposed to the rabies virus. This test may be performed on patients who are at

V

great risk for animal bites and have received the human diploid cell rabies vaccine. The rabies virus antibody test is also used in making the diagnosis of rabies in a patient suspected of having been exposed to the virus. PCR testing for nucleic acid is also available for skin biopsy, saliva, and CSF testing.

Rubella Virus

Screening for *rubella antibodies* is done to detect immunity to rubella. These tests detect the presence antibodies to rubella (the causative agent for *German measles*). These antibodies become elevated in patients with active rubella infection or with past infections. Children are vaccinated for rubella to prevent the effects of the disease and to minimize infection. Rubella testing documents immunity to rubella. Rubella immunity testing is suggested for all healthcare workers. Most importantly, however, it is done to verify the presence or absence of rubella immunity in pregnant women because congenital rubella infection in the first trimester of pregnancy is associated with congenital abnormalities of the fetus (heart defects, brain damage, deafness), abortion, or stillbirth. The term TORCH [p. 732] (toxoplasmosis, other, rubella, cytomegalovirus, herpes) has been applied to infections with recognized detrimental effects on the fetus.

Antirubella antibody testing is also used to diagnose rubella in infants (congenital rubella). Antibody testing is often used in children with congenital abnormalities that may have come from congenital rubella infection. Congenital infection may be confirmed by viral isolation from nasopharyngeal secretions and urine of the newborn. Rubella RNA can be detected in amniotic fluid, from the cord blood, or the placenta.

Rubeola Virus

The Rubeola *measles virus* is an RNA *paramyxovirus* and is not the same virus that causes the German measles; see rubella, above. Although it is most usually a self-limiting disease, the virus can easily be spread (by respiratory droplets) to nonimmune pregnant women and cause preterm delivery or spontaneous abortion. Testing for measles virus includes serologic identification of *measles rubeola antibodies.*

This test is used to diagnose measles in patients with a rash or viral syndrome when the diagnosis cannot be made clinically. Even more important, however, this test is used to establish and document immunity by previous measles infection or by previous vaccination. Populations commonly tested to document immunity include college students, health care workers, and pregnant women.

Varicella Virus

Varicella zoster virus (VZV) is a herpes virus that can cause acute, recurrent, or latent infection. Primary acute infection with VZV results in *chickenpox. Shingles* occurs when the virus becomes active again. Testing for VZV or the antibodies produced in response to VZV is not routinely used to diagnose active cases of chickenpox and shingles. It may be performed in pregnant women, newborns, in people before organ transplantation, and in those with HIV/AIDS. Testing may also be used to determine if someone has been previously exposed to VZV either through past infection or vaccination and has developed immunity to the disease. It can distinguish between an active or prior infection. It can determine whether someone with severe or atypical symptoms has an active VZV infection or has another condition with similar symptoms. The most frequent source of VZV viral DNA isolation is vesicular fluid. Serum is used for antibody testing.

Zika Virus

The Zika virus is transmitted to humans by an infected mosquito. Sexual transmission among humans has also been described. This testing is used to identify Zika infections in people who have symptoms of the infection and live in or who have traveled to an area where Zika is known to exist. In most cases, Zika virus infection causes a mild, self-limited illness including a rash, fever, arthralgia, headache, or conjunctivitis. Although Zika virus infection is generally well tolerated, infection in pregnant women can lead to microcephaly and other neurologic defects in fetuses.

Diagnosis of Zika virus infection is typically based on serologic tests that identify antibodies to Zika in the urine, serum, and CSF. Zika viral RNA can also be identified.

Interfering factors

- An inadequate specimen, the timing, or the choice of culture medium will cause false-negative test results.
- The use of a cotton swab or wooden applicator for specimen collection may destroy the virus.
- Antibody testing can cross react with other similar viruses causing false-positive results.
- False-negative results can occur in the early incubation stage or end-stage of infection.
- Immunosuppressed patients may have false-negative antibody tests.

V

Procedure and patient care

Before

- Fasting: no
- PT Explain the method of collection of the specimen.
- Obtain a history regarding the timing of symptoms.
- Maintain proper infection control and use recommended PPE.
- Tell women to refrain from intercourse, douching and tub bathing before the cervical swab is performed.
- Obtain an informed consent if required by the institution for all "opt-in" testing.
- If the patient wishes to remain anonymous, use a number with the patient's name; be sure to record it accurately.
- Accurately record the source of the specimen.

During

- Use a closed specimen system to obtain and transport the specimen to the laboratory.
- Transport the specimen immediately to the laboratory. Viruses in specimens quickly lose their vitality.
- Small-volume specimens such as tissue aspirates are often best transported in viral transport medium.
- To obtain a nasopharyngeal or oropharyngeal swab, use only sterile synthetic fiber swabs with plastic shafts. Insert the swab into the nostril or oropharynx until at desired location. Gently rub and roll the swab and leave it in place for a few seconds to absorb secretions before gently removing.
- To obtain saliva specimen, collect 1 to 5 mL into a sterile, leakproof container.
- To obtain a specimen from the skin, start by unroofing a vesicle, preferably a fresh fluid-filled vesicle, and then rubbing the base of a skin lesion with a polyester swab.
- For blood, collect whole blood in a serum separator tube.

After

- PT Explain that the patient may still be infectious and should continue to quarantine.
- Provide supportive care for symptoms.
- PT Explain to the patient and family when testing results will be available and how to obtain those results.

Abnormal findings

Viral infectious disease

vitamin B$_{12}$ (Cyanocobalamin and methylmalonic acid [MMA])

Type of test Blood; urine

Normal findings

Vitamin B$_{12}$: 160–950 pg/mL or 118–701 pmol/L (SI units)
MMA: < 3.6 µmol/mmol creatinine

Test explanation and related physiology

Vitamin B$_{12}$ is necessary for conversion of the inactive form of folate to the active form. This function is most notable in the formation and function of RBCs. Vitamin B$_{12}$ deficiency, like folic acid deficiency, causes anemia. The RBCs formed in light of these deficiencies consist of large megaloblastic RBCs. These RBCs cannot conform to the size of small capillaries. Instead, they fracture and hemolyze. The shortened life span ultimately leads to anemia.

In the stomach, gastric acid detaches vitamin B$_{12}$ from its binding proteins. Intrinsic factor (IF), which is necessary for vitamin B$_{12}$ absorption in the terminal ileum, is made in the stomach mucosa. Without IF, vitamin B$_{12}$ cannot be absorbed. Deficiency of IF is the most common cause of vitamin B$_{12}$ deficiency (pernicious anemia). The next most common cause of vitamin B$_{12}$ deficiency is lack of gastric acid to separate the ingested vitamin B$_{12}$ from its binding proteins. This is common in patients who have had gastric surgery. A third cause of vitamin B$_{12}$ deficiency is malabsorption caused by diseases of the small terminal ileum. Vitamin B$_{12}$ deficiency is common in poorly nourished elderly people and in vegetarians.

Serum B$_{12}$ is a measurement of recent B$_{12}$ ingestion. More prolonged B$_{12}$ deficiency is measured by *urinary methylmalonic acid (MMA)* measurement. Elevated serum MMA levels and urinary excretion of MMA are direct measures of tissue vitamin B$_{12}$ activity. The active form of B$_{12}$ is essential in the intracellular conversion of L-methylmalonyl coenzyme A (MMA CoA) to succinyl CoA. Without B$_{12}$, MMA CoA metabolism is diverted to make large quantities of MMA. MMA is then excreted by the kidneys. MMA testing is the most sensitive test for B$_{12}$ deficiency.

Higher plasma concentrations of vitamin B$_{12}$ have been associated with increased mortality especially in patients with chronic kidney disease.

Procedure and patient care

• See inside front cover for Routine Blood Testing.

V

- Fasting: verify with laboratory
- Blood tube commonly used: red
- PT Instruct the patient not to consume alcoholic beverages before the test. Check the time period with the physician or laboratory.
- Draw the specimen before starting vitamin B$_{12}$ therapy.

Abnormal findings

▲ **Increased levels**

Leukemia
Myeloproliferative disease
Polycythemia vera
Severe liver dysfunction

▼ **Decreased levels**

Achlorhydria
Atrophic gastritis
Folic acid deficiency
Inflammatory bowel disease
Intestinal worm infestation
Large proximal gastrectomy
Malabsorption syndromes
Pernicious anemia
Pregnancy
Resection of terminal ileum
Vitamin C deficiency
Zollinger-Ellison syndrome

notes

vitamin D (25-hydroxy vitamin D$_2$ and D$_3$; 1,25-dihydroxyvitamin D [1,25(OH)$_2$D])

Type of test   Blood

Normal findings

Total 25-hydroxy D (D$_2$ + D$_3$): 25–80 ng/mL
1,25(OH)$_2$D
    Males: 18–64 pg/mL
    Females: 18–78 pg/mL

Test explanation and related physiology

Vitamin D levels are calculated to ensure that postmenopausal women have adequate vitamin D levels to absorb dietary calcium. Because test results for vitamin D are quite variable and the benefits of vitamin D supplementation questionable, the role of this test is controversial. The two major forms of vitamin D are vitamin D$_2$ (or ergocalciferol) and vitamin D$_3$ (or cholecalciferol).

Vitamin D$_3$ is produced in skin exposed to sunlight, specifically ultraviolet B (UVB) radiation. After vitamin D is produced in the skin or consumed in food, it is converted in the liver and kidney to form 1,25-dihydroxy- vitamin D (1,25[OH]$_2$D). This is the chemical that is measured in vitamin D testing. Vitamin D regulates the calcium and phosphorus levels in the blood by promoting their absorption from food in the intestines and by promoting reabsorption of calcium in the kidneys. This enables normal mineralization of bone needed for bone growth and bone remodeling.

Procedure and patient care

- See inside front cover for Routine Blood Testing.
- Fasting: no
- Blood tube commonly used: red or green
- PT If the patient has a vitamin D deficiency, educate him or her about dietary sources and the need for sunlight.

V

Abnormal findings

▲ **Increased levels**

Excess dietary supplements
Williams syndrome

▼ **Decreased levels**

Acute inflammatory disease
Familial hypophosphatemic
    rickets
Gastrointestinal
    malabsorption syndromes
Inadequate dietary intake
Inadequate exposure to
    sunlight
Liver disease
Osteomalacia
Osteoporosis
Renal failure
Rickets

notes

white blood cell count and differential count (WBC and differential, Leukocyte count)

Type of test Blood

Normal findings

Total WBCs

Adult/child > 2 years: 5000–10,000/mm³ or 5–10 × 10⁹/L (SI units)

Child ≤ 2 years: 6200–17,000/mm³

Newborn: 9000–30,000/mm³

Differential count	%	Absolute (per mm³)
Neutrophils	55–70	2500–8000
Lymphocytes	20–40	1000–4000
Monocytes	2–8	100–700
Eosinophils	1–4	50–500
Basophils	0.5–1	25–100

Possible critical values

WBC count < 2500 or > 30,000/mm³

Test explanation and related physiology

The WBC count has two components. The first is a count of the total number of WBCs (leukocytes) in 1 mm³ of peripheral venous blood. The other component, the differential count, measures the percentage of each type of leukocyte present in the same specimen. Neutrophils and lymphocytes make up 75% to 90% of the total leukocytes. The total leukocyte count has a wide range of normal values, but many diseases may induce abnormal values.

An increased total WBC count (leukocytosis: WBC count > 10,000/mm³) usually indicates infection, inflammation, tissue necrosis, or leukemic neoplasia. Trauma or stress may increase the WBC count. A decreased total WBC count (leukopenia: WBC count < 4000/mm³) occurs in many forms of bone marrow failure (e.g., after antineoplastic chemotherapy or radiation therapy, marrow infiltrative diseases, overwhelming infections, dietary deficiencies, and autoimmune diseases).

The major function of the WBCs is to fight infection and react against foreign bodies or tissues. Five types of WBCs may easily be identified on a routine blood smear (p. 128). These cells,

W

in order of frequency, include neutrophils, lymphocytes, monocytes, eosinophils, and basophils.

WBCs are divided into granulocytes and nongranulocytes. Granulocytes include neutrophils, basophils, and eosinophils.

Neutrophils, the most common granulocyte, are produced in 7 to 14 days, and exist in the circulation for only 6 hours. The primary function of the neutrophil is phagocytosis (killing and digestion of bacterial microorganisms). Acute bacterial infections and trauma stimulate neutrophil production, resulting in an increased WBC count. Often when neutrophil production is significantly stimulated, early immature forms of neutrophils enter the circulation. These immature forms are called *band* or *stab* cells. This occurrence, referred to as a *shift to the left* in WBC production, is indicative of an ongoing acute bacterial infection. Neutrophils have multilobed nuclei and are sometimes referred to as polymorphonuclear leukocytes (PMNs or *polys*). The normal ranges for absolute counts depend on age, sex, and ethnicity.

Basophils (also called mast cells) and *eosinophils* are involved in the allergic reaction. Parasitic infestations also stimulate production of these cells. These cells are capable of phagocytosis of antigen–antibody complexes. As the allergic response diminishes, the eosinophil count decreases. Eosinophils and basophils do not respond to bacterial or viral infections.

Nongranulocytes (mononuclear cells) include lymphocytes, monocytes, and histiocytes. *Lymphocytes* are divided into two types: T-cells and B-cells. Whereas T-cells are primarily involved with cellular-type immune reactions, B-cells participate in humoral immunity (antibody production). The primary function of the lymphocytes is fighting chronic bacterial and acute viral infections. The differential count does not separate the T- and B-cells but rather counts the combination of the two.

Monocytes are phagocytic cells capable of fighting bacteria in a way very similar to that of neutrophils. However, monocytes can be produced more rapidly and can spend a longer time in the circulation than neutrophils.

The WBC count and differential counts are routinely measured as part of the complete blood count (p. 228). Serial WBC counts and differential counts have both diagnostic and prognostic value. For example, a persistent increase in the WBC count (particularly the neutrophils) may indicate a worsening of an infectious process (e.g., appendicitis). A dramatic decrease in the WBC count below the normal range may indicate marrow failure. In patients receiving chemotherapy, a reduced WBC count may delay further chemotherapy.

The absolute count is calculated by multiplying the differential count (%) by the total WBC count. For example, the *absolute neutrophil count (ANC)* is helpful in determining the patient's risk for infection. It is calculated by multiplying the WBC count by the percent of neutrophils and percent of bands; that is,

$$ANC = WBC \times (\% \text{ neutrophils} + \% \text{ bands})$$

If the ANC is less than 1000, the patient may need to be placed in protective isolation because he or she could be severely immunocompromised and at great risk for infection.

Interfering factors

- Physical activity and stress may cause an increase in WBC and differential values.
- Pregnancy and labor may cause increased WBC levels.
- Patients who have had a splenectomy have a persistent, mild elevation of WBC counts.

Procedure and patient care

- See inside front cover for Routine Blood Testing.
- Fasting: no
- Blood tube commonly used: lavender

Abnormal findings

▲ **Increased WBC count (leukocytosis)**

Infection
Inflammation
Leukemic neoplasia
Stress
Tissue necrosis
Trauma

▼ **Decreased WBC count (leukopenia)**

Autoimmune disease
Bone marrow failure
Bone marrow infiltration
  (e.g., myelofibrosis)
Congenital marrow aplasia
Dietary deficiency
Drug toxicity
Overwhelming infections

▲ ▼ **Increased/decreased differential count**

See Table W1.

W

TABLE W1 Causes of abnormalities in white blood cell (WBC) and differential counts

Type of WBC	Increased	Decreased
Basophils	*Basophilia* Leukemia Myeloproliferative disease (e.g., myelofibrosis, polycythemia rubra vera) Uremia	*Basopenia* Acute allergic reactions Hyperthyroidism Stress reaction
Eosinophils	*Eosinophilia* Allergic reactions Autoimmune diseases Eczema Leukemia Parasitic infections	*Eosinopenia* Increased adrenosteroid production
Lymphocytes	*Lymphocytosis* Chronic bacterial infection Infectious hepatitis Infectious mononucleosis Lymphocytic leukemia Multiple myeloma Radiation Viral infection (e.g., mumps, rubella)	*Lymphocytopenia* Drug therapy: adrenocorticosteroids, antineoplastics Immunodeficiency diseases Later stages of HIV infection Leukemia Radiation therapy Sepsis Systemic lupus erythematosus
Monocytes	*Monocytosis* Chronic inflammatory disorders Chronic ulcerative colitis Parasites (e.g., malaria) Tuberculosis Viral infections (e.g., infectious mononucleosis)	*Monocytopenia* Aplastic anemia Drug therapy: prednisone Hairy-cell leukemia

TABLE W1   Causes of abnormalities in white blood cell (WBC) and differential counts—cont'd

Type of WBC	Increased	Decreased
Neutrophils	*Neutrophilia* Acute suppurative infection Cushing syndrome Inflammatory disorders (e.g., rheumatic fever, thyroiditis, rheumatoid arthritis) Metabolic disorders (e.g., ketoacidosis, gout, eclampsia) Myelocytic leukemia Physical or emotional stress Trauma	*Neutropenia* Addison disease Aplastic anemia Dietary deficiency Drug therapy: myelotoxic drugs (i.e., chemotherapy) Overwhelming bacterial infection (especially in elderly patients) Radiation therapy Viral infections (e.g., hepatitis, influenza, measles)

notes

W

white blood cell scan (WBC scan, Inflammatory scan)

Type of test Nuclear scan

Normal findings

No signs of WBC localization outside the liver or spleen

Test explanation and related physiology

This test is based on the fact that WBCs are attracted to an area of infection or inflammation. When a patient is suspected of having had infection or inflammation yet the site cannot be localized, the injection of radiolabeled WBCs may identify and localize the area of inflammation or infection. This is especially helpful in patients who have a fever of unknown origin, suspected occult intraabdominal infection, or suspected (yet radiographically inapparent) osteomyelitis. The scan can differentiate infectious from noninfectious processes. For example, it is used to indicate whether an abnormal mass (e.g., a pancreatic pseudocyst) is infected. Areas of noninfectious inflammation (e.g., inflammatory bowel disease) also take up radiolabeled WBCs.

This scan requires drawing blood from the patient, separating out the WBCs, labeling the WBCs with technetium or indium, and reinjecting them back into the patient. Imaging of the whole body 4 to 24 hours later may show an area of increased radioactivity suggestive of accumulation of the radiolabeled WBCs in an area of infection or inflammation.

Procedure and patient care

Before

PT Explain the procedure to the patient. See p. xviii for radiation exposure and risks.

PT Assure the patient that he or she will not be exposed to large amounts of radioactivity because only tracer doses of the isotope are used.

PT Tell the patient that no preparation or sedation is required.

During

- Note the following procedural steps:
  1. Approximately 40 to 50 mL of blood is withdrawn from the patient, and the WBCs are extracted from the rest of the blood cells. The WBCs are suspended in saline and tagged with ^{99m}technetium (^{99m}Tc) or ^{111}indium (^{111}In) lipid-soluble product.
  2. The tagged WBCs are reinjected into the patient.

3. At 4, 24, and 48 hours after injection, a gamma ray detector/camera is placed over the body.
4. The patient is placed in supine, lateral, and prone positions so that all surfaces of the body can be visualized.
5. The radionuclide image is recorded on film.

After

PT Inform the patient that because only tracer doses of radioisotopes are used, no precautions need to be taken against radioactive exposure.

Abnormal findings

- Infection (e.g., abscess or osteomyelitis)
- Inflammation (e.g., inflammatory bowel disease, arthritis)

notes

W

D-**xylose absorption test** (Xylose tolerance test)

Type of test Blood; urine
Normal findings

Age	60-min plasma (mg/dL)	120-min plasma (mg/dL)	Urine (g/5 hr) [%]
Adult	20–57	30–58	>3.5–4 [>14]
Child	>15–20	>20	>4 [16–32]

Test explanation and related physiology

D-Xylose is a monosaccharide that is easily absorbed by the normal intestine. In patients with malabsorption, intestinal D-xylose absorption is diminished; as a result, blood levels and urine excretion are reduced. D-Xylose is not metabolized by the body. Its serum levels directly reflect intestinal absorption.

D-Xylose does not require pancreatic or biliary exocrine function. Its absorption is directly determined by the small intestine. This test is used to separate patients with diarrhea caused by maldigestion (pancreatic or biliary dysfunction) from those with diarrhea caused by malabsorption (sprue, Whipple disease, Crohn disease).

In this test, the patient is asked to drink a fluid containing a prescribed amount of D-xylose. Blood and urine levels are subsequently evaluated. Excellent gastrointestinal absorption is documented by high blood levels and good urine secretion of D-xylose. Poor intestinal absorption is marked by decreased blood levels and urine excretion.

Contraindications

- Patients with abnormal kidney function
- Patients who are dehydrated

Procedure and patient care

Before

PT Explain the procedure to the patient.
PT Instruct the adult patient to fast for 8 hours before testing.
PT Tell the pediatric patient or the parents that the patient should fast for at least 4 hours before testing.

During

- Collect a venous blood sample in a red-top tube before the patient ingests the D-xylose.
- Collect a first-voided morning urine specimen and send it to the laboratory.
- Ask the patient to drink the prescribed dose of D-xylose dissolved in 8 oz of water. Record the time of ingestion.
- Calibrate pediatric doses according to body weight.
- Repeat venipunctures to obtain blood in exactly 2 hours for an adult and 1 hour for a child.
- Collect urine for a designated time, usually 5 hours. Refrigerate the urine during the collection period.
- Observe the patient for nausea, vomiting, and diarrhea, which may occur as side effects of D-xylose.
- **PT** Instruct the patient to remain in a restful position. Intense physical activity may alter digestion and affect results.

After

- Apply pressure to the venipuncture site.
- **PT** Inform the patient that normal activity may be resumed after completion of the study.

Abnormal findings

▼ **Decreased levels**

Crohn disease
Enteropathy (e.g., radiation)
Giardia lamblia infestation
Hookworm
Lymphatic obstruction
Short-bowel syndrome
Small intestine bacterial overgrowth
Sprue
Viral gastroenteritis
Whipple disease

notes

X

zinc protoporphyrin (ZPP)

Type of test Blood

Normal findings

0–69 µmol/mol (mcg/dL)

Test explanation and related physiology

ZPP is sometimes used to evaluate iron deficiency anemia or lead poisoning. ZPP is found in red blood cells when heme production is inhibited by lead toxicity. Lead prevents iron, but not zinc, from attaching to the protoporphyrin. If there is iron deficiency, instead of incorporating a ferrous ion to form heme, protoporphyrin (the immediate precursor of heme) incorporates a zinc ion, forming ZPP. In addition to lead poisoning and iron deficiency, zinc protoporphyrin levels can be elevated as the result of a number of other conditions (e.g., sickle cell anemia).

Procedure and patient care

- See inside front cover for Routine Blood Testing.
- Fasting: yes (12 hours)
- Blood tube commonly used: verify with laboratory.

Abnormal findings

▲ **Increased levels**

   Anemia of chronic illness
   Hemodialysis
   Iron deficiency
   Lead poisoning
   Sickle cell anemia
   Sideroblastic anemia
   Vanadium exposure

notes

appendix A: list of tests by body system

Tests in this list are grouped by the following: cancer studies; cardiovascular, endocrine, gastrointestinal, hematologic, hepato-biliary, and immunologic systems; miscellaneous studies; and nervous, pulmonary, renal/urologic, reproductive, and skeletal systems.

CANCER STUDIES

Bence Jones protein, 112
Beta$_2$-microglobulin, 513
Bladder cancer markers, 122
Bone scan, 144
Breast cancer genetic testing, 369
Breast cancer genomics, 378
Breast cancer tumor analysis, 746
CA 15-3 and CA 27.29 tumor markers, 165
CA 19-9 tumor marker, 165
CA-125 tumor marker, 164, 165
Carcinoembryonic antigen, 165
Cathepsin D, 746
Cervical biopsy, 189
Colon cancer genetic testing, 369
Colo-rectal cancer tumor analysis, 221
Des gamma carboxy prothrombin, 165
DNA ploidy status, 746
Early prostate cancer antigen, 611
Estrogen receptor assay, 319
Gallium scan, 359

HER 2 protein, 746
Ki67 protein, 746
Liquid biopsy, 466
Mammography, 497
Melanoma genetic testing, 369
Microglobulin, 513
Neuron-specific enolase, 521
Octreotide scan, 531
Ovarian cancer genetic testing, 369
p53 protein, 746
Papanicolaou smear, 547
Progesterone receptor assay, 608
Prostate-specific antigen, 611
Salivary gland nuclear imaging, 651
Serotonin, 655
S-phase fraction, 746
Sputum cytology, 684
Thyroid cancer genetic testing, 369
Thyroid cancer genomic testing, 377
Thyroid fine-needle aspiration biopsy, 718
Tumor analysis, 746
Tumor markers, 164

CARDIOVASCULAR SYSTEM

Adenosine stress test, 176
Aldosterone, 19
Adiponectin, 5

Antimyocardial antibody, 67
Antistreptolysin O titer, 691
Apolipoproteins, 462

ENDOCRINE SYSTEM

GASTROINTESTINAL SYSTEM

HEMATOLOGIC SYSTEM

HEPATOBILIARY SYSTEM

IMMUNOLOGIC SYSTEM

MISCELLANEOUS STUDIES

list of tests by body system

NERVOUS SYSTEM

PULMONARY SYSTEM

RENAL/UROLOGIC SYSTEM

REPRODUCTIVE SYSTEM

SKELETAL SYSTEM

appendix B: list of tests by type

Tests in this list are grouped by the following types: blood, electrodiagnostic, endoscopy, fluid analysis, manometric, microscopic examinations, nuclear scans, other studies, sputum, stool, ultrasound, urine, and x-ray.

BLOOD TESTS

ELECTRODIAGNOSTIC TESTS

ENDOSCOPY

list of tests by type

FLUID ANALYSIS

MANOMETRIC TESTS

MICROBIOLOGIC EXAMINATIONS

NUCLEAR SCANS

OTHER STUDIES

SPUTUM TESTS

STOOL TESTS

ULTRASOUND TESTS

URINE TESTS

Adrenocorticotropic hormone stimulation test with metyrapone, 13
Albumin-creatinine ratio, 511
Aldosterone, 19
Amino acid profiles, 35
Amylase, 44
Appearance and color, 773
Bence Jones protein, 112
Beta$_2$-microglobulin, 513
11 Beta-prostaglandin F(2) alpha, 513
Bladder cancer markers, 122
Bone turnover markers, 146
Calcium, 159
Cortisol, 241
COVID-19 testing, 795
Creatinine clearance, 251
Crystals, 776
Culture and sensitivity, 783
Delta-aminolevulinic acid, 266
Dexamethasone suppression test, 268
Epithelial casts, 776
Estimated glomerular filtration rate, 251
Estriol excretion, 317
Estrogen fractions, 317
Ethanol, 320
Fatty casts, 776
Flow studies, 785
Fluorescence hybridization, 545
Fractional excretion of sodium, 678
Glucose, 774
Glucose tolerance test, 392
Granular casts, 776
HIV urine testing, 800
Hyaline casts, 776
17-Hydroxycorticosteroids, 430

5-Hydroxyindoleacetic acid, 431
Ketones, 775
17-Ketosteroids, 703
Kidney stone analysis, 450
Leucine aminopeptidase, 459
Leukocyte esterase, 774
Liquid biopsy, 466
Metyrapone test, 13
Microalbumin, 511
Nicotine and metabolites, 525
N-telopeptide, 146
Nitrites, 775
Odor, 773
Osmolality, 535
Pepsinogen, 559
pH, 773
Phenylketonuria test, 523
Porphyrins and porphobilinogens, 587
Potassium, 597
Prealbumin, 598
Pregnancy tests, 425
Pregnanediol, 601
Protein, 613
Pyridinium, 146
Red blood cells and casts, 776
Sodium, 678
Specific gravity, 774
Substance abuse testing, 693
Toxicology screening, 693
Tubular casts, 776
Uric acid, 769
Urinalysis, 772
Urinary methylmalonic acid, 805
Urine culture and sensitivity, 783
Vanillylmandelic acid and catecholamines, 790
Viral cultures, 796

list of tests by type

appendix C: disease and organ panels

This appendix includes groupings of tests commonly used either for screening or to evaluate disease situations. These panels may be modified or expanded in different clinical settings.

Anemia

Complete blood count (CBC), 228
Macrocytic anemia
  Folate, 352
  TSH, 716
  Vitamin B$_{12}$, 805
Microcytic anemia
  Reticulocyte index, 646
  Iron panel, 445
Normocytic anemia
  Reticulocyte index, 646
  Hemolysis profile, 237
Red blood cell (RBC) indices, 633
Reticulocyte count, 646

Arthritis

Antinuclear antibody (ANA), 70
C-reactive protein, 245
ESR (sedimentation rate), 306
Rheumatoid factor, 648
Uric acid, 769

Basic metabolic panel (BMP)

Blood urea nitrogen (BUN), 134
Calcium, 159
Carbon dioxide, 167
Chloride, 196
Creatinine, 249
Glucose, 386
Potassium, 595
Sodium, 676

Bone/joint

Albumin, 613
Alkaline phosphatase, 23
Calcium, 159
Osteocalcin, 146
Phosphorus, 564
Protein, total, 613
Uric acid, 769

Cardiac injury

Creatine kinase (CK), 247
CK-MB, 247
Myoglobin, 518
Troponin I, 741

Coagulation screening

Partial thromboplastin time (PTT), 557
Platelet count, 577
Prothrombin time (PT), 619

Coma

Alcohol, 320
Ammonia, 37
Anion gap, 50
Arterial blood gases, 89
Basic metabolic panel (BMP), 111
Calcium (total and ionized), 159
Ethyl alcohol, 320
Lactic acid, 452
Osmolality (serum), 533
Salicylate, 278
Toxicology screen, 693

appendix D: symbols and units of measurement

<	less than
≤	less than or equal to
>	greater than
≥	greater than or equal to
c (prefix)	centi (10^{-2})
C	celsius
cc	cubic centimeter
cg	centigram
cm	centimeter
cm H_2O	centimeter of water
cu	cubic
d (prefix)	deci (10^{-1})
dL	deciliter (100 mL)
f (prefix)	femto (10^{-15})
fL	femtoliter
fmol	femtomole
g	gram
hr	hour
IU	international unit
ImU	international milliunit
IμU	international microunit
k (prefix)	kilo (10^3)
kat	katal
kg	kilogram (1000 grams)
L	liter
m (prefix)	milli (10^{-3})
m	meter
m^2	square meter
m^3	cubic meter
mcg	microgram
mEq	milliequivalent
mEq/L	milliequivalent per liter
mg	milligram (1/1000 gram)
min	minute
mL	milliliter
mm	millimeter (1/10 centimeter)
mm^3	cubic millimeter
mM	millimole
mm Hg	millimeter of mercury
mm H_2O	millimeter of water

mmol	millimole
mol	mole
mOsm	milliosmole
mμ	millimicron
mU	milliunit
mV	millivolt
μ (prefix)	micro (10^{-6})
$μ^3$	cubic micron
μkat	microkatal
μL	microliter
μm	micrometer
$μm^3$	cubic micrometer
μmol	micromole
μU	microunit
n (prefix)	nano (10^{-9})
ng	nanogram
nkat	nanokatal
nm	nanometer
nmol	nanomole
p (prefix)	pico (10^{-12})
Pa	pascal
pg	picogram
pL	picoliter
pm	picometer
pmol	picomole
sec	second
SI units	International System of Units
U	unit
yr	year

Index

abbreviations for diagnostic and laboratory tests

A	AAT	Alpha$_1$-antitrypsin
	ABGs	Arterial blood gases
	ACE	Angiotensin-converting enzyme
	ACT	Activated clotting time
	ACTH	Adrenocorticotropic hormone
	ADH	Antidiuretic hormone
	AFB	Acid-fast bacilli
	AFP	Alpha-fetoprotein
	A/G ratio	Albumin/globulin ratio
	AIT	Agglutination inhibition test
	ALA	Aminolevulinic acid
	ALP	Alkaline phosphatase
	ALT	Alanine aminotransferase
	AMA	Antimitochondrial antibody
	ANA	Antinuclear antibody
	ANCA	Antineutrophil cytoplasmic antibody
	ANP	Atrial natriuretic peptide
	APCA	Antiparietal cell antibody
	APTT	Activated partial thromboplastin time
	ASMA	Antismooth muscle antibody
	ASO	Antistreptolysin O titer
	AST	Aspartate aminotransferase
B	BE	Barium enema
	BMC	Bone mineral content
	BMD	Bone marrow density
	BMP	Basic metabolic panel
	BNP	Brain natriuretic peptide
	BRCA	Breast cancer (gene)
	BSAP	Bone-specific alkaline phosphatase
	BTA	Bladder tumor antigen
	BUN	Blood urea nitrogen
C	C&S	Culture and sensitivity
	CBC	Complete blood count
	CC	Creatinine clearance
	CEA	Carcinoembryonic antigen
	CK	Creatine kinase
	CMP	Comprehensive metabolic panel
	CMV	Cytomegalovirus
	CO	Carbon monoxide
	CO$_2$	Carbon dioxide
	COHb	Carboxyhemoglobin test
	CPK, CP	Creatine phosphokinase
	CRP	C-reactive protein
	CSF	Cerebrospinal fluid
	CST	Contraction stress test
	CT	Computed tomography
	CTA	Computed tomography angiography
	cTnI	Cardiac troponin I
	cTnT	Cardiac troponin T
	CVB	Chorionic villus biopsy
	CVS	Chorionic villus sampling
	CXR	Chest x-ray

D	D&C	Dilation and curettage
	DEXA	Dual-energy x-ray absorptiometry
	DSA	Digital subtraction angiography
	DSMA	Disodium monomethane arsonate
	DST	Dexamethasone suppression test
E	EBV	Epstein-Barr virus
	ECG, EKG	Electrocardiography
	EEG	Electroencephalogram
	EGD	Esophagogastroduodenoscopy
	EIA	Enzyme immunoassay
	ELISA	Enzyme-linked immunosorbent assay
	EMG	Electromyography
	ENG	Electroneurography
	EP	Evoked potential
	EPCA	Early prostate cancer antigen
	EPO	Erythropoietin
	EPS	Electrophysiologic study
	ER	Estrogen receptor
	ERCP	Endoscopic retrograde cholangiopancreatography
	ESR	Erythrocyte sedimentation rate
	EUG	Excretory urography
F	FBS	Fasting blood sugar
	FDPs	Fibrin degradation products
	%FPSA	Percent free PSA
	FSH	Follicle-stimulating hormone
	FSPs	Fibrin split products
	FT_4	Thyroxin, free
	FTA-ABS	Fluorescent treponemal antibody absorption test
	FVL	Factor V Leiden
G	GE reflux	Gastroesophageal reflux scan
	GGT	Gamma-glutamyl transferase
	GGTP	Gamma-glutamyl transpeptidase
	GH	Growth hormone
	GHb, GHB	Glycosylated hemoglobin
	GI series	Gastrointestinal series
	GTT	Glucose tolerance test
H	HAA	Hepatitis-associated antigen
	HAI	Hemagglutination inhibition
	Hb, Hgb	Hemoglobin
	HCG	Human chorionic gonadotropin
	HCO_3	Bicarbonate
	Hct	Hematocrit
	Hcy	Homocysteine
	HDL	High-density lipoprotein
	5-HIAA	Hydroxyindoleacetic acid
	HIDA	Hepatic iminodiacetic acid
	HIV	Human immunodeficiency virus
	HLA-B27	Human lymphocyte antigen B27
	HTLV	Human T-cell lymphotrophic virus
I	IAA	Insulin autoantibody
	ICA	Islet cell antibody
	Ig	Immunoglobulin
	INR	International normalized ratio
	IV-GTT	Intravenous glucose tolerance test
	IVP	Intravenous pyelography
	IVU, IUG	Intravenous urography

K	KS	Ketosteroid
	KUB	Kidney, ureter, and bladder
L	LAP	Leucine aminopeptidase
	LATS	Long-acting thyroid stimulator
	LDH	Lactic dehydrogenase
	LDL	Low-density lipoprotein
	LFTs	Liver function tests
	LH	Luteinizing hormone
	LP	Lumbar puncture
	L/S ratio	Lecithin/sphingomyelin ratio
	LS spine	Lumbosacral spine
M	MA	Microalbumin
	MCH	Mean corpuscular hemoglobin
	MCHC	Mean corpuscular hemoglobin concentration
	MCV	Mean corpuscular volume
	MEG	Magnetic encephalography
	M/E ratio	Myeloid/erythroid ratio
	MMA	Methylmalonic acid
	MPG	Mean plasma glucose
	MPV	Mean platelet volume
	MRI	Magnetic resonance imaging
	MUGA	Multigated acquisition cardiac scan
N	NMP 22	Nuclear matrix protein 22
	NST	Nonstress test
	NT_x	N-telopeptide
O	O&P	Ova and parasites
	OB	Occult blood
	OCT	Oxytocin challenge test
	OGTT	Oral glucose tolerance test
	17-OHCS	17-Hydroxycorticosteroids
P	PAB	Prealbumin
	PAI-1	Plasminogen activator inhibitor-1
	PAP	Prostatic acid phosphatase
	P_{CO_2}	Partial pressure of carbon dioxide
	PCR	Polymerase chain reaction
	PET	Positron emission tomography
	PFTs	Pulmonary function tests
	pH	Hydrogen ion concentration
	PKU	Phenylketonuria
	PMN	Polymorphonuclear
	PNH	Paroxysmal nocturnal hemoglobinuria
	P_{O_2}	Partial pressure of oxygen
	PO_4	Phosphate
	PPBS	Postprandial blood sugar
	PPD	Purified protein derivative
	PPG	Postprandial glucose
	PR	Progesterone receptor
	PRA	Plasma renin assay
	PSA	Prostate-specific antigen
	PT	Prothrombin time
	PTH	Parathormone, parathyroid hormone
	PTHC, PTC	Percutaneous transhepatic cholangiography
	PTT	Partial thromboplastin time
	PYD	Pyridinium crosslink